ACSM's Resources for the Exercise Physiologist

A Practical Guide for the Health Fitness Professional

SECOND EDITION

ACSM's
Resources for the Exercise Physiologist

A Practical Guide for the Health Fitness Professional

SECOND EDITION

SENIOR EDITOR

Peter Magyari, PhD, FACSM, ACSM EP-C
University of North Florida
Jacksonville, Florida

ASSOCIATE EDITORS

Randi Lite, MA, ACSM-RCEP, ACSM-EIM3
Simmons College
Boston, Massachusetts

Marcus W. Kilpatrick, PhD, FACSM
University of South Florida
Tampa, Florida

James E. Schoffstall, EdD, FACSM, ACSM EP-C, ACSM-RCEP, ACSM/ NCHPAD CIFT, ACSM/NPAS PAPHS
Liberty University
Lynchburg, Virginia

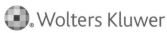. Wolters Kluwer

Philadelphia • Baltimore • New York • London
Buenos Aires • Hong Kong • Sydney • Tokyo

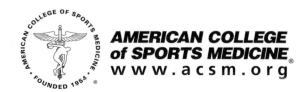

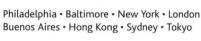

Executive Editor: Michael Nobel
Senior Product Development Editor: Amy Millholen
Editorial Coordinator: Lindsay Ries
Marketing Manager: Shauna Kelley
Senior Production Product Manager: Alicia Jackson
Design Coordinator: Stephen Druding
Manufacturing Coordinator: Margie Orzech
Compositor: Absolute Service, Inc.
ACSM Committee on Certification and Registry Boards Chair: William Simpson, PhD, FACSM
ACSM Publications Committee Chair: Jeffrey Potteiger, PhD, FACSM
ACSM Group Publisher: Katie Feltman

Second Edition

9 8 7 6 5 4 3 2 1

Printed in China

Library of Congress Cataloging-in-Publication Data

Names: Magyari, Peter, editor. | Lite, Randi, editor. | Kilpatrick, Marcus,
  editor. | Schoffstall, James, editor. | American College of Sports
  Medicine, issuing body.
Title: ACSM's resources for the exercise physiologist / senior editor, Peter
  Magyari ; associate editors, Randi Lite, Marcus Kilpatrick, James
  Schoffstall.
Other titles: American College of Sports Medicine's resources for the
  exercise physiologist | Resources for the exercise physiologist
Description: Second edition. | Philadelphia : Wolters Kluwer Health, [2018] |
  Includes bibliographical references and index.
Identifiers: LCCN 2017004011 | ISBN 9781496322869 (alk. paper)
Subjects: | MESH: Exercise Therapy | Exercise—physiology | Sports Medicine |
  Practice Guideline
Classification: LCC RM725 | NLM WB 541 | DDC 615.8/2—dc23 LC record
available at https://lccn.loc.gov/2017004011

DISCLAIMER

Care has been taken to confirm the accuracy of the information present and to describe generally accepted practices. However, the authors, editors, and publisher are not responsible for errors or omissions or for any consequences from application of the information in this publication and make no warranty, expressed or implied, with respect to the currency, completeness, or accuracy of the contents of the publication. Application of this information in a particular situation remains the professional responsibility of the practitioner; the clinical treatments described and recommended may not be considered absolute and universal recommendations.

The authors, editors, and publisher have exerted every effort to ensure that drug selection and dosage set forth in this text are in accordance with the current recommendations and practice at the time of publication. However, in view of ongoing research, changes in government regulations, and the constant flow of information relating to drug therapy and drug reactions, the reader is urged to check the package insert for each drug for any change in indications and dosage and for added warnings and precautions. This is particularly important when the recommended agent is a new or infrequently employed drug.

Some drugs and medical devices presented in this publication have Food and Drug Administration (FDA) clearance for limited use in restricted research settings. It is the responsibility of the health care provider to ascertain the FDA status of each drug or device planned for use in their clinical practice.

DEDICATION

This book is dedicated to all of the outstanding individuals, past and present, associated with the American College of Sports Medicine.

Acknowledgments

I could not have completed this project without the work of my associate editors Randi Lite, Jim Schoffstall, and Marcus Kilpatrick. I owe a special thanks to Randi Lite for stepping up to help me several times when I felt I was overwhelmed with this project. I give a well-deserved thank you to Walt Thompson for all he has done for me professionally over the years and his leadership in ACSM. Thank you to the publishing staff at ACSM (Katie Feltman and Angela Chastain), the production project manager from Wolters Kluwer (Alicia Jackson), and Harold Medina of Absolute Service, Inc., whose input was always both needed and appreciated. Finally, to my mom and dad (Judy and Don Magyari), my siblings (Trish, Don, and Tom), and my sons Myo and Rox, who have supported me throughout, I simply wish to acknowledge that "I love you."

Peter Magyari, Senior Editor

Foreword

ACSM's Committee on Certification and Registry Board (CCRB) consists of volunteers who focus on all aspects of certification, including the creation of exams and educational materials, oversight of all publications associated with certification, and job task analyses for all health fitness, clinical, and specialty certifications. For the past few years, the CCRB has engaged in strategic planning with the goal of advancing the profession of exercise science. In particular, the group focused on strategies to better establish and expand the role of exercise practitioners with a bachelor's or master's degree in exercise science.

One of the outcomes that emerged from the strategic planning was to establish a protected title that defines and describes the degreed exercise professional in terms that are recognized by the profession, medical community, employers, and the general public. After a great deal of debate and research, "Exercise Physiologist" emerged as the preferred title of degreed professionals in the area of health fitness. The title Exercise Physiologist clearly conveys a higher level of training and a demonstration of more advanced competencies compared to exercise professionals without a degree and is recognized by the U.S. Bureau of Labor Statistics. Ultimately ACSM's Board of Trustees approved changing the name of the Health Fitness Specialist (ACSM-HFS) certification to Certified Exercise Physiologist (ACSM EP-C).

As a result of this name change, this second edition of this book has a new name; ACSM's Resources for the Exercise Physiologist. It is a valuable study tool for degreed exercise professionals who aspire to attain this certification as well as an excellent evidence-based resource for those already practicing in the field. This edition provides updated information based on the latest scientific findings in every chapter. Of note, ACSM's new recommendations for exercise preparticipation health screening and a new chapter on functional movement are included in this edition.

I would like to personally thank past and present members of the CCRB for their hard work and dedication in maintaining ACSM certifications as the gold standard in the industry. The transition from ACSM-HFS to ACSM EP-C represents a bold step forward for the field and is a direct result of the commitment of many volunteers who worked together to advance our profession. I would like to acknowledge Dick Cotton, who served as ACSM director of certification from 2007 to 2017. He was committed to keeping ACSM certifications as the best in the industry and was a tireless advocate for both clinical and health fitness professionals. I wish Dick the best in his retirement.

To the editors — Dr. Peter Magyari, Randi Lite, Dr. Marcus W. Kilpatrick, and Dr. James E. Schoffstall — congratulations for creating a valuable and relevant resource that will benefit current and future exercise physiologists. Your commitment to the profession is an inspiration.

Deborah Riebe, PhD, FACSM, ACSM EP-C
Chair, ACSM Committee on Certification and
Registry Board, 2011–2015
Associate Dean, College of Health Sciences
Professor, Department of Kinesiology
University of Rhode Island
Kingston, Rhode Island

Preface

The purpose of this text is to serve as the key resource for certified exercise physiologists, with particular regard to the ACSM Certified Exercise Physiologist^{SM} (EP-C). To accomplish this, *ACSM's Resources for the Exercise Physiologist* provides information about the theory and practice that forms the basis of the EP-C scope of practice. This book is able to stand alone as a classroom text or serve as a supplement to many existing texts. The array and strength of the chapter contributors, many of whom are renowned experts in their fields, is a key aspect that adds to the value of this text.

The primary audience for *ACSM's Resources for the Exercise Physiologist* is the student or professional studying for the ACSM EP-C certification exam. Secondary markets include EP-Cs and personal trainers who wish to broaden their knowledge base. Other health care providers (nurses, physical therapists, etc.) looking to expand their understanding of exercise, exercise prescription, and best practices related to exercise also will find valuable information here.

Organization

This book is organized around the scope of practice domains identified for the ACSM EP-C. We begin with an introductory section focused on understanding exercise and physical activity along with preexercise screening. Part II includes assessment and programming for healthy populations. Part III covers a similar underlying theme but focuses on special populations, including those with metabolic disorders, pregnant women, children, and the elderly. Part IV includes counseling and behavioral strategies for encouraging and sustaining exercise, a critical need for all exercise professionals. The final section, Part V, covers legal, management, and professional issues relevant to all exercise professionals, especially those interested in owning a business or ascending the leadership ladder. The information within this text is based on *ACSM's Guidelines for Exercise Testing and Prescription, Tenth Edition*.

Features

Each of the chapters begins with **objectives** and ends with **open-ended questions** directly related to the objectives. Chapters contain **How To boxes**, which provide step-by-step instructions for different types of assessments an EP-C regularly encounters, and an **Exercise is Medicine Connection**, which describes research about the role of exercise in improving health. **Case Studies** (submitted by ACSM-certified individuals from around the country) are also a key feature as they detail real-life situations EP-Cs face, with suggestions on how to best address them. **Icons** highlight relevant video clips that are available on the book's Web site.

Additional Resources

ACSM's Resources for the Exercise Physiologist includes additional resources for students and instructors that are available on the book's companion Web site at http://thepoint.lww.com.

Students

- Video clips

Instructors

Approved adopting instructors will be given access to the following additional resources:

- Test generator
- PowerPoint presentations
- Image bank
- Case Study answers
- Angel/Blackboard/Moodle-ready cartridge

See the inside front cover of this text for more details, including the passcode you will need to gain access to the Web site.

Updates for the book can be found at http://certification.acsm.org/updates.

Contributors

Anthony A. Abbott, EdD, FACSM, ACSM-CPT, ACSM EP-C, ACSM-CEP, ACSM/ACS CET, ACSM/NCHPAD CIFT
Fitness Institute International, Inc.
Lighthouse Point, Florida
Chapter 14

John B. Bartholomew, PhD, FACSM
University of Texas at Austin
Austin, Texas
Chapter 13

Keith Burns, PhD, ACSM EP-C
Walsh University
North Canton, Ohio
Chapter 8

Katrina D. DuBose, PhD, FACSM
East Carolina University
Greenville, North Carolina
Chapter 7

J. Larry Durstine, PhD, FACSM
University of South Carolina
Columbia, South Carolina
Chapter 8

Gregory Dwyer, PhD, FACSM, ACSM-PD, ACSM-RCEP, ACSM-CEP, ACSM-ETT, EIM3
East Stroudsburg University
East Stroudsburg, Pennsylvania
Chapter 2

Avery D. Faigenbaum, EdD, FACSM, ACSM EP-C
The College of New Jersey
Ewing, New Jersey
Chapter 4

Mark D. Faries, PhD
Texas A&M University, AgriLife Extension Service
College Station, Texas
Chapter 12

Diana Ferris Dimon, MS
Praxair, Inc.
Danbury, Connecticut
Chapter 16

Charles J. Fountaine, PhD
University of Minnesota Duluth
Duluth, Minnesota
Chapter 3

Benjamin Gordon, PhD
University of North Florida
Jacksonville, Florida
Chapter 8

Sarah T. Henes, PhD, RD, LDN
Georgia State University
Atlanta, Georgia
Chapter 7

Josh Johann, MS, EIM1
The University of Tennessee at Chattanooga
Chattanooga, Tennessee
Chapter 8

Betsy Keller, PhD, FACSM, ACSM-ETT
Ithaca College
Ithaca, New York
Chapter 9

Marcus W. Kilpatrick, PhD, FACSM
University of South Florida
Tampa, Florida
Chapter 12

Matthew Kutz, PhD
Bowling Green State University
Bowling Green, Ohio
Chapter 15

Beth Lewis, PhD
University of Minnesota
Minneapolis, Minnesota
Chapter 11

Gary Liguori, PhD, FACSM, ACSM-CEP
The University of Rhode Island
Kingston, Rhode Island
Chapters 1 and 8

Randi Lite, MA, ACSM-RCEP, EIM3
Simmons College
Boston, Massachusetts
Chapter 18

Meir Magal, PhD, FACSM, ACSM-CEP
North Carolina Wesleyan College
Rocky Mount, North Carolina
Chapter 5

Peter Magyari, PhD, FACSM, ACSM EP-C
University of North Florida
Jacksonville, Florida
Chapter 2

Linda May, PhD
Eastern Carolina University
Greenville, North Carolina
Chapter 10

Jessica Meendering, PhD, ACSM EP-C
South Dakota State University
Brookings, South Dakota
Chapter 3

Laurie Milliken, PhD, FACSM
University of Massachusetts Boston
Boston, Massachusetts
Chapter 10

Nicole Nelson, MHS, LMT, ACSM EP-C
University of North Florida
Jacksonville, Florida
Chapter 6

Neal Pire, MA, FACSM, ACSM EP-C, ACSM-EIM2
Castle Connolly Private Health Partners, LLC
New York, New York
Chapter 16

Deborah Riebe, PhD, FACSM, ACSM EP-C
The University of Rhode Island
Kingston, Rhode Island
Chapter 7

James E. Schoffstall, EdD, FACSM, ACSM EP-C, ACSM-RCEP, ACSM/NCHPAD CIFT, ACSM/NPAS PAPHS
Liberty University
Lynchburg, Virginia
Chapter 17

John M. Schuna Jr., PhD
Oregon State University
Corvallis, Oregon
Chapter 1

Katie J. Schuver, PhD
University of Minnesota
Minneapolis, Minnesota
Chapter 11

John Sigg, PT, PhD
Ithaca College
Ithaca, New York
Chapter 9

Matthew Stults-Kolehmainen, PhD, ACSM EP-C
Yale-New Haven Hospital
New Haven, Connecticut
Teachers College Columbia University
New York, New York
Chapter 13

Kathleen S. Thomas, PhD, ACSM-CPT, ACSM EP-C
Norfolk State University
Norfolk, Virginia
Chapter 5

Reviewers

Cesar Alvarez, MA, ACSM EP-C
United States Air Force
Ramstein Air Base, Germany

Brigitte Baranek, ACSM EP-C
Magna International
Lansing, Michigan

Brian Garavaglia, PhD, ACSM-CPT, ACSM EP-C, ACSM/ACS CET, ACSM/NCHPAD CIFT, ACSM/NPAS PAPHS
Macomb Community College, Oakland Community College, St. Johns Hospital and Medical Center
Warren, Michigan

Karyn Gunnett-Shoval, PhD
Harvard University
Cambridge, Massachusetts

Allison Holm, BS, ACSM EP-C
EXOS
Lehi, Utah

Kamal Makkiya, BS, ACSM-RCEP, ACSM-CEP, ACSM EP-C
Westfield State University
Westfield, Massachusetts

Ashely Murchison, ACSM EP-C
Hamilton Health Care System
Dalton, Georgia

Allison Palisch, BS, BSN, RN, ACSM EP-C
St. Louis Children's Hospital
St. Louis, Missouri

Kevin Perrone, BS, ACSM EP-C, ACSM-EIM2
Legitimate Movement
Durham, North Carolina

Melissa Traynor, ACSM EP-C
Athletic Traynor Services
Toronto, Ontario, Canada

Kate Wheeler, BS, ACSM EP-C
Harris & Harris Express YMCAs
Charlotte, North Carolina

Jennifer Young, MA, ACSM EP-C
Cigna Onsite Enterprise
Houston, Texas

Contents

PART I

Overview

1

Understanding Physical Activity and Exercise

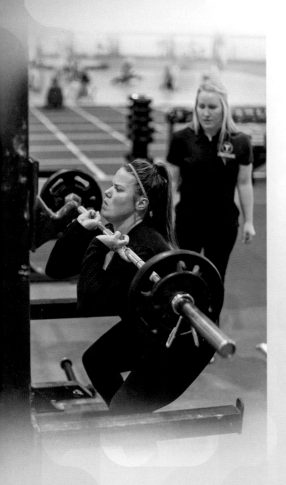

OBJECTIVES

- To define physical activity, exercise, health-related fitness, and skill-related fitness.

- To identify several key historical individuals and landmark research that were instrumental in building the current knowledge base regarding the health benefits of physical activity and physical fitness.

- To know how physical activity can positively impact health across the lifespan.

- To understand the general health risks associated with physical activity and exercise at different intensities and volumes.

INTRODUCTION

A practicing certified exercise physiologist (EP-C) should be able to distinguish between physical activity (PA), exercise, health-related fitness, and skill-related fitness. Although all of these are closely intertwined, they each have distinguishing features to make them unique. This chapter discusses some of these unique features, along with a review of important historical individuals and the landmarks in research in the evolution of fitness, leading to today's understanding of the health benefits and risks of exercise. Finally, there is an overview of current guidelines and recommendations for using exercise and PA to promote better health.

 ## Defining Physical Activity, Exercise, Health-Related Fitness, and Skill-Related Fitness

PA is by far the broadest of all the terms mentioned in the introduction. By definition, PA is any bodily movement produced by contracting skeletal muscles (voluntary muscle contractions), with a concomitant increase in energy expenditure (11). Although energy expenditure is increased during PA, it does not always reflect exercise, and it should not be confused with health- or skill-related fitness.

Voluntary muscle contractions, which are necessary during PA, can be static or dynamic. Static, or isometric, contractions produce no change in the affected joint angle, such as seen when pressing against a wall. With static contractions, muscle strength is gained in only one joint position, not across a range of motion, which limits the application of the strength. In addition, static strength gains are lost very quickly if not practiced daily. Conversely, a dynamic or isotonic contraction produces a change in the affected joint angle, such as a squat causing a change in knee angle or a pull-up resulting in a change in elbow angle. Dynamic movement also allows muscle strength gains to occur across the full range of motion and can better mimic daily activities or sporting movements, each of which can be characterized as displays of functional strength.

PA can be a blend of aerobic (oxygen dependent, *i.e.*, walking to the store, jogging) and anaerobic (oxygen independent, *i.e.*, moving furniture, lifting weights) activities, depending on the intensity. Within any one given activity, both aerobic and anaerobic processes may be present, as can both static and dynamic muscle contractions.

PA can also be categorized by its situational context outside of competitive level sport: leisure-time, occupational, household, and transportation. The purpose of any given bout of PA can vary by environment and can also change from day to day. For instance, transportation for some might mean using public transport and walking to and from the bus station and workplace. This type of PA is likely to provide some health-related benefits. Others might cycle vigorously to and from work at a more challenging pace. Both activities are transportation-related PA but are for a different purpose and with different outcomes.

One of the largest components of PA-related energy expenditure is occupational PA. A substantial portion of many Americans' waking day is spent working, with recent estimates indicating that employed individuals work an average of 7.5 hours $\cdot$ day^{-1} (88). However, during the past 50 years, there has been a dramatic reduction in the percentage of Americans working in occupations requiring moderate-intensity PA, as the nature of work has become less physically demanding (15). Moreover, it has been estimated that occupational energy expenditure has declined by more than 100 calories $\cdot$ day^{-1} over the past five decades. The increase in obesity prevalence among American adults may be partly related to this overall decrease in occupational PA.

Similar to occupational PA, observational evidence indicates that household PA in some population groups has also decreased over the past five decades (4). Gardening, home repairs, food preparation, cleaning (house and vehicle), and childcare are just some means of accumulating household PA throughout the day, and many have been made "easier" by technology.

Although there are numerous ways of accumulating PA (Table 1.1), and reaping the inherent health benefits, it remains difficult for many adults to find the necessary time (Table 1.2). Chapters 11 through 13 address different behavioral strategies and examples of ways to help initiate, accumulate, and sustain meaningful PA.

Exercise training may be considered a component of PA. Although exercise and PA are often used interchangeably, it is important to be able to clearly distinguish the two. Compared with PA, exercise is more specific to an end goal and quantifiable in its definition: any planned, structured, repetitive, and purposeful activity that seeks to improve or maintain any component of fitness for life or sport (11). Although exercise is certainly a form of PA, PA does not always include exercise. Household chores and using public transport are PAs, although typically not considered exercise. Conversely, daily 5-km training runs meet the definition of exercise and are also PA.

Physical fitness is a factor that directly relates to the quantity and type of PA an individual can perform. Physical fitness, however, includes different domains from health-related fitness. Physical fitness is defined as "a set of attributes that people have or achieve that relates to the ability to perform physical activity" (11). Physical fitness includes cardiorespiratory endurance; muscle strength, endurance, and power; flexibility; agility; balance; reaction time; and body composition. Physical fitness also implies specificity of training toward a particular goal. The majority of these attributes lend themselves to athletic performance or the subcomponent of physical fitness known as performance-related fitness.

Health-related fitness is another subcomponent of physical fitness. Although health- and performance-related fitness share certain attributes, they tend to appeal to individuals with very different interests and needs. In addition, health-related fitness is confined to cardiorespiratory fitness, muscular endurance, muscular strength, flexibility, and body composition.

Skill-related fitness is the third aspect of PA and can also be thought of as performance-related fitness. Skill-related fitness comprises agility, balance, coordination, power, reaction time, and speed and can result in an increased desire to participate in physical activities. Overall, skill-related fitness contributes to one's ability to function in a more skilled and efficient manner (44).

The underlying premise is that PA will maintain or improve health, with an emphasis on improving each kind of PA. This is in contrast to those individuals choosing to remain physically

Table 1.1	Popular Physical Activities and Common Barriers to Physical Activity
Popular Physical Activities	**Common Barriers to Physical Activity**
Walking	Lack of time/inconvenience
Gardening	Lack of motivation
Calisthenics	Not enjoyable/boring
Strength training	Fear of injury
Swimming	Lack of support/access
Yoga	Lack of self-esteem/self-conscious
Dancing	Lack of coordination
Jogging	Lack of encouragement

Table 1.2	Metabolic Equivalents (METs) Values of Common Physical Activities Classified as Light, Moderate, or Vigorous Intensity		
Very Light/Light (<3.0 METs)	**Moderate (3.0–5.9 METs)**		**Vigorous (≥6.0 METs)**

Very Light/Light (<3.0 METs)

Walking

Walking slowly around home, store, or office = 2.0^a

Household and Occupation

Standing performing light work, such as making bed, washing dishes, ironing, preparing food, or store clerk = 2.0–2.5

Leisure Time and Sports

Arts and crafts, playing cards = 1.5
Billiards = 2.5
Boating — power = 2.5
Croquet = 2.5
Darts = 2.5
Fishing — sitting = 2.5
Playing most musical instruments = 2.0–2.5

Moderate (3.0–5.9 METs)

Walking

Walking 3.0 mi · h^{-1} = 3.0^a
Walking at very brisk pace (4 mi · h^{-1}) = 5.0^a

Household and Occupation

Cleaning, heavy — washing windows, car, clean garage = 3.0
Sweeping floors or carpet, vacuuming, mopping = 3.0–3.5
Carpentry — general = 3.6
Carrying and stacking wood = 5.5
Mowing lawn — walk power mower = 5.5

Leisure Time and Sports

Badminton — recreational = 4.5
Basketball — shooting a round = 4.5
Dancing — ballroom slow = 3.0; ballroom fast = 4.5
Fishing from riverbank and walking = 4.0
Golf — walking pulling clubs = 4.3
Sailing boat, wind surfing = 3.0
Table tennis = 4.0
Tennis doubles = 5.0
Volleyball — noncompetitive = 3.0–4.0

Vigorous (≥6.0 METs)

Walking, Jogging, and Running

Walking at very, very brisk pace (4.5 mi · h^{-1}) = 6.3^a
Walking/hiking at moderate pace and grade with no or light pack (<10 lb) = 7.0
Hiking at steep grades and pack 10–42 lb = 7.5–9.0
Jogging at 5 mi · h^{-1} = 8.0^a
Jogging at 6 mi · h^{-1} = 10.0^a
Running at 7 mi · h^{-1} = 11.5^a

Household and Occupation

Shoveling sand, coal, etc. = 7.0
Carrying heavy loads, such as bricks = 7.5
Heavy farming, such as bailing hay = 8.0
Shoveling, digging ditches = 8.5

Leisure Time and Sports

Bicycling on flat — light effort (10–12 mi · h^{-1}) = 6.0
Basketball game = 8.0
Bicycling on flat — moderate effort (12–14 mi · h^{-1}) = 8; fast (14–16 mi · h^{-1}) = 10
Skiing cross-country — slow (2.5 mi · h^{-1}) = 7.0; fast (5.0–7.9 mi · h^{-1}) = 9.0
Soccer — casual = 7.0; competitive = 10.0
Swimming leisurely = 6.0^b
Swimming — moderate/hard = $8–11^b$
Tennis singles = 8.0
Volleyball — competitive at gym or beach = 8.0

^{a}On flat, hard surface.

^{b}MET values can vary substantially from individual to individual during swimming as a result of different strokes and skill levels.

Adapted from Ainsworth BE, Haskell WL, Whitt MC, et al. Compendium of physical activities: an update of activity codes and MET intensities. *Med Sci Sports Exerc.* 2000;32(9 Suppl):S498–504.

inactive and putting themselves at greater risk for premature morbidity and mortality. Therefore, when the EP-C develops an exercise prescription, or motivates an individual to initiate an exercise program, knowledge of these guiding principles is essential.

Historic Trends in Physical Activity

Ancient Times and the Rise of Exercise Physiology

The importance of PA as a means to promote health and well-being is not a new concept. In ancient China, records of exercise for health promotion date back to approximately 2500 BC (46). Following this, teachings of the Greek physician Hippocrates (30), of the fifth and fourth centuries BC, detailed the importance of exercise for health and well-being. Despite this ancient knowledge that PA confers health benefits, such teachings were generally based on inspirational beliefs and folk wisdom rather than empirical science (11). An understanding of the pathways and mechanisms through which PA influences health and well-being remained poorly understood until recent times. Much of our current understanding in these areas evolved out of advancements in human physiology, in particular, exercise physiology.

Moving forward from ancient times to the early 20th century, pioneers such as A.V. Hill and D.B. Dill, among many others, contributed vastly to the field of exercise physiology. Hill is perhaps best known for his work studying muscle mechanics and physiology, whereas Dill and numerous colleagues at the Harvard Fatigue Laboratory extensively studied exercise responses in varying environmental conditions. Collectively, developments in exercise physiology during this period laid the groundwork for our understanding of how PA and conditioning influences physical fitness.

T.K. Cureton and the Physical Fitness Movement

Building upon earlier advancements in the field of exercise physiology, T.K. Cureton's work during the 1940s focused on assessing physical fitness and the importance of physical conditioning. Cureton acted as a driving force behind the physical fitness movement in the United States while developing strong research and service programs at the University of Illinois. As a result, Cureton drew significant academic attention to the topics of physical fitness and physical conditioning (6). The cumulative contributions from Cureton and his graduate students provided much of the scientific basis for modern exercise prescription.

In addition to his scientific accomplishments, Cureton made a number of service contributions pertinent to the physical fitness movement. Several of his notable contributions included, but were not limited to, fitness training and testing of soldiers during World War II, assistance in the design of physical fitness training programs for Federal Bureau of Investigation trainees, and instrumental support in the development of the President's Council on Physical Fitness (6). Moreover, Cureton was one of the original 54 charter members of the American College of Sports Medicine (ACSM) at the time of its founding in 1954.

One of Cureton's many distinguished students who made substantial contributions to exercise physiology and the physical fitness movement was the late Michael Pollock. Pollock is perhaps most remembered as a prominent researcher who made notable contributions in the areas of exercise prescription and cardiac rehabilitation. Pollock was the lead author of the ACSM's first position statement regarding the mode and quantity of exercise necessary to elicit fitness improvements (2). In addition, Pollock was instrumental in legitimizing the role of cardiac rehabilitation as an integral part of medical treatment for patients with heart disease. Many of Pollock's significant contributions were made during his tenure at the well-known Cooper Institute for Aerobics Research in the mid-1970s.

Historical Evolution of Physical Activity Epidemiology

Although research developments in exercise physiology during the early to mid-20th century led to an improved understanding of how physical fitness could be impacted by PA, the relationships between PA and certain chronic conditions (*e.g.*, cardiovascular disease [CVD] and obesity) remained largely unknown. This was especially problematic considering the dramatic increase in CVD-related mortality that occurred during the first half of the 20th century. In an attempt to identify and understand the underlying causes of heart disease and other chronic conditions, a number of large-scale epidemiological studies (*e.g.*, Framingham Heart Study and Harvard Alumni Health Study) were initiated during the middle decades of the century.

The first epidemiological evidence indicating that greater amounts of PA were associated with reduced risks of CVD was presented by Morris and colleagues (56) after studying double-decker bus workers in London, England. The major finding from this line of research was that physically active bus conductors suffered roughly half the coronary events than did less active bus drivers. Further illustrating the potential health benefits of being physically active, later work by Paffenbarger and coworkers (64) demonstrated that work-related caloric expenditure and the risk of death from coronary heart disease were inversely related among longshoremen in San Francisco, California.

A number of subsequent large-scale epidemiological investigations demonstrated an inverse relationship between PA and CVD incidence and mortality (42,43,57,77,80). In general, these investigations showed a dose-response relationship as greater levels of PA were associated with reduced risks of developing CVD (Fig. 1.1).

Besides PA, research has shown that physical fitness is also inversely related to CVD incidence and mortality (8,19,41,75) (see Fig. 1.1). An important project related to this research area is the ongoing Aerobics Center Longitudinal Study (ACLS) conducted at the Cooper Clinic in Dallas, Texas. Men and women who visited the preventive medicine clinic completed a maximal treadmill test and were rated as having low, moderate, or high physical fitness based on their gender, age, and treadmill exercise time. Blair and colleagues (8) published one of the landmark papers in this research area using data from the ACLS, which demonstrated that higher levels of objectively measured physical fitness from the maximal treadmill test were associated with reduced risks of CVD mortality.

Development of Physical Activity Guidelines and Recommendations

The eventual accumulation of evidence pointing to the beneficial and protective role of PA on health-related outcomes resulted in the publication of a joint position statement by the ACSM and Centers for Disease Control and Prevention (CDC) in 1995 regarding PA and

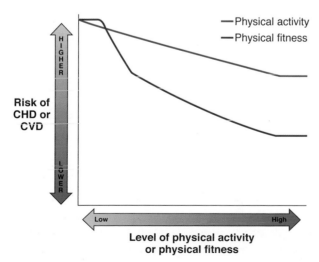

FIGURE 1.1. General relationships between PA or physical fitness level and relative risk of coronary heart disease (CHD) and cardiovascular disease (CVD). (Adapted with permission from Williams PT. Physical fitness and activity as separate heart disease risk factors: a meta-analysis. *Med Sci Sports Exerc.* 2001;33[5]:754–61.)

public health (65). Based on the current literature at the time, the joint position statement from the ACSM/CDC recommended that every adult accumulate 30 minutes or more of moderate-intensity PA on most, preferably all, days of the week. Soon to follow the ACSM/CDC joint position statement, the U.S. Department of Health and Human Services published the Surgeon General's Report on Physical Activity and Health in 1996 (90). This report presented a thorough review of the available evidence regarding PA and its relation to numerous health outcomes while restating the aerobic PA guidelines put forth by the joint ACSM/CDC position statement. Figure 1.2 shows the trend of US adults reporting no leisure-time PA, which has remained steady to slightly declining, since the release of the Surgeon General's Report on Physical Activity and Health in 1996.

Twelve years after the joint position statement by the ACSM/CDC, an update regarding PA and public health was issued in 2007 by the ACSM and the American Heart Association (AHA) (26). The updated position statement further clarified the recommendations made in 1995. One of the main changes was the more specific frequency recommendation for moderate-intensity PA as the "most, preferably all, days of the week" qualification was changed to "five days each week." In addition, the update incorporated guidelines for meeting the recommendation with vigorous PA and indicated that bouts of PA should last for at least 10 minutes in duration to be counted toward the 30-minute daily goal. Specifics relating to muscle strengthening were also incorporated into the updated recommendation.

One year after the updated ACSM/AHA PA recommendations, the U.S. Department of Health Human Services published the *2008 Physical Activity Guidelines for Americans* (91). This document represented the first comprehensive PA guidelines put forth by the US government. These guidelines presented recommendations for three different age groups (children and adolescents, adults, and older adults) and incorporated specifics regarding aerobic, muscle-strengthening, and flexibility activities. Unlike the 2007 ACSM/AHA guidelines, the *2008 Physical Activity Guidelines for Americans* did not specify a weekly frequency for aerobic activity (*e.g.*, ≥ 5 d $\cdot$ wk^{-1}). Instead, the guidelines simply called for an accumulation of 150 minutes of moderate-intensity PA on a weekly basis and suggested that the cumulative duration be spread throughout the week.

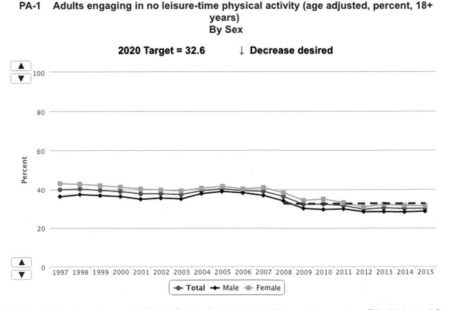

FIGURE 1.2. Trend line showing percentage of Americans completing no leisure-time PA. (Adapted from National Center for Heath Statistics, Centers for Disease Control and Prevention. [cited 2017 Mar 8]. Available from: https://www.healthypeople.gov/2020/topics-objectives/topic/physical-activity/national-snapshot)

Relationship between PA/Exercise and Health across the Lifespan

Until recently, attempts to quantify daily durations of PA in free-living conditions often relied on subjective self-report methods (*e.g.*, PA questionnaires and PA logs). However, the best estimates for county-by-county leisure-time PA were based on CDC self-report data and give a clear picture of which regions of the United States are least and most physically active (Fig. 1.3). In 2008, however, Troiano and colleagues (87) published a landmark paper detailing the first objective assessment of PA among a nationally representative sample of Americans during the 2003–2004 National Health and Nutrition Examination Survey. This objective assessment was conducted using specialized PA accelerometers, which can measure the duration and intensity of accumulated PA. Alarming among the findings from this assessment were the extremely low daily durations of moderate-to-vigorous PA (≥ 3 metabolic equivalents [METs]) across all ranges as less than 4% of American adults 20 years of age and older were meeting public health recommendations for PA (*i.e.*, a minimum of 30 min of moderate PA 5 or more days per week). Concurrent estimates of self-reported PA collected during the CDC's 2003 Behavioral Risk Factor Surveillance System indicated that 47.4% of American adults were meeting current PA recommendations (13). It is difficult to explain the discrepancy between the self-report and objective measures of PA; yet, this provokes concern that most Americans are not as active as they might think.

The low levels of PA demonstrated among the majority of Americans are particularly problematic, especially when considering the numerous health benefits associated with regular PA. Across the age continuum, PA can have positive impacts in biological, psychological, and social domains. Moreover, the therapeutic and prophylactic benefits of PA can often be obtained at little to no cost and in nearly any environment.

Physical Activity and Health in Children and Adolescents

In addition to healthy eating habits, incorporating regular PA into the lives of children and adolescents (17 years of age and younger) provides an early starting point to aid in the prevention of numerous chronic diseases. Chapters 11 through 13 discuss the importance of establishing positive health behaviors early in life as a means of lifelong healthy living. An increasingly prevalent chronic disease among America's youth is obesity. Data from the early 1970s indicated that 5.0% of 2- to 5-year-olds, 4.0% of 6- to 11-year-olds, and 6.1% of 12- to 19-year-olds were obese (62). However, two- to fourfold increases in obesity prevalence have been observed over

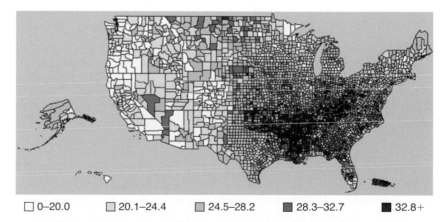

☐ 0–20.0   ☐ 20.1–24.4   ☐ 24.5–28.2   ■ 28.3–32.7   ■ 32.8+

FIGURE 1.3. 2013 estimates of leisure-time physical inactivity among adults 20 years of age or older. (Adapted from Centers for Disease Control and Prevention. *National Diabetes Surveillance System*. [cited 2017 Mar 8]. Available from: https://www.cdc.gov/diabetes/data/county.html)

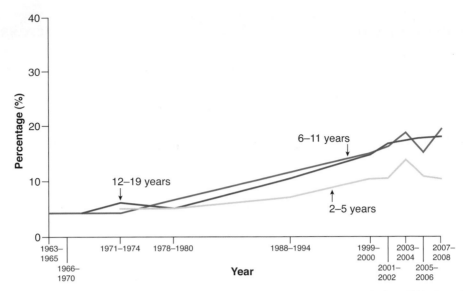

FIGURE 1.4. Childhood obesity trends since the early 1960s. (Adapted from Ogden C, Carroll M. *Prevalence of Obesity among Children and Adolescents: United States, Trends 1963–1965 through 2007–2008.* Hyattsville [MD]: Centers for Disease Control and Prevention, National Center for Health Statistics; 2010. 5 p.)

the past four decades as recent estimates indicate that 10.4% of 2- to 5-year-olds, 19.6% of 6- to 11-year-olds, and 18.1% of 12- to 19-year-olds are obese (Fig. 1.4). This has become a major health concern, as childhood obesity increases the risk for a host of other chronic diseases such as diabetes, hyperlipidemia, and hypertension (59). In addition, childhood obesity may result in detrimental behavioral, social, and economic effects (24,66,76). In fact, a 2015 U.S. Surgeon General public health report outlined the positive effects of enhancing both the physical and emotional health of adolescents in order to encourage the chances of a successful and healthy adulthood (58). The report noted that excessive consumption of sugary beverages (84% of adolescents), along with >7 hours of daily screen time (which displaces PA), are likely to lead to negative social, behavioral, and economic outcomes.

PA has been one of many modalities suggested as a means to address the rising obesity epidemic among children and adolescents. Among youth, lower levels of PA are associated with a greater risk of being overweight or obese (37,78). Moreover, evidence suggests that being physically active during childhood and adolescence positively influences metabolic risk factors related to Type 2 diabetes (40,71), which has become an emerging health problem among America's youth (1).

Adequate PA is also important for normal musculoskeletal development during childhood. An adequate stimulus via structured exercise and/or PA can help increase bone accretion during youth and adolescence (5). In turn, greater peak bone mineral density in early adulthood may be attained, which reduces the risk or delays the onset of osteoporosis in later adulthood (29).

Physical Activity and Health in Adults

Adults who engage in regular PA can enjoy many health benefits from being regularly physically active. Among adults, research has shown that increases in PA energy expenditure are associated with significant weight reduction (70,73,74,81). This has become especially pertinent, as approximately 69% of the US general population is either overweight or obese (63). However, regular PA carries health benefits regardless of any changes in body composition that occur as a result of increased PA energy expenditure (36). Additional health benefits of regular PA include, but are not limited to, reduced risks of Type 2 diabetes (32,50), hypertension (27,68), CVD (33,49), colon cancer (54), and all-cause mortality (34).

Of particular interest regarding PA among adults is the role it can play in the prevention of future CVD. The economic cost associated with CVD has grown substantially in recent times, with current estimates of the direct and indirect costs associated with CVD and stroke in the United States exceeding $500 billion in 2010 (45). Substantially increasing PA levels in the general population, and hence the proportion of adults meeting current PA guidelines, would undoubtedly have positive effects on CVD prevalence and its associated costs.

Physical Activity and Health in Older Adults

Recent evidence has shown that PA levels in America tend to decline as age increases and are lower among persons with chronic diseases (87). This age-related decline in PA may be partly attributable to limitations resulting from common chronic diseases. However, like younger adults and children, older individuals can also reap health benefits by being physically active (90,91). Interestingly, some research has demonstrated that leisure-time PA is a more important protective measure against heart disease in older adults (65 years of age and older) than in younger adults (84).

In comparison with younger individuals, older adults are more likely to have a chronic condition (*e.g.*, CVD). However, PA still confers health benefits on those individuals suffering from one or more chronic diseases. As an example, PA after first nonfatal myocardial infarction (MI) has been shown to reduce the risk for a second MI (82). In addition, regular PA has also been shown to be an effective treatment for osteoarthritis among older adults (10,67).

Particularly important to older adults, a physically active lifestyle can help them maintain physical function during later years (14). Much of this benefit is due to greater levels of functional capacity that can be achieved through PA (20). These higher levels of functional capacity can allow older individuals to live independently and make it easier to carry out activities of daily living. In addition, PA during later adulthood is associated with decreased risks of falls and osteoporotic fractures (21,28).

 ## General Risks Associated with Physical Activity/Exercise

It is the inherent responsibility of an EP-C to take reasonable precautions when working with individuals who wish to become physically active or to increase their current activity level. In physically inactive or symptom-free individuals, moderate-intensity exercise does not present a risk for CVD-related events (93). In addition, the *2008 Physical Activity Guidelines for Americans* emphasize the importance of regular PA across all age groups, almost regardless of current health status, as the benefits are far reaching (91).

Most physically inactive or symptom-free individuals can safely begin a low- to moderate-intensity PA program without the need for baseline exercise testing or prior medical clearance (see Chapter 2 for greater detail). The EP-C responsible for supervising vigorous-intensity exercise programs, regardless of the population, should have current training in basic and/or advanced cardiac life support and emergency procedures while also being keenly aware of the signs and symptoms of CVD.

Risks of Sudden Cardiac Death

Despite the known benefits of PA and exercise, inherent risk does exist. Sudden cardiac death associated with exercise is widely publicized, especially in children or adolescents. In truth, sudden cardiac death related to moderate exercise is extremely rare (79,86). For young individuals (younger than 30 years), the most common causes of sudden cardiac death are congenital and hereditary abnormalities; however, there is no clear consensus on the actual rate of sudden death in young individuals (18,51,92). High school and college athletes are typically required to have a preparticipation screening, which is one means of detecting potential cardiac issues.

Sudden cardiac death risk increases with age and prevalence of known or unknown CVD (23,25,55,79,85,93,95). Furthermore, the rates of sudden cardiac death, and acute MI are disproportionately higher in the least active individuals performing infrequent exercise (3), such as a generally inactive person shoveling heavy snow.

Although the exact mechanism of sudden cardiac death or MI remains elusive, there appears to be an acute arterial insult that dislodges already present plaque, resulting in platelet aggregation or thrombosis (7,12,16). The EP-C should have a basic understanding of this sequela and the inherent risks of sudden cardiac death or MI any one individual may carry. Appropriate screening is critical for minimizing this risk (see Chapter 2).

The Risk of Cardiac Events during Exercise Testing

A practicing EP-C is likely to suggest and perform baseline and follow-up exercise tests across a wide variety of individuals. Although submaximal exercise testing is generally considered safe for most, maximal- or vigorous-intensity exercise testing does pose some risk (22,38,53,72,83). Similar to exercise, exercise testing is also rather safe when performed properly. Overall, the risk of cardiac events during symptom-limited exercise testing in a clinical environment is low (6 cardiac events per 10,000 tests), and given proper screening and attention, most tests can be performed with a high degree of safety (60,61).

Musculoskeletal Injury Associated with Exercise

In addition to the acute risk of sudden cardiac death or MI, there is also an increased risk of musculoskeletal injury associated with exercise. Typically, the highest risk is associated with activities that are weight-bearing or involve repetitive motion: jogging, walking, cycling, weightlifting, and the like. The most common musculoskeletal injuries, regardless of gender, occur in the lower body, particularly at the knee or foot (31). The rate of musculoskeletal injury is highest in team and contact sports and includes injuries of all types, not just lower body injuries (12).

The annual rate of musculoskeletal injury associated with running and jogging is significant, ranging from 35% to 65% (39,47). However, only about 7% of US adults use jogging or running as their regular form of exercise. Walking for exercise, which is performed by approximately 30% of adults, is the most popular exercise in the United States (89). The musculoskeletal risk associated with walking is considerably lower than that with jogging, with about 1.5% of people reporting an injury in the previous month (69). Compared with joggers, walkers of both genders are at 25%–30% lower risk for incurring an acute or chronic musculoskeletal injury (17).

Aerobic dance and resistance training are two other popular types of exercise with a documented musculoskeletal injury rate. Resistance training includes weightlifting, body weight exercises, and the like, and was shown to have a 1-month injury rate of 2.4% (69).

Although certainly not life threatening, musculoskeletal injuries present a real and present issue. Preventing and minimizing injury will lead to greater opportunities to remain physically active, although, unfortunately, those previously injured from exercise are at higher risk for reinjury (35,39,48,52,94). Therefore, to minimize musculoskeletal injury from the outset, the EP-C should consider the following:

- Be diligent in choosing exercise modes and prescribing exercise that are based on an individual's current fitness level and desires, along with any past exercise experiences.
- Start at a low level of intensity, frequency, and duration and progress slowly.
- Be aware and make clients aware of early signs of potential injury (*i.e.*, increasing muscle soreness, bone and joint pain, excessive fatigue, and performance decrements). When noted, take appropriate precautions, which may include temporarily ceasing the activity, more frequent rest days, or simply decreasing the frequency, intensity, or duration of exercise.
- Set realistic exercise goals to avoid overexercising (see Chapter 12 for goal setting).

The Case of Rachel

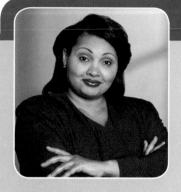

Submitted by **Kaitlin Teser, MS, EIM Level 2 Credentialed Certified Exercise Physiologist, Greater Boston Area, MA.**

Rachel is a 43-year-old moderately active mom with no cardiovascular, metabolic, or renal disease. Rachel's initial goal of losing 10 lb shifted to wanting to incorporate more active lifestyle habits into her daily routine.

Narrative

Rachel is a 43-year-old, low-risk woman who works 40 hours a week in a sedentary office job. Rachel's original goal was to lose 10 lb in 12 weeks. She was moderately active. Her two children, Zach, age 10 years, and Emily, age 8 years, are involved in karate. In addition to a walk around the local track with coworkers twice a week, Rachel also took a cardio kickboxing class on Saturday mornings.

Fitness Testing Results

The results of Rachel's fitness assessment were as follows:

Resting blood pressure	110/85 mm Hg	Good
Resting heart rate	81 bpm	Good
Body fat (%)	28.7	Fair
Body mass index	25.5	Average
Sit and reach (box)	29 cm	Fair
Muscular endurance (YMCA bench press)	16 reps	Low–average
Aerobic fitness (YMCA submaximal bike test)	$23.3 \text{ mL} \cdot \text{kg}^{-1} \cdot \text{min}^{-1}$	Very poor

Although Rachel's first wellness vision seemed like it related to active living, she was really focused on weight loss. I was careful to "meet her where she was" and encourage her use of the term *active living* in her wellness vision.

Rachel's First Wellness Vision

"My wellness vision is to be healthy, energetic, and vital. I am motivated by my desire to stay active with my children and continue to be active as I age. I am challenged by my demanding schedule and multiple commitments, but have been a regular exerciser in the past and know the importance of active living as a way of life. I am confident that with increased social support, a regular routine and a realistic weight management plan, I will achieve success."

Rachel's program followed the FITT principle and incorporated both health- and skill-related fitness components. She added another cardio kickboxing class to her week and convinced her coworkers to walk on the track an additional day. My work with Rachel focused on increasing strength and range of motion. I introduced Rachel to a variety of modalities that could be used both at home and at the office to provide brief workouts throughout the day. The more I put myself in Rachel's shoes and developed programs that were fun, efficient, and effective, the more she seemed to be engaged in the session. I learned that Rachel often went home and tried out a modified version of our activities with her children. After 4 weeks, Rachel's attitude started to shift. When talking about food, I heard less about her examples of "willpower," and more about healthy choices. Externally, one of the first changes I noticed was how she was dressed. Rachel had begun to wear work clothes that enabled her to perform a set of "tricep dips" at her desk. Her fitness indicators were all improving, and she genuinely seemed to have more pep in her step!

On completion of the 12-week program, Rachel had lost 6 lb and increased her strength, flexibility, and aerobic fitness. What was more exciting, however, was that Rachel had gained a real appreciation of the value of daily practices of active living. She was able to restructure her work schedule to allow her to walk to school once a week with her children. She incorporated stretch breaks into the start of every meeting at work. She used the stairs instead of the elevator and always opened a door with her own strength (without assistance from an automatic door). It was only in retrospect that Rachel realized that the choices she and her family were making for recreation had shifted from inside activities, such as shopping and the movies, to hiking, cycling, and swimming. Rachel also realized that her new choices had resulted in meeting new friends who shared similar interests in being active and enjoying family activities that involved movement.

Rachel's New Wellness Vision

"My wellness vision is to move and keep moving — to move freely through a full range of motion and to move in a way that enables me to do all the things that I need to do in my life and have energy left over. I want to move with and for my children and grandchildren. I may be challenged by old habits of acting on misguided priorities, but I know that with the help of my friends and family and by incorporating brief workout breaks into my day and committing to at least one act of active living every day, I will be able to sustain and maintain my newfound joy."

Rachel was able to achieve her new goal of moving more by small choices and daily practices that reflected a new attitude about exercise. She set an achievable goal of incorporating one act of active living into every day. Rachel also became willing to meet new people who were like-minded and would support her efforts to be active. To an outside observer, Rachel's changes may seem like minor adjustments in her schedule, but to anyone who really knows her, a seismic shift took place that will enable Rachel to realize her wellness vision and goals for the future.

QUESTIONS

- What did the EP-C do to support Rachel's goals? The EP-C had a key role in actively listening to Rachel. The EP-C was skilled in not only being able to identify Rachel's interest in losing weight but also wanting to incorporate active living. As a facilitator of motivation, the EP-C was able to encourage Rachel to identify ways in which active living techniques could be incorporated into daily life. The EP-C also provided a sound exercise program that encouraged competence, confidence, and relatedness.
- What role did social support play in Rachel's success? Rachel was able to establish herself as a leader and learner. She was encouraged to be creative in the completion of her goals. By including coworkers, Rachel was able to share the benefits of exercise and have support when she was challenged to work through lunch. Rachel was also able to enlist the help of her children by creating time for a walk to school morning.
- How can one act of active living a day make a difference in someone's life? A shift in attitude and expectations enabled Rachel to evaluate her original goals in a way that sustained her adherence to the program. By committing to one act of active living, Rachel was able to cultivate other habits of behavior around both exercise and nutrition that further aided her in reaching her weight loss and fitness goals.

References

1. Brownson RC, Eyler AA, King AC, Brown DR, Shyu Y, Sallis JF. Patterns and correlates of physical activity among US women 40 years and older. *Am J Public Health*. 2000;90(2):264–70.
2. Kerr J, Norman GJ, Sallis JF, Patrick K. Exercise aids, neighborhood safety, and physical activity in adolescents and parents. *Med Sci Sports Exerc*. 2008;40(7):1244–8.
3. Moore M, Tschannen-Moran B. *Coaching Psychology Manual*. Baltimore (MD): Lippincott Williams & Wilkins; 2009. 208 p.
4. Moustaka FC, Vlachopoulos SP, Kabitsis C, Theodorakis Y. Effects of an autonomy-supportive exercise instructing style on exercise motivation, psychological well-being, and exercise attendance in middle-age women. *J Phys Act Health*. 2012;9(1):138–50.

SUMMARY

As discussed earlier in this chapter, the notion that PA can improve and/or maintain health is by no means novel. However, it was not until substantial scientific advancements during the 20th century, in fields such as exercise physiology and epidemiology, that our understanding of how PA could treat and/or prevent common chronic diseases (*e.g.*, CVD, hypertension, and Type 2 diabetes mellitus) became known. Despite these advancements, there remain many unanswered questions regarding the exact pathways and mechanisms through which PA influences health. Along with that, there are also levels of uncertainty in terms of intensities and volume thresholds that can or should be performed to reap the greatest benefits without going too far.

Although there is still much to learn, the current evidence strongly indicates that regular PA and exercise can have tremendous benefits for an individual's physical, metabolic, and mental health. However, overexercising, doing too much too soon or for too long without adequate recovery methods, or exercising at an unsafe intensity can bring negative consequences, even as severe as sudden death. Although the risks associated with exercise are proportional to the amount and intensity of exercise, both acute and chronic, the benefits of habitual exercise far outweigh the risks.

This resource manual is intended to prepare the EP-C with the necessary tools to assess fitness and prescribe exercise for populations able to exercise without medical supervision. Although no manual is completely comprehensive, the information within should serve as an outstanding resource for both the new and the experienced exercise professional.

STUDY QUESTIONS

1. Compare and contrast PA, exercise, health-related fitness, and skill-related fitness.
2. Describe at least two individuals and two landmark research studies that made significant contributions to the current body of knowledge regarding PA/physical fitness and associated health benefits.
3. Describe the health benefits and health risks associated with acute and chronic PA.

REFERENCES

1. Amed S, Daneman D, Mahmud FH, Hamilton J. Type 2 diabetes in children and adolescents. *Expert Rev Cardiovasc Ther*. 2010;8(3):393–406.

2. American College of Sports Medicine. The recommended quality and quantity of exercise for developing and maintaining fitness in healthy adults. *Med Sci Sports Exerc*. 1978; 10(3):vii–x.

3. American College of Sports Medicine, American Heart Association. Exercise and acute cardiovascular events: placing the risks into perspective. *Med Sci Sports Exerc*. 2007;39(5): 886–97.

4. Archer E, Shook RP, Thomas DM, et al. 45-Year trends in women's use of time and household management energy expenditure. *PLoS One*. 2013;8(2):e56620.

5. Bailey DA, McKay HA, Mirwald RL, Crocker PRE, Faulkner RA. A six-year longitudinal study of the relationship of physical activity to bone mineral accrual in growing children: the University of Saskatchewan bone mineral accrual study. *J Bone Miner Res*. 1999;14(10):1672–9.

6. Berryman JW. Thomas K. Cureton, Jr.: pioneer researcher, proselytizer, and proponent for physical fitness. *Res Q Exerc Sport*. 1996;67(1):1–12.

7. Black A, Black MM, Gensini G. Exertion and acute coronary artery injury. *Angiology*. 1975;26(11):759–83.

8. Blair SN, Kohl HW III, Paffenbarger RS Jr, Clark DG, Cooper KH, Gibbons LW. Physical fitness and all-cause mortality: a prospective study of healthy men and women. *JAMA*. 1989;262(17):2395–401.

9. Blair SN, Morris JN. Healthy hearts — and the universal benefits of being physically active: physical activity and health. *Ann Epidemiol*. 2009;19(4):253–6.

10. Brosseau L, Pelland L, Wells G, Macleay L, Lamothe C, Michaud G. Efficacy of aerobic exercises for osteoarthritis. Part II. A meta-analysis. *Phys Ther Rev*. 2004;9:125–45.

11. Caspersen CJ, Powell KE, Christenson GM. Physical activity, exercise, and physical fitness: definitions and distinctions for health-related research. *Public Health Rep*. 1985;100(2): 126–31.

12. Centers for Disease Control and Prevention. Nonfatal sports- and recreation-related injuries treated in emergency departments — United States, July 2000–June 2001. *MMWR Morb Mortal Wkly Rep*. 2002;51(33):736–40

13. Centers for Disease Control and Prevention, National Center for Chronic Disease Prevention and Health Promotion, Division of Population Health. BRFSS Prevalence and Trends Data [Internet]. Atlanta (GA): Centers for Disease Control and Prevention; [cited 2015 Oct 3]. Available from: http://www.cdc.gov/brfss/brfssprevalence/

14. Chodzko-Zajko W, Schwingel A, Park CH. Successful aging: the role of physical activity. *Am J Lifestyle Med*. 2009;3(1):20–8.

15. Church TS, Thomas DM, Tudor-Locke C, et al. Trends over 5 decades in U.S. occupation-related physical activity and their associations with obesity. *PLoS One*. 2011;6(5):e19657.

16. Ciampricotti R, Deckers JW, Taverne R, el Gamal M, Relik-van Wely L, Pool J. Characteristics of conditioned and sedentary men with acute coronary syndromes. *Am J Cardiol*. 1994;73(4): 219–22.

17. Colbert LH, Hootman JM, Macera CA. Physical activity-related injuries in walkers and runners in the aerobics center longitudinal study. *Clin J Sport Med*. 2000;10(4):259–63.

18. Drezner JA, Chun JS, Harmon KG, Derminer L. Survival trends in the United States following exercise-related sudden cardiac arrest in the youth: 2000–2006. *Heart Rhythm*. 2008;5(6):794–9.

19. Ekelund LG, Haskell WL, Johnson JL, Whaley FS, Criqui MH, Sheps DS. Physical fitness as a predictor of cardiovascular mortality in asymptomatic North American men. The lipid research clinics mortality follow-up study. *N Engl J Med*. 1988;319(21):1379–84.

20. Evans WJ. Effects of exercise on body composition and functional capacity of the elderly. *J Gerontol A Biol Sci Med Sci*. 1995;50(Special Issue):147–50.

21. Feskanich D, Willett W, Colditz G. Walking and leisure-time activity and risk of hip fracture in postmenopausal women. *JAMA*. 2002;288(18):2300–6.

22. Gibbons L, Blair SN, Kohl HW, Cooper K. The safety of maximal exercise testing. *Circulation*. 1989;80(4):846–52.

23. Giri S, Thompson PD, Kiernan FJ, et al. Clinical and angiographic characteristics of exertion-related acute myocardial infarction. *JAMA*. 1999;282(18):1731–6.

24. Gortmaker SL, Must A, Perrin JM, Sobol AM, Dietz WH. Social and economic consequences of overweight in adolescence and young adulthood. *N Engl J Med*. 1993;329(14):1008–12.

25. Hammoudeh AJ, Haft JI. Coronary-plaque rupture in acute coronary syndromes triggered by snow shoveling. *N Engl J Med*. 1996;335(26):2001–2.

26. Haskell WL, Lee IM, Pate RR, et al. Physical activity and public health: updated recommendation for adults from the American College of Sports Medicine and the American Heart Association. *Med Sci Sports Exerc*. 2007;39(8):1423–34.

27. Hayashi T, Tsumura K, Suematsu C, Okada K, Fujii S, Endo G. Walking to work and the risk for hypertension in men: the Osaka Health Survey. *Ann Intern Med*. 1999;131(1):21–6.

28. Heesch KC, Byles JE, Brown WJ. Prospective association between physical activity and falls in community-dwelling older women. *J Epidemiol Community Health*. 2008;62(5):421–6.

29. Hernandez CJ, Beaupre GS, Carter DR. A theoretical analysis of the relative influences of peak BMD, age-related bone loss and menopause on the development of osteoporosis. *Osteoporos Int*. 2003;14(10):843–7.

30. Hippocrates. *Jones WHS, Translation*. Regimen I. Cambridge (MA): Harvard University Press; 1952. 229 p.

31. Hootman JM, Macera CA, Ainsworth BE, Addy CL, Martin M, Blair SN. Epidemiology of musculoskeletal injuries among sedentary and physically active adults. *Med Sci Sports Exerc*. 2002; 34(5):838–44.

32. Hu FB, Sigal RJ, Rich-Edwards JW, et al. Walking compared with vigorous physical activity and risk of type 2 diabetes in women: a prospective study. *JAMA*. 1999;282(15):1433–9.

33. Hu G, Tuomilehto J, Silventoinen K, Barengo NC, Jousilahti P. Joint effects of physical activity, body mass index, waist circumference and waist-to-hip ratio with the risk of cardiovascular disease among middle-aged Finnish men and women. *Eur Heart J*. 2004;25(24):2212–9.

34. Hu G, Tuomilehto J, Silventoinen K, Barengo NC, Peltonen M, Jousilahti P. The effects of physical activity and body mass index on cardiovascular, cancer and all-cause mortality among 47,212 middle-aged Finnish men and women. *Int J Obes.* 2005;29(8):894–902.

35. Jacobs SJ, Berson BL. Injuries to runners: a study of entrants to a 10,000 meter race. *Am J Sports Med.* 1986;14(2):151–5.

36. Janiszewski PM, Ross R. Physical activity in the treatment of obesity: beyond body weight reduction. *Appl Physiol Nutr Metab.* 2007;32(3):512–22.

37. Janssen I, Katmarzyk PT, Boyce WF, et al. Comparison of overweight and obesity prevalence in school-aged youth from 34 countries and their relationships with physical activity and dietary patterns. *Obes Rev.* 2005;6(2):123–32.

38. Knight JA, Laubach CA Jr, Butcher RJ, Menapace FJ. Supervision of clinical exercise testing by exercise physiologists. *Am J Cardiol.* 1995;75(5):390–1.

39. Koplan JP, Powell KE, Sikes RK, Shirley RW, Campbell CC. An epidemiologic study of the benefits and risks of running. *JAMA.* 1982;248(23):3118–21.

40. Ku CY, Gower BA, Hunter GR, Goran MI. Racial differences in insulin secretion and sensitivity in prepubertal children: role of physical fitness and physical activity. *Obes Res.* 2000; 8(7):506–15.

41. Lakka TA, Venäläinen JM, Rauramaa R, Salonen R, Tuomilehto J, Salonen JT. Relation of leisure-time physical activity and cardiorespiratory fitness to the risk of acute myocardial infarction. *N Engl J Med.* 1994;330(22):1549–54.

42. Lee IM, Paffenbarger RS Jr. Associations of light, moderate, and vigorous intensity physical activity with longevity: the Harvard alumni health study. *Am J Epidemiol.* 2000;151(3):293–9.

43. Leon AS, Connett J, Jacobs DR Jr, Rauramaa R. Leisure-time physical activity levels and risk of coronary heart disease and death: the multiple risk factor intervention trial. *JAMA.* 1987;258(17):2388–95.

44. Liguori G, Carroll-Cobb S. *FitWell: Questions and Answers.* New York (NY): McGraw-Hill; 2011. 66 p.

45. Lloyd-Jones D, Adams RJ, Brown TM, et al. Executive summary: heart disease and stroke statistics — 2010 update. *Circulation.* 2010;121(7):948–54.

46. Lyons AS, Petrucelli RJ. *Medicine: An Illustrated History.* New York (NY): Abradale Press; 1978. 130 p.

47. Lysholm J, Wiklander J. Injuries in runners. *Am J Sports Med.* 1987;15(2):168–71.

48. Macera CA, Pate RR, Powell KE, Jackson KL, Kendrick JS, Craven TE. Predicting lower-extremity injuries among habitual runners. *Arch Intern Med.* 1989;149(11):2565–8.

49. Manson JE, Hu FB, Rich-Edwards JW, et al. A prospective study of walking as compared with vigorous exercise in the prevention of coronary heart disease in women. *N Engl J Med.* 1999;341(9):650–8.

50. Manson JE, Nathan DM, Krolewski AS, Stampfer MJ, Willett WC, Hennekens CH. A prospective study of exercise and incidence of diabetes among US male physicians. *JAMA.* 1992;268(1):63–7.

51. Maron BJ, Doerer JJ, Haas TS, Tierney DM, Mueller FO. Sudden deaths in young competitive athletes: analysis of 1866 deaths in the United States, 1980–2006. *Circulation.* 2009;119(8):1085–92.

52. Marti B. Benefits and risks of running among women: an epidemiologic study. *Int J Sports Med.* 1988;9(2):92–8.

53. McHenry PL. Risks of graded exercise testing. *Am J Cardiol.* 1977;39(6):935–7.

54. McTiernan A, Ulrich C, Slate S, Potter J. Physical activity and cancer etiology: associations and mechanisms. *Cancer Causes Control.* 1998;9(5):487–509.

55. Mittleman MA, Maclure M, Tofler GH, Sherwood JB, Goldberg RJ, Muller JE. Triggering of acute myocardial infarction by heavy physical exertion. Protection against triggering by regular exertion. Determinants of Myocardial Infarction Onset Study Investigators. *N Engl J Med.* 1993; 329(23):1677–83.

56. Morris JN, Heady JA, Raffle PA, Roberts CG, Parks JW. Coronary heart-disease and physical activity of work. *Lancet.* 1953;265(6795):1053–7.

57. Morris JN, Pollard R, Everitt MG, Chave SPW, Semmence AM. Vigorous exercise in leisure-time: protection against coronary heart disease. *Lancet.* 1980;316(8206):1207–10.

58. Murthy VH. Surgeon General's perspectives: improving the physical and emotional health of adolescents to ensure success in adulthood. *Public Health Rep.* 2015;130(3):193–5.

59. Must A, Anderson SE. Effects of obesity on morbidity in children and adolescents. *Nutr Clin Care.* 2003;6(1):4–12.

60. Myers J, Prakash M, Froelicher V, Do D, Partington S, Atwood JE. Exercise capacity and mortality among men referred for exercise testing. *N Engl J Med.* 2002;346(11):793–801.

61. Myers J, Voodi L, Umann T, Froelicher VF. A survey of exercise testing: methods, utilization, interpretation, and safety in the VAHCS. *J Cardiopulm Rehabil.* 2000;20(4):251–8.

62. Ogden CL, Carroll MD. *Prevalence of Obesity among Children and Adolescents: United States, Trends 1963–1965 through 2007–2008.* Hyattsville (MD): Centers for Disease Control and Prevention, National Center for Health Statistics; 2010. 5 p.

63. Ogden CL, Carroll MD, Kit BK, Flegal KM. Prevalence of childhood and adult obesity in the United States, 2011-2012. *JAMA.* 2014;311(8):806–14.

64. Paffenbarger RS Jr, Laughlin ME, Gima AS, Black RA. Work activity of longshoremen as related to death from coronary heart disease and stroke. *N Engl J Med.* 1970;282(20): 1109–14.

65. Pate RR, Pratt M, Blair SN, et al. Physical activity and public health. A recommendation from the Centers for Disease Control and Prevention and the American College of Sports Medicine. *JAMA.* 1995;273(5):402–7.

66. Pediatrics Web site [Internet]. Elk Grove Village (IL): American Academy of Pediatrics; [cited 2011 May 15]. Available from: http://pediatrics.aappublications.org/

67. Pelland L, Brosseau L, Wells G, et al. Efficacy of strengthening exercises for osteoarthritis. Part I. A meta-analysis. *Phys Ther Rev.* 2004;9(2):77–108.

68. Pereira MA, Folsom AR, McGovern PG, et al. Physical activity and incident hypertension in black and white adults: the atherosclerosis risk in communities study. *Prev Med.* 1999; 28(3):304–12.

69. Powell KE, Heath GW, Kresnow MJ, Sacks JJ, Branche CM. Injury rates from walking, gardening, weightlifting, outdoor bicycling, and aerobics. *Med Sci Sports Exerc.* 1998; 30(8):1246–9.

70. Racette SB, Weiss EP, Villareal DT, et al. One year caloric restriction in humans: feasibility and effects on body composition and abdominal adipose tissue. *J Gerontol A Biol Sci Med Sci.* 2006;61(9):943–50.

71. Raitakari OT, Porkka KV, Taimela S, Telama R, Rasanen L, Viikari JS. Effects of persistent physical activity and inactivity on coronary risk factors in children and young adults. The cardiovascular risk in young Finns study. *Am J Epidemiol.* 1994;140(3):195–205.

72. Rochmis P, Blackburn H. Exercise tests. A survey of procedures, safety, and litigation experience in approximately 170,000 tests. *JAMA.* 1971;217(8):1061–6.

73. Ross R, Dagnone D, Jones PJ, et al. Reduction in obesity and related comorbid conditions after diet-induced weight loss or exercise-induced weight loss in men: a randomized, controlled trial. *Ann Intern Med.* 2000;133(2):92–103.

74. Ross R, Janssen I, Dawson J, et al. Exercise-induced reduction in obesity and insulin resistance in women: a randomized controlled trial. *Obes Res.* 2004;12(5):789–98.

75. Sandvik L, Erikssen J, Thaulow E, Erikssen G, Mundal R, Rodahl K. Physical fitness as a predictor of mortality among healthy, middle-aged Norwegian men. *N Engl J Med.* 1993;328(8):533–7.

76. Schwimmer JB, Burwinkle TM, Vami JW. Health-related quality of life of severely obese children and adolescents. *JAMA.* 2003;289(14):1813–9.

77. Sesso HD, Paffenbarger RS Jr, Lee IM. Physical activity and coronary heart disease in men. *Circulation.* 2000;102(9):975–80.

78 Singh GK, Kogan MD, Van Dyck PC, Siahpush M. Racial/ ethnic, socioeconomic, and behavioral determinants of childhood and adolescent obesity in the United States: analyzing independent and joint associations. *Ann Epidemiol.* 2008;18(9):682–95.

79. Siscovick DS, Weiss NS, Fletcher RH, Lasky T. The incidence of primary cardiac arrest during vigorous exercise. *N Engl J Med.* 1984;311(14):874–7.

80. Slattery ML, Jacobs DR Jr, Nichaman MZ. Leisure time physical activity and coronary heart disease death: the US railroad study. *Circulation.* 1989;79(2):304–11.

81. Slentz CA, Duscha BD, Johnson JL, et al. Effects of the amount of exercise on body weight, body composition, and measures of central obesity: STRRIDE — a randomized controlled study. *Arch Intern Med.* 2004;164(1):31–9.

82. Steffen-Batey L, Nichaman MZ, Goff DC Jr, et al. Change in level of physical activity and risk of all-cause mortality or reinfarction: the Corpus Christi Heart Project. *Circulation.* 2000;102(18):2204–9.

83. Stuart RJ Jr, Ellestad MH. National survey of exercise stress testing facilities. *Chest.* 1980;77(1):94–7.

84. Talbot LA, Morrell CH, Metter EJ, Fleg JL. Comparison of cardiorespiratory fitness versus leisure time physical activity as predictors of coronary events in men aged 65 years. *Am J Cardiol.* 2002;89(10):1187–92.

85. Thompson PD, Funk EJ, Carleton RA, Sturner WQ. Incidence of death during jogging in Rhode Island from 1975 through 1980. *JAMA.* 1982;247(18):2535–8.

86. Thompson PD, Stern MP, Williams P, Duncan K, Haskell WL, Wood PD. Death during jogging or running. A study of 18 cases. *JAMA.* 1979;242(12):1265–7.

87. Troiano RP, Berrigan D, Dodd KW, Mâsse LC, Tilert T, McDowell M. Physical activity in the United States measured by accelerometer. *Med Sci Sports Exerc.* 2008;40(1):181–8.

88. U.S. Bureau of Labor Statistics. *Economic News Release: American Time Use Survey —2010 Results.* Washington (DC): U.S. Bureau of Labor Statistics; [cited 2017 Feb]. Available from: http://www .bls.gov/news.release/atus.nr0.htm

89. U.S. Bureau of Labor Statistics. *Spotlight on Statistics: Sports and Exercise.* Washington (DC): U.S. Bureau of Labor Statistics; [cited 2017 Feb]. Available from: http://www.bls .gov/spotlight/2008/sports/pdf/sports_bls_spotlight.pdf

90. U.S. Department of Health and Human Services. *Physical Activity and Health: A Report of the Surgeon General* (DHHS Publication No. 017-023-00196-5). Washington (DC): U.S. Department of Health and Human Services; 1996. 292 p.

91. U.S. Department of Health and Human Services, Office of Disease Prevention & Health Promotion. *2008 Physical Activity Guidelines for Americans* (ODPHP Publication No. U0036). Washington (DC): U.S. Department of Health and Human Services; 2008. 76 p.

92. Van Camp SP, Bloor CM, Mueller FO, Cantu RC, Olson HG. Nontraumatic sports death in high school and college athletes. *Med Sci Sports Exerc.* 1995;27(5):641–7.

93. Vuori I. The cardiovascular risks of physical activity. *Acta Med Scand.* 1986;711:205–14.

94. Walter SD, Hart LE, McIntosh JM, Sutton JR. The Ontario cohort study of running-related injuries. *Arch Intern Med.* 1989;149(11):2561–4.

95. Willich SN, Lewis M, Lowel H, Arntz HR, Schubert F, Schroder R. Physical exertion as a trigger of acute myocardial infarction. Triggers and mechanisms of myocardial infarction study group. *N Engl J Med.* 1993;329(23):1684–90.

2

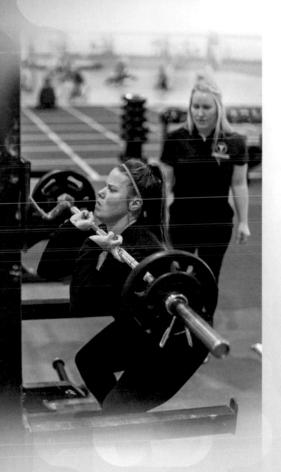

Preparticipation Physical Activity Screening Guidelines

OBJECTIVES

- To understand the process and outcomes of the American College of Sports Medicine (ACSM) Preparticipation Physical Activity Screening.

- To explore the importance of and issues with preparticipation physical activity screening as well as to investigate the various tools that may be used including the Physical Activity Readiness Questionnaire for Everyone (PAR-Q+) and a health history questionnaire.

- To determine course of action with a client once their risk has been established.

- To discuss the concept of absolute and relative contraindications to exercise testing.

INTRODUCTION

Ever since the increased promotion of physical activity in modern times, there has been an emphasis on preparticipation physical activity screening to ensure that the risks of an increased physical activity do not outweigh the benefits of this healthy behavior (6). The process of preparticipation physical activity screening has been increasingly professionalized over the years since its introduction. The American College of Sports Medicine (ACSM) is perhaps the best known organization in the area of preparticipation physical activity screening in the United States. The ACSM formally titled this process *risk stratification* in the 1990's in *ACSM's Guidelines for Exercise Testing and Prescription, Fourth Edition* (GETP) publication. This process was retitled *risk classification* in 2013 (3). With the release of 10th edition of GETP in 2017, there were some substantial changes to the preparticipation physical activity screening process including the elimination of the *risk stratification/classification* terminology (including low-, moderate-, and high-risk strata) and the nonuse of adding/subtracting ACSM risk factor thresholds for overall risk. This will be discussed further in this chapter.

The preparticipation physical activity screening process is also intimately tied to the contraindications for graded exercise testing discussed later in this chapter. This chapter will explore the preparticipation physical activity screening concept so the ACSM Certified Exercise Physiologist^{SM} (EP-C) can make informed decisions about the readiness of an individual to undertake a physically active lifestyle.

Importance of Preparticipation Physical Activity Screening

In order to reduce the likelihood of occurrence of any untoward or unwanted event(s) during a physical activity program, it is prudent to conduct some form of preparticipation physical activity screening on a client (24). Preparticipation physical activity screening, along with cardiovascular risk factor assessment discussed later in this chapter, may also be the first step in a health-related physical fitness assessment. Preparticipation physical activity screening involves gathering and analyzing demographic and health-related information on a client along with some medical/health assessments such as the presence of signs and symptoms in order to aid decision making on a client's physical activity future (3). The preparticipation physical activity screening is a dynamic process in that it may vary in its scope and components depending on the client's needs from a medical/health standpoint (*e.g.*, the client has some form of cardiovascular, metabolic, and/or renal disease, abbreviated as CMR) as well as the presence of signs and symptoms suggestive of CMR disease (*e.g.*, chest pain of an ischemic nature) and their physical activity program goals (they currently participate in moderate physical activity for the past 3 months).

The following is a partial list of the reasons why it is important to first screen clients for participation in physical activity programs (3,17):

- To identify those with medical contraindications (exclusion criteria) for performing physical activity
- To identify those who should receive a medical/physical evaluation/exam and clearance prior to performing a physical activity program
- To identify those who should participate in a medically supervised physical activity program
- To identify those with other health/medical concerns (*i.e.*, orthopedic injuries, *etc.*)

History of Preparticipation Physical Activity Screening

There are several national and international organizations that have made suggestions about just what these preparticipation physical activity screening guidelines should be including the ACSM (1,2,11,28). However, it is helpful to remember that these are just guidelines or suggestions. The prudent EP-C should devise a preparticipation physical activity screening scheme that best meets the needs of their client(s) and environment(s).

For instance, the U.S. Surgeon General in the 1996 report on *Physical Activity and Health* stated that (24)

> Previously inactive men over age 40, women over age 50, and people at high risk for CVD [CVD is an abbreviation for cardiovascular disease] should first consult a physician before embarking on a program of vigorous physical activity to which they are unaccustomed. People with disease should be evaluated by a physician first. . . .

In addition, a summary of the "cautions" listed on many pieces of exercise equipment as well as in exercise books and videos is to

- "First consult your physician before starting an exercise program."
- "This is especially important for
  - Men ≥45 years old; women ≥55 years old
  - Those who are going to perform vigorous physical activity
  - And for those who are new to exercise or are unaccustomed to exercise"

There is one major set of formal screening guidelines for individuals who wish to embark on a physical activity program. This set comes from the ACSM. The ACSM has published this set in their popular and often revised text, *ACSM's GETP* starting with their 4th edition in 1991. Several other professional organizations including the American Heart Association (AHA) have also published and revised their own set of preparticipation physical activity screening guidelines. The AHA guidelines were published most recently in their journal *Circulation* in 2001 (3,11).

As stated earlier, the ACSM, through its GETP text, has addressed preparticipation physical activity screening (3). In the past, the ACSM has listed these preparticipation physical activity screening guidelines often under the moniker, "Risk Stratification." Through the first eight editions (although risk stratification did not appear formally in the first three editions) of the GETP, there have been several revisions made to this risk stratification section. The ninth edition of the GETP terms this process as *risk classification*. The recent (2017) 10th edition of GETP has put forth major changes to the preparticipation physical activity screening process (3). We would categorize the revisions made to the GETP preparticipation physical activity screening process as mostly an elimination of the "strata" or levels used in risk classification as well as the elimination of the use of the ACSM risk factor thresholds for the process. In the place of the ACSM risk factor thresholds is the dependence on the physical activity history of the participant as well as the presence of CMR disease and the presence of signs and symptoms suggestive of CMR disease (3).

Levels of Screening

According to the ACSM, there are two basic approaches to preparticipation physical activity screening (3). One of these approaches can be performed by the individual wishing to become more physically active without direct input from an exercise professional (self-guided screening). Although the other approach involves interaction with an exercise professional such as an EP-C (professionally supervised screening). These two levels of screening are not mutually exclusive; for instance, an individual may first use the self-guided method before seeking an EP-C for professional guidance in preparticipation screening.

Self-Guided Screening

Self-guided approaches to preparticipation physical activity screening have been suggested by many organizations from the ACSM to the AHA as a minimum or starting point for the individual who wishes to increase his or her physical activity (3). The Physical Activity Readiness Questionnaire for Everyone (PAR-Q+) has been suggested for use in self-guided screening and is discussed next.

Physical Activity Readiness Questionnaire+

The Health History Questionnaire (HHQ) is generally thought of as being a comprehensive assessment of a client's medical and health history. Because the HHQ can be more information than is needed in some situations, the Physical Activity Readiness Questionnaire, or PAR-Q, was developed in Canada to be simpler in both scope and use (26). The original PAR-Q contains seven YES/NO questions that have been found to be both readable and understandable for an individual to answer. The PAR-Q was designed to screen out those clients from not participating in physical activities that may be too strenuous for them. The PAR-Q has been recommended as a minimal standard for entry into moderate-intensity exercise programs. Thus, the PAR-Q may be considered a useful tool for individuals to gauge their own "medical" readiness to participate in physical activity programs (3). However, since the PAR-Q may be best used to screen those who are at high risk for exercise and thus may need a medical exam, it may not be as effective in screening low- to moderate-risk individuals (28). Thus, the PAR-Q has recently morphed into the PAR-Q+ with some word changes among the seven YES/NO questions to better classify all individuals (3) (Fig. 2.1).

Thus, at the minimum, a prudent EP-C should consider suggesting to their clients that they fill out a PAR-Q+ prior to participation in any self-guided physical activity program (3,32).

The PAR-Q has been found to be a useful tool (26). In one article by de Oliveira Luz and colleagues (9), the PAR-Q was found to have a high (89%) sensitivity (producing many true positives) for picking up potential medical conditions that might impact an individual's exercise responses in older subjects. However, it should be noted that the specificity (or true negatives) of the PAR-Q in this subject pool was estimated at 42% (9). Thus, the PAR-Q may be quite good at detecting potential problems in clients before they occur in an exercise setting, but the form may also wrongly identify clients as having a potential problem when on further evaluation, there is no need for concern. This may not be a bad situation as the form errors of the side of caution. The prudent EP-C may therefore need to intervene in such cases as well as involve further health care professionals.

Because there are some potential problems noted with the PAR-Q as far as its ability to discern if an individual's potential adverse medical condition might impact his or her exercise response, the PAR-Q+ was developed. However, the PAR-Q+ is a very recent development and thus statistics related to the PAR-Q+ effectiveness are not yet available. It has been suggested by Jamnik and colleagues (16) that a qualified health/fitness professional (EP-C) may, using ACSM preparticipation physical activity screening process perform a thorough screening process.

ePARmed-X+Physician Clearance Follow-Up Questionnaire

The ePARmed-X+Physician Clearance Follow-Up Questionnaire was developed also in Canada as a tool that a physician can use to refer individuals to a professionally supervised physical activity program and make recommendations for that program. This form was designed to be used in those cases where a YES answer on one of the seven questions in the PAR-Q+ necessitates further medical clearance using the self-guided method. It is also worth noting, that not while required, the ePARmed-X+Physician Clearance Follow-Up Questionnaire (Fig. 2.2) could be used for medical clearance in a professionally supervised preparticipation physical activity screening.

2015 PAR-Q+

The Physical Activity Readiness Questionnaire for Everyone

The health benefits of regular physical activity are clear; more people should engage in physical activity every day of the week. Participating in physical activity is very safe for MOST people. This questionnaire will tell you whether it is necessary for you to seek further advice from your doctor OR a qualified exercise professional before becoming more physically active.

GENERAL HEALTH QUESTIONS

Please read the 7 questions below carefully and answer each one honestly: check YES or NO.	YES	NO
1) Has your doctor ever said that you have a heart condition ☐ OR high blood pressure ☐?	☐	☐
2) Do you feel pain in your chest at rest, during your daily activities of living, **OR** when you do physical activity?	☐	☐
3) Do you lose balance because of dizziness **OR** have you lost consciousness in the last 12 months? Please answer **NO** if your dizziness was associated with over-breathing (including during vigorous exercise).	☐	☐
4) Have you ever been diagnosed with another chronic medical condition (other than heart disease or high blood pressure)? **PLEASE LIST CONDITION(S) HERE:** _____	☐	☐
5) Are you currently taking prescribed medications for a chronic medical condition? **PLEASE LIST CONDITION(S) AND MEDICATIONS HERE:** _____	☐	☐
6) Do you currently have (or have had within the past 12 months) a bone, joint, or soft tissue (muscle, ligament, or tendon) problem that could be made worse by becoming more physically active? Please answer **NO** if you had a problem in the past, but it *does not limit your current ability* to be physically active. **PLEASE LIST CONDITION(S) HERE:** _____	☐	☐
7) Has your doctor ever said that you should only do medically supervised physical activity?	☐	☐

☑ **If you answered NO to all of the questions above, you are cleared for physical activity.**
  Go to Page 4 to sign the PARTICIPANT DECLARATION. You do not need to complete Pages 2 and 3.

  ▶ Start becoming much more physically active – start slowly and build up gradually.

  ▶ Follow International Physical Activity Guidelines for your age (www.who.int/dietphysicalactivity/en/).

  ▶ You may take part in a health and fitness appraisal.

  ▶ If you are over the age of 45 yr and **NOT** accustomed to regular vigorous to maximal effort exercise, consult a qualified exercise professional before engaging in this intensity of exercise.

  ▶ If you have any further questions, contact a qualified exercise professional.

⬤ **If you answered YES to one or more of the questions above, COMPLETE PAGES 2 AND 3.**

⚠ **Delay becoming more active if:**

  ✓ You have a temporary illness such as a cold or fever; it is best to wait until you feel better.

  ✓ You are pregnant - talk to your health care practitioner, your physician, a qualified exercise professional, and/or complete the ePARmed-X+ at **www.eparmedx.com** before becoming more physically active.

  ✓ Your health changes - answer the questions on Pages 2 and 3 of this document and/or talk to your doctor or a qualified exercise professional before continuing with any physical activity program.

FIGURE 2.1. Physical Activity Readiness Questionnaire for Everyone (PAR-Q+). (Reprinted with permission from the PAR-Q+ Collaboration and the authors of the PAR-Q+ [Dr. Darren Warburton, Dr. Norman Gledhill, Dr. Veronica Jamnik, and Dr. Shannon Bredin].) (*continued*)

2015 PAR-Q+

FOLLOW-UP QUESTIONS ABOUT YOUR MEDICAL CONDITION(S)

1.   Do you have Arthritis, Osteoporosis, or Back Problems?

If the above condition(s) is/are present, answer questions 1a-1c   If **NO** ☐ go to question 2

1a.	Do you have difficulty controlling your condition with medications or other physician-prescribed therapies? (Answer **NO** if you are not currently taking medications or other treatments)	YES ☐ NO ☐
1b.	Do you have joint problems causing pain, a recent fracture or fracture caused by osteoporosis or cancer, displaced vertebra (e.g., spondylolisthesis), and/or spondylolysis/pars defect (a crack in the bony ring on the back of the spinal column)?	YES ☐ NO ☐
1c.	Have you had steroid injections or taken steroid tablets regularly for more than 3 months?	YES ☐ NO ☐

2.   Do you have Cancer of any kind?

If the above condition(s) is/are present, answer questions 2a-2b   If **NO** ☐ go to question 3

2a.	Does your cancer diagnosis include any of the following types: lung/bronchogenic, multiple myeloma (cancer of plasma cells), head, and neck?	YES ☐ NO ☐
2b.	Are you currently receiving cancer therapy (such as chemotheraphy or radiotherapy)?	YES ☐ NO ☐

3.   Do you have a Heart or Cardiovascular Condition? *This includes Coronary Artery Disease, Heart Failure, Diagnosed Abnormality of Heart Rhythm*

If the above condition(s) is/are present, answer questions 3a-3d   If **NO** ☐ go to question 4

3a.	Do you have difficulty controlling your condition with medications or other physician-prescribed therapies? (Answer **NO** if you are not currently taking medications or other treatments)	YES ☐ NO ☐
3b.	Do you have an irregular heart beat that requires medical management? (e.g., atrial fibrillation, premature ventricular contraction)	YES ☐ NO ☐
3c.	Do you have chronic heart failure?	YES ☐ NO ☐
3d.	Do you have diagnosed coronary artery (cardiovascular) disease and have not participated in regular physical activity in the last 2 months?	YES ☐ NO ☐

4.   Do you have High Blood Pressure?

If the above condition(s) is/are present, answer questions 4a-4b   If **NO** ☐ go to question 5

4a.	Do you have difficulty controlling your condition with medications or other physician-prescribed therapies? (Answer **NO** if you are not currently taking medications or other treatments)	YES ☐ NO ☐
4b.	Do you have a resting blood pressure equal to or greater than 160/90 mmHg with or without medication? (Answer **YES** if you do not know your resting blood pressure)	YES ☐ NO ☐

5.   Do you have any Metabolic Conditions? *This includes Type 1 Diabetes, Type 2 Diabetes, Pre-Diabetes*

If the above condition(s) is/are present, answer questions 5a-5e   If **NO** ☐ go to question 6

5a.	Do you often have difficulty controlling your blood sugar levels with foods, medications, or other physician-prescribed therapies?	YES ☐ NO ☐
5b.	Do you often suffer from signs and symptoms of low blood sugar (hypoglycemia) following exercise and/or during activities of daily living? Signs of hypoglycemia may include shakiness, nervousness, unusual irritability, abnormal sweating, dizziness or light-headedness, mental confusion, difficulty speaking, weakness, or sleepiness.	YES ☐ NO ☐
5c.	Do you have any signs or symptoms of diabetes complications such as heart or vascular disease and/or complications affecting your eyes, kidneys, **OR** the sensation in your toes and feet?	YES ☐ NO ☐
5d.	Do you have other metabolic conditions (such as current pregnancy-related diabetes, chronic kidney disease, or liver problems)?	YES ☐ NO ☐
5e.	Are you planning to engage in what for you is unusually high (or vigorous) intensity exercise in the near future?	YES ☐ NO ☐

FIGURE 2.1. *(continued)*

2015 PAR-Q+

6.　Do you have any Mental Health Problems or Learning Difficulties? *This includes Alzheimer's, Dementia, Depression, Anxiety Disorder, Eating Disorder, Psychotic Disorder, Intellectual Disability, Down Syndrome*

If the above condition(s) is/are present, answer questions 6a-6b　　If **NO** ☐ go to question 7

6a.	Do you have difficulty controlling your condition with medications or other physician-prescribed therapies? (Answer **NO** if you are not currently taking medications or other treatments)	YES☐ NO☐
6b.	Do you **ALSO** have back problems affecting nerves or muscles?	YES☐ NO☐

7.　Do you have a Respiratory Disease? *This includes Chronic Obstructive Pulmonary Disease, Asthma, Pulmonary High Blood Pressure*

If the above condition(s) is/are present, answer questions 7a-7d　　If **NO** ☐ go to question 8

7a.	Do you have difficulty controlling your condition with medications or other physician-prescribed therapies? (Answer **NO** if you are not currently taking medications or other treatments)	YES☐ NO☐
7b.	Has your doctor ever said your blood oxygen level is low at rest or during exercise and/or that you require supplemental oxygen therapy?	YES☐ NO☐
7c.	If asthmatic, do you currently have symptoms of chest tightness, wheezing, laboured breathing, consistent cough (more than 2 days/week), or have you used your rescue medication more than twice in the last week?	YES☐ NO☐
7d.	Has your doctor ever said you have high blood pressure in the blood vessels of your lungs?	YES☐ NO☐

8.　Do you have a Spinal Cord Injury? *This includes Tetraplegia and Paraplegia*

If the above condition(s) is/are present, answer questions 8a-8c　　If **NO** ☐ go to question 9

8a.	Do you have difficulty controlling your condition with medications or other physician-prescribed therapies? (Answer **NO** if you are not currently taking medications or other treatments)	YES☐ NO☐
8b.	Do you commonly exhibit low resting blood pressure significant enough to cause dizziness, light-headedness, and/or fainting?	YES☐ NO☐
8c.	Has your physician indicated that you exhibit sudden bouts of high blood pressure (known as Autonomic Dysreflexia)?	YES☐ NO☐

9.　Have you had a Stroke? *This includes Transient Ischemic Attack (TIA) or Cerebrovascular Event*

If the above condition(s) is/are present, answer questions 9a-9c　　If **NO** ☐ go to question 10

9a.	Do you have difficulty controlling your condition with medications or other physician-prescribed therapies? (Answer **NO** if you are not currently taking medications or other treatments)	YES☐ NO☐
9b.	Do you have any impairment in walking or mobility?	YES☐ NO☐
9c.	Have you experienced a stroke or impairment in nerves or muscles in the past 6 months?	YES☐ NO☐

10.　Do you have any other medical condition not listed above or do you have two or more medical conditions?

If you have other medical conditions, answer questions 10a-10c　　If **NO** ☐ read the Page 4 recommendations

10a.	Have you experienced a blackout, fainted, or lost consciousness as a result of a head injury within the last 12 months **OR** have you had a diagnosed concussion within the last 12 months?	YES☐ NO☐
10b.	Do you have a medical condition that is not listed (such as epilepsy, neurological conditions, kidney problems)?	YES☐ NO☐
10c.	Do you currently live with two or more medical conditions?	YES☐ NO☐

PLEASE LIST YOUR MEDICAL CONDITION(S) AND ANY RELATED MEDICATIONS HERE: _____

_____

GO to Page 4 for recommendations about your current medical condition(s) and sign the PARTICIPANT DECLARATION.

FIGURE 2.1. *(continued)*

2015 PAR-Q+

☑ **If you answered NO to all of the follow-up questions about your medical condition, you are ready to become more physically active - sign the PARTICIPANT DECLARATION below:**

▶ It is advised that you consult a qualified exercise professional to help you develop a safe and effective physical activity plan to meet your health needs.

▶ You are encouraged to start slowly and build up gradually - 20 to 60 minutes of low to moderate intensity exercise, 3-5 days per week including aerobic and muscle strengthening exercises.

▶ As you progress, you should aim to accumulate 150 minutes or more of moderate intensity physical activity per week.

▶ If you are over the age of 45 yr and **NOT** accustomed to regular vigorous to maximal effort exercise, consult a qualified exercise professional before engaging in this intensity of exercise.

⬤ **If you answered YES to one or more of the follow-up questions** about your medical condition:

You should seek further information before becoming more physically active or engaging in a fitness appraisal. You should complete the specially designed online screening and exercise recommendations program - the **ePARmed-X+ at www.eparmedx.com** and/or visit a qualified exercise professional to work through the ePARmed-X+ and for further information.

⚠ **Delay becoming more active if:**

✓ You have a temporary illness such as a cold or fever; it is best to wait until you feel better.

✓ You are pregnant - talk to your health care practitioner, your physician, a qualified exercise professional, and/or complete the ePARmed-X+ **at www.eparmedx.com** before becoming more physically active.

✓ Your health changes - talk to your doctor or qualified exercise professional before continuing with any physical activity program.

⬤ You are encouraged to photocopy the PAR-Q+. You must use the entire questionnaire and NO changes are permitted.
⬤ The authors, the PAR-Q+ Collaboration, partner organizations, and their agents assume no liability for persons who undertake physical activity and/or make use of the PAR-Q+ or ePARmed-X+. If in doubt after completing the questionnaire, consult your doctor prior to physical activity.

PARTICIPANT DECLARATION

⬤ All persons who have completed the PAR-Q+ please read and sign the declaration below.

⬤ If you are less than the legal age required for consent or require the assent of a care provider, your parent, guardian or care provider must also sign this form.

I, the undersigned, have read, understood to my full satisfaction and completed this questionnaire. I acknowledge that this physical activity clearance is valid for a maximum of 12 months from the date it is completed and becomes invalid if my condition changes. I also acknowledge that a Trustee (such as my employer, community/fitness centre, health care provider, or other designate) may retain a copy of this form for their records. In these instances, the Trustee will be required to adhere to local, national, and international guidelines regarding the storage of personal health information ensuring that the Trustee maintains the privacy of the information and does not misuse or wrongfully disclose such information.

NAME _____   DATE _____

SIGNATURE _____   WITNESS _____

SIGNATURE OF PARENT/GUARDIAN/CARE PROVIDER _____

——— **For more information, please contact** ———
www.eparmedx.com
Email: eparmedx@gmail.com

Citation for PAR-Q+
Warburton DER, Jamnik VK, Bredin SSD, and Gledhill N on behalf of the PAR-Q+ Collaboration. The Physical Activity Readiness Questionnaire for Everyone (PAR-Q+) and Electronic Physical Activity Readiness Medical Examination (ePARmed-X+). Health & Fitness Journal of Canada 4(2):3-23, 2011.
Key References
1. Jamnik VK, Warburton DER, Makarski J, McKenzie DC, Shephard RJ, Stone J, and Gledhill N. Enhancing the effectiveness of clearance for physical activity participation; background and overall process. APNM 36(S1):S3-S13, 2011.
2. Warburton DER, Gledhill N, Jamnik VK, Bredin SSD, McKenzie DC, Stone J, Charlesworth S, and Shephard RJ. Evidence-based risk assessment and recommendations for physical activity clearance; Consensus Document. APNM 36(S1):S266-s298, 2011.

The PAR-Q+ was created using the evidence-based AGREE process (1) by the PAR-Q+ Collaboration chaired by Dr. Darren E. R. Warburton with Dr. Norman Gledhill, Dr. Veronica Jamnik, and Dr. Donald C. McKenzie (2). Production of this document has been made possible through financial contributions from the Public Health Agency of Canada and the BC Ministry of Health Services. The views expressed herein do not necessarily represent the views of the Public Health Agency of Canada or the BC Ministry of Health Services.

OSHF
Ontario Society for Health and Fitness

FIGURE 2.1. (*continued*)

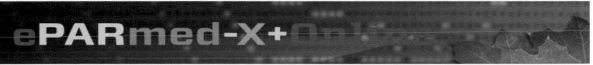

ePARmed-X+ Physician Clearance Follow-Up

This form is separated into three main sections:

A) Background information regarding the PAR-Q+ and ePARmed-X+ clearance process,
B) A brief history and demographic information regarding the participant, and
C) The physician's recommendations regarding the participant becoming more physically active.

At the end of this process, the participant is recommended to take this signed clearance form to a qualified exercise professional or other healthcare professional (as recommended in the ePARmed-X+) before becoming <u>more</u> physically active or engaging in a fitness appraisal.

A BACKGROUND INFORMATION REGARDING THE PAR-Q+ AND ePARMed-X+ CLEARANCE PROCESS

The ePARmed-X+ is an easy to follow interactive program (<u>www.eparmedx.com</u>) that can be used to determine an individual's readiness for increased physical activity participation or a fitness appraisal. The ePARmed-X+ supplements the paper and online versions of the new Physical Activity Readiness Questionnaire for Everyone (PAR-Q+).

Individuals who use the ePARmed-X+ have had a positive response to the PAR-Q+, or have been directed to the online program by a qualified exercise professional or another healthcare professional, owing to his/her current medical condition. At the end of the ePARmed-X+, it is possible that the participant is advised to consult a physician to discuss the various options regarding becoming <u>more</u> physically active. In this instance, the participant will be required to receive medical clearance for physical activity from a physician. Until this medical clearance is received, the participant is restricted to low intensity physical activity participation.

This document serves to assist both the participant and physician in the physical activity clearance process.

B PERSONAL INFORMATION

NAME: _____   SEX: ☐ M or ☐ F

ADDRESS: _____   BIRTHDATE (mm/dd/yy): _____
                       _____
                       _____

TELEPHONE: _____   HEALTH/MEDICAL NUMBER: _____

REASON FOR REFERRAL (SELECT ALL THAT APPLY):

☐ QUALIFIED EXERCISE PROFESSIONAL REFERRAL
☐ HEALTH CARE PROFESSIONAL REFERRAL
☐ ePARmed-X+ RECOMMENDATION

FIGURE 2.2. ePARmed-X+ Physician Clearance Follow-Up Questionnaire+. (Reprinted with permission from the PAR-Q+ Collaboration and the authors of the ePARmed-X+ [Dr. Darren Warburton, Dr. Norman Gledhill, Dr. Veronica Jamnik, and Dr. Shannon Bredin].) (*continued*)

ePARmed-X+ Online

C ePARmed-X+ PHYSICAL ACTIVITY READINESS PHYSICIAN REFERRAL FORM

Based on the current review of the health status of _____(name)
I recommend the following course of action:

☐ The participant should avoid engaging in physical activity at this time.

☐ The participant should engage in only a medically supervised physical activity/exercise program involving the supervision of a qualified exercise professional (or other appropriately trained health care professional) and overseen by a physician.

☐ The participant is cleared for intensity and mode appropriate physical activity/exercise training under the supervision of a qualified exercise professional.

☐ The participant is cleared for intensity and mode appropriate physical activity/exercise training with limited supervision (i.e., unrestricted physical activity).

The following precautions should be taken when prescribing exercise for the aforementioned participant:

o   With the avoidance of: _____
_____
_____
_____

o   With the inclusion of: _____
_____
_____
_____

NAME OF PHYSICIAN: _____

ADDRESS: _____

TELEPHONE: _____

Date of Medical Clearance (mm/dd/yy): _____

PHYSICIAN/CLINIC STAMP AND SIGNATURE

NOTE: This physical activity/exercise clearance is valid for a period of six months from the date it is completed and becomes invalid if the medical condition of the above named participant changes/worsens.

FIGURE 2.2. (*continued*)

Professionally Supervised Screening

Self-analysis of risk for physical activity is important with the large number of individuals who are currently not physically active but hopefully will become more active soon perhaps by self-guidance. Thus, they will need to, or should, use some means to determine their physical readiness, like the PAR-Q+. However, many individuals will seek the knowledge and guidance of an EP-C for this service. Professional readiness, under the guidance of an EP-C, may involve collecting a health history on an individual (and possibly medical clearance, if warranted) while following the ACSM preparticipation physical activity process (3). The EP-C may be involved in professional screening at the "lower" levels of risk, whereas professionals such as the ACSM Certified Clinical Exercise Physiologist® (CEP) will be more likely involved with individuals at a higher risk. In the following section, we discuss the HHQ as well as the medical evaluation/clearance.

Health History Questionnaire

Some form of an HHQ is necessary to use with a client to establish his or her medical/health risks for participation in a physical activity program (13,28). The HHQ, along with other medical/health data, is also used in the process of preparticipation physical activity screening. The HHQ should be tailored to fit the needs of the program as far as asking for the specific information needed from a client. In general, the HHQ should minimally assess a client's (3)

- Family history of CMR disease
- Personal history of various diseases and illnesses including CMR disease
- Surgical history
- Past and present health behaviors/habits (such as history of cigarette smoking and physical activity)
- Current use of various drugs/medications
- Specific history of various signs and symptoms suggested of CMR disease among other things

The current edition of the GETP contains a more detailed list of the specifics of the health and medical evaluations (including desirable laboratory tests) (3). Again, the prudent EP-C should tailor the HHQ to their client's specific needs. A sample HHQ is included in this chapter (Fig. 2.3).

Medical Examination/Clearance

A medical examination led by a physician (or other qualified health care professional) may also be necessary or desirable to help evaluate the health and/or medical status of your client prior to a physical activity program. The suggested components of this medical examination can be found in the most current edition of the GETP (3). In addition to a medical examination, it may be desirable to perform some routine laboratory assessments (*i.e.*, fasting blood cholesterol and/or resting blood pressure) on your client prior to physical activity programming (28). Clients who are at a higher risk for exercise complications may need (it is recommended) a medical clearance prior to participation in a physical activity program.

Preparticipation Physical Activity Screening Process

The process for screening prior to participation in a physical activity program has been altered significantly from past iterations of this process from the ACSM (3). Essentially, only three items need to be considered to complete the process, as is spelled out in Figure 2.4. Perhaps the first item to consider in the process is the individual's past physical activity history. The individual can be queried about his or her physical activity history using the HHQ and/or by questioning. Next, the individual should be evaluated for the presence of known CMR disease. This, too, can be assessed using the HHQ and/or by questioning. Finally, in the process is the assessment of the individual's presence of signs and symptoms that can be suggestive of CMR disease. The ACSM in its recent GETP provides a form for the assessment of all three of these components of the process. This form can be found in Figure 2.5.

HEALTH HISTORY QUESTIONNAIRE

NAME_____AGE_____DATE_____DATE OF BIRTH_____
      First   M.I.   Last   day/month/yr   day/month/yr

ADDRESS_____
      Street   City/State/Zip

TELEPHONE (home)_____(business)_____(cell)_____

OCCUPATION_____PLACE OF EMPLOYMENT_____

MARITAL STATUS: (circle one)   SINGLE   MARRIED   DIVORCED   WIDOWED

SPOUSE:_____

EDUCATION: (check highest level)   ELEMENTARY_____ HIGH SCHOOL_____ COLLEGE_____

GRADUATE_____

ETHNICITY:_____ PERSONAL PHYSICIAN_____

LOCATION_____

Reason for last doctor visit?_____ Date of last physician exam_____

Have you previously been tested for an exercise Program?   YES_____   NO_____   YEAR(s)_____

LOCATION OF TEST_____

Person to contact in case of an emergency_____ Phone #_____

(relationship)_____

PLEASE CHECK YES or NO

PAST (Have you ever had?)	YES	NO
High blood pressure	☐	☐
Heart problems	☐	☐
Disease of the arteries	☐	☐
Varicose veins	☐	☐
Lung disease	☐	☐
Asthma	☐	☐
Kidney disease	☐	☐
Hepatitis	☐	☐
Diabetes	☐	☐
Orthopedic problems	☐	☐
Arthritis	☐	☐

FAMILY (Have any immediate family or grandparents had?)	YES	NO
Heart attacks	☐	☐
High blood pressure	☐	☐
High cholesterol	☐	☐
Stroke	☐	☐
Diabetes	☐	☐
Congenital heart defect	☐	☐
Heart operations	☐	☐
Early death	☐	☐
Other family illness _____		
_____		
_____		

PRESENT SYMPTOMS (Have you recently had?)	YES	NO
Chest pain/discomfort	☐	☐
Shortness of breath	☐	☐
Dizzy spells	☐	☐
Skipped heart beats	☐	☐
Trouble sleeping	☐	☐
Ankle swelling	☐	☐
Leg pain/cramping	☐	☐
Frequent headaches	☐	☐
Frequent colds	☐	☐
Back pain	☐	☐
Orthopedic problems	☐	☐

(FOR STAFF COMMENTS)

_____
_____
_____

FIGURE 2.3. Health History Questionnaire used at East Stroudsburg University. (*continued*)

HEALTH HISTORY QUESTIONNAIRE

HOSPITALIZATIONS: Please list recent hospitalizations (Women: do not list normal pregnancies)

Year	Location	Reason

Any other medical problems/concerns not already identified? Yes_____ No_____ (Please list below)

_____

Have you ever had your cholesterol measures? Yes_____ No_____; If yes, (value)_____ (Date)_____

Are you taking any Prescription or Non-Prescription medications? Yes_____ No_____ (include birth control pills)

Medication	Reason for Taking	For How Long?

Do you currently smoke? Yes_____ No_____ If so, what? Cigarettes_____ Cigars_____ Pipe_____

How much per day: < .5 pack_____   0.5 to 1pack_____   1.5 to 2 packs_____   > 2 packs_____

Have you ever quit smoking? Yes_____ No_____ When?_____ How many years and how

much did you smoke?_____

Do you drink any alcoholic beverages? Yes_____ No_____ If Yes, how much in 1 week?

Beer_____(cans)   Wine_____(glasses)   Hard liquor_____(drinks)

Do you drink any caffeinated beverages? Yes_____ No_____ If Yes, how much in 1 week?

Coffee_____(cups)   Tea_____(glasses)   Soft drinks_____(cans)

ACTIVITY LEVEL EVALUATION

What is your occupational activity level?   sedentary_____; light_____; moderate_____; heavy_____

Do you currently engage in vigorous physical activity on a regular basis? Yes_____ No_____

If so, what type?_____ How many days per week?_____

How much time per day? (check one)   < 15 min_____   15–30 min_____   30–45 min_____   > 60 min_____

Do you ever have an uncomfortable shortness of breath during exercise? Yes_____ No_____

Do you ever have chest discomfort during exercise? Yes_____ No_____ If so, does it go away with rest?_____

Do you engage in any recreational or leisure-time physical activities on a regular basis? Yes_____ No_____

If so, what activities?_____

On average: How often?_____times/week;   For how long?_____time/session

FIGURE 2.3. (*continued*)

HEALTH HISTORY QUESTIONNAIRE

Are you currently following a weight reduction diet plan? Yes_____ No_____ Name:_____

If so, how long have you been dieting? _____months   Is the plan prescribed by your doctor? Yes_____ No_____

Have you used weight reduction diets in the past? Yes_____ No_____;   If yes, how often and which type(s)?

_____

Please indicate the reasons why you want to join the exercise program.

To lose weight _____ Doctor's recommendation_____ For good health _____ Enjoyment_____

Release of tension_____ Improve physical appearance _____ Other _____

<u>**FOR STAFF USE:**</u>

_____

_____

FIGURE 2.3. (*continued*)

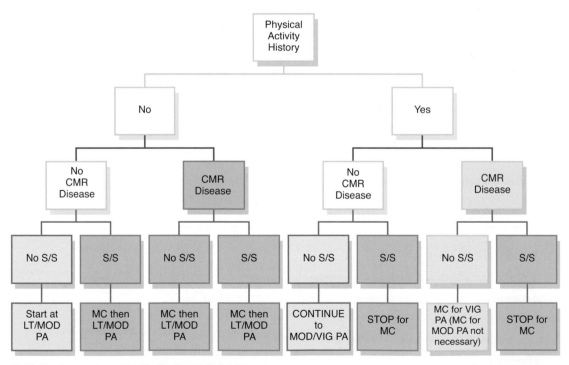

CMR: Cardiovascular, metabolic, and/or renal disease
S/S: Signs and symptoms suggestive of CMR disease
MC: Medical clearance
LT/MOD PA: Light to moderate physical activity
VIG PA: Vigorous physical activity

FIGURE 2.4. Decision tree for preparticipation screening; simplified algorithm.

Exercise Preparticipation Health Screening Questionnaire for Exercise Professionals

Assess your client's health needs by marking all *true* statements.

Step 1

SYMPTOMS
Does your client experience:
_____ chest discomfort with exertion
_____ unreasonable breathlessness
_____ dizziness, fainting, blackouts
_____ ankle swelling
_____ unpleasant awareness of a forceful, rapid or irregular heart rate
_____ burning or cramping sensations in your lower legs when walking short distance

If you **did** mark any of these statements under the symptoms, **STOP**, your client should should seek medical clearance before engaging in or resuming exercise. Your client may need to use a facility with a **medically qualified staff**.

If you **did not** mark any symptoms, continue to steps 2 and 3.

Step 2

CURRENT ACTIVITY
Has your client performed planned, structured physical activity for at least 30 min at moderate intensity on at least 3 days per week for at least the last 3 months?

Yes ☐ No ☐

Continue to Step 3.

Step 3

MEDICAL CONDITIONS
Has your client had or do they currently have:
_____ a heart attack
_____ heart surgery, cardiac catheterization, or coronary angioplasty
_____ pacemaker/implantable cardiac defibrillator/rhythm disturbance
_____ heart valve disease
_____ heart failure
_____ heart transplantation
_____ congenital heart disease
_____ diabetes
_____ renal disease

Evaluating Steps 2 and 3:

- If you **did not mark any of the statements in Step 3**, medical clearance is not necessary.
- If you marked Step 2 **"yes"** and **marked any of the statements in Step 3**, your client may continue to exercise at light to moderate intensity without medical clearance. Medical clearance is recommended before engaging in vigorous exercise.
- If you marked Step 2 **"no"** and **marked any of the statements in Step 3**, medical clearance is recommended. Your client may need to use a facility with a **medically qualified staff**.

FIGURE 2.5. Preparticipation physical activity screening questionnaire for exercise professionals.

It is important to note that the process of ACSM preparticipation physical activity screening has been divorced from the concept of the need for and supervisory qualifications of a graded exercise test and other health-related physical fitness assessments. Recent professional society opinions and research have devalued the use of graded exercise testing for many adults as part of the diagnostic workup for cardiovascular disease (3). Thus, preparticipation physical activity screening is about participating in a physical activity program not about exercise testing. We will discuss all three components of the preparticipation physical activity screening process in the following section.

PHYSICAL ACTIVITY (OR EXERCISE) HISTORY

An individual who currently engages in physical activity is considered to be at lower risk for a cardiovascular event during exercise than one who is sedentary. Current physical activity is considered to be within the last 3 months. The threshold dose of physical activity that is necessary to lower one's risk, according to the ACSM, is 30 minutes or more of at least moderate physical activity on at least 3 days $\cdot$ week^{-1}. Moderate physical activity has several descriptors associated with it including exercise at a level that is between 40% and 60% of the individual's heart rate reserve or maximal oxygen uptake reserve. Moderate-intensity physical activity or exercise is further described as between 3 and 6 metabolic equivalents (METs) and at a rating of perceived exertion (RPE) of around 12–13 on the traditional 6–20 scale. Also, moderate-intensity causes noticeable increases in heart rate and breathing.

KNOWN CARDIOVASCULAR, METABOLIC, AND/OR RENAL DISEASE

Clients with any of the CMR diseases are at a higher risk for an untoward event during exercise. Thus, the presence of a CMR disease will influence the level of preparticipation physical activity screening. A listing of the specific diseases and/or conditions covered are as follows:

- Heart attack
- Heart surgery, cardiac catheterization, or coronary angioplasty
- Pacemaker/implantable cardiac defibrillator/rhythm disturbance
- Heart valve disease
- Heart failure
- Heart transplantation
- Congenital heart disease (*congenital* refers to birth)
- Diabetes, type 1 and 2
- Renal disease such as renal failure

Those of you familiar with "older" systems of risk classification will note the absence of pulmonary diseases from this list of diseases and/or conditions. Pulmonary disease has been shown to be less likely to cause untoward events during exercise than CMR disease and thus has been removed from the list (3).

ACSM MAJOR SIGNS OR SYMPTOMS SUGGESTIVE OF CARDIOVASCULAR DISEASE

There are several outward signs or symptoms that may indicate a client has current CMR disease. These signs and symptoms can be found in the following sections along with further discussion of these signs or symptoms. If a client has any of these signs or symptoms, then he or she is considered at a higher risk, and it is recommended that you seek medical clearance before they participate in a physical activity program. It is important to remember that these signs or symptoms must be interpreted within the clinical context in which they appear because they are not all specific for CMR disease.

Discussion of ACSM Signs or Symptoms

There are eight signs and symptoms suggestive of CMR disease which include:

- Pain or discomfort in the chest, neck, jaw, arms, or other areas that may be due to ischemia or lack of oxygenated blood flow to the tissue, such as the heart (27). Remember that chest pain or angina is not always located in the chest area of a client. Women in particular may experience low back pain or feelings of indigestion as opposed to chest pain. Some key features of this pain that *favors an ischemic origin* include the following:

- *Character*: The pain is felt as constricting, squeezing, burning, "heaviness," or "heavy feeling."
- *Location*: The pain is substernal, across the midthorax, anteriorly; in one or both arms or shoulders; in neck, cheeks, or teeth; or in forearms, fingers, and/or in the interscapular region.
- *Provoking factors*: The pain comes on with exercise or exertion, excitement, other forms of stress, cold weather, or after meals (3).

- *Dyspnea* is the medical term for shortness of breath (27). Dyspnea is expected in most individuals during moderate to severe exertion such as stair climbing. However, shortness of breath at rest or with mild exertion may indicate cardiac and/or pulmonary disease and should be examined by a physician. Dyspnea (defined as an abnormally uncomfortable awareness of breathing) is one of the principal symptoms of cardiac and pulmonary disease. It commonly occurs during strenuous exertion in healthy, well-trained individuals and during moderate exertion in healthy, untrained individuals. However, it should be regarded as abnormal when it occurs at a level of exertion that is not expected to evoke this symptom in a given individual. Abnormal exertional dyspnea suggests the presence of cardiopulmonary disorders, in particular, left ventricular dysfunction or chronic obstructive pulmonary disease (3).

- Syncope, or fainting, and dizziness during exercise may indicate poor blood flow to the brain due to inadequate cardiac output from a number of cardiac disorders (27). However, syncope and dizziness upon sudden cessation of exercise is relatively common even among healthy individuals due to a sudden decrease in venous return and consequent reduction in blood flow to the brain. Cardiac disorders that are associated with syncope and dizziness are potentially life-threatening and include severe coronary artery disease, hypertrophic cardiomyopathy, aortic stenosis, and malignant ventricular dysrhythmias. Although dizziness or syncope shortly *after* cessation of exercise should not be ignored, these symptoms may occur even in healthy individuals as a result of a reduction in venous return to the heart (3).

- Orthopnea refers to trouble breathing while lying down. Paroxysmal nocturnal dyspnea refers to difficulty breathing while asleep, beginning usually 2–5 hours after the onset of sleep, which may be relieved by sitting on the side of the bed or getting out of bed (27). Both are indicative of poor left ventricular function. Patients with these conditions often report sleeping in recliners to lessen the symptoms of this disorder. Orthopnea is relieved promptly by sitting upright or standing. Although nocturnal dyspnea may occur in individuals with chronic obstructive pulmonary disease, it differs in that it is usually relieved following a bowel movement rather than specifically by sitting up (3).

- Ankle edema, or swelling, that is not due to injury is suggestive of heart failure, a blood clot, insufficiency of the veins, or a lymph system blockage (27). Generalized edema (known as anasarca) occurs in individuals with the nephrotic (from the kidneys) syndrome, severe heart failure, or hepatic (from the liver) cirrhosis. Bilateral ankle edema that is most evident at night is a characteristic sign of heart failure or bilateral chronic venous insufficiency. Unilateral edema of a limb often results from venous thrombosis or lymphatic blockage in the limb (3).

- Palpitations and tachycardia both refer to rapid beating or fluttering of the heart (27). The client may report a feeling of unpleasantness associated with the unusual heart rhythm. Palpitations (defined as an unpleasant awareness of the forceful or rapid beating of the heart) may be induced by various disorders of cardiac rhythm. These include tachycardia, bradycardia of sudden onset, ectopic beats, compensatory pauses, and accentuated stroke volume resulting from valvular regurgitation. Palpitations also often result from anxiety states and high cardiac output (or hyperkinetic) states, such as anemia, fever, thyrotoxicosis, arteriovenous fistula, and the so-called idiopathic hyperkinetic heart syndrome (3).

- Intermittent claudication refers to severe calf pain when walking (27). This pain indicates a lack of oxygenated blood flow to the working muscles similar in origin to chest pain. The pain does not occur with standing or sitting, is reproducible from day to day, is more severe when walking upstairs or up a hill, and is often described as a cramp, which disappears within 1–2 minutes after stopping exercise. Coronary artery disease is more prevalent in individuals with intermittent claudication. Patients with diabetes are at increased risk for this condition (3).

■ Heart murmurs are unusual sounds caused by blood flowing through the heart (27). Although some murmurs may be innocent, heart murmurs may indicate valvular or other cardiovascular disease. From an exercise safety standpoint, it is especially important to exclude hypertrophic cardiomyopathy and aortic stenosis as underlying causes because these are among the more common causes of exertion-related sudden cardiac death. Unless previously diagnosed and determined to be safe, all murmurs should be evaluated by a physician (3).

■ Unusual fatigue or shortness of breath that occurs during light exertion or normal activity and not during strenuous activity (27). Although there may be benign origins for these symptoms, they also may signal the onset of or change in the status of cardiovascular and/or metabolic disease (3).

WHAT TO DO ONCE RISK IS ESTABLISHED?

Figure 2.4 is our attempt to clarify some of the decisions aided by the ACSM preparticipation physical activity screening process. The EP-C should always keep in mind that the ACSM preparticipation physical activity screening process is a guideline and may need to be modified based on several issues such as local medical practice or custom.

Essentially, Figure 2.4 represents a paradigm shift in preparticipation screening from previous ACSM screening paradigms, and we have chosen to colorize the figure to aid the EP-C with this decision tree. Medical clearance, which may include a medical examination by a health care professional including a physician, is suggested and recommended to be a part of the preparticipation physical activity screening workup if your client has signs and symptoms suggestive of CMR disease. We have denoted this outcome using the color blue in Figure 2.4. In fact, individuals who meet these criteria (signs and symptoms suggestive of CMR disease) should only participate after getting medical clearance to do so. Individuals who may be free of signs and symptoms but have the presence of CMR disease may benefit from medical clearance, and thus, we have used the color yellow for caution in Figure 2.4. This is very true in your clients who currently do not participate in a physical activity program. However, in most "apparently healthy" clients (free of CMR disease and signs and symptoms suggestive of CMR disease), it is acceptable to get them started in a moderate-intensity physical activity program without the need for previous medical clearance. We have used the color green for this outcome in Figure 2.4.

As you can see in Figure 2.4, the current physical activity history of a client does influence these decisions. For instance, if your client has not been physically active in the recent past (last 3 mo), then you are more likely to recommend medical clearance to start a low to moderate physical activity program, whereas the previously physically active client may be able to proceed to a more moderate to vigorous physical activity program.

The prudent EP-C would always err on the side of caution when there are uncertainties and request full medical clearance. The ePARmed-X+Physician Clearance Follow-Up Questionnaire may be used for medical clearance.

Vigorous exercise is often defined as greater than or equal to 60% of your client's functional capacity (≥ 6 METs, ≥ 14 on a 6–20 RPE scale, and cause substantial increases in heart rate and breathing), whereas low to moderate exercise programs would be less than 60% of functional capacity (5,12,15,23).

Two previous features of the ACSM Risk Stratification/Classification process were the use and supervision of graded exercise testing. Nondiagnostic exercise testing is generally performed for exercise prescriptive and/or functional capacity purposes, whereas diagnostic exercise testing may be performed to assess the presence or impact of cardiovascular disease (34). Submaximal exercise testing may also be useful in individualizing your client's exercise prescription as well as gaining functional capacity information as is discussed in other chapters of this textbook. Research and expert opinion has recently questioned the value of the diagnostic exercise test (12,19).

The supervision criterion of exercise testing has also undergone much revision in recent years. Training in exercise testing administration is required and includes certification in emergency care (*i.e.*, AHA Advanced Cardiac Life Support Certification) as well as experience in exercise testing interpretation and emergency plan practice (12,18,19).

Thus, a competent EP-C may oversee the judicious use of the preparticipation physical activity screening and graded exercise test for exercise prescription purposes in their lower risk clients. However, other personnel may need to become involved if the preparticipation physical activity screening suggests the need for medical clearance (3,25).

American Association of Cardiovascular and Pulmonary Rehabilitation (AACVPR) Risk Stratification

Other professional organizations have also published guidelines that address risk stratification and preparticipation physical activity screening (1–3,10,15,34). Most prominently among these are AHA and AACVPR. Similar to the recent changes in ACSM preparticipation exercise screening, other guidelines have been modified to reduce impediments to begin or continue safe and effective exercise programming.

The AACVPR has contributed to the field of preparticipation physical activity screening and risk stratification with guidelines revised most recently in 2013 (1–3,34). The AACVPR risk stratification scheme continues to utilize Low, Moderate, and High risk categories to identify level of risk of physical activity triggering an untoward event.

The AACVPR risk stratification scheme may serve as a nice bridge toward offering services and programming to more "risky" or diseased clients as might be found in clinical exercise programs such as cardiac rehabilitation or medical fitness facilities, perhaps supervised by a CEP or ACSM Registered Clinical Exercise Physiologist® (RCEP). The AACVPR risk stratification guidelines are listed in Figure 2.6 (3,34).

Pitfalls of ACSM Preparticipation Physical Activity Screening

Perhaps the greatest pitfall of ACSM preparticipation physical activity screening is overlooking a sign or symptom of ongoing cardiovascular disease and then the client has a cardiac event while under your direction. Although the incidence of such events are rare (see "Exercise is Medicine" box), the prudent EP-C should exercise caution in minimizing such risk (14,29–31). To reduce the risk of such an event, the EP-C should obtain as much medical history information as possible through the HHQ and client interviews. When in doubt, particularly in a moderately risky client who may, in actuality, be of a higher risk client, the ACSM recommends consulting with a health care professional for advice on how to proceed. Remember, it is better to be conservative and prudent than to endanger your client's health (12).

Of course, this conservatism in preparticipation physical activity screening must be balanced by the public health argument of putting up too many obstacles or barriers to participation in the way of your client that you drive your client away from adopting a physically active, and healthy, lifestyle. Thus, your client might be encouraged to begin a low- to moderate-intensity program, where the overall risks of untoward events are minimal, before they undergo further medical evaluation (3). It is perhaps important for all individuals beginning a physical activity program that the initial intensity be low to moderate and increase gradually in a progressive overload fashion as discussed in other chapters in this text and the ACSM GETP (3,25).

Recommendations versus Requirements

It is important to remember that the goal of GETP is to provide direction on how to screen participants and proceed with physical activity programming. In all cases, the EP-C should exercise caution and use their best judgment when handling an individual client. When in doubt, referring a client for a medical evaluation and clearance is always in good judgment.

LOWEST RISK

Characteristics of patients at lowest risk for exercise participation (all characteristics listed must be present for patients to remain at lowest risk)

- Absence of complex ventricular dysrhythmias during exercise testing and recovery

- Absence of angina or other significant symptoms (*e.g.*, unusual shortness of breath, light-headedness, or dizziness, during exercise testing and recovery)

- Presence of normal hemodynamics during exercise testing and recovery (*i.e.*, appropriate increases and decreases in heart rate and systolic blood pressure with increasing workloads and recovery)

- Functional capacity ≥7 metabolic equivalents (METs)

Nonexercise Testing Findings

- Resting ejection fraction ≥50%

- Uncomplicated myocardial infarction or revascularization procedure

- Absence of complicated ventricular dysrhythmias at rest

- Absence of congestive heart failure

- Absence of signs or symptoms of postevent/postprocedure myocardial ischemia

- Absence of clinical depression

MODERATE RISK

Characteristics of patients at moderate risk for exercise participation (any one or combination of these findings places a patient at moderate risk)

- Presence of angina or other significant symptoms (*e.g.*, unusual shortness of breath, light-headedness, or dizziness occurring only at high levels of exertion [≥7 METs])

- Mild-to-moderate level of silent ischemia during exercise testing or recovery (ST-segment depression <2 mm from baseline)

- Functional capacity <5 METs

FIGURE 2.6. American Heart Association risk stratification. (Reprinted from Williams MA. Exercise testing in cardiac rehabilitation. Exercise prescription and beyond. *Cardiol Clin.* 2001;19[3]:415–31, with permission from Elsevier.) (*continued*)

Nonexercise Testing Findings

- Rest ejection fraction 40%–49%

HIGHEST RISK

Characteristics of patients at high risk for exercise participation (any one or combination of these findings places a patient at high risk)

- Presence of complex ventricular dysrhythmias during exercise testing or recovery

- Presence of angina or other significant symptoms (*e.g.*, unusual shortness of breath, light-headedness, dizziness at low levels of exertion [<5 METs] or during recovery)

- High level of silent ischemia (ST-segment depression ≥2 mm from baseline) during exercise testing or recovery

- Presence of abnormal hemodynamics with exercise testing (*i.e.*, chronotropic incompetence or flat or decreasing systolic blood pressure with increasing workloads) or recovery (*i.e.*, severe postexercise hypotension)

Nonexercise Testing Findings

- Rest ejection fraction <40%

- History of cardiac arrest or sudden death

- Complex dysrhythmias at rest

- Complicated myocardial infarction or revascularization procedure

- Presence of congestive heart failure

- Presence of signs or symptoms of postevent/postprocedure myocardial ischemia

- Presence of clinical depression

FIGURE 2.6. (*continued*)

It is important to note that to date, there are no published reports on the effectiveness of the ACSM preparticipation physical activity screening or the AACVPR risk classification schemes. Thus, although it is prudent to recommend that the EP-C follow or adopt such a preparticipation screening scheme, it is difficult to suggest this as a requirement to follow for a quality exercise program because it is lacking an evidence base (16).

 ## Contraindications to Exercise Testing

The process of evaluating risk (through a medical exam/health history and the ACSM preparticipation physical activity screening) may identify clinical characteristics of an individual that make physical activity risky and, thus, contraindicated. There are a host of clinical characteristics that have been identified and published by ACSM (as well as other organizations, such as the AHA) that are termed *contraindications*. These contraindications generally refer to exercise testing. This list can be found in Figure 2.7 (3). As you can see, many of these contraindications are cardiovascular disease–related only to be known by consultation with a physician and likely sophisticated medical testing. However, the resting blood pressure relative contraindication criterion (>200 mm Hg systolic blood pressure or 110 mm Hg diastolic blood pressure) is likely to be known by the EP-C during basic health-related physical fitness testing.

Absolute Contraindications

- Acute myocardial infarction within 2 days
- Ongoing unstable angina
- Uncontrolled cardiac arrhythmia with hemodynamic compromise
- Active endocarditis
- Symptomatic severe aortic stenosis
- Decompensated heart failure
- Acute pulmonary embolism, pulmonary infarction, or deep venous thrombosis
- Acute myocarditis or pericarditis
- Acute aortic dissection
- Physical disability that precludes safe and adequate testing

Relative Contraindications

- Known obstructive left main coronary artery stenosis
- Moderate to severe aortic stenosis with uncertain relationship to symptoms
- Tachyarrhythmias with uncontrolled ventricular rates
- Acquired advanced or complete heart block
- Recent stroke or transient ischemia attack
- Mental impairment with limited ability to cooperate
- Resting hypertension with systolic >200 mm Hg or diastolic >110 mm Hg
- Uncorrected medical conditions, such as significant anemia, important electrolyte imbalance, and hyperthyroidism

REF: Fletcher GF, Ades PA, Kligfield P, et al. Exercise standards for testing and training: a scientific statement from the American Heart Association. *Circulation.* 2013;128(8):873–934.

FIGURE 2.7. Contraindications to exercise testing.

What Does Contraindication Really Mean?

Just like ACSM preparticipation physical activity screening, these are guidelines that may be followed. A contraindication is a clinical characteristic that individuals may have that may make physical activity and thus, exercise testing, more risky than if the individual did not have that clinical characteristic. For instance, if an individual has unstable angina, or chest pain (unstable angina refers to chest pain that is not well controlled or predictable), then if they exercise their heart may become ischemic which could lead to a myocardial infarction, or heart attack. Although it is important to note that the incidence of cardiovascular complications is rare during exercise, a prudent EP-C would be advised to follow the contraindications listed to minimize this incidence (3,25,31). As previously discussed, many of the contraindications listed are not common, but the EP-C should protect the individual from all known and likely risks.

Absolute versus Relative

The list of contraindications is often divided between those that are *absolute* and those that are *relative*. Essentially, absolute refers to those criteria that are absolute contraindications; individuals with those biomarkers should not be allowed to participate in any form of physical activity program and/or exercise test. However, those individuals with clinical contraindications that are listed as relative may be accepted or allowed into a physical activity assessment and/or program if it is deemed that the benefits for the individual outweigh the risks to the individual (24,25). For instance, if your client has a resting blood pressure of 210/105 mm Hg, it may be decided to allow your client (medical director decision, likely) into the physical activity program because the benefits to the individual may outweigh the risks of exercising with such as high blood pressure because the individual is controlled and stable in terms of their blood pressure.

Repurposing Risk Factor Assessment and Management

As mentioned previously, the ACSM CVD Risk Assessment is no longer a mandatory component for determining if medical clearance is warranted before individuals begin an exercise program. However, identifying and controlling CVD risk factors remains an important objective of disease prevention and management. Therefore, under the new recommendations, the EP-C is encouraged to complete a CVD risk factor analysis with their patients and clients. The goal has simply shifted from using the ACSM CVD risk factor assessment as a tool for preparticipation health screening and risk stratification to identifying and managing CVD risk in patients and clients. As will be addressed later in this textbook, CVD risk factors may significantly impact exercise prescription.

Another important reason to provide CVD Risk Assessment is to help educate and inform the client about his or her need to make lifestyle modifications such as increasing physical activity and incorporating more healthful food choices in his or her diets.

Review of ACSM Atherosclerotic Cardiovascular Disease (CVD) Risk Factors and Defining Criteria

Using the client's health history (and basic health evaluation data such as resting blood pressure), simply total the number of positive ACSM Coronary Artery Disease Risk Factor Thresholds the person meets. Having one or none of these indicates a low risk of future cardiovascular disease, whereas two or more risk factors indicate an increased risk of disease. Note that only one positive factor is assigned per ACSM Risk Factor Thresholds. For instance, in obesity, a body mass index (BMI) greater than 30 kg $\cdot$ m^{-2} and a waist circumference of 105 cm (for men) would count as only one positive factor. Likewise, having both high systolic and high diastolic resting blood pressure readings would result in only one positive factor. If a client is taking a medication for hypertension or high cholesterol, he or she is considered positive for the associated risk factor regardless of his or her actual resting blood pressure or blood cholesterol measurements. There is also one negative factor (having high high-density lipoprotein [HDL-C]) that would offset one positive risk factor. The following is a detailed list of the ACSM Atherosclerotic Cardiovascular Disease (CVD) Risk Factors and Defining Criteria (3, Table 3.1):

- Client's age of 45 years or older for males and 55 years or older for females (24)
- Family history of specific cardiovascular events including myocardial infarction (heart attack), coronary revascularization (bypass surgery or angioplasty), or sudden cardiac death. This applies to first-degree relatives only. First-degree relatives are biological parents, siblings, and children. The risk factor threshold is met when at least one male relative has had one of the three specific events prior to age 55 years or before age 65 years in a female relative (33).
- If the client currently smokes cigarettes, quit smoking within the last 6 months, or if he or she is exposed to secondhand smoke on a regular basis. Secondhand smoke exposure can be assessed by the presence of cotinine in your client's urine (11,20).
- A sedentary lifestyle is defined as not participating in a regular exercise program nor meeting the minimal recommendations of 30 minutes or more of moderate physical activity on 3 days $\cdot$ week^{-1} for a least 3 months (22).
- Obesity is defined as a BMI greater than or equal 30 kg $\cdot$ m^{-2} or a waist circumference of greater than 102 cm ($\sim$40 in) for men and greater than 88 cm ($\sim$35 in) for women. If available, body fat percentage values could also be used with appropriate judgment of the EP-C (11).
- Hypertension refers to having a resting blood pressure equal to or above 140 mm Hg systolic or equal to or above 90 mm Hg diastolic or if the client is currently taking any of the numerous antihypertensive medications. Very importantly, these resting blood pressures must have been assessed on at least two separate occasions (7,8).
- Dyslipidemia refers to having a low-density lipoprotein cholesterol (LDL-C) equal or above 130 mg $\cdot$ dL^{-1}, an HDL-C of less than 40 mg $\cdot$ dL^{-1}, or if the client is taking a lipid-lowering medication. Use equal or greater than 200 mg $\cdot$ dL^{-1} if only the total blood cholesterol measurement is available (21). Although not explicitly stated in the ACSM guidelines, the cholesterol risk factor is similar to the measurement of blood pressure in that it should be abnormal on at least two separate occasions to be counted as a risk factor. Also, LDL-C is typically not measured but rather estimated from HDL-C, total cholesterol (TC), and triglycerides (3).
- Diabetes is defined as having a fasting plasma glucose $\geq$126 mg $\cdot$ dL^{-1} (7.0 mmol $\cdot$ L^{-1}) or 2 h plasma glucose values in oral glucose tolerance test (OGTT) $\geq$200 mg $\cdot$ dL^{-1} (11.1 mmol $\cdot$ L^{-1}) or HbA1C $\geq$6.5%. There must be at least two separate abnormal results for the risk factor to be counted. Remember, FBG of 126 mg $\cdot$ dL^{-1} or greater would indicate the individual has diabetes which would automatically place him or her in the high-risk level (4).
- High-serum HDL-C equal or greater than 60 mg $\cdot$ dL^{-1} (this is a negative risk factor that would offset one positive risk factor). HDL-C participates in reverse cholesterol transport and thus may lower the risk of cardiovascular disease. Although it is not stated in the ACSM guidelines, it is suggested that a client have had his or her HDL-C measured on at least two separate occasions (3).

Comparing the clients personal data to the ACSM Atherosclerotic Cardiovascular Disease (CVD) Risk Factors and Defining Criteria outlined above will help the EP-C to educate the client about his or her current health risk and evaluate the effectiveness of the exercise protocol at managing and/or attenuating this risk.

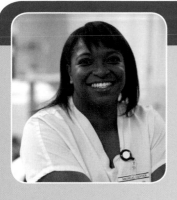

Case Studies

Below are listed three case studies using one individual (Sam J.) for the purposes of exploring further the processes of ACSM preparticipation physical activity screening, contraindications to exercise, and ACSM Risk Factor Thresholds.

ACSM Preparticipation Physical Activity Screening Case Study

The following case study is presented as an example of how to perform ACSM preparticipation physical activity screening:

Sam J., your client, decides he wants to exercise in your program. You take him through your routine preactivity screening. He presents to you with the following information: His father died of a heart attack at the age of 52 yr. His mother was put on medication for hypertension 2 yr ago at the age of 69 yr. He presents no signs or symptoms of CMR disease and is a nonsmoker. His personal data shows that he is 38 yr old. He weighs 170 lb and is 5 ft 8 in tall. His body fat percentage was measured at 22% via skinfolds. His cholesterol is 270 mg · dL^{-1}, HDL is 46 mg · dL^{-1}, and his resting blood glucose is 84 mg · dL^{-1}. His resting heart rate is 74 bpm, and his resting blood pressure measured 132/82 and 130/84 mm Hg on two separate occasions. He has a sedentary job in a factory and stands on his feet all day. He complains that as a supervisor on the job, he never gets a rest throughout his shift and often is required to work overtime. He routinely plays basketball once each week with his work buddies and then goes out for a few beers.

Physical Activity History

He plays some basketball once a week and thus is not physically active by the ACSM definition.

Presence of Cardiovascular, Metabolic, and/or Renal Disease

None noted.

Major Symptoms or Signs suggestive of Cardiovascular, Metabolic, and/or Renal Disease

None noted.

ACSM Preparticipation Physical Activity Screening Status

Medical clearance is not necessary before starting a physical activity program of a light to moderate intensity. He may progress to more vigorous-intensity exercise following ACSM GETP (3,25).

Contraindications Case Study

Sam J. has a medical evaluation with his personal physician prior to joining your vigorous exercise program. His physician performs a medical evaluation (physical exam) and reports the following: Sam J. has no signs and symptoms of CMR disease and has the known risk factors you already uncovered (dyslipidemia and sedentary lifestyle as well as a family history). His physical exams results are unremarkable except for the relative contraindications listed below.

Absolute Contraindications

None.

Relative Contraindications

Sam suffers some from rheumatoid arthritis that is not usually made worse by exercise. In addition, Sam suffered a musculoskeletal injury to his low back last year that forced him to miss 1 wk of work. However, his low back area has been problem free as of the last 6 mo.

Contraindication Analysis

Sam may not suffer from any technical contraindications that would prevent him from performing an exercise test for exercise prescription purposes as well as participating in an exercise program. Remember, relative contraindications are considered in terms of cost and benefit to your client. Certainly, as a prudent EP-C, you will want to conduct the exercise test for prescriptive purposes being careful not to exacerbate Sam's previous back injury. In addition, Sam having rheumatoid arthritis should signal you to take it easy with your client. A cautious physical activity program should be recommended for him that limits his use of his core and lower back muscles.

ACSM CVD Risk Factors History

	ACSM Coronary Artery Disease Risk Factor Thresholds	Comment
−	Age	
+	Family History	Father had heart attack (myocardial infarction) at age 52 yr old; mother with hypertension does not count
−	Cigarette Smoking	Okay, nonsmoker (not sure about passive smoke)
−	Hypertension	Okay, blood pressures measured are "fine" (132/84 mm Hg)
+	Dyslipidemia	$TC = 270$ mg $\cdot$ dL^{-1} (LDL-C unknown)
−	Diabetes	Okay ($FBG = 82$ mg $\cdot$ dL^{-1})
−	Obesity	Okay ($BMI = 25.8$ kg $\cdot$ m^{-2})
+	Sedentary Lifestyle	Sedentary
	High HDL-C	Not positive ($HDL = 46$ mg $\cdot$ dL^{-1})
3	(+) Risk Factors	

ACSM Risk Factor Analysis

Sam has a risk factor profile that is hyperlipidemic or dyslipidemic (his total cholesterol is 270 mg $\cdot$ dL^{-1} or mg%). In addition, he is currently sedentary. Thus, a prudent EP-C would stress to this client the importance of adopting a physically active lifestyle with moderate physical activity to start. In addition a health care provider may wish to explore further Sam's dyslipidemia and treatment.

EXERCISE IS MEDICINE

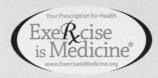

"Don't exercise too much, you may have a heart attack." How often have you heard that before. Dr. Paul Thompson and his colleagues from around the world have conducted many studies over the years to help refute that claim. In one particular study published back in 1996 in the *Archives of Internal Medicine*, Dr. Thompson studied the complications that may occur from participation in exercise (29). That study found that only 6 per 100,000 men die of exertion each year. In this article, Dr. Thompson suggested that the routine use of cardiovascular exercise tests has little diagnostic value for cardiovascular disease because of the rarity of sudden cardiac death in the population. In a scientific statement from the American Heart Association published in *Circulation* in 2007, the writing team (Dr. Thompson and his colleagues) further suggested that the risk of sudden death from exercise is greatest in those least accustomed to physical activity (31). This lends further support to the concepts of performing diagnostic exercise tests only on those at high risk for cardiovascular disease as well as using the principle of progressive overload in exercise training by starting those who are unaccustomed to exercise at a lower exercise load (intensity and duration) and gradually increasing the exercise load as they become more accustomed to exercise. Thus, the incidence of sudden cardiac death is lessened in your client. From this study and others, you can see the influence on the current ACSM preparticipation physical activity screening guidelines (3,25).

SUMMARY

Preparticipation physical activity screening is a process that may include health/medical history and informed consent of an individual client. The process is one where the client is prepared for the upcoming physical activity program. Although there are several examples or models that can be followed for the preparticipation physical activity screening process, the bottom line is the need to evaluate a client's medical readiness to undertake the physical activity program planned for them. Thus, the preparticipation physical activity screening gives the relative assurance that the client is ready and able (based on national guidelines, such as from ACSM) to participate in the rigors of the physical activity training process. It is thus important that the EP-C perform the preparticipation physical activity screening on their client.

STUDY QUESTIONS

1. Discuss each individual ACSM Risk Factor Threshold. Specifically, how do the individual ACSM Risk Factor Thresholds match up with the modifiable and nonmodifiable risk factors for coronary heart disease listed by the AHA?
2. Given the 2013 scientific statement from the AHA as well as the *2008 Physical Activity Guidelines for Americans*, does the ACSM preparticipation physical activity screening guidelines aid or hinder the concept of increasing physical activity behavior of all Americans?
3. Diabetes is relatively stressed in the ACSM preparticipation physical activity screening guidelines. (Diabetes is a CMR disease.) What are some of the complications of diabetes that justifies its inclusion in the preparticipation guidelines?

REFERENCES

1. American Association of Cardiovascular and Pulmonary Rehabilitation. *Guidelines for Cardiac Rehabilitation and Secondary Prevention Programs.* 4th ed. Champaign (IL): Human Kinetics; 2004. 288 p.

2. American Association of Cardiovascular and Pulmonary Rehabilitation. *Guidelines for Pulmonary Rehabilitation Programs.* 3rd ed. Champaign (IL): Human Kinetics; 2004. 200 p.

3. American College of Sports Medicine. *ACSM's Guidelines for Exercise Testing and Prescription.* 10th ed. Philadelphia (PA): Wolters Kluwer; 2018.

4. American Diabetes Association. Diagnosis and classification of diabetes mellitus. *Diabetes Care.* 2007;30(Suppl 1):S42–7.

5. Brawner CA, Vanzant MA, Ehrman JK, et al. Guiding exercise using the talk test among patients with coronary artery disease. *J Cardiopulm Rehabil.* 2006;26(2):72–7.

6. Buchner DM. Physical activity to prevent or reverse disability in sedentary older adults. *Am J Prev Med.* 2003;25(3 Suppl 2):214–5.

7. Cardiovascular Risk Reduction Guidelines in Adults: Cholesterol Guideline Update (ATP IV) Hypertension Guideline Update (JNC 8) Obesity Guideline Update (Obesity 2) Integrated Cardiovascular Risk Reduction Guideline: timeline for release of updated guidelines [Internet]. Bethesda (MD): National Heart, Lung and Blood Institute, National Institutes of Health; [cited 2011 Jul 7]. Available from: http://www.nhlbi.nih.gov/guidelines/cvd_adult/background.htm

8. Chobanian AV, Bakris GL, Black HR, et al. The Seventh Report of the Joint National Committee on Prevention, Detection, Evaluation, and Treatment of High Blood Pressure: the JNC 7 report. *JAMA.* 2003;289(19):2560–72.

9. de Oliveira Luz LG, de Albuquerque Maranhao Neto G, de Tarso Veras Farinatti P. Validity of the Physical Activity Readiness Questionnaire (PAR-Q) in elder subjects. *Rer Brasileira de Cine Desempenho Hun.* 2007;9(4):366–71.

10. Executive summary of the clinical guidelines on the identification, evaluation, and treatment of overweight and obesity in adults. *Arch Intern Med.* 1998;158(17):1855–67.

11. Fletcher GF, Ades PA, Kligfield P, et al. Exercise standards for testing and training: a scientific statement from the American Heart Association. *Circulation.* 2013;128(8):873–934.

12. Garber CE, Blissmer B, Deschenes MR, et al. American College of Sports Medicine stand. Quantity and quality of exercise for developing and maintaining cardiorespiratory, musculoskeletal, and neuromotor fitness in apparently healthy adults: guidance for prescribing exercise. *Med Sci Sports Exer.* 2011;43(7):1334–59.

13. Gibbons RJ, Balady GJ, Bricker JT, et al. ACC/AHA 2002 guideline update for exercise testing: summary article. A report of the American College of Cardiology/American Heart Association Task Force on Practice Guidelines (Committee to Update the 1997 Exercise Testing Guidelines). *J Am Coll Cardiol.* 2002;40(8):1531–40.

14. Giri S, Thompson PD, Kiernan FJ, et al. Clinical and angiographic characteristics of exertion-related acute myocardial infarction. *JAMA.* 1999;282(18):1731–6.

15. Haskell WL, Lee IM, Pate RR, et al. Physical activity and public health: updated recommendation for adults from the American College of Sports Medicine and the American Heart Association. *Circulation.* 2007;116(9):1081–93.

16. Jamnik VK, Gledhill N, Shephard RJ. Revised clearance for participation in physical activity: greater screening responsibility for qualified university-educated fitness professionals. *Appl Physiol Nutr Metab.* 2007;32(6):1191–7.

17. Kaminsky LA, editor. *ACSM's Health-Related Physical Fitness Assessment Manual.* 4th ed. Philadelphia (PA): Lippincott Williams & Wilkins; 2013. 192 p.

18. Kern KB, Halperin HR, Field J. New guidelines for cardiopulmonary resuscitation and emergency cardiac care: changes in the management of cardiac arrest. *JAMA.* 2001;285(10):1267–9.

19. Lahav D, Leshno M, Brezis M. Is an exercise tolerance test indicated before beginning regular exercise? A decision analysis. *J Gen Intern Med.* 2009;24(8):934–8.

20. Maron BJ, Araújo CG, Thompson PD, et al. Recommendations for preparticipation screening and the assessment of cardiovascular disease in masters athletes: an advisory for healthcare professionals from the working groups of the World Heart Federation, the International Federation of Sports Medicine, and the American Heart Association Committee on Exercise, Cardiac Rehabilitation, and Prevention. *Circulation.* 2001;103(2):327–34.

21. National Cholesterol Education Program (NCEP) Expert Panel on Detection, Evaluation, and Treatment of High Blood Cholesterol in Adults (Adult Treatment Panel III). Third Report of the National Cholesterol Education Program (NCEP) Expert Panel on Detection, Evaluation, and Treatment of High Blood Cholesterol in Adults (Adult Treatment Panel III) final report. *Circulation.* 2002;106(25):3143–421.

22. Pate RR, Pratt M, Blair SN, et al. Physical activity and public health. A recommendation from the Centers for Disease Control and Prevention and the American College of Sports Medicine. *JAMA.* 1995;273(5):402–7.

23. Persinger R, Foster C, Gibson M, Fater DC, Porcari JP. Consistency of the talk test for exercise prescription. *Med Sci Sports Exerc.* 2004;36(9):1632–6.

24. *Physical Activity and Health: A Report of the Surgeon General.* Atlanta (GA): U.S. Department of Health and Human Services, Centers for Disease Control and Prevention, National Center for Chronic Disease Prevention and Health Promotion; 1996. 278 p.

25. Riebe D, Franklin BA, Thompson PD, et al. Updating ACSM's recommendations for exercise preparticipation health screening. *Med Sci Sports Exerc.* 2015;47(11):2473–79.

26. Shephard RJ, Thomas S, Weller I. The Canadian Home Fitness Test. 1991 update. *Sports Med.* 1991;11(6):358–66.

27. Stedman, editor. *Stedman's Medical Dictionary for the Health Professions and Nursing.* 5th ed. Baltimore (MD): Lippincott Williams & Wilkins; 2005. 2154 p.

28. Swain DP. *ACSM's Resource Manual for Guidelines for Exercise Testing and Prescription.* 7th ed. Philadelphia (PA): Lippincott Williams & Wilkins; 2013. 896 p.

29. Thompson PD. The cardiovascular complications of vigorous physical activity. *Arch Intern Med.* 1996;156(20):2297–302.

30. Thompson PD, Buchner D, Pina IL, et al. Exercise and physical activity in the prevention and treatment of atherosclerotic cardiovascular disease: a statement from the Council on Clinical

Cardiology (Subcommittee on Exercise, Rehabilitation, and Prevention) and the Council on Nutrition, Physical Activity, and Metabolism (Subcommittee on Physical Activity). *Circulation.* 2003;107(24):3109–16.

31. Thompson PD, Franklin BA, Balady GJ, et al. Exercise and acute cardiovascular events placing the risks into perspective: a scientific statement from the American Heart Association Council on Nutrition, Physical Activity, and Metabolism and the Council on Clinical Cardiology. *Circulation.* 2007;115(17):2358–68.

32. U.S. Department of Health and Human Services. *2008 Physical Activity Guidelines for Americans.* Washington (DC): U.S. Department of Health and Human Services; 2008 [cited 2015 Oct 30]. Available from: http://health.gov/paguidelines /guidelines

33. U.S. Preventive Services Task Force. Screening for coronary heart disease: recommendation statement. *Ann Intern Med.* 2004;140(7):569–72.

34. Williams MA. Exercise testing in cardiac rehabilitation. Exercise prescription and beyond. *Cardiol Clin.* 2001;19(3):415–31.

Assessments and Exercise Programming for Apparently Healthy Participants

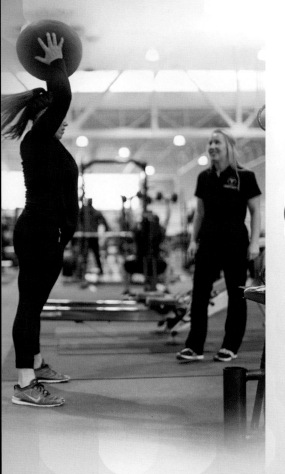

Cardiorespiratory Fitness Assessments and Exercise Programming for Apparently Healthy Participants

OBJECTIVES

- To understand basic anatomy and physiology of the cardiovascular and pulmonary systems as they relate to cardiorespiratory fitness.

- To select appropriate cardiorespiratory fitness assessments.

- To utilize the FITT-VP framework to develop cardiorespiratory fitness.

- To understand how the effect of environment, medications, and musculoskeletal injuries may contraindicate some individuals ability to exercise.

INTRODUCTION

Cardiorespiratory fitness (CRF) may be defined as the ability of the circulatory and respiratory systems to supply oxygen to the muscles to perform dynamic physical activity (41,97). High CRF is associated with increase health benefits (41), and it has been well established that individuals who do moderate- or vigorous-intensity aerobic physical activity have significantly lower risk of cardiovascular disease than inactive people (97). A dose-response relationship exists between aerobic fitness and health outcomes, as increased levels of CRF are associated with numerous positive health outcomes and reductions in chronic disease and all-cause mortality (11,41).

Therefore, the principal role of the American College of Sports Medicine (ACSM) Certified Exercise Physiologist^{SM} (EP-C) is to provide the development and maintenance of CRF to clientele. To provide safe, evidence-based instruction, the EP-C needs a firm science foundation in the physiology of the cardiovascular and pulmonary systems. Once this groundwork has been established, the EP-C can then begin the art of individualized exercise prescription.

 ## Basic Anatomy and Physiology of the Cardiovascular and Pulmonary Systems as They Relate to Cardiorespiratory Fitness

Goal of the Cardiovascular and Respiratory Systems

The cardiovascular and respiratory systems work in synchrony to provide oxygen and remove waste from the body. The respiratory system supports gas exchange, promoting the movement of oxygen and carbon dioxide from the environment into the blood and from the blood back into the environment. The cardiovascular system is responsible for the delivery of oxygenated blood and nutrients to the cell to make energy in the form of adenosine triphosphate (ATP). The cardiovascular system is also responsible for the removal of "waste" from the cell, so it can be transported to its appropriate destination for elimination or recycling (Fig. 3.1).

Anatomy and Physiology of the Cardiovascular and Respiratory Systems

The main components of the cardiovascular system are the heart and vasculature. The heart is a four-chambered muscular pump composed of the right and left atria (upper chambers) and the right and left ventricles (lower chambers). Specifically, the right ventricle is responsible for pumping deoxygenated blood to the lungs for oxygen loading and carbon dioxide unloading. After gas exchange occurs in the pulmonary circulation, blood returns to the left atria. The left ventricle is then responsible for generating the force necessary to drive the blood out of its chamber and through the vasculature. The right and left atria act to provide support to their respective ventricles, serving as a reservoir of blood that eventually moves into the ventricles. The vasculature consists of arteries, arterioles, capillaries, venules, and veins; they can be thought of as a series of tubes that branch and become smaller in diameter as they move away from the heart (see Fig. 3.1).

In the systemic circulation (aorta to vena cava), the arteries and arterioles carry oxygenated blood, whereas in the pulmonary circulation (pulmonary artery to pulmonary vein), the arteries and arterioles carry "deoxygenated blood," or blood that contains less oxygen than arterial blood. As the vasculature is more distal from the heart, arteries branch into smaller arterioles, which in turn branch and merge with

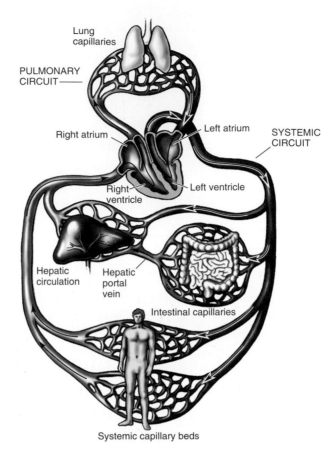

FIGURE 3.1. Schematic representation of the integration between the cardiovascular system and the respiratory system. (Reproduced from Swain D, editor. *ACSM's Resource Manual for Guidelines for Exercise Testing and Prescription.* 7th ed. Baltimore [MD]: Lippincott Williams & Wilkins; 2014. 896 p.)

the capillaries. The capillary is the smallest and most numerous of the blood vessels and is the location of gas and nutrient exchange. Deoxygenated blood and metabolic byproducts move out of capillaries into venules, which consolidate into veins as they move closer to the heart. Veins are responsible for delivering the deoxygenated blood back to the right side of the heart, where the cycle then repeats endlessly. In overview, blood moves through the major components of the heart and circulatory system in the following order: right atrium, right ventricle, pulmonary artery, lungs, pulmonary vein, left atrium, left ventricle, aorta, organs and tissues, and finally the vena cava, before returning back to the right atrium.

Adenosine Triphosphate Production

ATP is an energy-bearing molecule composed of carbon, hydrogen, nitrogen, oxygen, and phosphorus atoms and is found in all living cells. Nervous transmission, muscle contractions, formation of nucleic acids, and many other energy-consuming reactions of metabolism are possible because of the energy in ATP molecules.

Cells break down the food we eat with the ultimate goal of producing ATP, which is the cellular form of energy used within the body to fuel work. Muscle cells are very limited in the amount of ATP they can store. To support muscle contraction during continuous exercise, cells must continuously create ATP at a rate equal to ATP use through a combination of three primary metabolic systems: creatine phosphate (CP), anaerobic glycolysis, and the oxidative system.

The most immediate source of ATP is the CP system. Small amounts of CP are stored within each cell, and one CP donates a phosphate group to adenosine diphosphate (ADP) to create one

ATP, or a simple one-to-one trade-off. This simplicity allows for the rapid production of ATP within the cell; however, this production is short-lived. Because of this, the CP system can provide ATP to fuel work only during short-intense bouts of exercise, owing to the limited storage capacity of CP within each cell. Therefore, the CP system is the primary source of ATP during very short, intense movements, such as discus throw, shot put, and high jump, and any maximal-intensity exercise lasting less than approximately 10 seconds.

Anaerobic glycolysis is the next most immediate energy source and consists of a metabolic pathway that breaks down carbohydrates (glucose or glycogen) into pyruvate. The bond energy produced from the breakdown of glucose and glycogen is used to phosphorylate ADP and create ATP. The net energy yield for anaerobic glycolysis, without further oxidation through the subsequent oxidative systems, is two ATPs if glucose is the substrate and three ATPs if glycogen is the substrate. When oxygen is available in the mitochondria of the cell, pyruvate continues to be broken down to acetyl-coenzyme A (acetyl-CoA) and enters the aerobic energy system. Alternatively, in the absence of adequate oxygen supply, pyruvate is converted to lactic acid, which gradually builds up in muscle cells and the blood. Anaerobic glycolysis is the primary source of ATP during medium-duration, intense exercise, such as the 200-m and 400-m sprint events or any exercise of an intensity that cannot be continued for more than approximately 90 seconds.

Anaerobic energy systems can produce ATP quickly, but they are limited in the duration for which they can continue to produce ATP. For longer duration exercise or low-intensity exercise regardless of duration, the body relies most heavily on the oxidative metabolic energy systems. The aerobic or oxidative energy system does not contribute much energy at the onset of exercise but is able to sustain energy production for a longer duration. As exercise intensity decreases, allowing for longer exercise duration, the relative contribution of the anaerobic energy systems decreases and the relative contribution of the aerobic energy systems increases (Fig. 3.2).

The oxidative system includes two metabolic pathways: the Krebs cycle (aerobic glycolysis) and the electron transport chain. Unlike the anaerobic energy systems mentioned earlier, the oxidative systems require the presence of oxygen to produce ATP, which takes place in the mitochondria of the cell. This is why the mitochondria are known as the "powerhouse of the cell," as that is where the majority of ATP is generated.

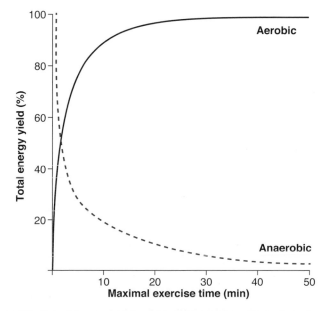

FIGURE 3.2. Relative contribution of the anaerobic and aerobic energy systems based on duration of exercise. (Reproduced from Swain D, editor. *ACSM's Resource Manual for Guidelines for Exercise Testing and Prescription.* 7th ed. Baltimore [MD]: Lippincott Williams & Wilkins; 2014. 896 p.)

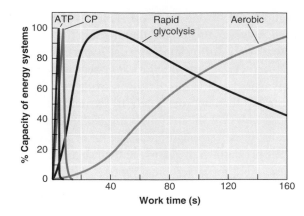

FIGURE 3.3. Relative contribution of the CP system, glycolysis, and the aerobic oxidative system to total energy production based on duration of exercise. (From Swain D, editor. *ACSM's Resource Manual for Guidelines for Exercise Testing and Prescription.* 7th ed. Baltimore [MD]: Lippincott Williams & Wilkins; 2014. 896 p.)

The Krebs cycle requires the presence of carbohydrates, proteins, or fats. These macronutrients are broken down through a series of chemical reactions with their subsequent energy collected and used to create ATP independently and within the electron transport chain. This oxidative system is the primary source of ATP used during low- to moderate-intensity aerobic exercise lasting longer than 1 to 2 minutes all the way up to long-distance endurance events.

The anaerobic and aerobic energy systems work together to create ATP to fuel exercise. The ATP stored within the muscle cell will be used during the first few seconds of exercise onset. As stored ATP decreases, the contribution of ATP production via the CP system increases. Subsequently, as the stores of CP are reduced, anaerobic glycolysis becomes the primary contributing energy system to ATP creation. Aerobic ATP production becomes the primary fuel source in exercise lasting more than approximately 1 to 2 minutes. Figure 3.3 depicts the relative contribution of each source for exercise lasting between 1 and 160 seconds. Although the contribution of energy production differs on the basis of intensity and duration of exercise within the CP system, anaerobic glycolysis, and the oxidative systems, all of these primary metabolic pathways work in synchrony to produce the energy required to sustain the biological work of the human body.

The EP-C should be familiar with the metabolic pathways used to create energy in the body and the link between the oxidative metabolic pathways, the cardiovascular system, and the respiratory system. Within this context, anaerobic metabolism can be called upon even during long-duration exercise, particularly when using interval training consisting of intermittent high-intensity bouts.

Overview of Cardiorespiratory Responses to Acute Graded Exercise of Conditioned and Unconditioned Participants

Oxygen Uptake Kinetics during Submaximal Single-Intensity Exercise

As discussed in the previous section, oxygen is required to create ATP via the oxidative energy system. As workload increases, so does the energy requirement, and more oxygen is required to make ATP. Therefore, the volume of oxygen the body consumes volume of oxygen consumed per unit time ($\dot{V}O_2$) is proportional to workload. Upon the transition from rest to submaximal exercise, $\dot{V}O_2$ increases and reaches a steady state in 1–4 minutes (81). Steady state is the point at which $\dot{V}O_2$ plateaus during submaximal aerobic exercise, and energy production via the aerobic energy systems is equal to the energy required to perform the set intensity of work. Prior to steady state, $\dot{V}O_2$ is lower than required to create adequate energy for the given task primarily via the oxidative energy

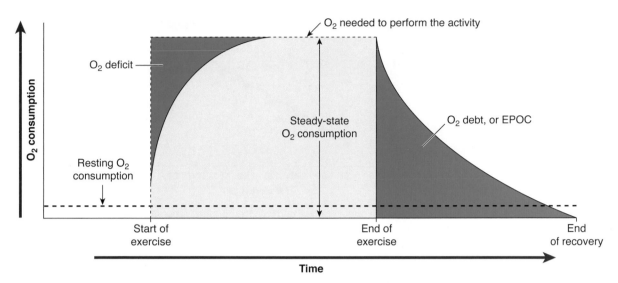

FIGURE 3.4. Oxygen uptake kinetics upon transition from rest to exercise, during submaximal single-intensity exercise, and upon transition from exercise back to a resting condition. (From Kraemer W, Fleck S, Deschenes M. *Exercise Physiology: Integrating Theory and Application*. Philadelphia [PA]: Lippincott Williams & Wilkins; 2012. 512 p.)

systems. This period of inadequate oxygen consumption has been termed *the oxygen deficit* (71). During this period, the anaerobic energy systems are responsible for providing the energy to make up for the difference between the energy produced via the aerobic energy systems and the energy required to perform the work required (37). The time required to reach steady state is influenced by the training state and the magnitude of the increase in exercise intensity (52,81). Aerobic exercise training decreases the time required to reach steady-state, thus reducing the oxygen deficit. This is beneficial because less ATP production will be required and therefore less anaerobic byproducts from the anaerobic energy systems at the start of exercise and upon transition to a higher workload of exercise (52,81).

After cessation of exercise, $\dot{V}O_2$ remains elevated because of the increased work associated with the resynthesis of ATP and CP within muscle cells, lactate removal, and elevated body temperature, hormones, heart rate (HR), and respiratory rate (40). This elevation after exercise was first called *oxygen debt* (54) but is now commonly referred to as *excess postexercise oxygen consumption* (EPOC). Figure 3.4 provides a visual representation of the oxygen uptake kinetics upon transition from rest to exercise and depicts oxygen deficit, steady state, and EPOC.

Oxygen Uptake Kinetics during Graded Intensity Exercise

Graded exercise testing is used in many settings to determine baseline fitness and relevant health risks. Typically, the EP-C will use either maximal or submaximal graded exercise testing to determine baseline fitness, which can be compared at future time points for assessing fitness improvements. It is important for the EP-C conducting graded exercise tests to be well aware of the normal and abnormal hemodynamic response to incremental exercise, as described in the sections that follow.

During incremental exercise, $\dot{V}O_2$ increases slowly within the first few minutes of exercise and eventually reaches a steady state at each submaximal exercise intensity. Steady-state $\dot{V}O_2$ continues to increase linearly as workload increases (Fig. 3.5) until maximal $\dot{V}O_2$ ($\dot{V}O_{2max}$) is reached. $\dot{V}O_{2max}$ is the highest volume of oxygen the body can consume. It is often used as an indicator of aerobic fitness and endurance exercise performance because a higher $\dot{V}O_{2max}$ indicates a greater capacity to create ATP via oxidative energy production and a greater ability to supply the energy required to support higher intensity exercise workloads.

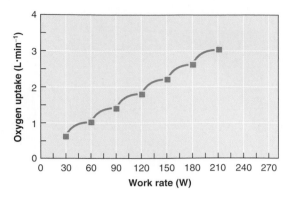

FIGURE 3.5. Relationship between oxygen uptake and workload during graded intensity exercise. (From Swain D, editor. *ACSM's Resource Manual for Guidelines for Exercise Testing and Prescription.* 7th ed. Baltimore [MD]: Lippincott Williams & Wilkins; 2014. 896 p.)

The Fick equation can be used to determine $\dot{V}O_{2max}$. The Fick principle states that $\dot{V}O_{2max} = HR_{max} \times SV_{max} \times$ a-$\dot{V}O_2$ difference max, where $\dot{V}O_2$ = oxygen consumption (mL $\cdot$ kg^{-1} $\cdot$ min^{-1}), HR = heart rate (bpm), SV = stroke volume (mL $\cdot$ beat^{-1}), and a-$\dot{V}O_2$ difference = arteriovenous oxygen difference. This equation demonstrates that $\dot{V}O_{2max}$ is dictated by maximal cardiac output (SV$_{max} \times$ HR$_{max}$) and maximal arteriovenous oxygen difference.

Arteriovenous Oxygen Difference Response to Graded Intensity Exercise

The a-$\dot{V}O_2$ difference reflects the difference in oxygen content between the arterial and the venous blood. The a-$\dot{V}O_2$ difference provides a measure of the amount of oxygen taken up by the working muscles from the arterial blood. Resting oxygen content is approximately 20 mL $\cdot$ dL^{-1} in arterial blood and 15 mL $\cdot$ dL^{-1} in venous blood, yielding an a-$\dot{V}O_2$ of about 5 mL $\cdot$ dL^{-1}. During exercise, venous oxygen content decreases as a result of the increased consumption of oxygen by the working muscles, thus resulting in an increase in a-$\dot{V}O_2$ difference with increasing exercise intensity.

Heart Rate, Stroke Volume, and Cardiac Output Responses to Graded Intensity Exercise

HR increases linearly with increasing workload until HR maximum is reached, which is also typically the point of exercise maximum. Although maximal HR (HR$_{max}$) declines with age (19), trained athletes have lower resting HRs throughout the lifespan. Training itself has little impact on HR$_{max}$. However, training can decrease an individual's HR at a given submaximal workload from pre- to postaerobic exercise training as a sign of increased fitness. SV is the volume of blood the heart ejects with each beat. Similar to HR, SV increases with workload but only up to approximately 40%–60% of $\dot{V}O_{2max}$ in the general population (18,55). Beyond 40%–60% of $\dot{V}O_{2max}$, SV has been shown to decrease slightly in sedentary individuals (30,53) while continuing to increase beyond 40%–60% of $\dot{V}O_{2max}$ in highly trained individuals (49,105). As SV increases with training, resting HR tends to decrease, as more blood being pumped per beat allows the heart to beat less often at rest.

Cardiac output is the product of SV and HR and is also a measure of blood pumped per minute. Cardiac output increases steadily during graded intensity exercise because of the linear rise in HR and curvilinear rise in SV. Increases in cardiac output beyond ~50% of $\dot{V}O_{2max}$ are primarily mediated by increases in HR in untrained individuals. Trained individuals also have the capacity to increase cardiac output via increases in HR, but because they can see continued increase in SV past that of an untrained individual, they have a greater capacity to increase cardiac output (19). See Figure 3.6 for a visual comparison of HR, SV, and cardiac output responses to graded exercise intensity between trained and untrained individuals.

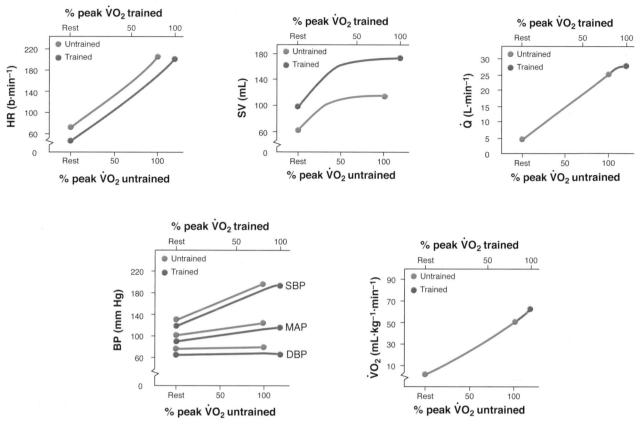

FIGURE 3.6. Cardiovascular responses to graded intensity exercise in trained and untrained individuals. (From Kraemer W, Fleck S, Deschenes M. *Exercise Physiology: Integrating Theory and Application*. Philadelphia [PA]: Lippincott Williams & Wilkins; 2012. 512 p.)

Pulmonary Ventilation Response to Graded Intensity Exercise

Pulmonary ventilation is the volume of air inhaled and exhaled per minute. It is calculated by multiplying the frequency of breathing by the volume of air moved per breath (tidal volume). Pulmonary ventilation increases linearly with work rate until 50%–80% of $\dot{V}O_{2max}$, at which point it reaches the ventilatory threshold and ventilation begins to increase exponentially (99). Ventilatory threshold has been used as an indicator of performance and training intensity; trained subjects can reach higher workloads than untrained subjects before reaching their ventilatory threshold (34).

Blood Pressure Response to Graded Intensity Exercise

Blood pressure (BP) is proportional to the product of cardiac output and total peripheral resistance (TPR) (the overall resistance to blood flow by the blood vessels). Systolic blood pressure (SBP) is the pressure in the arteries during ventricular contraction, or systole, and is heavily influenced by changes in cardiac output. Thus, just as cardiac output increases linearly with increasing workload, so does SBP. Diastolic blood pressure (DBP) is the pressure in the arteries when the heart is relaxed, or diastole and is heavily influenced by TPR. During dynamic, large muscle mass exercise, vascular beds within active muscle vasodilate, decreasing resistance within these blood vessels. In contrast, blood vessels in less metabolically active tissues constrict, increasing resistance within these blood vessels. TPR is determined by the systemic resistance throughout the entire vasculature and is thus determined by the relative proportion of the vasculature that has undergone vasodilation versus vasoconstriction during exercise. During graded exercise, TPR may drop slightly because of the large muscle vasodilation. As a result of this and the contrasting increase in cardiac output, DBP remains relatively stable (85).

Mean arterial pressure (MAP) is the average BP in the arterial system over one complete cardiac cycle (MAP = DBP + 0.33 [SBP − DBP]). MAP is not a critical value to assess during regular exercise and instead is more commonly used in a clinical or diagnostic setting. However, it is worth noting that as a result of training, SBP, DBP, and MAP are all reduced slightly at submaximal workloads (61). See Figure 3.6 for a visual comparison of the BP responses to graded exercise intensity between trained and untrained individuals.

In summary, the EP-C should understand that HR, pulmonary ventilation, a-$\dot{V}O_2$ difference, SV, cardiac output, SBP, and mean arterial BP increase during graded intensity exercise, whereas DBP remains stable or decreases slightly during aerobic type exercise. These cardiovascular and pulmonary adaptations support greater oxygen uptake to allow for the increase in aerobic energy production required during exercise.

Measuring Blood Pressure and Heart Rate before, during, and after Graded Exercise

Blood Pressure and Heart Rate Assessment

Visit thePoint to watch video 3.1 about blood pressure management.

To determine whether clients have an appropriate cardiovascular response to graded exercise, the EP-C should assess BP and HR before, during, and after exercise. (See previous section for a description of the expected HR and BP response to graded intensity exercise.) Prior to exercise, BP and HR should be assessed while resting in the exercise position that will subsequently be used for exercise testing. HR can be accessed via multiple techniques, such as radial and carotid pulse palpation, auscultation with a stethoscope, or the use of a reliable HR monitor. If using pulse palpation, the pulse should be counted for a minimum of 15 seconds and multiplied by 4 to calculate HR in units of beats per minute (bpm). Counting HR for less than 15 seconds reduces the accuracy and reliability of this technique. If the pulse palpation technique is to be used during and after exercise to assess HR, palpation of the radial artery may be a superior choice to the carotid artery because of the possibility of activating the carotid baroreceptors and inducing a reduction in HR, SV, TPR, and MAP (9). BP is typically assessed via brachial artery auscultation. To obtain accurate and reliable BP readings, the EP-C should practice standard BP assessment techniques as specified in the box titled "How to Assess Resting Blood Pressure" (79,98).

During graded exercise testing, BP and HR should be assessed at each exercise intensity. For some tests, it is important for HR to reach a steady state before advancing, and, therefore, HR should be assessed at least two times at each stage to ensure that it is appropriate to move to the next workload. Generally, this is done at the end of each of the last 2 minutes of each exercise stage. BP should also be assessed during the last minute of each exercise stage. Taking accurate HR and BP assessments during exercise is a skill that requires significant practice by the EP-C in order to be completed accurately and in a timely manner while the client continues to exercise. When performing exercise HR and BP assessments, the EP-C needs to ensure that the clients arm is relaxed, at heart level, and not touching any exercise equipment. After completion of exercise, BP and HR should be assessed for a minimum of 5 minutes of recovery or until each become stable (9).

Rate Pressure Product

In addition to checking for appropriate cardiovascular responses, the EP-C can use these data to calculate an individual's "rate pressure product" (RPP). RPP, also referred to as double product, is the product of HR and SBP that occurs concomitantly and serves as an estimate of myocardial oxygen demand ($M\dot{V}O_2$) (RPP = HR × SBP). At rest, the heart consumes approximately 70% of the oxygen delivered to the cardiac muscle. During exercise, the cardiac muscle performs more work because of increased HR and increased contractility, and thus, $M\dot{V}O_2$ increases during exercise in

HOW TO   Assess Resting Blood Pressure

1. Patients should be seated quietly for at least 5 min in a chair with back support (rather than on an examination table) with their feet on the floor and their arm supported at heart level. Patients should refrain from smoking cigarettes or ingesting caffeine for at least 30 min preceding the measurement.

2. Measuring supine and standing values may be indicated under special circumstances.

3. Wrap cuff firmly around upper arm at heart level; align cuff with brachial artery.

4. The appropriate cuff size must be used to ensure accurate measurement. The bladder within the cuff should encircle at least 80% of the upper arm. Many adults require a large adult cuff.

5. Place stethoscope chest piece below the antecubital space over the brachial artery. Bell and diaphragm side of chest piece seem to be equally effective in assessing BP (15). Avoid using the thumb to secure the stethoscope against the arm as this may allow the evaluators pulse to be detected through the stethoscope.

6. Quickly inflate cuff pressure to 20 mm Hg above first Korotkoff sound.

7. Slowly release pressure at rate equal to 2–5 mm Hg $\cdot$ s^{-1}.

8. SBP is the point at which the first of two or more Korotkoff sounds is heard (phase 1), and DBP is the point before the disappearance of Korotkoff sounds (phase 5).

9. At least two measurements should be made (minimum of 1 min apart), and the average should be taken.

10. BP should be measured in both arms during the first examination. Higher pressure should be used when there is consistent interarm difference.

11. Provide to patients, verbally and in writing, their specific BP numbers and BP goals.

Modified from American College of Sports Medicine. *ACSM's Guidelines for Exercise Testing and Prescription*. 9th ed. Philadelphia (PA): Lippincott Williams & Wilkins; 2013. 480 p. For additional, more detailed recommendations, see American College of Sports Medicine. *ACSM's Health-Related Physical Fitness Assessment Manual*. 3rd ed. Philadelphia (PA): Lippincott Williams & Wilkins; 2009. 192 p.

direct proportion to exercise intensity (12). Therefore, if HR and SBP are lower at a given submaximal exercise intensity, the $M\dot{V}O_2$ will be lower, indicating increased fitness. The RPP can be useful to the EP-C when performing exercise testing or prescribing exercise to clients with cardiovascular disease who have been medically cleared for exercise (10).

Selecting Appropriate Cardiorespiratory Fitness Assessments for Healthy Populations, Including Pregnant Women

Cardiorespiratory Fitness Assessments Benefits

CRF is an umbrella term that serves as an indicator of the functional capacity of the heart, lungs, blood vessels, and muscles to work in synchrony to support dynamic, large muscle mass exercise (10). CRF assessment is regularly performed in both healthy and clinical populations. In clinical populations, CRF testing is used for screening, diagnosis, and prognosis of medical conditions. CRF testing is also used in both clinical and healthy populations to gain insight into the most appropriate frequency, intensity, duration, and mode of exercise to prescribe when creating individualized exercise programs, and as a motivational tool to help track progress and continually set obtainable, short-term goals (12).

Types of Cardiorespiratory Fitness Assessments

Visit thePoint to watch video 3.2 about determining the correct seat height on a cycle ergometer.

CRF can be assessed through a variety of step tests, field tests, and submaximal $\dot{V}O_2$ prediction tests. The wide variety of well-respected and widely used CRF tests allows the EP-C the opportunity to select an assessment that provides the desired physiological informational while adhering to the needs of the client and the resources available. Table 3.1 provides an organizational chart of the most popular CRF tests for your reference. A detailed description of the most popular cardiorespiratory testing protocols can be found in the *ACSM's Health-Related Physical Fitness Assessment Manual* (10), and additional references are listed in the Table 3.1.

The gold standard used to measure CRF is the assessment of $\dot{V}O_{2max}$ via open circuit spirometry during maximal-intensity, aerobic exercise. Open circuit spirometry requires the collection of expired air from the client during a graded intensity exercise test to maximal exertion. The volume and content of oxygen and carbon dioxide in the expired air is analyzed with a highly specific gas analyzer. These data allow for the calculation of oxygen consumption at each workload of a graded exercise test. As discussed previously, $\dot{V}O_2$ will increase linearly as workload increases until $\dot{V}O_2$ plateaus, and $\dot{V}O_{2max}$ is reached. Although assessment of $\dot{V}O_{2max}$ with gas analysis is the gold standard of CRF assessment, it requires expensive equipment, technical expertise, and maximal intensity exercise performance by the client. These requirements limit the use of $\dot{V}O_{2max}$ testing using open circuit spirometry to primarily clinical laboratory and research settings (9).

Submaximal oxygen uptake ($\dot{V}O_2$) estimates $\dot{V}O_{2max}$ from the HR response to submaximal single stage or graded exercise. Therefore, precise assessment of HR is a critical factor in determining $\dot{V}O_{2max}$ and should be a well-developed skill by the EP-C. HR can easily be affected by environmental, dietary, and behavioral factors, and the EP-C should do his or her best to control these factors during submaximal $\dot{V}O_2$ testing. Because submaximal testing relies on predictions, there is an increased chance of error because of a variety of factors, such as estimations on resting and maximum HR. To minimize the error of prediction, the following assumptions must be met during submaximal exercise testing: (a) steady-state HR is achieved within 3–4 minutes at each

Table 3.1	**Cardiorespiratory Fitness Assessments**		
Cardiorespiratory Fitness Assessment Techniques			
Type of Test	**Intensity**	**Specific Test Protocols**	**Major Equipment Needed**
Maximal oxygen uptake $\dot{V}O_{2max}$	Maximal	Open circuit spirometry during graded exercise test to volitional fatigue (1)	Treadmill, cycle ergometer, arm ergometer, etc.
Submaximal oxygen uptake	Submaximal	Astrand-Rhyming Cycle Ergometer Test (20)	Cycle ergometer
		YMCA Cycle Ergometer Test (104)	Cycle ergometer
Step tests	Maximal or submaximal	Queens College/McArdle Step Test (70)	Aerobic step or specific height bench, metronome
		Harvard Step Test (22)	
		Astrand-Rhyming Step Test (20)	
Field tests	Maximal or submaximal	Rockport Walk (60)	Level walking/running surface
		12-Minute Walk/Run Test (32,33)	
		1.5-Mile Run Test (10)	

workload, (b) HR increases linearly with work rate, (c) a consistent work rate should be maintained throughout each stage of testing, and (d) estimation/prediction of should be accurate (10). Unfortunately, estimation/prediction of HR_{max} is not an exact science and is highly variable. If true HR_{max} differs significantly from predicted HR_{max}, this assumption may introduce a source of error into the prediction of $\dot{V}O_{2max}$ via submaximal $\dot{V}O_2$ testing (16).

Step tests are a widely utilized form of CRF assessment because of the practicality of this technique. They are short in duration, require little equipment yet are easily portable, and allow for assessment of large groups. Various step test protocols range from submaximal to maximal, giving the EP-C a wide range of choices that he or she should critically assess before determining which is most appropriate for the client. Intensity is determined by step height and step cadence. Most step tests predict $\dot{V}O_{2max}$ from recovery HR (20,22,70), whereas some step tests use steady-state exercise HR to estimate CRF (69). The lower the exercise HR and the greater the rate of recovery, the higher the estimated $\dot{V}O_{2max}$.

Field tests are also widely utilized to assess CRF. The most common forms of field tests include assessment of the amount of time required to cover a set distance or assessment of the distance covered in a set amount of time. Field tests are versatile, in that they can utilize many modes of exercise, such as walking, running, cycling, and swimming. Field tests have many of the same benefits as step tests, in that they are short in duration, require little equipment, can be used for large groups, and can be performed wherever a safe, flat, known distance is available. However, field tests can be more subjective in nature, largely because of the dependency on client effort, and therefore are not as reliable as laboratory tests for assessing CRF.

Selecting the Appropriate Cardiorespiratory Fitness Assessment

When choosing which cardiorespiratory assessment to utilize, the EP-C should consider intensity, length, and expense of the test; type and number of personnel needed; equipment and facilities needed; physician supervision needs and safety concerns; information required as a result of the assessment; required accuracy of results; appropriateness of mode of exercise; and the willingness of the participant to perform the test (10). The EP-C should review the Physical Activity Readiness Questionnaire, health history, and risk assessment documents collected during the prescreening visit to help determine which assessment will be best (see Chapter 2 on prescreening and risk classification). On the basis of the client's risk classification category, the intent of the exercise test, and the other considerations, the EP-C should think critically to determine whether a submaximal or maximal test is most appropriate on a case-by-case basis and to avoid a "one size fits all" approach. Although maximal testing may be quite precise, it has many drawbacks, including first and foremost the increased risk of exercising to exhaustion, especially in clients presenting with any level of risk other than "low" (9). Other drawbacks to maximal testing include increased costs and time, specialized personnel and supplies, and the discomfort of asking the client to exercise to complete exhaustion. Submaximal tests may therefore be more appropriate for many individuals and, when conducted appropriately, result in a reasonable estimate of $\dot{V}O_{2max}$ (17).

Cardiorespiratory Fitness in Pregnant Women

Exercise is beneficial to both mother and baby during pregnancy (7,36), and therefore, pregnant women should be encouraged to maintain an active lifestyle during pregnancy and the postpartum period. The EP-C should be aware that pregnant women are considered a special population, and thus, the exercise testing and prescription guidelines for pregnant women differ slightly from the general guidelines given to nonpregnant women. The ACSM supports the exercise guidelines for

HOW TO   Assess Cardiorespiratory Fitness in Adults of Low Fitness Level: The Rockport Walking Test

Equipment Needed

1. Track or level surface
2. Stopwatch
3. HR monitor (optional)
4. Scale to measure body weight
5. Clipboard, recording sheet, and pencil
6. Calculator

Important Information and Tips

1. Although many CRF assessments require the individual to run/jog, these types of tests may be contraindicated for individuals with orthopedic concerns or of low fitness level. Therefore, the EP-C may choose to utilize the Rockport Walking Test to assess maximal aerobic capacity.

2. The procedure for the Rockport Walking Test is as follows:

   a. Locate a level surface, preferably a track and determine the distance or lap that is equivalent to 1 mile.

   b. After a proper warm-up, instruct the client to walk 1 mile as fast as possible, without jogging or running.

   c. Immediately after 1 mile has been completed, record the walk time in minutes.

   d. If the individual is wearing an HR monitor, record the HR achieved immediately upon reaching the 1-mile mark. If an HR monitor is not available, upon completion of the mile, take the client's pulse for 15 seconds and multiply by 4 to determine peak HR.

   e. Data may now be entered into the following formula:

   $\dot{V}O_{2max}$ (mL $\cdot$ kg^{-1} $\cdot$ min^{-1}) 5 = 132.853 − (0.0769 × body weight in lb) − (0.3877 × age in yr) + (6.315 × gender [1 for men, 0 for women]) − (3.2649 × 1 mile walk time in minutes) − (0.1565 × HR)

   f. Data may be compared with normative tables listed in Suggested Reading.

Example

1. What is the predicted maximal aerobic capacity for a 64-yr-old woman, who weighs 155 lb, completes the Rockport test in 16 min with an HR of 142 bpm?

$$\dot{V}O_{2max} = 132.853 − (0.0769 × 155) − (0.3877 × 64) + (6.315 × 0) − (3.2649 × 16)$$
$$− (0.1565 × 142) = 21.7 \text{ mL} \cdot \text{kg}^{-1} \cdot \text{min}^{-1}$$

2. Normative data suggest that this individual would be rated as "low average" for her age.

Reference

Kline GM, Porcari JP, Hintermeister R, et al. Estimation of VO_{2max} from a one-mile track walk, gender, age, and body weight. *Med Sci Sports Exerc*. 1987;19(3):253–9.

Suggested Reading

Morrow JR Jr, Jackson AW, Disch JG, Mood DP. *Measurement and Evaluation in Human Performance*. 4th ed. Champaign (IL): Human Kinetics; 2011. 472 p.

pregnancy set forth by the American College of Obstetricians and Gynecologists (7), which provide absolute and relative contraindications for exercise participation during pregnancy (7). If exercise is not contraindicated, pregnant women can follow the ACSM and Surgeon General's recommendations to accumulate a minimum of 150 minutes of moderate-intensity exercise weekly (7,97). Exercise intensities of 60%–70% of HR_{max} or 50%–60% of $\dot{V}O_{2max}$ (on the low end of moderate-intensity exercise) are advised for pregnant women who were not physically active before pregnancy. Women who were active before exercise can exercise at a higher workload (15). If exercise testing is warranted in a pregnant woman, maximal exercise testing should be avoided unless absolutely necessary for medical reasons. Although submaximal exercise testing is more appropriate for this population (9), there is usually little need to conduct fitness assessments in pregnant women. Special consideration should be given to the mode of exercise to ensure that the subject feels comfortable and that there is low risk of injury and falls. The EP-C should also ensure that exercise testing is performed in a thermoneutral environment and during a state of adequate hydration (9). During testing, the EP-C should closely monitor the pregnant woman so as not to miss any test termination signs or symptoms (7).

Interpreting Results of Cardiorespiratory Fitness Assessments, Including Determination of $\dot{V}O_2$ and $\dot{V}O_{2max}$

After completing cardiopulmonary exercise assessment, the EP-C should interpret the results of the assessment and share the information with his or her client. To maximize client understanding of CRF testing, individual $\dot{V}O_{2max}$ data are often compared with established criterion-referenced and normative standards. Criterion-referenced standards classify individuals into categories or groups, such as "excellent" or "needs improvement," on the basis of external criteria. In contrast, normative standards provide percentiles from data collected within a specific population. The EP-C can use either type of standard when interpreting data and may find it helpful to present data to clients using both types of standards, as one may have more impact with a client on the basis of his or her perspective. Care should be taken when using normative standards to ensure that the client population and the normative standard population are similar. If there is discrepancy within the populations, normative data are not appropriate for comparisons (12). Table 3.2 provides both normative and criterion-referenced $\dot{V}O_{2max}$ data specific to age and sex.

Low CRF levels have been shown to be an independent predictor of cardiovascular disease and all-cause mortality (21,100). The EP-C should discuss this relationship with clients, as it may bring added meaning to the test results and help motivate clients to improve their CRF. Both maximal and submaximal tests can be used to evaluate CRF at a given point in time as well as changes in CRF that result from physical activity participation (9). A higher $\dot{V}O_{2max}$, lower HR at a given intensity of submaximal exercise, or a lower recovery HR indicates an overall improvement in CRF.

Metabolic Calculations as They Relate to Cardiorespiratory Exercise Programming

Metabolic calculations can be a tremendous asset to the EP-C. An EP-C can use these calculations to determine calorie expenditure for clients interested in weight control, along with helping other clients reach daily and weekly goals for exercise.

| Table 3.2 | Fitness Categories for Maximal Aerobic Power for Men and Women by Age | | | | | | | |

%		Balke Treadmill (time)	Maximal $\dot{V}O_2$ (mL $\cdot$ kg^{-1} $\cdot$ min^{-1})	12-Min Run (miles)	1.5-Mile Run (time)	Balke Treadmill (time)	Maximal $\dot{V}O_2$ (mL $\cdot$ kg^{-1} $\cdot$ min^{-1})	12-Min Run (miles)	1.5-Mile Run (time)
					Men (n = 15,771)				
			Age 20–29 (n = 2,463)				Age 30–39 (n = 13,308)		
99	Superior	31:03	59.8	1.98	8:35	30:00	58.3	1.93	8:49
95		28:01	55.4	1.86	9:18	27:02	54.0	1.82	9:34
90	Excellent	26:40	53.5	1.80	9:40	25:22	51.6	1.75	10:02
85		25:30	51.8	1.75	10:00	24:12	49.9	1.70	10:24
80		25:00	51.1	1.73	10:09	23:03	48.3	1.66	10.47
75	Good	23:09	48.4	1.66	10:45	22:10	47.0	1.62	11:06
70		22:30	47.5	1.63	10:59	21:30	46.0	1.59	11:22
65		22:00	46.8	1.61	11:10	21:00	45.3	1.57	11:33
60		21:05	45.4	1.58	11:31	20:05	44.0	1.54	11:56
55	Fair	20:30	44.6	1.55	11:45	20:00	43.9	1.53	11:58
50		20:00	43.9	1.53	11:58	19:00	42.4	1.49	12:25
45		19:02	42.5	1.49	12:23	18:05	41.1	1.46	12:50
40		18:30	41.7	1.47	12:38	17:39	40.5	1.44	13:04
35	Poor	18:00	41.0	1.45	12:53	17:00	39.5	1.41	13:24
30		17:15	39.9	1.42	13:16	16:20	38.6	1.39	13:46
25		16:31	38.8	1.39	13:40	15:41	37.6	1.36	14:09
20		15:46	37.8	1.36	14:06	15:00	36.7	1.33	14:34
15	Very poor	15:00	36.7	1.33	14:34	14:01	35.2	1.29	15:13
10		13:31	34.5	1.27	15:35	13:00	33.8	1.25	15:58
5		11:18	31.3	1.18	17:22	11:11	31.1	1.18	17:29
1		7:40	26.1	1.04	21:25	8:00	26.5	1.05	20:58
					Men (n = 31,259)				
			Age 40–49 (n = 19,566)				Age 50–59 (n = 11,693)		
99	Superior	28:30	56.1	1.87	9:10	27:00	54.0	1.81	9:34
95		26:00	52.5	1.77	9:51	23:31	49.0	1.67	10:38
90	Excellent	24:00	49.7	1.69	10:28	24:56	46.7	1.61	11:11

Continued

Table 3.2		Fitness Categories for Maximal Aerobic Power for Men and Women by Age (continued)							
%		Balke Treadmill (time)	Maximal $\dot{V}O_2$ (mL · kg^{-1} · min^{-1})	12-Min Run (miles)	1.5-Mile Run (time)	Balke Treadmill (time)	Maximal $\dot{V}O_2$ (mL · kg^{-1} · min^{-1})	12-Min Run (miles)	1.5-Mile Run (time)
Men (n = 31,259)									
		Age 40–49 (n = 19,566)				**Age 50–59 (n = 11,693)**			
85		23:00	48.2	1.65	10:48	20:31	44.6	1.55	11:45
80		21:44	46.4	1.60	11:16	19:39	43.4	1.52	12:07
75	Good	20:41	44.9	1.56	11:41	18:36	41.9	1.48	12:36
70		20:01	43.9	1.53	11:58	18:00	41.0	1.45	12:53
65		19:30	43.2	1.51	12:11	17:14	39.9	1.42	13:17
60		19:00	42.4	1.49	12:25	16:45	39.2	1.40	13:32
55	Fair	18:00	41.0	1.45	12:53	16:01	38.1	1.37	13:57
50		17:25	40.1	1.43	13:11	15:29	37.4	1.35	14:16
45		17:00	39.5	1.41	13:24	15:00	36.7	1.33	14:34
40		16:15	38.5	1.38	13:49	14:16	35.6	1.30	15:03
35	Poor	15:45	37.7	1.36	14:07	13:52	35.0	1.29	15:20
30		15:01	36.7	1.33	14:34	13:00	33.8	1.25	15:58
25		14:30	35.9	1.31	14:53	12:30	33.0	1.23	16:21
20		13:48	34.9	1.28	15:22	12:00	32.3	1.21	16:46
15	Very poor	13:00	33.8	1.25	15:58	11:00	30.9	1.17	17:38
10		12:00	32.3	1.21	16:46	10:00	29.4	1.13	18:38
5		10:01	29.5	1.13	18:37	8:20	27.0	1.07	20:53
1		7:01	25.1	1.01	22:20	5:25	22.8	0.95	25:01
Men (n = 3,752)									
		Age 60–69 (n = 3,285)				**Age 70–79 (n = 467)**			
99	Superior	25:00	51.1	1.73	10:09	24:00	49.7	1.69	10:28
95		21:18	45.8	1.59	11:26	18:45	42.1	1.48	12:31
90	Excellent	19:08	42.6	1.50	12:21	17:00	39.5	1.41	13:24
85		18:00	41.0	1.45	12:53	16:00	38.1	1.37	13:58
80		17:01	39.6	1.41	13:23	15:00	36.7	1.33	14:34
75	Good	16:07	38.3	1.38	13:53	14:01	35.2	1.29	15:13
70		15:29	37.4	1.35	14:16	13:05	33.9	1.26	15:54

Continued

| Table 3.2 | Fitness Categories for Maximal Aerobic Power for Men and Women by Age (continued) |

%		Balke Treadmill (time)	Maximal $\dot{V}O_2$ (mL $\cdot$ kg^{-1} $\cdot$ min^{-1})	12-Min Run (miles)	1.5-Mile Run (time)	Balke Treadmill (time)	Maximal $\dot{V}O_2$ (mL $\cdot$ kg^{-1} $\cdot$ min^{-1})	12-Min Run (miles)	1.5-Mile Run (time)
		Men ($n = 3,752$)							
		Age 60–69 ($n = 3,285$)				Age 70–79 ($n = 467$)			
65		15:00	36.7	1.33	14:34	12:33	33.1	1.23	16:19
60		14:14	35.5	1.30	15:04	12:01	32.3	1.21	16:45
55	Fair	13:45	34.9	1.28	15:25	11:26	31.5	1.19	17:15
50		13:02	33.8	1.25	15:56	10:51	30.7	1.17	17:47
45		12:30	33.0	1.23	16:21	10:21	29.9	1.15	18:16
40		12:00	32.3	1.21	16:46	10:00	29.4	1.13	18:38
35	Poor	11:30	31.6	1.19	17:11	9:04	28.1	1.09	19:39
30		11:00	30.9	1.17	17:38	8:52	27.8	1.09	19:53
25		10:05	29.6	1.14	18:32	8:05	26.7	1.06	20:51
20		9:30	28.7	1.11	19:10	7:24	25.7	1.03	21:47
15	Very poor	8:36	27.4	1.08	20:12	6:39	24.6	1.00	22:54
10		7:26	25.7	1.03	21:44	5:30	22.9	0.95	24:52
5		6:00	23.7	0.97	23:58	4:01	20.8	0.89	27:56
1		3:05	19.4	0.85	6:18	2:15	18.2	0.82	32:46
		Women ($n = 6,039$)							
		Age 20–29 ($n = 1,397$)				Age 30–39 ($n = 4,642$)			
99	Superior	27:19	54.4	1.83	9:29	26:00	52.5	1.77	9:51
95		24:00	49.7	1.69	10:28	22:27	47.4	1.63	11:00
90	Excellent	22:00	46.8	1.61	11:10	21:00	45.3	1.57	11:33
85		21:00	45.3	1.57	11:33	20:00	43.9	1.53	11:58
80		20:01	43.9	1.53	11:58	19:00	42.4	1.49	12:25
75	Good	19:00	42.4	1.49	12:25	18:00	41.0	1.45	12:53
70		18:01	41.0	1.45	12:53	17:01	39.6	1.41	13:23
65		18:00	41.0	1.45	12:53	16:19	38.6	1.39	13:47
60		17:00	39.5	1.41	13:24	15:49	37.8	1.37	14:04
55	Fair	16:15	38.5	1.38	13:49	15:18	37.1	1.34	14:23
50		15:45	37.7	1.36	14:07	15:00	36.7	1.33	14:34

Continued

Table 3.2		**Fitness Categories for Maximal Aerobic Power for Men and Women by Age** (continued)						
%		Balke Treadmill (time)	Maximal $\dot{V}O_2$ (mL $\cdot$ kg^{-1} $\cdot$ min^{-1})	12-Min Run (miles)	1.5-Mile Run (time)	Balke Treadmill (time)	Maximal $\dot{V}O_2$ (mL $\cdot$ kg^{-1} $\cdot$ min^{-1})	12-Min Run (miles)	1.5-Mile Run (time)

Women (n = 6,039)								
		Age 20–29 (n = 1,397)				**Age 30–39 (n = 4,642)**		
45		15:01	36.7	1.33	14:34	14:00	35.2	1.29	15:14
40		14:36	36.0	1.32	14:50	13:26	34.4	1.27	15:38
35	Poor	14:00	35.2	1.29	15:14	13:00	33.8	1.25	15:58
30		13:08	34.0	1.26	15:52	12:09	32.5	1.22	16:38
25		12:24	32.9	1.23	16:26	12:00	32.3	1.21	16:46
20		12:00	32.3	1.21	16:46	11:00	30.9	1.17	17:38
15	Very poor	11:00	30.9	1.17	17:49	10:01	29.5	1.13	18:37
10		10:01	29.5	1.13	18:37	9:01	28.0	1.09	19:43
5		8:21	27.1	1.07	20:31	7:35	25.9	1.30	21:31
1		6:00	23.7	0.97	23:58	5:27	25.9	0.95	24:57

Women (n = 11,248)								
		Age 40–49 (n = 6,709)				**Age 50–59 (n = 4,539)**		
99	Superior	25:00	51.1	1.73	10:09	21:30	46.0	1.59	11:22
95		21:01	45.3	1.57	11:32	18:03	41.1	1.46	12:52
90	Excellent	20:00	43.9	1.53	11:58	17:00	39.5	1.46	13:24
85		18:04	41.1	1.46	12:51	15:29	37.4	1.35	14:16
80		17:05	39.7	1.42	13:22	15:00	36.7	1.33	14:34
75	Good	16:45	39.2	1.40	13:32	14:04	35.3	1.30	15:11
70		16:00	38.1	1.37	13:58	13:30	34.5	1.27	15:35
65		15:03	36.7	1.33	14:32	12:59	33.7	1.25	15:58
60		14:45	36.3	1.32	14:44	12:30	33.0	1.23	16:21
55	Fair	14:01	35.2	1.29	15:13	12:00	32.3	1.21	16:46
50		13:46	34.9	1.28	15:24	11:29	31.6	1.19	17:13
45		13:01	33.8	1.25	15:57	11:01	30.9	1.17	17:38
40		12:30	33.0	1.23	16:21	10:30	30.2	1.15	18:07
35	Poor	12:00	32.3	1.21	16:46	10:01	29.5	1.13	18:37
30		11:18	31.3	1.18	17:22	9:40	29.0	1.12	18:59
25		10:40	30.4	1.16	17:58	9:00	28.0	1.09	19:44

Continued

| Table 3.2 | Fitness Categories for Maximal Aerobic Power for Men and Women by Age (continued) |

%		Balke Treadmill (time)	Maximal $\dot{V}O_2$ (mL · kg^{-1} · min^{-1})	12-Min Run (miles)	1.5-Mile Run (time)	Balke Treadmill (time)	Maximal $\dot{V}O_2$ (mL · kg^{-1} · min^{-1})	12-Min Run (miles)	1.5-Mile Run (time)
		Women (n = 11,248)							
		Age 40–49 (n = 6,709)				Age 50–59 (n = 4,539)			
20		10:00	29.4	1.13	18:38	8:20	27.0	1.07	20:32
15	Very poor	9:10	28.2	1.10	19:32	7:35	25.9	1.03	21:31
10		8:08	26.7	1.06	20:47	6:46	24.8	1.00	22:43
5		7:00	25.1	1.01	22:22	5:35	23.1	0.95	24:42
1		5:00	22.2	0.93	25:49	3:43	20.4	0.88	28:39
		Women (n = 1,500)							
		Age 60–69 (n = 1,313)				Age 70–79 (n = 187)			
99	Superior	20:00	43.9	1.53	11:58	20:00	43.9	1.53	11:58
95		15:47	37.8	1.36	14:05	15:01	36.7	1.33	14:34
90	Excellent	14:30	35.9	1.31	14:53	12:30	33.0	1.23	16:21
85		13:31	34.5	1.27	15:35	11:43	31.9	1.20	17:00
80		12:30	33.0	1.23	16:21	11:00	30.9	1.17	17:38
75	Good	12:00	32.3	1.21	16:46	10:23	30.0	1.15	18:14
70		11:19	31.3	1.18	17:21	10:01	29.5	1.13	18:37
65		11:00	30.9	1.17	17:38	10:00	29.4	1.13	18:38
60		10:25	30.0	1.15	18:12	9:05	28.1	1.10	19:38
55	Fair	10:00	29.4	1.13	18:38	8:59	28.0	1.09	19:44
50		9:46	29.1	1.12	18:52	8:37	27.4	1.08	20:11
45		9:16	28.4	1.10	19:25	8:01	26.6	1.05	20:56
40		8:41	27.5	1.08	20:06	7:33	25.9	1.03	21:34
35	Poor	8:09	26.8	1.06	20:46	7:01	25.1	1.01	22:20
30		7:43	26.1	1.04	21:20	6:49	24.8	1.00	22:38
25		7:05	25.2	1.01	22:14	6:29	24.4	0.99	23:10
20		6:45	24.7	1.00	22:44	6:07	23.8	0.98	23:46
15	Very poor	6:15	24.0	0.98	23:32	5:15	22.6	0.94	25:20
10		5:33	23.0	0.95	24:46	4:30	21.5	0.91	26:51
5		4:45	21.9	0.92	26:19	3:15	19.7	0.86	29:51
1		3:07	19.5	0.86	30:13	1:17	16.8	0.78	36:12

Adapted with permission from The Cooper Institute, Dallas, Texas. Updated 2013. For more information: www.cooperinstitute.org.

Energy Units and Conversion Factors

Energy can be presented using many different terms in the field of exercise physiology, such as absolute oxygen consumption ($L \cdot min^{-1}$ or $mL \cdot min^{-1}$), relative oxygen consumption ($mL \cdot kg^{-1} \cdot min^{-1}$), metabolic equivalents (METs), and kilocalories. The EP-C should possess a firm understanding of the different terms used to express energy expenditure to allow for easy conversion of data from one term to another.

Oxygen consumption refers to the rate at which oxygen is consumed by the body. It can be expressed in absolute ($L \cdot min^{-1}$) or relative ($mL \cdot kg^{-1} \cdot min^{-1}$) terms. Absolute oxygen consumption is the raw volume of oxygen consumed by the body, whereas relative oxygen consumption is the volume of oxygen consumed relative to body weight and can serve as a useful measure of fitness between individuals.

METs present the energy cost of exercise in a simple format that can be easily used by the general public to gauge exercise intensity. One MET is equal to the relative oxygen consumption at rest, which is approximately $3.5 \ mL \cdot kg^{-1} \cdot minute^{-1}$. Using METs as energy cost units allows for the energy cost of exercise to be presented in multiples of rest. For example, if an individual is working at an energy cost of 10 METs, he or she is completing approximately 10 times the amount of work and using 10 times the amount of energy of that at rest. The Compendium of Physical Activity provides a list of the energy cost for different forms of physical activity using METs (2–4). In addition, METs can be used to calculate energy expenditure over time ($[MET \times kg \times 3.5] / 200 = kcal \cdot min^{-1}$).

Kilocalorie is an estimate of energy cost that can be related directly to physical activity and exercise, and the EP-C can calculate the number of kilocalories expended during an exercise bout if oxygen consumption is measured or estimated using previously mentioned methods. The EP-C can then estimate weight gain, loss, or maintenance, depending on a client's goal, remembering that 3,500 kcal equals 1 lb of fat.

As an EP-C, understanding the conversion of energy between units is crucial. The flowchart in Figure 3.7 provides a visual tool to help the EP-C understand the link between energy units and serves as a helpful guide when practicing unit conversions.

ACSM Metabolic Formula

Although open circuit spirometry is the gold standard technique used to assess oxygen consumption and estimate energy cost during exercise, it is not accessible and/or feasible in all applications. The ACSM provides metabolic formula (9) to allow the EP-C an alternative method of energy cost estimation for popular modes of physical activity. The metabolic formula calculates gross energy expenditure, which refers to the sum of energy used at rest and during exercise (Table 3.3). In contrast, net energy expenditure refers to the energy cost of exercise that exceeds the energy required to support the body at rest. Thus, the energy costs calculated from the metabolic formula will represent the amount of energy required to complete the exercise task, including the energy required to support resting energy requirements. After energy cost is estimated, the conversion factors discussed earlier can be used to convert into the appropriate energy expression required for application purposes, such as weight loss or weight gain goals.

Examples

Tracy, a 58-kg woman, would like to begin an exercise program.

1. You advise Tracy to walk at 3.0 mph on a treadmill at 10% grade. What is her $\dot{V}O_2$?

   Walking $\dot{V}O_2 \ mL \cdot kg^{-1} \cdot minute^{-1} = (0.1 \times speed) + (1.8 \times speed \times fractional \ grade) + 3.5 \ mL \cdot kg^{-1} \cdot minute^{-1}$

   $3.0 \ mph \times 26.8 = 80.4 \ m \cdot minute^{-1}$

   $10\% \ grade = 0.10$

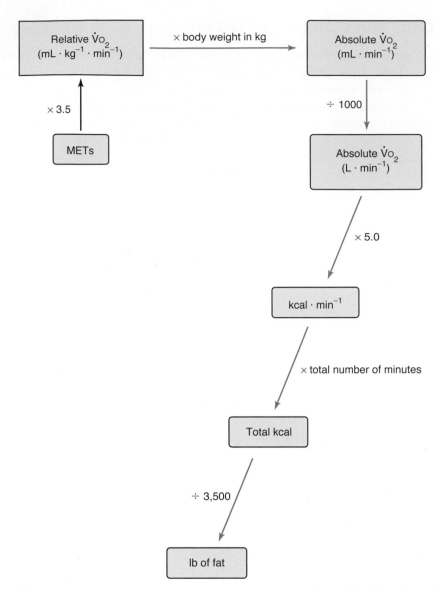

FIGURE 3.7. The energy equivalency chart: the seven energy expressions. (From Bibi KW, editor. *ACSM's Certification Review*. 3rd ed. Baltimore [MD]: Lippincott Williams & Wilkins; 2010. 320 p.)

Walking $\dot{V}O_2$ mL · kg^{-1} · minute^{-1} = (0.1 × 80.4) + (1.8 × 80.4 × 0.10) + 3.5 mL · kg^{-1} · minute^{-1}

Walking $\dot{V}O_2$ mL · kg^{-1} · minute^{-1} = 26 mL · kg^{-1} · minute^{-1}

2. How many METs is this exercise intensity?

METs = $\dot{V}O_2$ mL · kg^{-1} · minute^{-1} / 3.5

METs = 26 mL · kg^{-1} · minute^{-1} / 3.5

METs = 7.432

3. Tracy decides that she would rather ride a stationary bicycle. What would be the equivalent work rate on the cycle ergometer?

Leg cycling $\dot{V}O_{2max}$ mL · kg^{-1} · minute^{-1} = (1.8 × work rate / body weight) + (3.5) + (3.5 mL · kg · minute^{-1})

26 mL · kg^{-1} · minute^{-1} = (1.8 × work rate / 58) + (3.5) + (3.5 mL · kg^{-1} · minute^{-1})

Table 3.3	Metabolic Calculations for the Estimation of Energy Expenditure ($\dot{V}O_2$ [mL $\cdot$ kg^{-1} $\cdot$ min^{-1}]) during Common Physical Activities			
	Sum These Components			
Activity	**Resting Component**	**Horizontal Component**	**Vertical Component/ Resistance Component**	**Limitations**
Walking	3.5	0.1 × speed[a]	1.8 × speed[a] × grade[b]	Most accurate for speeds of 1.9–3.7 min $\cdot$ h^{-1} (50–100 m $\cdot$ min^{-1})
Running	3.5	0.2 × speed[a]	0.9 × speed[a] × grade[b]	Most accurate for speeds >5 min $\cdot$ h^{-1} (134 m $\cdot$ min^{-1})
Stepping	3.5	0.2 × steps $\cdot$ min^{-1}	1.33 × (1.8 × step height[c] × steps $\cdot$ min^{-1})	Most accurate for stepping rates of 12–30 steps $\cdot$ min^{-1}
Leg cycling	3.5	3.5	(1.8 × work rate[d]) / body mass[e]	Most accurate for work rates of 300–1,200 kg $\cdot$ m $\cdot$ min^{-1} (50–200 W)
Arm cycling	3.5		(3 × work rate[d]) / body mass[e]	Most accurate for work rates between 150–750 kg $\cdot$ m $\cdot$ min^{-1} (25–125 W)

[a]Speed in m $\cdot$ min^{-1}.

[b]Grade is percentage grade expressed in decimal format (*e.g.*, 10% = 0.10).

[c]Step height in meter.

Multiply by the following conversion factors:

lb to kg: 0.454; in to cm: 2.54; ft to m: 0.3048; m to km: 1.609; min $\cdot$ h^{-1} to m $\cdot$ min^{-1}: 26.8; kg $\cdot$ m $\cdot$ min^{-1} to W: 0.164; W to kg $\cdot$ m $\cdot$ min^{-1}: 6.12; $\dot{V}O_{2max}$ L $\cdot$ min^{-1} to kcal $\cdot$ min^{-1}: 4.9; $\dot{V}O_{2max}$ mL $\cdot$ kg^{-1} $\cdot$ min^{-1} to MET: 3.5.

[d]Work rate in kilogram meters per minute (kg $\cdot$ m $\cdot$ min^{-1}) is calculated as resistance (kg) × distance per revolution of flywheel × pedal frequency per minute. Note: Distance per revolution is 6 m for Monark leg ergometer, 3 m for the Tunturi and BodyGuard ergometers, and 2.4 m for Monark arm ergometer.

[e]Body mass in kilogram.

Adapted from American College of Sports Medicine. *ACSM's Resource Manual for Guidelines for Exercise Testing and Prescription.* 5th ed. Philadelphia (PA): Lippincott Williams & Wilkins; 2006. 896 p.

$$19 \text{ mL} \cdot \text{kg}^{-1} \cdot \text{minute}^{-1} = (1.8 \times \text{work rate} / 58)$$
$$612 \text{ kg} \cdot \text{m} \cdot \text{minute}^{-1} = \text{work rate}$$

4. If Tracy exercises as prescribed for 30 minutes, 5 days $\cdot$ week^{-1}, for 5 weeks, how much fat mass weight will Tracy lose? (Assume that her caloric intake stays consistent.)

$$30 \text{ minutes} \cdot \text{day}^{-1} \times 5 \text{ days} \cdot \text{week}^{-1} = 150 \text{ minutes} \cdot \text{week}^{-1}$$
$$150 \text{ minutes} \cdot \text{week}^{-1} \times 5 \text{ weeks} = 750 \text{ total minutes}$$
$$\dot{V}O_2 = 26 \text{ mL} \cdot \text{kg}^{-1} \cdot \text{minute}^{-1}$$
$$26 \text{ mL} \cdot \text{kg}^{-1} \cdot \text{minute}^{-1} \times 58 \text{ kg} = 1,450 \text{ mL} \cdot \text{minute}^{-1}$$
$$1,450 \text{ mL} \cdot \text{minute}^{-1} / 1,000 = 1.450 \text{ L} \cdot \text{minute}^{-1}$$
$$1.450 \text{ L} \cdot \text{minute}^{-1} \times 5 \text{ kcal} = 7.25 \text{ kcal} \cdot \text{minute}^{-1}$$
$$7.25 \text{ kcal} \cdot \text{minute}^{-1} \times 750 \text{ minutes} = 5,437.5 \text{ kcal}$$
$$5,437.5 / 3,500 = 1.55 \text{ lb of fat}$$

EXERCISE IS MEDICINE CONNECTION

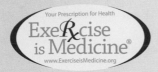

Morris JN, Heady JA, Raffle PAB, Roberts CG, Parks JW. Coronary heart disease and physical activity of work. *Lancet.* 1953;265(6795):1053–7.

Famed British epidemiologist Dr. Jeremy Morris was one of the pioneers in helping establish a link between physical activity and coronary heart disease (CHD). In his landmark 1953 study (74), Morris and colleagues compared the incidence of CHD between conductors and drivers in London transport employees. Morris's main findings showed that the physically active conductors, whose job duties required climbing the stairs of London's fabled double-decker buses, had a different pattern of CHD from that of the bus drivers, who were sedentary for the majority of their workday. The physically active conductors had lower rates of CHD than the bus drivers, displayed symptoms of CHD at a much later age than the drivers, which were less severe, and had a substantially lower mortality rate of fatal myocardial infarction. Morris's findings that physical activity was protective against CHD were met with heavy skepticism from the prevailing conventional wisdom of the day, yet Morris pressed on, replicating his findings in future studies of postal workers and civil servants, consistently demonstrating the protective effects of regular physical activity and exercise in work and/ or recreational pursuits. Dr. Morris's work also lends credence to the hazards of sedentary behavior, which have come under increased focus with the advent of inactivity physiology research. Thanks to the efforts of Dr. Morris, the EP-C can enthusiastically educate clients that Exercise is Medicine.

FITT-VP Framework for the Development of Cardiorespiratory Fitness in Apparently Healthy People

The acronym FITT-VP (F = frequency, I = intensity, T = time or duration, T = type or mode, V = volume or amount of exercise, P = progression or advancement) provides the framework to establish an exercise prescription in healthy individuals (Table 3.4). Given the wide array of fitness levels the EP-C may encounter, the FITT-VP principle may be customized to meet the unique goals and needs of the individual.

The CRF components of the FITT-VP principle have been adopted from the most recent recommendations from the ACSM, American Heart Association, and the *2008 Physical Activity Guidelines for Americans.*

The evidence-based recommendations for CRF following the FITT-VP principle are as follows (9,41,51,97):

Frequency

Moderate-intensity aerobic exercise should be done at least 5 days · week^{-1}, *or* vigorous-intensity aerobic exercise done at least 3 days · week^{-1}, *or* a combination of moderate- and vigorous-intensity aerobic exercise done at least 3–5 days · week^{-1}.

Table 3.4	Aerobic (Cardiovascular Endurance) Exercise Evidence-Based Recommendations
FITT-VP	**Evidence-Based Recommendation**
Frequency	■ $\geq$5 d · wk^{-1} of moderate exercise, or $\geq$3 d · wk^{-1} of vigorous exercise, or a combination of moderate and vigorous exercise on $\geq$3–5 d · wk^{-1} is recommended.
Intensity	■ Moderate and/or vigorous intensity is recommended for most adults. ■ Light- to moderate-intensity exercise may be beneficial in deconditioned persons.
Time	■ 30–60 min · d^{-1} of purposeful moderate exercise, or 20–60 min · d^{-1} of vigorous exercise, or a combination of moderate and vigorous exercise per day is recommended for most adults. ■ <20 min of exercise per day can be beneficial, especially in previously sedentary persons.
Type	■ Regular, purposeful exercise that involves major muscle groups and is continuous and rhythmic in nature is recommended.
Volume	■ A target volume of $\geq$500–1,000 MET-min · wk^{-1} is recommended. ■ Increasing pedometer step counts by $\geq$2,000 steps · d^{-1} to reach a daily step count $\geq$7,000 steps · d^{-1} is beneficial. ■ Exercising below these volumes may still be beneficial for persons unable or unwilling to reach this amount of exercise.
Pattern	■ Exercise may be performed in one (continuous) session per day, or in multiple sessions of $\geq$10 min, to accumulate the desired duration and volume of exercise per day. ■ Exercise bouts of <10 min may yield favorable adaptations in very deconditioned individuals.
Progression	■ A gradual progression of exercise volume by adjusting exercise duration, frequency, and/or intensity is reasonable until the desired exercise goal (maintenance) is attained. ■ This approach may enhance adherence and reduce risks of musculoskeletal injury and adverse coronary heart disease events.

Adapted from Garber CE, Blissmer B, Deschenes MR, et al. American College of Sports Medicine position stand. Quantity and quality of exercise for developing and maintaining cardiorespiratory, musculoskeletal, and neuromotor fitness in apparently healthy adults: guidance for prescribing exercise. *Med Sci Sports Exerc.* 2011;43(7):1334–59.

Intensity

A combination of moderate- (40%–59% $\dot{V}O_2R$) and/or vigorous-intensity (60%–84% $\dot{V}O_2R$) exercise is recommended for most healthy individuals. Intensity may be prescribed using multiple methods such as, but not limited to, HR reserve (HRR), rating of perceived exertion (RPE), percentage $\dot{V}O_{2max}$, and percentage of age-predicted maximal HR.

Time

For substantial health benefits, individuals should accrue at least 150 minutes · week^{-1} of moderate-intensity exercise *or* 75 minutes · week^{-1} of vigorous-intensity exercise *or* an equivalent combination of moderate and vigorous aerobic exercise. For additional and more substantial health benefits such as weight management or fitness goals, moderate-intensity exercise may be increased to at least 300 minutes · week^{-1}, *or* vigorous-intensity exercise may be increased to at least 150 min · week^{-1}, *or* an equivalent combination of moderate and vigorous physical activity.

Type

All types of physical activity are beneficial as long as they are of sufficient intensity and duration. Rhythmic, continuous exercise that involves major muscle groups is the most typical choice; however, for more advanced individuals, intermittent exercise such as interval training or stop-and-go sports may be used to accumulate the recommended frequency, intensity, and time needed for CRF.

Volume

Exercise volume is the product of the FIT (frequency, intensity, time) components of exercise prescription. A dose-response relationship exists between physical activity and health outcomes, in which greater amounts of physical activity are associated with greater health benefits. Recommended target volumes include $\geq$500–1,000 MET-min $\cdot$ week^{-1}, which is roughly equivalent to an energy expenditure of 1,000 kcal $\cdot$ week^{-1}.

Progression

The recommended rate of progression of an exercise program is dependent on the individual's health status, physical fitness, training responses, and exercise program goals. Therefore, progression may consist of increasing any of the components of the FITT-VP principles as tolerated by the individual. Any progression should be made gradually, avoiding large increases in any of the FITT-VP components to minimize risks. The progression of exercise may be from a single session per day, or in multiple sessions of $\geq$10 minutes. An increase in exercise time/duration per session of 5–10 minutes every 1–2 weeks is reasonable to advance toward the recommended quantity and quality of exercise.

Inherent within the FITT-VP framework are the following principles of training that the EP-C must consider when prescribing cardiorespiratory exercise:

Progressive Overload

The overload principle is at the foundation of all exercise prescription. To improve CRF, the individual must exercise at a level greater than accustomed to induce adaptation. The EP-C can implement the overload principle by manipulating the frequency, intensity, or time of the exercise prescription. For example, if an EP-C is working with a client who typically runs on a treadmill at 75% HR$_{max}$, for 30 minutes, 3 days $\cdot$ week^{-1}, the overload principle may be adhered to by increasing the intensity of the run to 80% of HR$_{max}$, increasing the time spent running to 40 minutes, or increasing running to 4 days $\cdot$ week^{-1}. It is important for the EP-C to understand that all variables should not be increased simultaneously, as small incremental progression allows the body to adapt, which is key to reducing the risk of overuse injuries (96).

Reversibility

The principle of reversibility can be viewed as the opposite of the overload principle. Commonly referred to as the "use it or lose it" principle, the reversibility principle dictates that once cardiorespiratory training is decreased or stopped for a significant period (2–4 weeks), previous improvements will reverse and decrease, and the body will readjust to the demands of the reduced physiological stimuli (80). Hard-earned gains in CRF can be lost if the training stimulus is removed, and the EP-C should be aware that prior gains made with clients who have taken long breaks from training will necessitate readjusting previous exercise prescriptions.

Individual Differences

The principle of individual differences states that all individuals will not respond similarly to a given training stimulus (70). The EP-C will encounter a wide range of individuals of varying age and fitness levels, each of whom will demonstrate varied responses to a given exercise stimulus. Within an exercise prescription for CRF, the EP-C will encounter high and low responders because of the large genetic component that affects the degree of potential change in $\dot{V}O_{2max}$ (103). The variation in fitness levels necessitates a personalized exercise prescription based on the unique needs of the individual.

Specificity of Training

The specificity principle, also known as the SAID (specific adaptations to imposed demands) principle, is dependent on the type and mode of exercise. The specificity principle states that specific exercise elicits specific adaptations, creating specific training effects (70). For example, if an EP-C is working with a client who wishes to improve his or her time in an upcoming half-marathon, the principle of specificity dictates that in order to improve, the EP-C needs to select a training stimulus specific to the activity in question. Thus, running would be the appropriate mode to select, as activities such as cycling or swimming do not train the specific muscles and movement patterns needed to complete a half-marathon.

Safe and Effective Exercises Designed to Enhance Cardiorespiratory Fitness

As discussed in the introduction to the FITT-VP framework, when designing an exercise program to develop CRF, the type of exercise that is generally prescribed to improve health and fitness is rhythmic and continuous and uses large muscle groups (9). Given the nearly unlimited number of ways to be physically active, there is no shortage of exercise options for the EP-C to choose from when prescribing physical activity to enhance CRF. Exercise options can be viewed on a continuum, ranging from the relatively simple, such as brisk walking, to much more complex and vigorous, such as repeat 400-m interval sprints approaching 100% $\dot{V}O_{2max}$. Although the options to improve CRF may seem overwhelming at times, the ACSM has created a classification scheme to help the EP-C make an appropriate exercise selection that matches the fitness level and unique interests of the clientele an EP-C may be serving (9). Cardiovascular endurance exercises may be divided into four categories (Table 3.5):

Type A: endurance exercises requiring minimal skill or physical fitness to perform, such as walking or water aerobics
Type B: vigorous-intensity endurance exercises requiring minimal skill, such as running or spinning
Type C: endurance activities requiring skill to perform, such as cross-country skiing or in-line skating
Type D: recreational sports, such as tennis or basketball

Subsequently, the EP-C can modify any activity from the four categories to best accommodate the skill level, physical fitness stage, and personal preferences of the individual or groups the EP-C may be serving.

An additional method of classifying cardiorespiratory exercise that may be useful to the EP-C is by weight-bearing or non–weight-bearing activities. Weight-bearing activities cause muscles and bones to work against gravity, such as jogging or aerobic dance, versus non–weight-bearing activities in which the stress on the bones, joints, and muscles is lessened, such as in cycling or swimming. Although some weight-bearing physical activity is important for bone health (26), many individuals may have orthopedic limitations that may necessitate the need to choose more nonimpact physical activity options. In addition, low-impact physical activity has a third or less of the injury risk of higher impact activities (97). Table 3.6 highlights five of the most popular exercise modalities (76) and the advantages and disadvantages of each.

Table 3.5	Modes of Aerobic (Cardiorespiratory Endurance) Exercises to Improve Physical Fitness		
Exercise Group	Exercise Description	Recommended for	Examples
A	Endurance activities requiring minimal skill or physical fitness to perform	All adults	Walking, leisurely cycling, aqua-aerobics, slow dancing
B	Vigorous-intensity endurance activities requiring minimal skill	Adults (as per the preparticipation screening guidelines in Chapter 2) who are habitually physically active and/or at least average physical fitness	Jogging, running, rowing, aerobics, spinning, elliptical exercise, stepping exercise, fast dancing
C	Endurance activities requiring skill to perform	Adults with acquired skill and/or at least average physical fitness levels	Swimming, cross-country skiing, skating
D	Recreational sports	Adults with a regular exercise program and at least average physical fitness	Racquet sports, basketball, soccer, downhill skiing, hiking

Adapted from Armstrong LE, Brubaker PH, Whaley MH, Otto RM, American College of Sports Medicine. *ACSM's Guidelines for Exercise Testing and Prescription.* 7th ed. Baltimore (MD): Lippincott Williams & Wilkins; 2005. 366 p.

Table 3.6	Advantages and Disadvantages of Different Exercises	
Exercise	Advantages	Disadvantages
Walking	Does not require expensive equipment, special skill, or special facilities; can be done indoors or outdoors (63)	Potential safety concerns of walking environment (78)
Jogging/running	Easily accessible and large caloric expenditure; promotes bone health	Increased injury risk because of higher impact, environmental concerns
Bicycling	Reduced impact on bones and joints	Cost of bicycle, weather, safety of cycling environment
Swimming	Buoyancy provides great alternative for individuals with joint pain	Skill level needed; chlorinated pool may aggravate respiratory conditions, and warm moist air may benefit asthmatics
Aerobic machines	Multiple options allowing exercise, regardless of weather; many provide low-impact workout option	Ownership and maintenance costs of home aerobic machines, use of aerobic machines may necessitate membership at fitness facility

Interval Training

The implementation of interval training to improve CRF and/or metabolic health is an additional method of ExRx that the EP-C may wish to consider. Interval training is broadly defined as when a period of intense activity is interspersed with a period of low to moderate activity (70). Interval training, traditionally in the form of sprints ranging from 10 s to 5 min, has long been utilized in the conditioning of athletes for energy system development and performance enhancement purposes (48,62). However, the use of interval training within sedentary or recreationally active populations has been growing in popularity among fitness professionals (94). From an exercise efficiency standpoint, the lower exercise volume and subsequent time commitment needed for interval training could be very appealing to individuals with limited time, a common barrier to exercise participation (43,95).

When prescribing interval training, the EP-C is encouraged to consider the interval training nomenclature first proposed by Weston *et al.* that differentiate high-intensity interval training (HIIT) from sprint interval training (SIT) (102). HIIT is traditionally performed at an intensity that is greater than the anaerobic threshold and is often performed at an intensity close to that which elicits $\geq$80–100% peak heart rate, whereas SIT is characterized by an all-out, supramaximal effort equal to or greater than the pace that elicits $\geq$100% $\dot{V}O_{2peak}$ (24,25,44,62,68). Of potential great interest to the EP-C is a recent systematic review and meta-analysis of HIT of patients with lifestyle-induced chronic diseases, which recommended that a 4 $\times$ 4 protocol (work = 4 intervals at 4 min at 85%–95% peak HR; rest = 3 intervals at 3 min at 70% peak HR, 3 d/wk) demonstrated the biggest changes in $\dot{V}O_{2peak}$, was well tolerated, and had excellent adherence (102). Furthermore, there is emerging research for the EP-C to consider as to the value of low volume interval training (LVIT), in which a total exercise time commitment of >15 min can provide a potent stimulus to physiological adaptations associated with improved health (45). LVIT protocols range from the extraordinarily demanding (8 bouts of all-out 20 s efforts with 10 s rest in between, 4 d/wk) (67,90,91) to much less severe protocols (2–3 bouts of all-out 20 s efforts with 2–3 min rest in between, 3 d/wk), (6,46,47,72) all of which yielded significant changes in indices of metabolic health and aerobic capacity.

When prescribing interval training, the EP-C can manipulate at least nine different variables that could impact the desired metabolic, cardiopulmonary, or neuromuscular responses (24); however, the primary factors of interest concern (a) the intensity and duration of the exercise and recovery interval and (b) the total number of intervals performed (24,70). Consistent with the principles of ExRx and FITT-VP framework, the decision for the EP-C to implement interval training will be dependent on initial CRF assessments, the specific goals of the clientele, and selecting the exercise modality that will best lead to exercise adherence and self-efficacy (95).

Determining Exercise Intensity

The EP-C has multiple options to determine the appropriate exercise intensity when prescribing physical activity to improve CRF. Options range from direct measurements in clinical or laboratory settings to more subjective ratings based on feelings of exertion or fatigue. The precision needed to determine exercise intensity will be dependent on the unique conditions, needs, and preferences of the clientele the EP-C may be serving. The EP-C may consider using any of the following methods to determine exercise intensity:

Heart Rate Reserve Method

HRR, or Karvonen method, requires the EP-C to determine the resting HR and maximum HR of the client. Resting HR is optimally measured in the morning while the client is in bed before rising (70), whereas maximum HR is best measured during a progressive maximal exercise test but can also be estimated via age-predicted formulas (9). The HRR is the difference between maximum HR and resting HR. Target HR will be determined by considering the habitual physical activity, exercise level, and goals of the client (9). To assign a target HR, use the following formula:

$$\text{Target HR} = [(\text{Maximum HR} - \text{Resting HR}) \times \% \text{ intensity desired}] + \text{Resting HR}$$

For example, if your client has a maximum HR of 200 bpm and a resting HR of 60 bpm, and wishes to exercise at 65%–75% of HRR, the HR range would be 151–165 bpm:

$$[(200 - 60) \times 65\%] + 60 = \text{Target HR of 151 bpm}$$
$$[(200 - 60) \times 75\%] + 60 = \text{Target HR of 165 bpm}$$

Peak Heart Rate Method

The peak HR method requires the EP-C to determine the client's HR_{max}. This may be accomplished from direct measurement, such as a $\dot{V}O_{2max}$ treadmill test, or maximum HR may be estimated from age-predicted formulas. Common estimation equations that the EP-C may consider include the following:

- Maximum HR = 220 − age in years
- Maximum HR = 207 − (0.7 × age in years) (61)
- Maximum HR = 200 − (0.5 × age in years) (73)
- Maximum HR = 208 − (0.7 × age in years) (92)
- Maximum HR = 206.9 − (0.67 × age in years) (42).

The EP-C should be aware that each of the earlier equations might overestimate maximum HR in certain populations, while underestimating in others (9). The EP-C is advised to use maximal HR estimations only as a guide and to realize that estimates may not be accurate for certain individuals. Once HR_{max} has been determined, the EP-C may assign a target HR by following the formula:

$$\text{Target HR} = \text{Maximum HR} \times \% \text{ intensity desired}$$

For example, if a client is 40 years old and has a selected workload of 85% of maximum HR, and the EP-C chooses the equation, Maximum HR = 206.9 − (0.67 × age) to estimate maximum HR, the calculations would be as follows:

$$206.9 - (0.67 \times 40) = \text{Estimated maximum HR of 180 bpm}$$
$$180 \times 85\% = \text{Target HR of 153 bpm}$$

Peak $\dot{V}O_2$ Method

The peak $\dot{V}O_2$ method may be used if the EP-C has measured or estimated the $\dot{V}O_{2max}$ of the client in a laboratory or field setting. However, one should be cautious when assigning workload on the basis of estimated because of the expected error in extrapolating HR (*e.g.*, 220 − age = standard deviation of 12–15 bpm) (9). Once the $\dot{V}O_{2max}$ has been determined, the formula below may be followed:

$$\text{Target } \dot{V}O_2 = \dot{V}O_{2max} \times \% \text{ intensity desired}$$

For example, an EP-C working with an individual with a measured $\dot{V}O_{2max}$ of 60 mL $\cdot$ kg^{-1} $\cdot$ minute^{-1}, with an exercise prescription of 90% maximum, would calculate the target $\dot{V}O_2$ as follows:

$$60 \times 90\% = \text{Target } \dot{V}O_{2max} \text{ of 54 mL} \cdot \text{kg}^{-1} \cdot \text{min}^{-1}$$

Peak Metabolic Equivalent Method

In some instances, the EP-C may choose the peak MET method to guide intensity. Whereas $\dot{V}O_{2max}$ is a relative measure of intensity, METs provide an absolute measure, allowing the intensity of various physical activity options to be compared with each other. Resources such as the Compendium of Physical Activity (2–4) feature extensive MET listings for a wide array physical activity options. Because 1 MET is equivalent to $3.5 \text{ mL} \cdot \text{kg}^{-1} \cdot \text{minute}^{-1}$, an individual's peak MET level can be determined simply by dividing one's measured or estimated $\dot{V}O_{2max}$ by 3.5. For example, an individual with a $\dot{V}O_{2max}$ of 35 would have a peak MET level of 10 METs. Once an individual's peak MET has been determined, the EP-C can prescribe exercise at an appropriate workload by using a target MET level. The formula for determining target METs is as follows (12):

$$\text{Target METs} = (\% \text{ intensity desired}) \, [(\dot{V}O_{2max} \text{ in METs}) - 1] + 1$$

For example, for an individual with a $\dot{V}O_{2max}$ of $35 \text{ mL} \cdot \text{kg}^{-1} \cdot \text{minute}^{-1}$ and who wants to exercise at an intensity of 70% the target METs can be calculated as follows:

Step 1: $\dot{V}O_{2max}$ in METs = $35 \text{ mL} \cdot \text{kg}^{-1} \cdot \text{minute}^{-1} / 3.5 \text{ mL} \cdot \text{kg}^{-1} \cdot \text{minute}^{-1}$ = 10 METs
Step 2: Target METs = $(0.70) \, (10 - 1) + 1$
Step 3: Target METs = $(0.70) \, (9) + 1$
Step 4: Target METs = $6.3 + 1 = 7.3$ METs

Thus, the EP-C could select activities from the compendium of physical activities that correspond with a MET level between 7.0 and 7.5.

$\dot{V}O_{2max}$ Reserve Method

The $\dot{V}O_2$ reserve ($\dot{V}O_2R$) method may be used when the EP-C has directly measured or estimated the client's $\dot{V}O_{2max}$ and resting $\dot{V}O_2$ in a laboratory setting. The $\dot{V}O_2R$ is the difference between $\dot{V}O_{2max}$ and resting $\dot{V}O_2$. Target $\dot{V}O_2R$ will be dependent on the goals of the client:

$$\text{Target } \dot{V}O_2R = [(\dot{V}O_{2max} - \dot{V}O_{2rest}) + \text{intensity desired}] + \dot{V}O_{2rest}$$

For example, for a client with a $\dot{V}O_{2max}$ of $35 \text{ mL} \cdot \text{kg}^{-1} \cdot \text{minute}^{-1}$, a resting $\dot{V}O_2$ of $3.5 \text{ mL} \cdot \text{kg}^{-1} \cdot \text{minute}^{-1}$, and a selected workload of 60% $\dot{V}O_2R$, the calculation would be as follows:

$$[(35 - 3.5) \times 60\%] + 3.5 = \text{Target } \dot{V}O_2R \text{ of } 22.4 \text{ mL} \cdot \text{kg}^{-1} \cdot \text{min}^{-1}$$

Talk Test Method

The talk test is a simple and convenient method to determine exercise intensity, especially for individuals who may be unaccustomed to physical activity. The talk test is a subjective measure of relative intensity, which helps differentiate between moderate and vigorous physical activity. If an individual is able to talk, but not sing, the physical activity is considered moderate. However, once the intensity of the activity increases to a point at which an individual is not able to say more than a few words without pausing for breath, the intensity would be considered vigorous (27,97). Once comfortable speech is no longer possible, the vigorousness of the exercise may be outside the range for the individual to sustain, and the EP-C can instruct the client to stop or reduce the level of effort.

Perceived Exertion Method

The perceived exertion method is another subjective rating of how hard one may be working. Perceived exertion is most commonly measured through Borg's RPE Scale, which ranges from 6 to 20, 6 meaning no exertion at all, and 20 meaning maximal exertion (27). The RPE range of 11–16 is recommended to improve CRF (8).

An additional perceived exertion scale for the EP-C to be familiar with is Borg's Category Ratio Scale, commonly abbreviated as CR-10. The CR-10 uses a scale of 0–10, in which sitting is 0 and the highest level of effort possible is 10 (97). A CR-10 range of 5–8 corresponds with moderate- (CR 5–6) and vigorous-intensity (CR 7–8) physical activity.

Abnormal Responses to Exercise

Increases in HR, SBP, and ventilation, from rest, are normal responses to cardiorespiratory exercise in healthy individuals. Although the benefits and overall safety of cardiorespiratory exercise have been well established (9,41), the EP-C should be aware of potential abnormal responses to exercise that may necessitate the termination of exercise session and possibly require medical assistance. The "How to Read the Signs: Stopping an Exercise Test" box provides general indications for stopping an exercise session (9). The EP-C should consider that individuals who are detrained, returning from injury, or unaccustomed to physical activity may have a very low tolerance and capacity for exercise, and thus, in addition to the general indications highlighted in the box, the EP-C should be judicious in the design of initial exercise prescriptions and communicate with his or her clients at all times.

Contraindications to Cardiovascular Training Exercises

The EP-C will undoubtedly encounter individuals with physical or clinical limitations in which the risks of exercise testing and subsequent prescription may outweigh any potential benefits (9). Individuals with cardiac, respiratory, metabolic, or musculoskeletal disorders should be supervised by clinically trained personnel when beginning an exercise program (see Chapter 8 for more details on these populations). A thorough preexercise screening, obtaining informed consent, and review of medical history are necessary for the EP-C to identify potential contraindications and to ensure

---

HOW TO   **Read the Signs: Stopping an Exercise Test**

The following lists general indications the EP-C should watch for when giving an exercise test; being able to recognize these will avoid injury or problems.

- Onset of angina or angina-like symptoms
- Drop in SBP of ≥10 mm Hg with an increase in work rate, or if SBP decreases below the value obtained in the same position before testing
- Excessive rise in BP: SBP >250 mm Hg and/or DBP >115 mm Hg
- Shortness of breath, wheezing, leg cramps, or claudication
- Signs of poor perfusion: light-headedness, confusion, ataxia, pallor, cyanosis, nausea, or cold and clammy skin
- Failure of HR to increase with increased exercise intensity
- Noticeable change in heart rhythm by palpation or auscultation
- Participant requests to stop
- Physical or verbal manifestations of severe fatigue
- Failure of the testing equipment

the safety of the client (9). Chapter 2 provides greater detail on properly assessing risk factors along with Chapter 34, "Exercise Prescription and Medical Considerations," in *ACSM's Resource Manual for Guidelines for Exercise Testing and Prescription* (12). However, it is inevitable that the EP-C will encounter apparently healthy clients who develop chest pain, breathing difficulty, musculoskeletal distress, or other worrisome symptoms during an exercise session. The EP-C should immediately stop exercise, ensure client safety, and then refer the client to the appropriate health care professional.

Effect of Common Medications on Cardiorespiratory Exercise

It is not uncommon for the EP-C to work with clients who may be taking prescribed and over-the-counter (OTC) medications. Whereas it is never the role of the EP-C to administer, prescribe, or educate clients on the use or effects of medications (31), it is important for the EP-C to understand the potential complex interactions of medication and exercise (75). Medications may alter HR, BP, and/or exercise capacity (9), and therefore, clients taking medication should be strongly encouraged to communicate any changes in medication routines to the EP-C (31). Please refer to Chapter 8 for the effect common OTC and prescription medications have on exercise.

Signs and Symptoms of Common Musculoskeletal Injuries Associated with Cardiorespiratory Exercise

Although a properly designed CRF prescription results in minimal risk (96), the EP-C should be aware of the signs and symptoms of common musculoskeletal injuries associated with exercise (57).

- Exquisite point tenderness
- Pain that persists even when the body part is at rest
- Joint pain
- Pain that does not go away after warming up
- Swelling or discoloration
- Increased pain with weight-bearing activities or with active movements
- Changes in normal bodily functions

Previous research suggests the risk of injury is directly related to the increase in the amount of physical activity performed (96), and thus, the chance for musculoskeletal injury increases as the individual performs exercise at greater levels of frequency and intensity (57). The individuals with whom the EP-C may work will come from varied backgrounds, presenting a wide array of potential intrinsic and extrinsic risk factors that may predispose clients to injury (11). Common risk factors that the EP-C may encounter are listed as follows (modified from 84):

Intrinsic Risk Factors

History of previous injury
Inadequate fitness or conditioning
Body composition
Bony alignment abnormalities
Strength or flexibility imbalances
Joint or ligamentous laxity
Predisposing musculoskeletal disease

Extrinsic Risk Factors

Excessive load on the body
Type of movement
Speed of movement
Number of repetitions
Footwear
Surface
Training errors
Excessive distances
Fast progression
High intensity
Running on hills
Poor technique
Fatigue
Adverse environmental conditions
Air quality
Darkness
Heat or cold
High humidity
Altitude
Wind
Worn or faulty equipment

Once the EP-C has addressed potential risks, strategies to minimize injury may be employed, especially in at-risk individuals. The EP-C should consider the age, level of fitness, and prior experience of potential clients when individualizing exercise prescriptions (97). It is recommended that the EP-C use an intensity relative to a client's fitness level to usher in a desired level of effort, while slowly increasing the duration and frequency of physical activity before increasing intensity (97). Previous research suggests that the injury risk is increased in individuals who run, participate in sports, and engage in more than 1.25 hours · week^{-1} of physical activity (56). Therefore, when working with clients who may fit this profile, the EP-C should take steps to minimize potential risk via proper assessment, client education, and exercise program design. In addition, the EP-C should closely monitor increases in physical activity, especially in previously sedentary individuals, as the larger the overload to one's baseline physical activity, the greater the chance of injury (96).

Effects of Heat, Cold, or High Altitude on the Physiologic Response to Exercise

Hot, cold, and high-altitude environments alter the typical physiological response to exercise. These extreme environments have the ability to stress our physiological systems to their maximal capacity and may negatively impact exercise performance before acclimatization (89). The EP-C should be aware of the major challenges of exercise in hot, cold, and/or high-altitude environments and the impact of these environments on the physiological response to exercise.

Heat Stress

Hot environments reduce the body's ability to dissipate heat and thus promote an increase in core body temperature. In an effort to maintain a neutral body temperature when exposed to a hot environment, sweat rate and skin blood flow increase to promote heat loss (59). Although critical for heat dissipation, increased sweat rates and skin blood flow challenge the capacity of the cardiovascular system and may be the primary performance limiting factors during exercise in a hot environment (28). Increased sweat rates can cause a reduction in plasma volume and increase the risk of dehydration (86). Furthermore, increased sweat rates may lead to a decrease in SV, which then prompts an increase in HR to maintain cardiac output at submaximal workloads. This "HR drift," or elevated HR at submaximal loads, can decrease performance dramatically in a hot environment. Increased blood flow to the skin circulation comes at the expense of reduced blood flow to the working muscle (85). In addition to these primary cardiovascular limiting factors, other physiological changes occur during exercise in the heat that may contribute to reduced performance capacity, such as diminished central nervous system function and increased muscle glycogen utilization (28). The EP-C should expect higher HR values at a given workload during exercise in the heat compared with exercise in a thermoneutral environment. HR may not reach a steady state during prolonged, submaximal intensity exercise because of the increased sweat rate, leading to cardiovascular drift. During cardiovascular drift, HR climbs over time, thereby decreasing overall performance (39,58). Staying well hydrated during exercise may help attenuate cardiovascular drift.

Cold Stress

Exercise in a cold environment facilitates heat loss produced during exercise. However, long duration exercise events in a cold environment increase the risk of hypothermia. If core temperature is challenged, the body attempts to increase heat production and limit heat loss via shivering and vasoconstriction of blood vessels in the skin (28). Individuals with greater subcutaneous fat mass have an advantage at limiting heat loss in cold environments, as their thicker subcutaneous fat layer acts as form of insulation or barrier between the warm blood and the cold environment (87). The HR and cardiac output responses to exercise in a cold environment are similar to those of a thermoneutral environment (38); however, respiratory rate is higher at a given submaximal intensity and $\dot{V}O_{2max}$ may be slightly lower. The primary barrier to maximal performance in a cold environment may simply be the extra work associated with wearing bulky clothing during exercise. Bulky clothing increases the energy cost of exercise because of the extra weight of the clothing, alterations in movement resulting in augmented extraneous work, and increased friction as layers of clothing slide against each other during exercise (77,93). Overall, the effect on $\dot{V}O_{2max}$ in a cold environment is negligible compared with that in a hot environment.

Altitude

Barometric pressure decreases with ascent to altitude. The partial pressure of oxygen (PO_2) is equal to the product of barometric pressure and the percentage of oxygen in the air. For example, the partial pressure at sea level is 760 mm Hg and the percentage of oxygen in dry air is 20.93%. Thus, the PO_2 at sea level is approximately 159 mm Hg ($PO_2 = 760 \times .2093$). If, however, you are at an altitude at which barometric pressure is only 550 mm Hg, the PO_2 now decreases to 115 mm Hg ($PO_2 = 760 \times .2093$). It is a common misconception that the "thin air" at altitude has less oxygen than the air at sea level; the percentage of oxygen in the air remains the same at all elevations in the stratosphere. It is the change in barometric pressure that causes the PO_2 to decrease at altitude and reduces our ability to provide oxygen to working muscles. In response to lower PO_2 at altitude, pulmonary ventilation increases. During the initial days of high-altitude exposure, SV decreases (5,83) yet HR increases (50) to a greater extent, causing an increase in cardiac output at a given submaximal exercise intensity (101). There is typically no change noted in BP (83). Other changes that could affect performance when transferring to altitude include weight loss (82) and sleep disturbances (101). To stay at the same relative intensity of exercise (*e.g.*, submaximal HR), unacclimatized individuals will have to reduce the absolute intensity of exercise at a higher altitude because of the greater difficulty of doing exercise at the higher altitude. The time it takes to become acclimatized to altitude varies greatly between individuals and also depends on the local altitude. It is best for the EP-C to assume that there will need to be a significant reduction in intensity and duration of exercise during the initial days of altitude adjustment, but that over time, exercise should become more comfortable.

Acclimatization When Exercising in a Hot, Cold, or High-Altitude Environment

Acclimatization is the process of physiological adaptation that occurs in response to changes in the natural environment. Acclimation is a related term but refers to the process of physiological adaptation that occurs in response to experimentally induced changes in climate, such as an environmental chamber in a research laboratory (28). Both acclimatization and acclimation can improve exercise performance in extreme environments.

Heat acclimatization has been shown to elicit many favorable physiological responses that may improve exercise performance in a hot environment (13,14,29), such as lower core body temperature, lower skin temperature, higher sweat rate, higher plasma volume, lower HR at a specific workload, lower perception of effort, and improved conservation of sodium. As a whole, these physiological adaptations improve heat dissipation from the body to the environment and limit cardiovascular strain.

In general, heat acclimatization requires gradual exposure to exercise in the heat on consecutive days. In order for complete adaptation to occur, 2 to 4 hours of moderate- to high-intensity exercise in a hot environment for 10 consecutive days is suggested (66). Partial acclimation to the heat can also be completed by training athletes wearing additional layers of clothing in a cool environment (35). Although the acclimation benefits of this technique will never reach the magnitude of true acclimatization, it may serve a purpose when the alternative choice is no acclimation. The first few days of exercise in a hot or humid environment should be light in intensity with frequent rest periods provided. The intensity of exercise should gradually build to the length and intensity desired for performance. The benefits of acclimation decrease after only days of exposure to another climate (64) and completely dissipate after approximately 2–3 weeks (14). Thus, acclimatization to the heat occurs annually in individuals living in areas where there is a wide variation in climate across the course of the year.

Cold acclimatization causes the shivering threshold to be reset to a lower mean skin temperature. This is a positive adaptation as it suggests cold acclimatization enhances the ability to maintain heat production through means besides shivering (23). In addition, cold acclimatization has also been shown to improve maintenance of hand and feet temperatures (88), potentially attenuating the loss of dexterity that normally accompanies cold extremities.

Altitude acclimatization requires adjusting to the lower PO_2. The lower PO_2 at altitude stimulates the production of additional red blood cells (erythropoiesis) to increase the oxygen-carrying capacity of the blood. Within hours of ascent to altitude, the kidneys increase the release of the hormone erythropoietin to stimulate erythropoiesis, but this process takes time, and the full benefits of erythropoiesis may not take effect for 4 or more weeks (28). After the oxygen-carrying capacity of the blood is restored via erythropoiesis, the HR, SV, cardiac output, and pulmonary ventilation responses to exercise revert back to more typical conditions. Today, many endurance athletes use altitude training to improve their athletic performance by practicing the "live high, train low" strategy (65), which is a unique strategy of gaining the benefits of high altitude acclimatization ("live high") and the maintenance of high-intensity training at sea level ("train low") to occur in synchrony. After returning to sea level, the benefits of altitude acclimatization have been shown to last up to 3 weeks (65).

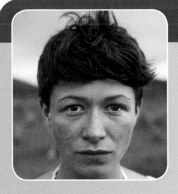

The Case of Sylvia

Submitted by **Leah Hantman, BS, ACSM EP-C, Franklin, MA, and Sarah Burnham, BS, ACSM EP-C, Somers, CT**

Sylvia is a 35-year-old single college professor who is challenged by adhering to a regular exercise routine. She needs variety to stay motivated. Teaching Sylvia about ways to use intensity and duration as a means of providing variety increased her ability to stay active. Sylvia's goal was to run the local Hot Chocolate 5K road race without walking.

Physical Data

Resting BP: 109/77 mm Hg
Resting HR: 78 bpm
Weight: 163 lb
Height: 66 in
Body mass index: 26.34 kg $\cdot$ m^{-2}
Body fat percentage measured by calipers: 33.4
CRF measured by submaximal bike test: $\dot{V}O_{2max}$: 21.3 mL $\cdot$ kg^{-1} $\cdot$ min^{-1}
ACSM Risk Classification (1): Low

Psychosocial Assessment Data (3)

Sylvia viewed wellness as having the energy to complete her daily tasks and enough extra energy for extracurricular activities as well. Wellness for Sylvia involved feeling well rested, relaxed, and energetic. The most important thing to Sylvia when making her journey toward wellness was to increase her stamina to run a 5K race without stopping. She believed that by keeping a picture of her healthy self in mind and reminding herself that this journey is doing something truly good for herself and those she loves, she can overcome any obstacles. One of the biggest obstacles that Sylvia faced was time management. She was afraid that she would feel overwhelmed or tired and want to give up completely. She also got bored very quickly. Sylvia was very aware that she had control over her schedule and that she could use her stubborn nature to stick to a goal. Sylvia liked gadgets as a mechanism to help her stay on track. She also had a strong social support network of friends who were willing to help her reach her goals.

Sylvia's Program

Cardiorespiratory

Cardio will be done 3 days a week — 1 day interval and 2 days of free cardio like a group exercise class or a jog.

Interval
F: 1 day a week
I: 3 minutes HR$_{max}$ 70%–90% and RPE is 12–15 out of 20 (breath should be elevated and carrying on a conversation very difficult); 2 minutes of active recovery HR$_{max}$ 50%–60% and RPE is at 6–10 (can carry on a conversation and breathing is easier)
T: 30–45 minutes with warm-up and cool-down
T: intervals, cardio drills and plyometrics

Free Cardio
F: 2 days a week
I: 60%–80% HR$_{max}$ and RPE 10–12
T: goal of continual movement of 45–60 minutes by week 10
T: jogging either outside or on a treadmill, a cardio group exercise class such as Zumba

Progression for Sylvia included a basic couch to 5K running program that included a progression of walk/runs to slow jog/runs to jog/runs to running at 60%–80% HR_{max} for 45 minutes. It also incorporated hill workouts.

Muscular Fitness

F: 2 days a week
I: reach muscle fatigue by 10 to 12 reps
T: 30 minutes or however long it takes to get through one set
T: free weights, medicine balls, body weight, and machines

At first, a workload of 70% intensity was suggested but proved to be too high to start. Given Sylvia's $\dot{V}O_2$ of $21 \text{ mL} \cdot \text{kg}^{-1} \cdot \text{minute}^{-1}$ and her goals, interval training was suggested to burn calories and increase endurance while allowing Sylvia to ebb in and out of her comfort zone. Short bursts of high-intensity exercise (65%–85% of maximum HR) followed by lower intensity recovery periods (50%–65% of maximum HR) proved to be more effective.

These target values of $\%HR_{max}$ provided a means of quantifying exercise intensity to optimize training results. If the optimal training intensity is 60%–80% $\dot{V}O_{2max}$, then, according to the ACSM, the corresponding optimal training HR is 70%–85% maximum HR (1). The theory of SAID and the 10% rule were applied throughout the program to ensure steady progression, avoid overtraining, and maintain self-efficacy in performance.

Sylvia completed the Hot Chocolate Run in just over 37 minutes. Her e-mail after the race showed the importance of using HR and RPE as useful feedback for training.

After the Race

Sylvia sent an e-mail after the race:

"I just wanted to thank you for your help over the last few weeks. I finished the Hot Chocolate Run faster than I anticipated. I think calibrating my RPE against my actual heart rate on Friday was HUGELY helpful. I ran further than I probably would have without stopping because I knew I was in a good workout range. When I did stop to walk (which I only did a few times), I timed myself, knowing from Friday's cardio workout that I only needed about 2 minutes max to lower my heart rate. I even kicked out the jams a little in the home stretch, sprinting to the finish line. Thanks."

QUESTIONS

- What is and how is it significant in cardiovascular fitness?
- What physiological adaptations and mental advantages come with interval training?
- In regard to what biometric traits might be correlated with physiological effect of lower levels of cardio fitness?
- What principle governs the 10% rule?

References

1. American College of Sports Medicine. *ACSM's Guidelines for Exercise Testing and Prescription*. 10th ed. Baltimore (MD): Lippincott Williams & Wilkins; 2018.
2. Bayati M, Farzad B, Gharakhanlou R, Agha-Alinejad H. A practical model of low-volume high-intensity interval training induces performance and metabolic adaptations that resemble "all-out" sprint interval training. *J Sports Sci Med*. 2011;10(3):571–6.
3. Charkoudian N. Physiologic considerations for exercise performance in women. *Clin Chest Med*. 2004;25:247–55.
4. Mannie K. Strategies for overload and progression. *Coach Athletic Dir*. 2006;75(9):8–12.
5. Moore M, Tschannen-Moran R. *Coaching Psychology Manual*. Baltimore (MD): Lippincott Williams & Wilkins; 2009. 208 p.

SUMMARY

Assessing and prescribing exercise is both an art and science; it should be taken as a serious responsibility by the EP-C. There are numerous means of assessing CRF so that the EP-C can accommodate a wide range of clientele safely. Also, the FITT-VP principle provides a framework of prescribing exercise that also allows for tremendous individual variation.

Properly assessing and prescribing exercise can play a significant role in helping individuals initiate an enjoyable exercise program. Using the most appropriate assessment and prescription techniques limits all types of risk and provides the individual with a solid foundation to begin his or her lifetime of physical activity.

STUDY QUESTIONS

1. Maximal oxygen uptake is commonly used as a marker of aerobic exercise capacity. Explain the science behind this concept. In other words, how is oxygen used in the body and why does a greater maximal oxygen uptake equate to greater aerobic exercise capacity?
2. Write out the Fick equation. Define each term within the Fick equation and discuss how each component of the equation changes with exercise training.
3. A 165-lb woman is walking on the treadmill at 3 mph at 2% grade for 30 minutes. Calculate the $\dot{V}O_2$, METs, and estimated caloric expenditure of this activity.
4. Using the HRR method, what is the target HR range for a 55-year-old man with a resting HR of 72 bpm, with an exercise prescription of 60%–70% of HRR?
5. Describe your cardiorespiratory exercise options for a 55-year-old obese woman with a history of lower back, knee, and ankle pain. What exercises may be contraindicated for this person and what are some alternative choices?

REFERENCES

1. Adams GM, Beam WC. *Exercise Physiology: Laboratory Manual.* 5th ed. New York (NY): McGraw-Hill; 2008. 320 p.

2. Ainsworth BE, Haskell WL, Herrmann SD, et al. 2011 Compendium of physical activities: a second update of codes and MET values. *Med Sci Sports Exerc.* 2011;43(8):1575–81.

3. Ainsworth BE, Haskell WL, Leon AS, et al. Compendium of physical activities: classification of energy costs of human physical activities. *Med Sci Sports Exerc.* 1993;25(1):71–80.

4. Ainsworth BE, Haskell WL, Whitt MC, et al. Compendium of physical activities: an update of activity codes and MET intensities. *Med Sci Sports Exerc.* 2000;32(Suppl 9):S498–516.

5. Alexander JK, Hartley LH, Modelski M, Grover RF. Reduction of stroke volume during exercise in man following ascent to 3,100 m altitude. *J Appl Physiol.* 1967;23(6):849–58.

6. Allison MK, Baglole JH, Martin BJ, MacInnis MJ, Gurd BJ, Gibala MJ. Brief intense stair climbing improves cardiorespiratory fitness. *Med Sci Sports Exerc.* 2017;49(2):298–307.

7. American College of Obstetricians and Gynecologists. Exercise during pregnancy and the postpartum period. ACOG Committee Opinion No 267. *Obstet Gynecol.* 2002; 99(1):171–3.

8. American College of Sports Medicine. *ACSM's Guidelines for Exercise Testing and Prescription.* 7th ed. Philadelphia (PA): Lippincott Williams & Wilkins; 2006. 366 p.

9. American College of Sports Medicine. *ACSM's Guidelines for Exercise Testing and Prescription.* 9th ed. Philadelphia (PA): Lippincott Williams & Wilkins; 2013. 480 p.

10. American College of Sports Medicine. *ACSM's Health-Related Physical Fitness Assessment Manual.* 3rd ed. Philadelphia (PA): Lippincott Williams & Wilkins; 2009. 192 p.

11. American College of Sports Medicine. *ACSM's Resource Manual for Guidelines for Exercise Testing and Prescription.* 5th ed. Philadelphia (PA): Lippincott Williams & Wilkins; 2006. 898 p.

12. American College of Sports Medicine. *ACSM's Resource Manual for Guidelines for Exercise Testing and Prescription.* 6th ed. Philadelphia (PA): Lippincott Williams & Wilkins; 2010. 868 p.

13. Armstrong LE, Costill DL, Fink WK. Changes in body water and electrolytes during heat acclimation: effects of dietary sodium. *Aviat Space Environ Med.* 1987;58(2):143–8.

14. Armstrong LE, Maresh CM. The induction and decay of heat acclimatization in trained athletes. *Sports Med.* 1991;12(5): 302–12.

15. Artal R, O'Toole M. Guidelines of the American College of Obstetricians and Gynecologists for exercise during pregnancy and the postpartum period. *Brit J Sports Med.* 2003;37(1):6–12.

16. Astrand PO. Aerobic work capacity in men and women with specific reference to age. *Acta Physiol Scand.* 1960;49(Suppl 169):45–60.

17. Astrand PO. Principles of ergometry and their implications in sport practice. *Int J Sports Med.* 1984;5:102–5.

18. Astrand PO, Cuddy TE, Saltin B, Stenberg J. Cardiac output during submaximal and maximal work. *J Appl Physiol.* 1964; 19:268–74.

19. Astrand PO, Rodahl K, Dahl HA, Stromme SB. *Textbook of Work Physiology: Physiological Bases of Exercise.* 4th ed. Champaign (IL): Human Kinetics; 2003. 656 p.

20. Astrand PO, Ryhming I. A nomogram for calculation of aerobic capacity (physical fitness) from pulse rate during submaximal work. *J Appl Physiol.* 1954;7(2):218–21.

21. Blair SN, Kohl HW, Barlow CE, Paffenbarger RS, Gibbons LW, Macera CA. Changes in physical fitness and all-cause mortality: a prospective study of healthy and unhealthy men. *JAMA.* 1995;273:1093–8.

22. Brouha L. The step test: a simple method of measuring physical fitness for muscular work in young men. *Res Quart Exerc Sport.* 1991;14:31–6.

23. Bruck K. Basic mechanisms in longtime thermal adaptation. In: Szelenyi Z, Szekely M, editors. *Advances in Physiological Science. Vol. 23.* Oxford (England): Pergamon Press; 1980. 263 p.

24. Buchheit M, Laursen PB. High-intensity interval training, solutions to the programming puzzle: part I: cardiopulmonary emphasis. *Sports Med.* 2013;43(5):313–38.

25. Buchheit M, Laursen PB. High-intensity interval training, solutions to the programming puzzle: part II: anaerobic energy, neuromuscular load and practical applications. *Sports Med.* 2013;43(10):927–54.

26. Centers for Disease Control and Prevention Web site [Internet]. Atlanta (GA): Centers for Disease Control and Prevention; [cited 2011 Aug 3]. Available from: http://www.cdc.gov/physicalactivity/everyone/health/index.html#StrengthenBonesMuscles

27. Centers for Disease Control and Prevention Web site [Internet]. Atlanta (GA): Centers for Disease Control and Prevention; [cited 2011 Aug 11]. Available from: http://www.cdc.gov/physicalactivity/everyone/measuring/index.html

28. Cheung SS. *Advanced Environmental Exercise Physiology.* Champaign (IL): Human Kinetics; 2010. 272 p.

29. Cheung SS, McLellan TM. Influence of heat acclimation, aerobic fitness, and hydration effects on tolerance during uncompensable heat stress. *J Appl Physiol.* 2000;84(5): 1731–9.

30. Christie J, Sheldahl LM, Tristani FE, Sagar KB, Ptacin JJ, Wann S. Determination of stroke volume and cardiac output during exercise: comparison of two-dimensional and Doppler echocardiography, Fick oximetry, and thermodilution. *Circulation.* 1987;76:539–47.

31. Clark MA, Lucett S, Corn RJ. *NASM Essentials of Personal Fitness Training.* 3rd ed. Philadelphia (PA): Lippincott Williams & Wilkins; 2008. 552 p.

32. Cooper KH. A means of assessing maximal oxygen intake. Correlation between field and treadmill testing. *JAMA.* 1968; 203(3):201–4.

33. Cooper KH. Testing and developing cardiovascular fitness within the United States Air Force. *J Occup Med.* 1968;10(11): 636–9.

34. Dawson B. Exercise training in sweat clothing in cool conditions to improve heat tolerance. *Sports Med.* 1994;17(4):233–44.

35. Davis JH. Anaerobic threshold: review of the concept and directions for future research. *Med Sci Sports Exerc.* 1985;17(1):6–21.

36. Dempsey FC, Butler FL, Williams FA. No need for a pregnant pause: physical activity may reduce the occurrence of gestational diabetes mellitus and preeclampsia. *Exerc Sports Sci Rev.* 2005;33(3):141–9.

37. Di Prampero P, Boutellier U, Pietsch P. Oxygen deficit and stores at onset of muscular exercise in humans. *J Appl Physiol.* 1983;55(1 Pt 1):146–53.

38. Doubt TJ. Physiology of exercise in the cold. *Sport Med.* 1991;11(6):367–81.

39. Ekelund LG. Circulatory and respiratory adaptation during prolonged exercise of moderate intensity in the sitting position. *Acta Physiol Scand.* 1967;69(4):327–40.

40. Gaesser G, Brooks G. Metabolic bases of excess post exercise oxygen consumption: a review. *Med Sci Sports Exerc.* 1984;16(1):29–43.

41. Garber CE, Blissmer B, Deschenes MR, et al. American College of Sports Medicine position stand. Quantity and quality of exercise for developing and maintaining cardiorespiratory, musculoskeletal, and neuromotor fitness in apparently healthy adults: guidance for prescribing exercise. *Med Sci Sports Exerc.* 2011;43(7):1334–59.

42. Gellish RL, Goslin BR, Olson RE, McDonald A, Russi GD, Moudgil VK. Longitudinal modeling of the relationship between age and maximal heart rate. *Med Sci Sports Exerc.* 2007;39(5):822–9.

43. Gibala MJ. High-intensity interval training: a time-efficient strategy for health promotion? *Curr Sports Med Rep.* 2007;6(4):211–3.

44. Gibala MJ, McGee SL. Metabolic adaptations to short-term high-intensity interval training: a little pain for a lot of gain? *Exerc Sport Sci Rev.* 2008;36(2):58–63.

45. Gillen JB, Gibala MJ. Is high-intensity interval training a time-efficient exercise strategy to improve health and fitness? *Appl Physiol Nutr Metab.* 2014;39(3):409–12.

46. Gillen JB, Martin BJ, MacInnis MJ, Skelly LE, Tarnopolsky MA, Gibala MJ. Twelve weeks of sprint interval training improves indices of cardiometabolic health similar to traditional endurance training despite a five-fold lower exercise volume and time commitment. *PLoS One.* 2016;11(4):e0154075.

47. Gillen JB, Percival ME, Skelly LE, Martin BJ, Tan RB, Tarnopolsky MA, Gibala MJ. Three minutes of all-out intermittent exercise per week increases skeletal muscle oxidative capacity and improves cardiometabolic health. *PLoS One.* 2014;9(11):e111489.

48. Gist NH, Fedewa MV, Dishman RK, Cureton KJ. Sprint interval training effects on aerobic capacity: a systematic review and meta-analysis. *Sports Med.* 2014;44(2):269–79.

49. Gledhill N, Cox D, Jamnik V. Endurance athletes' stroke volume does not plateau: major advantage is diastolic function. *Med Sci Sports Exerc.* 1994;26(9):1116–21.

50. Grover R, Reeves JT, Grover EB, Leathers JE. Muscular exercise in young men native to 3,100 m altitude. *J Appl Physiol.* 1967;22(3):555–64.

51. Haskell WL, Lee IM, Pate RR, et al. Physical activity and public health: updated recommendation for adults from the American College of Sports Medicine and the American Heart Association. *Med Sci Sports Exerc.* 2007;39(8):1423–34.

52. Hickson RC, Bomze HA, Holloszy JO. Faster adjustment of O_2 update to the energy requirement of exercise in the trained state. *J Appl Physiol.* 1978;44(6):877–81.

53. Higginbotham MB, Morris KG, Williams RS, McHale PA, Coleman RE, Cobb FR. Regulation of stroke volume during submaximal and maximal upright exercise in normal man. *Circ Res.* 1986;58(2):281–91.

54. Hill A. The oxidative removal of lactic acid. *J Physiol.* 1914; 48:x–xi.

55. Holmgren A, Johnson B, Sjostrand T. Circulatory data in normal subjects at rest and during exercise in recumbent position, with special reference to the stroke volume at different work intensities. *Acta Physiol Scand.* 1960;49:343–63.

56. Hootman JM, Macera CA, Ainsworth BE, Martin M, Addy CL, Blair SN. Association among physical activity level, cardiorespiratory fitness, and risk of musculoskeletal injury. *Am J Epidemiol.* 2001;154(3):251–8.

57. Howley ET, Franks BD. *Health Fitness Instructor's Handbook.* 4th ed. Champaign (IL): Human Kinetics; 2003. 573 p.

58. Johnson JM, Rowell LB. Forearm and skin vascular responses to prolonged exercise in man. *J Appl Physiol.* 1975;39(6):920–92.

59. Kenney WL, Munce T. Aging and human temperature regulation. *J Appl Physiol.* 2003;95:2598–603.

60. Kline GM, Porcari JP, Hintermeister R, et al. Estimation of VO_{2max} from a one-mile track walk, gender, age, and body weight. *Med Sci Sports Exerc.* 1987;19(3):253–9.

61. Kraemer, WJ, Fleck SJ, Deschenes MR. *Exercise Physiology: Integrating Theory and Application.* Philadelphia (PA): Lippincott Williams & Wilkins; 2012. 512 p.

62. Laursen PB, Jenkins DG. The scientific basis for high-intensity interval training: optimising training programmes and maximising performance in highly trained endurance athletes. *Sports Med.* 2002;32(1):53–73.

63. Lee IM, Buchner DM. The importance of walking to public health. *Med Sci Sports Exerc.* 2008;40(7 Suppl):S512–8.

64. Lee SM, Williams WJ, Schneider SM. Role of skin blood flow and sweating rate in exercise thermoregulation after bed rest. *J Appl Physiol.* 2002;92(5):2026–34.

65. Levine BD, Stray-Gundersen J. "Living high-training low": effect of moderate-altitude acclimatization with low-altitude training on performance. *J Appl Physiol.* 1997;83(1):102–12.

66. Lind AR, Bass DE. Optimal exposure time for development of acclimatization to heat. *Fed Proc.* 1963;22:704–8.

67. Ma JK, Scribbans TD, Edgett BA, Boyd C, Simpson CA, Little JP, Gurd BJ. Extremely low-volume, high-intensity interval training improves exercise capacity and increases mitochondrial protein content in human skeletal muscle. *Open J Mol Integr Physiol.* 2013;3(4):202–10.

68. MacInnis MJ, Gibala MJ. Physiological adaptations to interval training and the role of exercise intensity. *J Physiol.* 2016 [Epub ahead of print]. doi:10.1113/JP273196.

69. Mariz JS, Morrison JF, Peter J. A practical method of estimating an individual's maximal oxygen uptake. *Ergonomics.* 1961;4:97–122.

70. McArdle WD, Katch FI, Katch VL. *Exercise Physiology: Nutrition, Energy, and Human Performance.* 7th ed. Philadelphia (PA): Lippincott Williams & Wilkins; 2010. 1104 p.

71. Medbø JI, Mohn AC, Tabata I, Bahr R, Vaage O, Sejersted OM. Anaerobic capacity determined maximal accumulated O2 deficit. *J Appl Physiol.* 1988;64(1):50–60.

72. Metcalfe RS, Babraj JA, Fawkner SG, Vollaard NBJ. Towards the minimal amount of exercise for improving metabolic health: beneficial effects of reduced-exertion high-intensity interval training. *Eur J Appl Physiol.* 2012;112(7):2767–75.

73. Miller WC, Wallace JP, Eggert KE. Predicting max HR and the HR-VO2 relationship for exercise prescription in obesity. *Med Sci Sports Exerc.* 1993;25(9):1077–81.

74. Morris JN, Heady JA, Raffle PA, Roberts CG, Parks JW. Coronary heart disease and physical activity of work. *Lancet*. 1953;265(6795):1053–7.

75. Muse T. Cardiovascular medication and your client. IDEA Health and Fitness Association Web site [Internet]. 2006 [cited 2011 Aug 12]. Available from: http://www.ideafit.com/files/pdf/fitness-library/cardiovascular-medication-and-your-client-0

76. National Sporting Goods Association. 2010 Participation — Ranked by Total Participation [Internet]. 2011 [cited 2011 Aug 18]. Available from: http://www.nsga.org/files/public/2010 Participation_Ranked_by_TotalParticipation_4Web.pdf

77. Patton JF. The effects of acute cold exposure on exercise performance. *J Appl Sport Sci Res*. 1988;2:72–8.

78. Phillips EM, Capell J, Jonas S. Getting started as a regular exerciser. In: Jonas S, Phillips EM, editors. *Exercise is Medicine: A Clinician's Guide to Exercise Prescription*. Philadelphia (PA): Lippincott Williams & Wilkins; 2009. 272 p.

79. Pickering TG, Hall JE, Appel LJ, et al. Recommendations for blood pressure measurement in humans and experimental animals: part 1: blood pressure measurement in humans: a statement for professionals from the Subcommittee of Professional and Public Education of the American Heart Association Council on High Blood Pressure Research. *Hypertension*. 2005;45:142–61.

80. Plowman SA, Smith DL. *Exercise Physiology for Health, Fitness, and Performance*. 3rd ed. Philadelphia (PA): Lippincott Williams & Wilkins; 2011. 744 p.

81. Powers S, Dodd S, Beadle R. Oxygen update kinetics in trained athletes differing in VO2max. *Eur J Appl Physiol*. 1985;54(3):306–8.

82. Pugh LG. Physiological and medical aspects of the Himalayan Scientific and Mountaineering Expedition, 1960-61. *BMJ*. 1962;2:621–33.

83. Reeves JT, Groves BM, Sutton JR, et al. Operation Everest II: Preservation of cardiac function at extreme altitude. *J Appl Physiol*. 1987;63:531–9.

84. Renstrom P, Kannus P. Prevention of sports injuries. In: Strauss RH, editor. *Sports Medicine*. Philadelphia (PA): WB Saunders; 1992. p 307–29.

85. Rowell LB. *Human Cardiovascular Control*. New York (NY): Oxford University Press; 1993. 500 p.

86. Shirreffs SM, Armstrong LE, Cheuvront SN. Fluid and electrolyte needs for preparation and recovery from training and competition. *J Sports Sci*. 2004;22:57–63.

87. Smith RM, Hanna JM. Skinfolds and resting heat loss in cold air and water: temperature equivalence. *J Appl Physiol*. 1975;39:93–102.

88. Stocks J, Taylor N, Tipton M, Greenleaf J. Human physiological responses to cold exposure. *Aviat Space Environ Med*. 2004;75(5):444–57.

89. Suzuki Y. Human physical performance and cardiorespiratory responses to hot environments during submaximal upright cycling. *Ergonomics*. 1980;23(6):527–42.

90. Tabata I, Irisawa K, Kouzaki M, Nishimura K, Ogita F, Miyachi M. Metabolic profile of high intensity intermittent exercise. *Med Sci Sports Exerc*. 1997;29(3):390–95.

91. Tabata I, Nishimura K, Kouzaki M, Hirai Y, Ogita F, Miyachi M, Yamamoto K. Effects of moderate-intensity endurance and high intensity intermittent training on anaerobic capacity and VO2max. *Med Sci Sports Exerc*. 1996;28(10):1327–30.

92. Tanaka HK, Monahan KD, Seals DR. Age-predicted maximal heart rate revisited. *J Am Coll Cardiol*. 2001;37(1):153–6.

93. Teitlebaum A, Goldman RF. Increased energy cost with multiple clothing layers. *J Appl Physiol*. 1972;32(6):743–4.

94. Thompson WR. Worldwide survey of fitness trends for 2016: 10th anniversary edition. *ACSM's Health Fitness J*. 2015;19(6):9–18.

95. Trost SG, Owen N, Bauman AE, Sallis JF, Brown W. (2002). Correlates of adults' participation in physical activity: review and update. *Med Sci Sport Exerc*. 2002;34(12):1996–2001.

96. U.S. Department of Health and Human Services. *Physical Activity Guidelines Advisory Committee Report 2008 (ODPHP Publication No. U0049)*. Washington (DC): 2008. 683 p.

97. U.S. Department of Health and Human Services. *2008 Physical Activity Guidelines for Americans (ODPHP Publication No. U0036)*. Washington (DC): 2008. 76 p.

98. U.S. Department of Health and Human Services. *The Seventh Report of the Joint National Committee on Prevention, Detection, Evaluation, and Treatment of High Blood Pressure — Complete Report*. Bethesda (MD): National Heart, Lung, and Blood Institute; 2004. 104 p.

99. Wasserman K, Whipp BJ, Koyal SN, Beaver WL. Anaerobic threshold and respiratory gas exchange during exercise. *J Appl Physiol*. 1973;35(2):236–43.

100. Wei M, Kampert JB, Barlow CE, et al. Relationship between low cardiorespiratory fitness and mortality in normal-weight, overweight, and obese men. *JAMA*. 1999;282(16):1547–53.

101. West JB. Physiology of extreme altitude. In: Fregly MJ, Blatteis CM, editors. *Handbook of Physiology: Section 4: Environmental Physiology, Volume II*. New York (NY): Oxford University Press; 1996. 1586 p.

102. Weston KS, Wisløff U, Coombes JS. High-intensity interval training in patients with lifestyle-induced cardiometabolic disease: a systematic review and meta-analysis. *Br J Sports Med*. 2014;48(16):1227–34.

103. Wilmore JH, Costill DL, Kenney WL. *Physiology of Sport and Exercise*. 4th ed. Champaign (IL): Human Kinetics; 2008. 592 p.

104. *YMCA Fitness Testing and Assessment Manual*. Champaign (IL): Human Kinetics; 1989.

105. Zhou B, Conlee RK, Jensen R, Fellingham GW, George JD, Fisher AG. Stroke volume does not plateau during graded exercise in elite male distance runners. *Med Sci Sports Exerc*. 2001;33:1849–54.

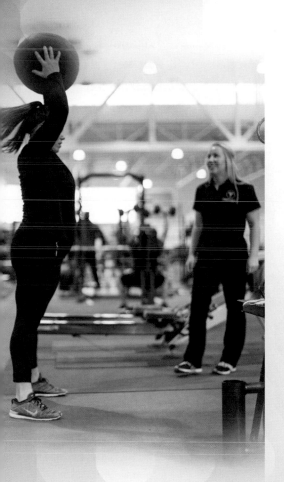

Muscular Strength and Muscular Endurance Assessments and Exercise Programming for Apparently Healthy Participants

- To understand the importance of muscular strength and endurance for health and fitness.

- To describe the basic structure and function of muscle.

- To explain the fundamental principles of resistance training.

- To identify resistance training program variables.

- To compare different resistance exercise modalities.

- To design resistance training programs for apparently healthy adults and individuals with medically controlled disease.

INTRODUCTION

The development of muscular strength and muscular endurance is an essential component of health-related physical fitness. There has been a tremendous increase in the number of scientific publications on this topic, and resistance training has become a top 10 worldwide fitness trend (32,61,76). Like aerobic exercise, regular participation in a training program designed to enhance muscular strength and muscular endurance can improve the quality of life for men and women of all ages and abilities (25,27,72,80). The American College of Sports Medicine (ACSM) recommends participating in a comprehensive fitness program that includes resistance exercise, and the World Health Organization recognizes the potential benefits of muscle-strengthening activities for healthy children and adults (2,25,82).

In addition to enhancing all components of muscular fitness (i.e., muscular strength, muscular endurance, and muscular power), higher levels of muscular fitness are associated with significantly better cardiometabolic risk profiles, lower risk of all-cause mortality, and fewer cardiovascular disease events (4,16,24,37,38,52). Resistance training can improve body composition as well as selected health-related biomarkers including blood glucose levels and blood pressure in individuals with mild or moderate hypertension (2,31,41,80). Regular participation in muscle-strengthening activities can lower the risk of developing Type 2 diabetes (31) and can improve glycemic control and insulin sensitivity in adults with this condition (29). Furthermore, an increase in lean body mass as a result of resistance training can contribute to the maintenance of, or increase in, resting or basal metabolic rate (3).

EXERCISE IS MEDICINE CONNECTION

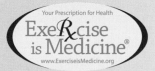

Handgrip Strength Predicts Cardiovascular Risk
Leong D, Teo K, Rangarajan S, et al. Prognostic value of grip strength: findings from the Prospective Urban-Rural Epidemiology (PURE) study. *Lancet.* 2015;386(9990):266–73.

Although reduced levels muscle strength have been associated with an increased risk of all-cause and cardiovascular mortality, the prognostic value of grip strength with respect to cardiovascular disease and mortality is unknown. Leong and colleagues (48) assessed grip strength in almost 140,000 adults enrolled in the Prospective Urban Rural Epidemiology study which is a large, longitudinal population study done in 17 countries of varying incomes and sociocultural settings. Grip strength data were collected before and after a median follow-up of 4 years. Grip strength was inversely associated with all-cause mortality, cardiovascular mortality, noncardiovascular mortality, myocardial infarction, and stroke. Grip strength was a stronger predictor of all-cause and cardiovascular mortality than systolic blood pressure. These findings indicate that grip strength can be a simple, quick, and inexpensive method for assessing an individual's risk of death and cardiovascular disease (48).

Resistance training over months or years can increase bone mass and has proven to be a valuable measure for preventing the loss of bone mass in people with osteoporosis (42). Importantly, regular participation in a resistance training program can contribute to an improved health-related quality of life by enhancing physical function, attenuating age-related weight gain, and enabling people to do what they enjoy while maintaining their independence (27,40,51).

This chapter provides a basic overview of muscle structure and function, highlights the fundamental principles of resistance exercise, and outlines program design considerations for developing, implementing, and progressing resistance training programs that are consistent with individual needs, goals, and abilities. In this chapter, the term *resistance training* (also known as *strength training*) refers to a specialized method of physical conditioning that involves the progressive use of a wide range of resistive loads and a variety of training modalities designed to enhance muscular fitness. The term *resistance training* should be distinguished from the terms *bodybuilding* and *powerlifting* which are competitive sports.

 ## Basic Structure and Function

An understanding of the basic structure and function of the muscular system is important for designing fitness programs and optimizing training adaptations. Many of the fundamental principles of resistance training discussed later in this chapter are grounded in an understanding of muscle structure and function. Although the body has more than 600 skeletal muscles that vary in shape and size, the basic purpose of skeletal muscle, especially during resistance training, is to provide force to move the joints of the body in different directions.

The smallest contractile unit within a muscle is called a sarcomere, which is made up of different proteins. A myofibril consists of many sarcomeres, and groups of myofibrils make up a single muscle fiber or muscle cell. Different types of connective tissue called fascia surround these structures and create a stable, yet flexible, environment. The connective tissue in muscle is like a rubber band that stretches and recoils to provide added force to a muscle contraction.

The muscles that are the primary movers of a joint are called the agonists, and the muscles that assist in that movement are called synergists. Antagonists are muscles that oppose a movement. For example, during the biceps curl exercise, the biceps brachii and brachialis are the agonists for that movement, the brachioradialis is the synergist, and the triceps brachii is the antagonist. Only the parts of a muscle that are used during an exercise will adapt to the training stress; furthermore, different training loads stimulate different amounts of muscle. That is why it is important to understand muscle structure and be aware that different training loads recruit different muscle fibers.

Muscle Fiber Types and Recruitment

Although skeletal muscle is made up of thousands of muscle fibers, there are generally two types of muscle fibers. Type I fibers (also called slow twitch fibers) have a high oxidative capacity and a lower contractile force capability and are better for endurance activities. Type II fibers (also called fast twitch fibers) have a high glycolytic capacity and a higher contractile force capability and are better for strength and power activities. Although each muscle fiber type has various subtypes (type IIa, IIx), the ratio of type I and type II fibers in the body varies for each person and depends mainly on hereditary factors. Regular resistance training may cause a small change in fiber type composition, but these changes are primarily from one subgroup of fiber to another subgroup of fiber. Thus, resistance training will not convert type I fibers to type II fibers, but different training loads and different movement speeds can alter the involvement of different types of muscle fibers in a given movement (22).

Because muscle fibers that are not stimulated will not reap the benefits of training, it is important to understand how muscle fibers are recruited for action. Muscle fibers are innervated by a motor neuron, and this neuromuscular gathering is called a motor unit. Although each motor unit is composed of either all type I or all type II fibers, the size of a motor unit as well as the number of fibers within a motor unit varies within different muscles. The size principle of motor unit activation states that motor units are recruited from the smallest to the largest, depending on the force production demands. Smaller or low-threshold motor units (mostly type I fibers) are recruited first, and larger or high-threshold motor units (mostly type II fibers) are recruited later, depending on the demands of the exercise (22) (Fig. 4.1).

Training with heavy loads that can be lifted only four to six times (*e.g.*, a 4–6 repetition maximum [RM]) will activate higher threshold motor units than training with a load that can be lifted 12–15 times (*e.g.*, a 12- to 15-RM) (11,22). However, even if heavy loads are lifted, low-threshold motor units will be recruited first, and then high-threshold motor units will be activated as needed to produce the necessary force. Although exceptions exist, to recruit high-threshold motor units, specific types of resistance exercise that involve lifting heavy loads, moving lighter loads at a fast velocity, or both are needed to achieve a training effect in these muscle fibers (22). The concept of training periodization or program variation (discussed later in this chapter) is based on the principle that different training loads and power requirements recruit different types and numbers of motor units (62).

Types of Muscle Action

Muscles can perform different types of muscle actions. When a weight is lifted, the involved muscles normally shorten and this is called a concentric muscle contraction, and when a weight is lowered, the involved muscles lengthen and this is called an eccentric muscle action. For example, when an individual extends the hips and knees from a parallel squat position to the standing phase, the gluteus maximus and vastus lateralis perform concentric muscle contractions (Fig. 4.2). The gluteus maximus and vastus lateralis perform eccentric muscle action when the weight is lowered from the standing phase to the parallel squat position. If a muscle is activated but no movement at the joint takes place, the muscle action is called isometric (or static). This type of muscle action takes place during the standing phase of the squat exercise when the weight is held stationary and no visible movement occurs. Isometric muscle actions also occur when the weight is too heavy to lift any further (61). This typically happens during the "sticking point" of an exercise when the force produced by the muscle equals the resistance (61).

The amount of force produced by a muscle is dependent on a number of factors, including the type of muscle action. The highest force produced occurs during an eccentric muscle action, and maximal force produced during an isometric muscle action is greater than that seen during a

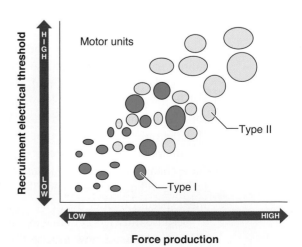

FIGURE 4.1. Size principle of motor unit recruitment. (Reproduced with permission from Haff G, Triplett N, editors. *Essentials of Strength Training and Conditioning.* 4th ed. Champaign [IL]: Human Kinetics; 2016. 752 p.)

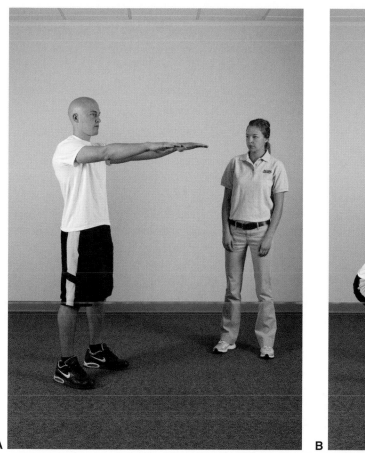
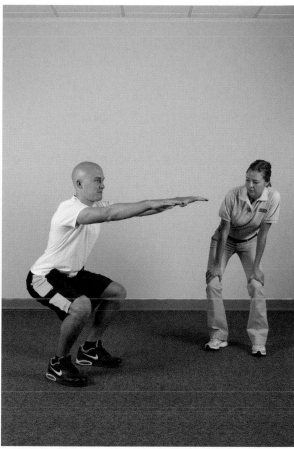

FIGURE 4.2. Squat without weights starting position **(A)** and squat position **(B)**.

concentric contraction. Furthermore, as the velocity of movement increases, the amount of force that is generated decreases during a concentric muscle contraction and increases during an eccentric muscle action (22) (Fig. 4.3). This is an important consideration when designing resistance training programs because high force development during maximal eccentric muscle actions has been linked to muscle soreness (33). Although eccentric muscle actions are a potent stimulus for increases in muscle size and strength (19), a gradual and progressive introduction to resistance

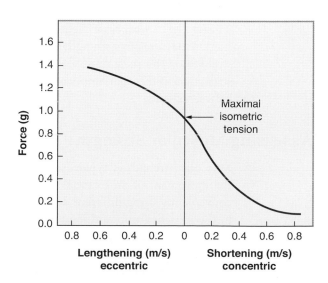

FIGURE 4.3. Force–velocity relationship. (From Ratamess N. *ACSM's Foundations of Strength Training and Conditioning.* Baltimore [MD]: Lippincott Williams & Wilkins; 2012:25.)

training is warranted to reduce the risk of a muscle strain. Even trained individuals who accentuate the eccentric phase of a lift can experience muscle soreness for several days after an exercise session (57). Moreover, extended periods of eccentric training with very heavy loads can result in serious complications such as rhabdomyolysis, which may harm kidney function (13).

 ## Assessment Protocols

Muscular fitness can be assessed by a variety of laboratory and field-based measures. Results from muscular fitness tests can provide valuable information about an individual's baseline fitness and can be used to design individualized resistance training programs that target muscle weaknesses and imbalances. Moreover, data from periodic muscular fitness assessments can be used to highlight a client's progress and provide positive feedback that can promote exercise adherence. For safety purposes, physically inactive adults with known cardiovascular, metabolic, and/or renal disease or any signs or symptoms suggestive of these diseases should seek medical clearance before beginning a resistance training program (68). Physically active asymptomatic adults may begin a light to moderate-intensity resistance training program without medical clearance and progress gradually as tolerated (68). More information on exercise preparticipation health screening can be found in Chapter 2.

Muscular fitness tests are specific to the muscle groups being assessed, the velocity of movement, the joint range of motion (ROM), and the type of equipment available (61). Furthermore, no single test exists for evaluating total body muscular fitness, so professionals need to carefully select and supervise the most appropriate muscular fitness tests for each client. Also, individuals should participate in several familiarization/practice sessions before testing and adhere to a specific protocol (including repetition duration and ROM) to obtain a reliable fitness score that can be used to track fitness changes over time. Because an acute bout of static stretching may have adverse effects on subsequent strength and power performance, large amplitude dynamic movements (also known as dynamic stretching) and test-specific activities should precede muscular fitness testing (6).

An initial assessment of muscular fitness and a change in muscular strength or muscular endurance over time can be based on the absolute value of the weight lifted or the total number of repetitions performed with proper technique. Although population-specific norms are available for most health-related muscular fitness tests, when strength comparisons are made between individuals, the values should be expressed as relative values (per kilogram of body weight) (2). For example, a client who weighs 100 kg and lifts 75 kg on the chest press exercise has a relative strength score of $0.75 \text{ kg} \cdot \text{kg}^{-1}$, whereas a client who weighs 80 kg and lifts the same amount of weight on the same exercise has a relative strength score of $0.94 \text{ kg} \cdot \text{kg}^{-1}$. Although both clients have the same absolute strength on the chest press exercise, the lighter client has a higher measure of relative upper body strength, and this is an important consideration when comparing individual strength performance between clients.

Assessing Muscular Strength

Muscular strength is typically assessed in fitness facilities with dynamic measures that involve the movement of an external load or body part. Although isometric strength can be measured conveniently using different devices such as handgrip dynamometers, these measures are specific to the muscle group and joint angle and therefore provide limited information regarding overall muscular strength. The 1-RM, which is the heaviest weight that can be lifted only once using proper technique, is the standard muscular strength assessment (61). However, a multiple RM such as a 10-RM can also be used to assess muscular strength and provide valuable information regarding

HOW TO — Assess One-Repetition Maximum (1-RM) Strength

1. Warm up for 5–10 min with low-intensity aerobic exercise and dynamic stretching.
2. Perform a specific warm-up with several repetitions with a light load.
3. Select an initial weight that is within the subject's perceived capacity (~50%–70% of capacity).
4. Attempt a 1-RM lift; if successful, rest approximately 3–5 min before the next trial.
5. Increase resistance progressively (*e.g.*, 2.5–20 kg) until the subject cannot complete the lift. A 1-RM should be obtained within four sets to avoid excessive fatigue.
6. The 1-RM is recorded as the heaviest weight lifted successfully through the full ROM with proper technique.

an individual's training program. For example, if a client was training with an 8- to 12-RM weight, the performance of a 10-RM strength test could provide an index of strength changes over time.

Procedures for administering 1-RM (or multiple RM) strength tests after the familiarization period and an adequate warm-up are outlined in the "How to" box. A familiarization period is particularly important for individuals with no prior resistance exercise experience because they need to learn proper exercise technique and be taught how to produce maximal effort during the test. A proper familiarization period (*e.g.*, 3–4 practice sessions for each exercise) will likely achieve appropriate familiarization and reliability for RM strength testing (22,61). Moreover, communication between the certified exercise physiologist (EP-C) and the client can help determine a progression pattern of loading with reasonable accuracy. In terms of safety, properly trained spotters are needed to enhance strength testing procedures, particularly during the performance of free weight exercises such as the bench press and back squat.

Normative data for the chest press and leg press exercises are available in *ACSM's Guidelines for Exercise Testing and Prescription* (2). However, additional research is needed to provide norms for different exercises and different types of resistance training equipment because 1-RM performance is significantly greater on weight machines than free weights (50).

Assessing Muscular Endurance

Muscular endurance is the ability to perform repeated contractions over a period and is typically assessed with field measures such as the push-up tests (Fig. 4.4). This test can be used independently or in combination with other tests of muscular endurance to screen for muscle weaknesses and aid

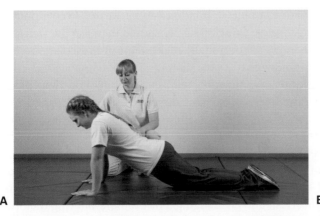
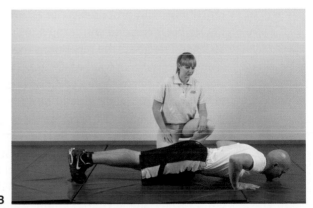

FIGURE 4.4. Proper positioning for the push-up test: **(A)** the starting position for women and **(B)** the downward position for men.

in the exercise prescription. Procedures for administering the push-up test is described in the "How to" box. Normative data for the push-up test is available in *ACSM's Guidelines for Exercise Testing and Prescription* (2). Of note, overweight individuals may find this test difficult to perform, and poor results obtained during testing may discourage participation in an exercise program. EP-Cs should carefully consider which tests are appropriate for each individual and most likely to yield beneficial information.

Fundamental Principles of Resistance Training

Simply engaging in resistance training does not ensure that muscular fitness gains will occur. Training programs need to be based on fundamental training principles and carefully prescribed to optimize training outcomes and maximize exercise adherence. Although factors such as initial level of fitness, heredity, age, sex, nutritional status, and health habits (*e.g.*, sleep) will influence the rate and magnitude of adaptation that occurs, seven fundamental principles that determine the effectiveness of all resistance training programs are the principles of (a) *Progression*, (b) *Regularity*, (c) *Overload*, (d) *Creativity*, (e) *Enjoyment*, (f) *Specificity*, and (g) *Supervision*. These basic principles can be remembered as the PROCESS of resistance training program design (21).

Principle of Progression

The principle of progression refers to the fact that the demands placed on the body must be continually and progressively increased over time to achieve long-term gains in muscular fitness. This does not mean that heavier weights should be used every workout but rather that over time, the physical stress placed on the body should gradually become more challenging to continually stimulate adaptations. Without a more challenging exercise stimulus that is consistent with individual needs, goals, and abilities, the human body has no reason to adapt any further. This principle is particularly important after the first few months of resistance training when the threshold for training-induced adaptations in conditioned individuals is higher (2).

At the start of a resistance training program, the 10-RM on the leg press might be 50 kg, which is likely an adequate stimulus to promote adaptations. But as training progresses, 10 repetitions with 50 kg would be suboptimal for stimulating gains in muscle fitness strength as 50 kg "feels easy" for 10 repetitions. If the training load is not increased at a rate that is compatible with the training-induced adaptations that are occurring, no further gains in muscular fitness will occur. A reasonable guideline for a beginner is to increase the training weight about $5\%–10\% \cdot week^{-1}$ and decrease the repetitions by 2–4 when a given load can be performed for the desired number of repetitions with proper exercise technique. For example, if an adult can perform 12 repetitions of the leg press exercise with proper exercise technique using 50 kg, he should increase the weight to 55 kg and decrease the repetitions to 8 if he wants to continually make gains in muscular strength. A more conservative approach would be to follow the "2 plus 2" rule (5). That is, once this client can perform two or more additional repetitions over the assigned repetition goal on two consecutive workouts, weight should be added to the leg press exercise during the next training session. Alternatively, he could increase the number of sets, increase the number of repetitions, or add another leg exercise to his exercise routine (5).

Individuals who have achieved a desired level of muscular fitness may not need to progress the training program to maintain that level of performance. However, program variation is important for exercise adherence, and experienced exercisers may benefit from periodically changing program variables to keep the training stimulus fresh and challenging. For example, altering the order of exercises or mode of resistance training can limit training plateaus (62).

Visit thePoint to watch video 4.2, which demonstrates the push-up test for men and women.

HOW TO	**Assess Upper Body Strength and Endurance with the Push-Up Test**

1. Explain the purpose of the test to the client (to determine how many push-ups can be completed to reflect upper body muscular strength and endurance).

2. Inform clients of proper breathing technique (to exhale with the effort, which occurs when pushing away from the floor).

3. The push-up test usually is administered with men starting in the standard "down" position (hands pointing forward and under the shoulder, back straight, and head up, using the toes as the pivotal point). For women, the modified knee push-up position is often used, with legs together, lower leg in contact with mat, ankles plantarflexed, back straight, hands shoulder width-apart, and head up, using the knees as the pivotal point. (Note: Some men will need to use the modified position, and some women can use the full-body position.)

4. The subject must raise the body by straightening the elbows and return to the "down" position, until the chin touches the mat. The stomach should not touch the mat.

5. For both men and women, the subject's back must be straight at all times and the subject must push-up to a straight-arm position.

6. Demonstrate the test and allow the client to practice if desired.

7. Remind the client that the maximal number of push-ups performed consecutively without rest is counted as the score.

8. Begin the test when the client is ready. Stop the test when the client strains forcibly or is unable to maintain the appropriate exercise technique within two repetitions.

Descriptions of procedures are adapted from the American College of Sports Medicine. *ACSM's Guidelines for Exercise Testing and Prescription.* 10th ed. Philadelphia (PA): Wolters Kluwer; 2018.

Principle of Regularity

Resistance training must be performed regularly several times per week to make continual gains in muscular fitness. Although the optimal training frequency may depend on training status and program design, two to three training sessions per week on nonconsecutive days are reasonable for most adults. Inconsistent training will result in only modest training adaptations, and periods of inactivity will result in a loss of muscular strength and size (47). The adage "use it or lose it" is appropriate for resistance exercise because training-induced adaptations cannot be stored. Although adequate recovery is needed between resistance training sessions, the principle of regularity states that long-term gains in muscular fitness will be realized only if the program is performed on a consistent basis.

Principle of Overload

The overload principle is a basic tenet of all resistance training programs. The overload principle simply states that to enhance muscular fitness, the body must exercise at a level beyond that at which it is normally stressed (43). For example, an adult who can easily complete 10 repetitions with 20 kg while performing a chest press exercise must increase the weight, the repetitions, or the number of sets if she wants to increase her upper body strength. Otherwise, if the training stimulus is not increased beyond the level to which the muscles are accustomed, she will not maximize training adaptations even if other aspects of the training program are well designed. Although overload is typically manipulated by changing the exercise intensity, duration, or frequency, adding more advanced exercises to a training program is another way to place greater overload on the body (61,62). For example, progressing from a weight machine leg press to a free weight back squat can place a new training demand on the body which is needed for long-term gains.

Principle of Creativity

The creativity principle refers to the imagination and ingenuity that can help to optimize training-induced adaptations and enhance exercise adherence. Because an intimidating gym environment and a lack of confidence in using exercise equipment may be a barrier to attendance (56), creative approaches for designing and implementing exercise programs are needed. For example, the provision of exercise variety and technology-based exercise interventions have been found to provide a creative means for promoting physical activity in adults (75). In order for clients to remain engaged and interested in resistance training, fitness professionals need to reflect on past experiences and use creative thinking to facilitate the development of training programs that are safe, effective, and challenging. By sensibly incorporating novel exercises and new training equipment into the training program, professionals can help clients overcome barriers and maintain interest in resistance exercise (61,62,77). Depending on each client's needs and abilities and goals, EP-Cs can incorporate medicine balls, kettlebells, or suspension trainers into resistance training programs to optimize strength gains, enhanced adherence, and stimulate an ongoing interest in this type of exercise (61).

Although the quantitative aspects of resistance training and its physiological adaptations are important considerations, the qualitative aspects of exercise program design should not be overlooked (58). This is where the art and science of designing resistance training programs come into play because the principles of exercise science need to be balanced with imagination and creativity. Sharing experiences with other EP-Cs can help to foster creative expression and spark an appreciation for original ideas related to the design of resistance training programs. By taking time to reflect on the design and implementation of resistance training programs, EP-Cs can fuel their creativity to generate answers to challenging situations. Notwithstanding the critical importance of exercise safety and proper technique, novelty and training variety are important for stimulating strength development (34,61).

Principle of Enjoyment

Enjoyment of physical activity is an important determinant of long-term participation in recreational fitness activities and structured exercise programs (46,54,55). The principle of enjoyment states that participants who genuinely enjoy exercising are more like to adhere to the exercise program and achieve training goals. Although encouragement from fitness professionals and support from family and friends can influence exercise behaviors (79), the enjoyment an individual feels during and after an exercise session can facilitate the sustainability of the desired behavior.

Although resistance training programs should be challenging, clients should have the competence and confidence in their physical abilities to perform the exercises or activities with energy and vigor. As such, enjoyment can be defined as a balance between skill and challenge (18). If the resistance training program is too advanced, clients will be anxious and will lose interest. Conversely, if the training program is too easy, then clients will become bored. Resistance training programs should be matched with the physical abilities of the participants in order for the training experience to be enjoyable. EP-Cs who provide immediate and meaningful feedback on challenging exercises can help clients negotiate demanding situations and therefore maintain a state of enjoyment while training.

Principle of Specificity

The principle of specificity refers to the distinct adaptations that take place as a result of the training program. For example, the adaptations to resistance training are specific to the muscle actions, velocity of movement, exercise ROM, muscle groups trained, energy systems involved, and intensity and volume of training (11,65). The principle of specificity is often referred to as the SAID principle (which stands for specific adaptations to imposed demands). In terms of designing resistance training programs, only muscle groups that are trained will make desired adaptations in selected parameters of muscular fitness. Exercises such as the squat and leg press can be used to enhance lower body strength, but these exercises will not affect upper body strength.

In addition, the adaptations that take place in a muscle or muscle group will be as simple or as complex as the stress placed on them. For example, because basketball requires multiple-joint and multiplanar movements in the sagittal (*i.e.*, left to right), frontal (*i.e.*, front to back), and transverse (*i.e.*, upper to lower) planes, it seems prudent for basketball players to include muscle actions and complex movements that closely mimic the demands of their sport. Anatomical views of the sagittal, frontal, and transverse planes of the human body are shown in Figure 4.5. An understanding of basic biomechanics and exercise movements that take place in these planes will help EP-Cs select exercises that are consistent with specific movement patterns, muscle actions, and joint angles that need to be trained.

It is also important that the exercises and joint ranges of motion in the training program are consistent with the demands of the target activity. Hence, the specificity principle also applies to the design of resistance training programs for individuals who want to enhance their abilities to perform activities of daily life such as stair climbing and yard work, which require multiple-joint and multiplanar movements. Observations of a sport or activity (with or without video analysis) can provide the EP-Cs with information regarding the relevant movements and appropriate ranges of motion that are particularly important to train. The potential benefits of movement-specific resistance training are highlighted by the growing popularity of medicine balls, stability balls, kettlebells, and other exercise devices that are often used to enhance rotational strength, muscle power, postural control, and agility.

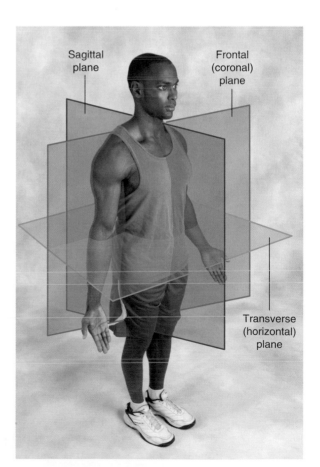

FIGURE 4.5. Anatomical planes of the human body. (From Bushman B, editor. *ACSM's Resources for the Personal Trainer.* 4th ed. Baltimore [MD]: Lippincott Williams & Wilkins; 2014. 592 p.)

Principle of Supervision

The principle of supervision states that the safety and efficacy of exercise programs are maximized when qualified fitness professionals supervise activities while providing instruction and encouragement (60,61). Not only does supervised training reduce the risk of injury, but clients who participate in supervised resistance training programs are likely to make greater gains in muscular fitness and performance than unsupervised training (17,26,53). Indeed, qualified supervision is a critical component of any resistance training program, particularly for beginners who need guidance and instruction.

Adults who participate in supervised resistance training programs tend to self-select higher training loads and, consequently, have higher levels of maximal strength (63). Because most men and women tend to self-select resistance training loads that are only 40%–56% of their 1-RM on a given exercise (20,23,28), they are likely training at an intensity that is suboptimal for muscle and strength development. Resistance training programs are most effective when they are designed and supervised by qualified fitness professionals who understand the PROCESS of exercise program design (21).

 ## Program Design Considerations

Because most adults are not meeting current muscle strengthening recommendations, tailored interventions and qualified supervision and instruction and are warranted (49,78). Resistance training programs should be based on a participant's health status, current fitness level, personal interests, and individual goals. By assessing the needs of each participant and applying the fundamental principles of training to the program design, safe and effective resistance training programs can be developed for each individual. Of note, the health status of each participant should be assessed before participating in a resistance training program because it is important to identify "at-risk" individuals who may need medical clearance and a modification of their exercise prescription (2).

An important factor to consider when designing resistance training programs is the participant's current fitness status or previous experience resistance training. Those who have the least experience resistance training tend to have a greater capacity for improvement compared with those who have been resistance training for several years. Although any reasonable resistance training program can be used to increase the muscle strength of untrained individuals, more advanced programs are needed to produce desirable adaptations in trained individuals. This is based on the observation that the potential for adaptation gradually decreases as training experience increases. Thus, as individuals gain experience with resistance training, more complex programs are needed to make continual gains in muscular fitness (14,61).

Types of Resistance Training

Different types of resistance training have proven to be effective for enhancing muscular fitness (9,22,61). Although each type of resistance exercise has advantages and disadvantages, there are several important factors to consider when selecting one type of training over another or including multiple types within a given training program. The most common types of resistance training include dynamic constant external resistance (DCER) training, variable resistance training, isokinetics, and plyometrics.

Dynamic Constant External Resistance Training

DCER training is the most common method of resistance training for enhancing muscular fitness. DCER describes a type of training in which the weight lifted does not change during the lifting (concentric) and lowering (eccentric) phase of an exercise. Although the term *isotonic* was traditionally used to describe this type of training, this term literally means constant (*iso*)tension (*tonic*).

Because tension exerted by a muscle as it shortens varies with the mechanical advantage of the joint and the length of the muscle fibers at a particular joint angle, the term *isotonic* does not accurately describe this method of resistance exercise.

Different types of training equipment, including free weights (*e.g.*, barbells and dumbbells) and weight machines, and endless combinations of sets and repetitions can be used for DCER training. Weight machines generally limit the user to fixed planes of motion. However, they are easy to use and are ideal for isolating muscle groups. Free weights are less expensive and can be used for a wide variety of different exercises that require greater proprioception, balance, and coordination. In addition to improving health and fitness, DCER training is commonly used to enhance motor performance skills and sports performance. For example, weightlifting exercises such as the power clean (Fig. 4.6) and snatch are recognized as some of the most effective exercises for increasing muscle power because they require explosive movements and a more complex neural activation pattern than do traditional strength-building exercises such as the chest press or leg extension (15).

During DCER training, the weight lifted does not change throughout the ROM. Because muscle tension can vary significantly when a DCER exercise is performed, the heaviest weight that can be lifted throughout a full ROM is limited by the strength of a muscle at the weakest joint angle. As a result, DCER exercise provides enough resistance in some parts of the movement range but not enough resistance in others. For example, during the barbell bench press exercise, more weight can be lifted during the last part of the exercise than in the first part of the movement when the barbell is being pressed off the chest.

In an attempt to overcome this limitation, mechanical devices that operate through a lever arm or cam have been designed to vary the resistance throughout the exercise's ROM. These devices are known as variable resistance machines and theoretically force the muscle to contract maximally throughout the ROM by varying the resistance to match the exercise strength curve. These machines can be used to train all the major muscle groups, and by automatically changing the resistive force throughout the movement range, they provide proportionally less resistance in weaker segments of the movement and more resistance in stronger segments of the movement. Like all weight

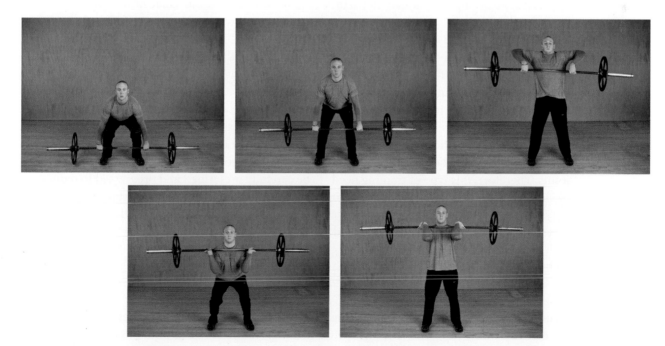

FIGURE 4.6. The clean: beginning, first pull, transition, second pull, and catch positions. (From Ratamess N. *ACSM's Foundations of Strength Training and Conditioning*. Baltimore [MD]: Lippincott Williams & Wilkins; 2012:356.)

machines, variable resistance machines provide a specific movement path that makes the exercise easier to perform, compared with free weight exercises, which require balance, coordination, and the involvement of stabilizing muscle groups.

Isokinetics

Isokinetic training involves dynamic muscular actions that are performed at a constant angular limb velocity. This type of training requires specialized equipment, and most isokinetic devices are designed to train only single-joint movements. Isokinetic machines generally are not used in fitness centers, but this type of training is used by physical therapists and certified athletic trainers for injury rehabilitation. Unlike other types of resistance training, the speed of movement — rather than the resistance — is controlled during isokinetic training. If the purpose of the exercise program is to increase strength at higher velocities (*e.g.*, for enhanced sports performance), performing high-speed isokinetic training appears prudent. Because data from isokinetic studies support velocity specificity (22,61), the best approach may be to perform isokinetic training at slow, intermediate, and fast velocities to develop increased strength and power at different movement speeds.

Plyometric Training

Plyometric training refers to a specialized method of conditioning designed to enhance neuromuscular performance (12). Unlike traditional strength-building exercises such as the bench press and squat, plyometric training is characterized by quick, powerful movements that involve a rapid stretch of a muscle (eccentric muscle action) immediately followed by a rapid shortening of the same muscle (concentric muscle action). This type of muscle action provides a physiological advantage because the muscle force generated during the concentric muscle action is potentiated by the preceding eccentric muscle action (69). Although both concentric and eccentric muscle actions are important for plyometric training, the amount of time it takes to change direction from the eccentric to the concentric phase of the movement is a critical factor in plyometric training. This period is called the amortization phase, which should be as short as possible (<0.1 s) to maximize training adaptations. Individuals can achieve significant gains in muscular fitness from a training program that includes plyometrics provided the exercises are sensibly progressed and performed with proper technique (12).

Exercises that involve jumping, skipping, hopping, and other explosive movements with medicine balls can be considered a type of plyometric training. Although plyometric exercises are often associated with high-intensity drills such as depth jumps (*i.e.*, jumping from a box to the ground and then immediately jumping upward; Fig. 4.7), less intense activities such as double leg hops and jumping jacks can also be considered a type of plyometric exercise because every time the feet hit the ground, the quadriceps go through a stretch-shortening cycle. Of practical importance, plyometric exercises can place a great amount of stress on the involved muscles, connective tissues, and joints. Therefore, this type of training needs to be carefully prescribed and progressed to reduce the likelihood of musculoskeletal injury. The importance of starting with basic movements (*e.g.*, double leg jump and freeze) or establishing an adequate baseline of strength before participating in a plyometric program should not be overlooked by the EP-C.

It is reasonable for individuals to begin plyometric training with one or two sets of six to eight repetitions of lower intensity drills and gradually progress to several sets of higher intensity exercises over time as technical competence improves. Plyometrics are not a stand-alone fitness program and should be incorporated into a training session that includes other types of resistance training. To optimize training adaptations, performance of more than 40 repetitions per session appears to be the most beneficial plyometric training volume (69). For example, a trained individual with experience performing plyometric exercises could perform two sets of six repetitions on four different lower body movements. Other considerations for plyometric training include proper footwear and a shock-absorbing landing surface (*e.g.*, suspended floor or grass playing field).

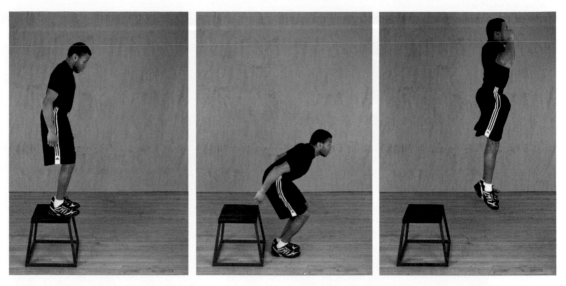

FIGURE 4.7. Depth jump. (From Ratamess N. *ACSM's Foundations of Strength Training and Conditioning.* Baltimore [MD]: Lippincott Williams & Wilkins; 2012:356.)

Modes of Resistance Training

Almost any mode of resistance training can be used to enhance muscular fitness provided that the fundamental principles of training are adhered to and the program is sensibly progressed over time. Some types of equipment are relatively easy to use, whereas others require balance, coordination, and high levels of skill. A decision to use a certain mode of resistance training should be based on an individual's health status, training experience, and personal goals. The major modes of resistance training are weight machines, free weights, body weight exercises, and a broadly defined category of balls, bands, and elastic tubing.

Single-joint exercises such as the biceps curl target a specific muscle group and require less skill to perform, whereas multiple-joint exercises such as the barbell squat involve more than one joint or major muscle group and require more balance and coordination. Although both single- and multiple-joint exercises are effective for enhancing muscular fitness, multiple-joint exercises are generally considered more effective for increasing muscle strength because they involve a greater amount of muscle mass and therefore enable a heavier weight to be lifted (36,61). Multiple-joint exercises have also been shown to have the greatest acute metabolic and anabolic (*e.g.*, testosterone and growth hormone) hormonal response, which could have a favorable impact on the design of resistance training programs targeting improvements in muscle size and body composition (44).

Weight machines are designed to train all the major muscle groups and can be found in most fitness centers. Both single-joint (*e.g.*, leg extension) and multiple-joint (*e.g.*, leg press) exercises can be performed on weight machines, which are relatively easy to use because the exercise motion is controlled by the machine and typically occurs in only one anatomical plane. This may be particularly important to consider when designing resistance training programs for sedentary or inexperienced individuals. Weight machines are designed to fit the average male or female, although a seat pad or back pad can be used to adjust the body position of individuals who are smaller or larger. Two examples of multiple-joint exercises performed on weight machines are shown in Figures 4.8 (lat pull-down) and 4.9 (pull-up).

Free weights are also popular in fitness centers and come in a variety of shapes and sizes. Although it typically takes longer to learn proper exercise technique when using free weights compared with weight machines, there are several advantages of free weight training. For example, free weights offer a greater variety of exercises than weight machines because they can be moved in many different directions. Another important benefit of using free weights is that they require the use of additional stabilizing and assisting muscles to hold the correct body position during an

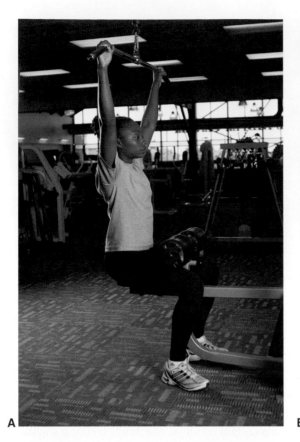
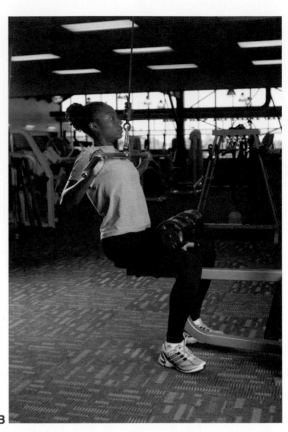

FIGURE 4.8. Pull-down: starting position **(A)** and pull-down position **(B)**.

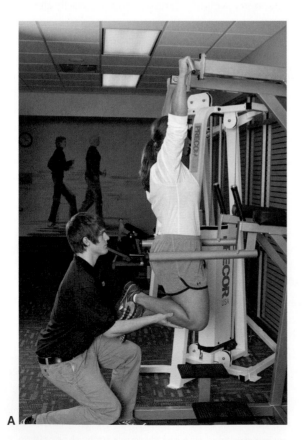
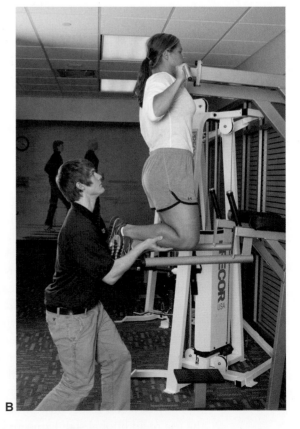

FIGURE 4.9. Assisted lat pull-up: starting position **(A)** and pull-up position **(B)**.

exercise. Instruction on proper exercise technique, sensible starting weights, and the appropriate use of a spotter are needed to reduce the risk of an accident (39,59).

Total body free weight exercises, including modified cleans, pulls, and presses, can be incorporated into a training program provided that qualified instruction is available and safety measures are in place (*e.g.*, a safe lifting environment and appropriate loads) (32,61). However, the EP-C should be aware of the extra time it takes to teach advanced free weight exercises and should be knowledgeable of the progression from basic exercises (*e.g.*, front squat) to skill-transfer exercises (*e.g.*, overhead squat), and finally to weightlifting movements (*e.g.*, clean and jerk).

Visit thePoint to watch videos 4.3 through 4.5, which demonstrate a curl-up, a labile push-up, and a pull-up/chin-up, respectively.

Body weight exercises such as push-ups and curl-ups are some of the oldest modes of resistance training. Obviously, a major advantage of body weight training is that equipment is not needed and a variety of exercises can be performed. Conversely, a limitation of body weight training is the difficulty in adjusting the body weight to the individual's strength level. Sedentary or overweight participants may not be strong enough to perform even one repetition of a body weight exercise. In such cases, using exercise machines and training devices that allow individuals to perform body weight exercises such as pull-ups and dips by using a predetermined percentage of their body weight is desirable. This type of equipment provide an opportunity for participants of all abilities to incorporate body weight exercises into their resistance training program and feel good about their accomplishments.

Stability balls, medicine balls, and elastic tubing are effective training modes that are used by fitness professionals and therapists. Stability balls are lightweight, inflatable balls (about 45–75 cm in diameter) that add the elements of balance and coordination to any exercise while targeting selected muscle groups. Medicine balls come in different shapes and sizes (about 1–>10 kg) and are an effective alternative to free weights and weight machines; Figure 4.10 shows an underhand medicine ball toss;

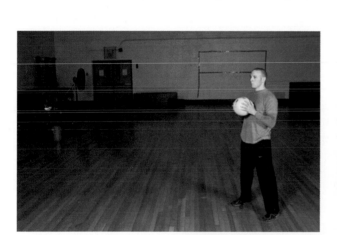
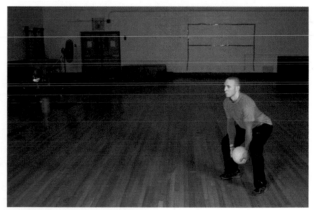
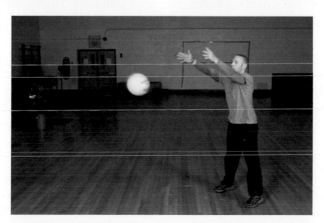

FIGURE 4.10. Underhand medicine ball toss. (From Ratamess N. *ACSM's Foundations of Strength Training and Conditioning.* Baltimore [MD]: Lippincott Williams & Wilkins; 2012:363.)

Table 4.1	Comparison of Different Modes of Resistance Training			
	Weight Machines	**Free Weights**	**Body Weight**	**Balls and Cords**[a]
Cost	High	Low	None	Very low
Portability	Limited	Variable	Excellent	Excellent
Ease of use	Excellent	Variable	Variable	Variable
Muscle isolation	Excellent	Variable	Variable	Variable
Functionality	Limited	Excellent	Excellent	Excellent
Exercise variety	Limited	Excellent	Excellent	Excellent
Space requirements	High	Variable	Low	Low

[a]Medicine balls, stability balls, and elastic cords.

others include the side-to-side toss, chest pass, overhead throw, back throw, vertical throw, slams, pullover pass, side toss, and front rotation throw. Resistance training with an elastic rubber cord involves performing an exercise against the force required to stretch the cord and then returning it to its unstretched state. Stability balls, medicine balls, and elastic tubing are not only relatively inexpensive but are also being used more and more commonly as tools to enhance strength, muscular endurance, and power. In addition, exercises performed with these devices can be proprioceptively challenging, which carries added benefit. Table 4.1 summarizes the advantages and disadvantages of different modes of resistance training.

Safety Concerns

Although all resistance training activities have some degree of medical risk, the chance of injury can be reduced by following established training guidelines and safety procedures. In addition, due to interindividual variability in the response to resistance training, an EP-C needs to monitor the ability of all participants to tolerate the stress of strength and conditioning programs. Without proper supervision and instruction, injuries that require medical attention can happen.

In an evaluation of resistance training–related injuries presenting to emergency departments in the United States, researchers reported that men suffered more trunk injuries than women, whereas women had more accidental injuries compared with men (59). Figure 4.11 illustrates the percentage of resistance training–related injuries at each body part for men and women between the ages of 14 and 30 years who presented to US emergency departments.

Although there have not been any prospective trials that have focused specifically on measures to prevent resistance training–related injuries, an EP-C who understands resistance training guidelines and acknowledges individual differences should provide supervision and instruction. This is particularly important for beginners who need to receive instruction on proper exercise technique as well as basic education on resistance training procedures (*e.g.*, weight room etiquette, appropriate spotting procedures, and the proper storage of equipment). All exercises should be performed in a controlled manner through the full ROM of the joint using proper breathing techniques (*i.e.*, exhalation during the concentric phase and inhalation during the eccentric phase) avoiding the Valsalva maneuver. Individuals with orthopedic injuries or pain should use a symptom-limited ROM when performing selected resistance exercises. Modifiable risk factors associated with resistance training injuries that can be reduced or eliminated with qualified supervision and instruction are outlined in Table 4.2.

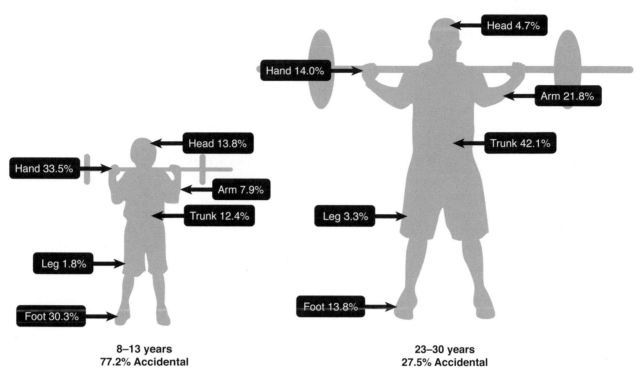

FIGURE 4.11. Resistance training–related injuries presenting to US emergency rooms.

EP-Cs should be able to correctly perform the exercises they prescribe and should be able to modify exercise form and technique if necessary. When working in a fitness facility, the staff should be attentive and should try to position themselves with a clear view of the training center so that they can have quick access to individuals who need assistance. The resistance training area should be well lit and large enough to handle the number of individuals exercising in the facility at any given time. The facility should be clean, and the equipment should be well maintained. In addition, EP-Cs are responsible for enforcing safety rules (*e.g.*, proper footwear and safe storage of weights) and ensuring that individuals are training effectively.

Table 4.2	Modifiable Risk Factors Associated with Resistance Training Injuries that Can Be Reduced (or Eliminated) with Qualified Supervision and Instruction
Risk Factor	**Modification by Qualified EP-C**
Health-related concern	Communicate with treating clinician and modify program
Unsafe exercise environment	Adequate training space and proper equipment layout
Improper use of equipment	Clear instruction on exercise technique and training
Excessive load and volume	Gradual progression of training program
Poor trunk control	Targeted resistance exercises for core musculature
Muscle imbalances	Include agonist and antagonist exercises for selected muscle groups
Inadequate recuperation	Modify training program and consider lifestyle factors such as proper nutrition and adequate sleep

Resistance Training Program Variables

Despite various claims about the best resistance training program, there is not one *optimal* combination of sets, repetitions, and exercises that will promote long-term adaptations in muscular fitness for all individuals. Rather, many program variables need to be systematically altered over time to achieve desirable outcomes (22,62). Clearly, resistance training programs need to be individualized and based on one's health history, training experience, and personal goals.

The program variables that should be considered when designing a resistance training program include (a) choice of exercise, (b) order of exercise, (c) resistance used, (d) training volume (total number of sets and repetitions), (e) rest intervals between sets and exercises, (f) repetition velocity, and (g) training frequency (22). By varying one or more of these program variables, a limitless number of resistance training programs can be designed. But because individuals will respond differently to the same resistance training program, sound decisions must be made on the basis of an understanding of resistance exercise, individual needs, and personal goals. Table 4.3 summarizes ACSM's FITT principles for resistance training for apparently healthy adults (2).

Choice of Exercise

A limitless number of exercises can be used to enhance muscular fitness. It is important to select exercises that are appropriate for an individual's exercise technique experience and training goals. Also, the choice of exercises should promote muscle balance across joints and between opposing

Table 4.3	Summary of ACSM's FITT Guidelines for Resistance Training
Frequency	Resistance train 2–3 nonconsecutive days per week.
Intensity	Sedentary persons should start resistance training with 40%–50% 1-RM. Intermediate exercisers should use ~60%–80% 1-RM to improve muscular strength. Experienced exercisers can use heavier loads (≥80% 1-RM) to improve muscular strength. Lighter loads (<50% 1-RM) and shorter rest periods between sets should be used to improve local muscular endurance.
Time	No specific resistance training duration has been identified.
Type	Include multiple-joint exercises for the major muscle groups. Target agonist and antagonist muscle groups to avoid muscle imbalances. Different types of equipment and body weight exercises can be used.
Repetitions	8–12 repetitions are recommended to improve muscular strength in most adults. 10–15 repetitions are recommended for improving strength in deconditioned and older individuals. 15–20 repetitions are recommended to improve muscular endurance.
Sets	2–4 sets are recommended to improve strength and power in most adults. A single set can be effective for novices and older individuals.
Pattern	Rest intervals of 2–3 min between each set are effective. A recovery period of 48 h between sessions for a muscle group is recommended.
Progression	A gradual progression of greater resistance, repetitions, and frequency is recommended.

Adapted with permission from American College of Sports Medicine. *ACSM's Guidelines for Exercise Testing and Prescription.* 10th ed. Philadelphia (PA): Wolters Kluwer; 2018.

Visit thePoint to watch videos 4.6 through 4.10, which demonstrate a wood chop, squats, lunges, and a dumbbell bench press.

Visit thePoint to watch videos 4.11 and 4.12, which demonstrate plank and a side bridge, respectively.

muscle groups (*i.e.*, agonists and antagonists) such as the quadriceps and hamstrings or the chest and upper back. Exercises generally can be classified as single-joint (*i.e.*, body-part specific) or multiple-joint (*i.e.*, structural). Although single-joint exercises that isolate muscle groups can be incorporated into a resistance training program, it is important to eventually include multiple-joint exercises to promote the coordinated use of multiple-joint movements (2).

Exercises can also be classified as closed kinetic chain or open kinetic chain. Closed kinetic chain exercises are those in which the distal joint segment is stationary (*e.g.*, squat), whereas open chain exercises are those in which the terminal joint is free to move (*e.g.*, leg extension). Closed kinetic chain exercises more closely mimic everyday activities and include more functional movement patterns (61).

Another important issue regarding the choice of exercise is the inclusion of exercises for the lumbopelvic hip complex, which is commonly referred to as the core musculature (1). Strengthening the abdominals, hip, and low back enhances body control and may also reduce the risk of injury during athletic events and activities of daily life (7,8,30). If individuals lack proper postural control during the performance of a resistance exercise, they will not be able to transfer energy efficiently to the distal segments and will be more susceptible to an injury. Thus, prehabilitation exercises for the core musculature should be included in resistance training programs. That is, exercises that may be prescribed for the rehabilitation of an injury should be prescribed beforehand as a preventive health measure.

Exercises such as planks and bridges are effective for core conditioning. Multidirectional exercises that involve rotational movements and diagonal patterns performed with one's own body weight or a medicine ball can also be effective in strengthening the core musculature. In addition, research has indicated that the progressive introduction of greater instability during resistance training with devices such as stability balls might have application for reducing lower back pain, increasing joint stability, and enhancing core muscle activation (7). Depending on the needs and goals of the individual, other prehabilitation exercises (*e.g.*, internal and external rotation for the rotator cuff musculature) can be incorporated into the training session. For example, researchers reported that 4–8 weeks of prehabilitation resistance training before total knee arthroplasty improved strength and function in older adults with severe osteoarthritis (74).

Order of Exercise

There are many ways to arrange the sequence of exercises in a training session. Traditionally, beginners perform total body workouts that involve multiple exercises stressing all major muscle groups each session. In this type of workout, large muscle group exercises should be performed before smaller muscle group exercises and multiple-joint exercises should be performed before single-joint exercises. Following this exercise order will allow heavier weights to be used on the multiple-joint exercises because fatigue will be less of a factor. It is also helpful to perform more challenging exercises earlier in the workout when the neuromuscular system is less fatigued. Thus, power exercises such as plyometrics and weightlifting movements should be performed before more traditional strength exercises such as a back squat or bench so that an individual can train for maximal power without undue fatigue (61).

Individuals with resistance training experience may modify their training programs by performing a split routine program. For example, they could perform upper body exercises only during one workout and lower body exercises only during the following workout. Although different training programs are effective for enhancing muscular strength and performance, individual goals, time available for training, and personal preference should determine the exercise program that is used.

Resistance Load Used

One of the most important variables in the design of a resistance training program is the amount of resistance used for an exercise. Gains in muscular fitness are influenced by the amount of weight lifted, which is highly dependent on other program variables such as exercise order, training volume, repetition speed, and rest interval length (22). In an investigation that examined changes in muscle size and muscle composition in response to resistance exercise with light and heavy loads, the adaptive changes in muscle were significantly smaller after nonexhaustive light load training than after heavy-load training (11). These data as well as other reports demonstrate that adaptations to resistance training are linked to the intensity of the training program (36,70,73). Thus, to maximize gains in muscle strength and performance, it is recommended that training sets be performed to muscle fatigue but not to exhaustion using the appropriate resistance.

The use of RM loads is a relatively simple method to prescribe resistance training intensity. Research studies suggest that RM loads of 6 or less have the greatest effect on developing muscle strength, whereas RM loads of 20 or more have the greatest effect on developing local muscular endurance (22). Although novices can make significant gains in muscle strength with lighter loads, individuals with resistance training experience need to train periodically with heavier loads (62).

Accordingly, repetitions ranging between 8 and 12 (~60%–80% 1-RM) are commonly used to enhance muscular fitness in novice to intermediate exercises (2). Experienced exercisers may train at intensities greater than 80% 1-RM to achieve the desired gains in muscle strength (2). Using lighter weights (*e.g.*, <50% 1-RM; 15–20 repetitions) will have less effect on muscular strength but more effect on muscular endurance. Because each repetition zone (*e.g.*, 3–6, 8–12, or 15–20) has its advantages, the best approach may be to systematically vary the resistance used to avoid training plateaus and optimize training adaptations (62). Furthermore, consistent training at high intensities increases the risk of overtraining (61).

A percentage of an individual's 1-RM can also be used to determine the resistance training intensity. If the 1-RM on the leg press exercise is 100 kg, a training intensity of 60% would be 60 kg. It is reasonable for beginners or deconditioned individuals to use a resistance training intensity of approximately 40%–50% 1-RM for 10–15 repetitions because they are mostly improving motor performance at this stage, and proper exercise technique is of paramount importance. As individuals get stronger and gain training experience, heavier resistances will be needed to make continual gains in muscular strength and performance. Meta-analytical procedures have found that 60% of 1-RM and 80% of 1-RM produced the largest strength increases in untrained and training adults, respectively (67). Obviously, this method of prescribing resistance exercise requires the frequent evaluation of the 1-RM. In many cases, this is not realistic because of the time required to perform 1-RM testing correctly on different exercises. Furthermore, maximal resistance testing for small muscle group assistance exercises is not typically performed.

The EP-Cs should be knowledgeable about the relationship between the percentage of the 1-RM and the number of repetitions that can be performed. In general, most individuals can perform about 10 repetitions using 75% of their 1-RM. However, the number of repetitions that can be performed at a given percentage of the 1-RM varies with the amount of muscle mass required to perform the exercise. For example, research has shown that at a given percentage of the 1-RM, adults can perform more repetitions on a large muscle group exercise such as the back squat compared with a smaller muscle group exercise such as the arm curl (71). Therefore, prescribing a resistance training intensity of 70% of 1-RM on all exercises warrants additional consideration because at 70% of 1-RM, an individual may be able to perform 20 or more repetitions on a large muscle group exercise, which may not be ideal for enhancing muscular strength (71). If a percentage of the 1-RM is used for prescribing resistance exercises, the prescribed percentage of the 1-RM for each exercise may need to be changed to maintain a desired training range (*e.g.*, 8- to 10-RM).

Training Volume

The number of exercises performed per session, the repetitions performed per set, and the number of sets performed per exercise all influence the training volume (22). The ACSM recommends that apparently healthy adults should train each muscle group for two to four sets to achieve muscular fitness goals (2). For example, the chest muscles can be trained with four sets of the bench press or two sets of the bench press and two sets of dumbbell flys. It is important to remember that every training session does not need to be characterized by the same number of sets, repetitions, and exercises.

Although untrained individuals can respond favorably to single set training, meta-analytical data have shown that multiple set training is more effective than single set training for strength enhancement in untrained and in trained populations (10,45,66). However, program variation characterized by periods of low-volume training can provide needed recovery for individuals who have been participating in a high-volume training program for a prolonged period. Because recovery is an integral part of any training program, high-volume training needs to be balanced with low-volume sessions to facilitate recovery. In addition, low-volume sessions provide a learning opportunity for the EP-C to reinforce proper exercise technique on specific movement patterns.

Rest Intervals between Sets

The length of the rest period between sets will influence energy recovery and the training adaptations that take place (64,81). For example, if the primary goal of the program is to maximize gains in muscular strength, heavier weights and longer rest intervals (*e.g.*, 2–3 min) are required, whereas if the goal is muscular endurance, lighter weights and shorter rest periods (*e.g.*, <1 min) are required. As previously noted with other program variables, the same rest interval does not need to be used for all exercises. In addition, fatigue resulting from a previous exercise should be considered when prescribing the rest interval if maximal gains in muscular strength are desired.

Repetition Velocity

The velocity or cadence at which a resistance exercise is performed can affect the adaptations to a training program because gains in muscular fitness are specific to the training velocity. For example, fast-velocity plyometric training or weightlifting exercises are more likely to enhance speed and power than slower velocity resistance exercise on a weight machine (12,15). In any case, beginners need to learn how to perform each exercise correctly and develop an adequate level of strength before optimal gains in power performance are realized. As individuals improve muscular strength and gain experience performing higher velocity movements, heavier loads or more complex exercises may be used to optimize training adaptations. It is likely that the performance of different training velocities and the integration of numerous training techniques may provide the most effective training stimulus (22,61).

Training Frequency

A resistance training frequency of two to three times per week on nonconsecutive days is recommended for beginners (2). A resistance training frequency of once per week may maintain muscle strength as long as the resistance training intensity is adequate, but more frequent training sessions are needed to optimize adaptations (2). A training frequency of two to three times per week on nonconsecutive days will allow for adequate recovery between sessions (48–72 h) and has proven to be effective for enhancing muscular fitness (25). However, trained individuals who perform more advanced programs may need a longer period of recovery time between sessions. Factors such as the training volume, training intensity, exercise selection, nutritional intake, and sleep habits may influence one's ability to recover from and adapt to the training program. For example, trained individuals who perform a split routine may resistance train four times a week, but they train each muscle group only twice a week. Although an increase in training experience does not necessitate an increase in training frequency, a higher training frequency does allow for greater specialization characterized by more exercises and a higher weekly training volume.

Periodization

Periodization is a concept that refers to the systematic variation in training program design. Because it is impossible to continually improve at the same rate over long-term training, properly varying the training variables can limit training plateaus, maximize performance gains, and reduce the likelihood of overtraining (9). The underlying concept of periodization is based on Selye's general adaptation syndrome, which proposes that after a certain period, adaptations to a new stimulus will no longer take place unless the stimulus is altered (43,62). In essence, periodization is a process whereby an EP-C regularly changes the training stimulus to keep it effective. Although the concept of periodization has been part of resistance training program design for many years, our understanding of the benefits of periodized training programs compared with nonperiodized programs continues to be explored in the literature (34,35).

The concept of periodization is not just for elite athletes but also for individuals with different levels of training experience who want to enhance their health and fitness. By periodically varying program variables such as the choice of exercise, training resistance, number of sets, rest periods between sets, or any combination of these, long-term performance gains will be optimized and the risk of "overuse" injuries may be reduced (9). Moreover, it is reasonable to suggest that individuals who participate in well-designed programs and continue to improve their health and fitness may be more likely to adhere to an exercise program for the long term.

For example, if a trained individual's lower body routine typically consists of the leg press, leg extension, and leg curl exercises, performing the back squat and dumbbell lunge exercises on alternate workout days will likely increase the effectiveness of the training program and reduce the likelihood of staleness and boredom. Furthermore, varying the training weights, number of sets, and/or rest interval between sets can help prevent training plateaus, which are not uncommon among fitness enthusiasts. Many times, a strength plateau can be avoided by periodically varying the exercises or varying the training intensity and training volume to allow for ample recover. In the long term, program variation with adequate recovery will allow an individual to make even greater gains because the body will be challenged to adapt to even greater demands (62).

The general concept of periodization is to prioritize training goals and then develop a long-term plan that varies throughout the year (62). In general, the year is divided into specific training cycles (*e.g.*, a macrocycle, a mesocycle, and a microcycle), with each cycle having a specific goal (*e.g.*, hypertrophy, strength, or power). One model of periodization is referred to as a linear model because the volume and intensity of training gradually change over time (61). For example, at the start of a macrocycle, the training volume may be high and the training intensity may be low. As the year progresses, the volume is decreased as the intensity of training increases. Although this type of training originally was designed for athletes who attempted to peak for a specific competition, it can be modified by an EP-C for enhancing health and fitness. For example, individuals who routinely perform the same combination of sets and repetitions on all exercises will benefit from gradually increasing the weight and decreasing the number of repetitions as strength improves.

A second model of periodization is referred to as an undulating (nonlinear) model because of the daily fluctuations in training volume and intensity (61). For example, on the major exercises, a trained individual may perform two or three sets with 8- to 10-RM loads on Monday, three or four sets with 4- to 6-RM loads on Wednesday, and one or two sets with 12- to 15-RM loads on Friday. Whereas the heavy training days will maximally activate the trained musculature, selected muscle fibers will not be maximally taxed on light and moderate training days. By alternating training volume and intensity, the participant can minimize the risk of overtraining and maximize the potential for strength and power enhancement (9,62).

General Recommendations

Resistance training has the potential to offer unique benefits to men and women of all ages and abilities. Regular participation in a progressive resistance training program can enhance muscular fitness and improve an individual's health status. However, the design of resistance training programs can be complex, and program variables including the choice of exercise, order of exercise, training intensity, training volume, repetition velocity, and rest period between sets and exercises need to be systematically varied over time to optimize gains in muscle fitness and performance. In addition, resistance training programs need to be individualized and consistent with personal goals to maximize outcomes and exercise adherence. Ultimately, knowledge of muscle structure and function along with an understanding of resistance training principles will determine the effectiveness of the training program.

In addition to understanding the science of resistance exercise, EP-Cs need to appreciate the art of prescribing exercise. Resistance training programs need to be individualized and consistent with personal needs, goals, and abilities. A key factor for safe and effective resistance training is proper program design that includes exercise instruction, sensible progression, and periodic evaluations to assess progress toward training goals. This requires effective leadership, realistic goal setting, and a solid understanding of training-induced adaptations that take place in both beginners and experienced exercisers.

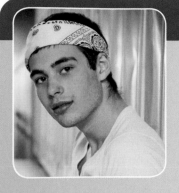

The Case of Jeremy

Submitted by **Benjamin Gleason, ACSM-HFS, NSCA-CSCS, US Air Force, Niceville, FL**
Jeremy is a former high school athlete, now 23 years old and apparently healthy.

Narrative

Jeremy's body composition is within normal ranges, as are his BP and heart rate. He cites no family history of disease. He works out in the local gym for four sessions per week and spends 1 to 2 hours per session. This has been his primary mode of regular exercise since high school, and he plays recreational sports in the local city league in his free time. He wishes to continue his current exercise pattern but has come to see you to discuss some issues he's been having lately. He casually complains to you during his fitness screening that he suffers mild knee pain and low back pain during and after his workouts. On observing him in a gym session, you notice that when he performs the squat, he rounds his back and places most of his weight on the balls of his feet. He also rounds his back slightly when he performs the deadlift and hyperextends his spine at the end of the lift. During standing overhead pressing movements, he leans back to force out a few extra reps. He has been suffering from mild pain in his knees and back for some time now, and says his high school sports coach used to tell him "No pain, no gain!" when he brought it up from time to time several years ago. He asks you if this pain is normal and says he doesn't want to sound like a wimp to the other guys in the gym. His typical weight program involves three or four sets of 6 to 12 repetitions on every exercise, and he performs at least three exercises for each body part in his program. Mondays he does chest and triceps, Tuesday he does legs, Thursday he does back and biceps, and Friday he does shoulders. He includes some light cardio on a stationary bike or a treadmill after most workouts.

Analysis

Jeremy's workout program is a typical one used by many bodybuilders, but his attention to detail on form leaves much to be desired. Apparently, he was not taught the proper exercise technique by his coach in high school or the fitness center staff, and Jeremy has developed some movement pattern disorders. To reduce the likelihood of knee and back pain during the squat and deadlift, he should keep the majority of his bodyweight on his heels as he descends and rises throughout the ROM and keep his back in the neutral position. It will take time to break old habits, and Jeremy will need to use a lighter load to learn proper technique on these free weight exercises. Jeremy should visit a medical professional to address any possible injuries beyond the minor pain he experiences during exercise. His habits of hyperextending his back at the top of the deadlift and arching his back to get more reps on overhead presses are likely contributors to his back pain and serve no practical advantage in resistance training as they are high-risk methods. A deadlift is complete when the lifter returns to the standing position only and not beyond (hyperextension). The posterior chain musculature (low back, gluteals, hamstrings) requires considerable attention in an effective training program, and the correct initiation of movement is imperative to reduce the risk of injury and produce the desired performance effects.

QUESTIONS

- Discuss Jeremy's tendency to round his back during deadlifts and how it may be causing his low back pain.
- Why is knee pain common in individuals who squat in an anterior-dominant manner?
- Provide at least three exercises to address Jeremy's apparent posterior chain deficiency.
- Suggest two core stability exercises that may help Jeremy hold spinal stability better.

References

1. Bird S, Barrington-Higgs S. Exploring the deadlift. *Strength Cond J.* 2010;32(2):46–51.
2. Chiu L. A teaching progression for squatting exercises. *Strength Cond J.* 2011;33(2):46–54.
3. Gamble P. An integrated approach to training core stability. *Strength Cond J.* 2007;29(1):58–68.
4. McGill S. *Low Back Disorders, Evidence-Based Prevention and Rehabilitation.* Champaign (IL): Human Kinetics; 2002. 295 p.

SUMMARY

In this chapter, the benefits and importance of muscular strength and endurance for health and fitness were described. An overview of the basic structure and function of the muscle was also provided. Fundamental principles relating to resistance training for health and fitness were reviewed. The primary variables of a resistance training program were described. The role of the EP-C in designing a resistance program for apparently healthy adults and individuals with controlled disease was discussed. Tools for developing an individualized resistance training program from assessment to implementation to evaluation were provided.

STUDY QUESTIONS

1. Describe the size principle of motor unit recruitment and explain its practical application to resistance exercise program design.
2. Discuss seven fundamental principles that influence the effectiveness of resistance training programs.
3. Compare and contrast three different modes of resistance training and discuss the advantages and disadvantages of each method.
4. List and describe program variables that should be considered when designing a resistance training program.
5. Design a resistance training program for an untrained healthy adult and include recommendations for participant safety, program progression, and exercise adherence.

REFERENCES

1. Akuthota V, Ferreiro A, Moore T, Fredericson M. Core stability exercise principles. *Curr Sports Med Rep.* 2008;7(1):39–44.

2. American College of Sports Medicine. *ACSM's Guidelines for Exercise Testing and Prescription.* 10th ed. Philadelphia (PA): Wolters Kluwer; 2018.

3. Aristizabal JC, Freidenreich DJ, Volk BM, et al. Effect of resistance training on resting metabolic rate and its estimation by a dual-energy x-ray absorptiometry metabolic map. *Eur J Clin Nutr.* 2015;69(7):831–6.

4. Artero EG, Lee DC, Lavie CJ, et al. Effects of muscular strength on cardiovascular risk factors and prognosis. *J Cardiopulm Rehabil Prev.* 2012;32(6):351–8.

5. Baechle T, Earle R. Learning how to manipulate training variables to maximize results. In: *Weight Training: Steps to Success.* 4th ed. Champaign (IL): Human Kinetics; 2011. p. 177–88.

6. Behm DG, Chaouachi A. A review of the acute effects of static and dynamic stretching on performance. *Eur J Appl Physiol.* 2011;111(11):2633–51.

7. Behm DG, Drinkwater EJ, Willardson JM, Cowley PM. The role of instability rehabilitation resistance training for the core musculature. *Strength Cond J.* 2011;33(3):72–81.

8. Bihdanna T, Hewett T, Reeves P, Goldberg B, Cholewicki J. Deficits in neuromuscular control of the trunk. *Am J Sports Med.* 2007;35(7):1123–30.

9. Bompa T, Haff G. *Periodization — Theory and Methodology of Training.* 5th ed. Champaign (IL): Human Kinetics; 2009. 424 p.

10. Borde R, Hortobágyi T, Granacher U. Dose-response relationships of resistance training in healthy old adults: a systematic review and meta-analysis. *Sports Med.* 2015;45(12):1693–720.

11. Campos GE, Luecke TJ, Wendeln HK, et al. Muscular adaptations in response to three different resistance-training regimens: specificity of repetition maximum training zones. *Eur J Appl Physiol.* 2002;88(1–2):50–60.

12. Chu D, Myer G. *Plyometrics.* Champaign (IL): Human Kinetics; 2013. 248 p.

13. Clarkson P. Exertional rhabdomyolysis and acute renal failure in marathon runners. *Sports Med.* 2007;37:361–3.

14. Conlon J, Newton R, Tufano J, et al. Periodization strategies in older adults: impact on physical function and health. *Med Sci Sports Exerc.* 2016;48(12):2426–36.

15. Cormie P, McGuigan MR, Newtown RU. Developing maximal neuromuscular power: part 2 — training considerations for improving maximal power production. *Sports Med.* 2011; 41(2):125–146.

16. Cornelissen V, Fagard R, Coeckelberghs E, Vanhees L. Impact of resistance training on blood pressure and other cardiovascular risk factors. *Hypertension.* 2011;58(5):950–8.

17. Coutts A, Murphy A, Dascombe B. Effect of direct supervision of a strength coach on measures of muscular strength and power in young rugby league players. *J Strength Cond Res.* 2004;18(2):316–23.

18. Csikszentmihalyi M, Abuhamdeh S, Nakamura J. Flow. In: Elliot A, Dweck CS, editors. *Handbook of Competence and Motivation.* New York (NY): Guilford Press; 2005. p. 598–698.

19. Dudley G, Tesch P, Miller B, Buchanan P. Importance of eccentric actions in performance adaptations to resistance training. *Aviat Space Envir Med.* 1991;62(6):543–50.

20. Elsangedy H, Krause M, Krinski K, Alves R, Hsin Nery Chao C, da Silva S. Is the self-selected resistance exercise intensity by older women consistent with the American College of Sports Medicine guidelines to improve muscular fitness? *J Strength Cond Res.* 2013;27(7):1877–84.

21. Faigenbaum A, McFarland J. Resistance training for kids: right from the start. *ACSM Health Fitness J.* 2016;20(5):16–22.

22. Fleck S, Kraemer W. *Designing Resistance Training Programs.* 4th ed. Champaign (IL): Human Kinetics; 2014. 520 p.

23. Focht BC. Perceived exertion and training load during self-selected and imposed-intensity resistance exercise in untrained women. *J Strength Cond Res.* 2007;21(1):183–7.

24. Gale C, Martyn C, Cooper C, Sayer A. Grip strength, body composition and mortality. *Int J Epidemiol.* 2007;36(1):228–35.

25. Garber C, Blissmer B, Deschenes M, et al. American College of Sports Medicine position stand. Quantity and quality of exercise for developing and maintaining cardiorespiratory, musculoskeletal, and neuromotor fitness in apparently healthy adults: guidance for prescribing exercise. *Med Sci Sports Exerc.* 2011;43(7):1334–59.

26. Gentil P, Bottaro M. Influence of supervision ratio on muscle adaptations to resistance training in nontrained subjects. *J Strength Cond Res.* 2010;24(3):639–43.

27. Gielen S, Laughlin MH, O'Conner C, Duncker DJ. Exercise training in patients with heart disease: review of beneficial effects and clinical recommendations. *Prog Cardiovasc Dis.* 2015;57(4):347–55.

28. Glass SC, Stanton DR. Self-selected resistance training intensity in novice weightlifters. *J Strength Cond Res.* 2004;18(2):324–7.

29. Gordon BA, Benson AC, Bird SR, Fraser SF. Resistance training improves metabolic health in type 2 diabetes: a systematic review. *Diabetes Res Clin Pract.* 2009;83(2):157–75.

30. Granacher U, Gollhofer A, Hortobágyi T, Kressig RW, Muehlbauer T. The importance of trunk muscle strength for balance, functional performance, and fall prevention in seniors: a systematic review. *Sports Med.* 2013;43(7):627–41.

31. Grøntved A, Pan A, Mekary RA, et al. Muscle-strengthening and conditioning activities and risk of type 2 diabetes: a prospective study in two cohorts of US women. *PLoS Med.* 2014;11(1):e1001587.

32. Haff G, Triplett T. *Essentials of Strength and Conditioning.* 4th ed. Champaign (IL): Human Kinetics; 2016. 752 p.

33. Hamlin M, Quigley B. Quadriceps concentric and eccentric exercise 2: differences in muscle strength, fatigue and EMG activity in eccentrically-exercised sore and non-sore muscles. *J Sci Med Sport.* 2001;4(1):104–15.

34. Harries SK, Lubans DR, Callister R. Systematic review and meta-analysis of linear and undulating periodized resistance training programs on muscular strength. *J Strength Cond Res.* 2015;29(4):1113–25.

35. Hartmann H, Wirth K, Keiner M, Mickel C, Sander A, Szilvas E. Short-term periodization models: effects on strength and speed-strength performance. *Sports Med.* 2015;45(10):1373–86.

36. Holm L, Reitelseder S, Pedersen T, et al. Changes in muscle size and MHC composition in response to resistance exercise with heavy and light loading intensity. *J Appl Physiol.* 2008;105(5):1454–61.

37. Jurca R, LaMonte M, Barlow C, Kampert J, Church T, Blair S. Association of muscular strength with incidence of metabolic syndrome in men. *Med Sci Sports Exerc*. 2005;37(11):1849–55.

38. Kamiya K, Masuda T, Tanaka S, et al. Quadriceps strength as a predictor of mortality in coronary artery disease. *Am J Med*. 2015;128(11):1212–9.

39. Kerr Z, Collins C, Comstock R. Epidemiology of weight training-related injuries presenting to United States emergency departments, 1990 to 2007. *Am J Sports Med*. 2010; 38(4):765–71.

40. Kim YH, Kim KI, Paik NJ, Kim KW, Jang HC, Lim JY. Muscle strength: a better index of low physical performance than muscle mass in older adults. *Geriatr Gerontol Int*. 2016;16(5):577–85.

41. Klimcakova E, Polak J, Moro C, et al. Dynamic strength training improves insulin sensitivity without altering plasma levels and gene expression of adipokines in subcutaneous adipose tissue in obese men. *J Clin Endocrinol Metab*. 2006;91(12): 5107–12.

42. Kohrt W, Bloomfield S, Little K, Nelson M, Yingling V. American College of Sports Medicine position stand: physical activity and bone health. *Med Sci Sports Exerc*. 2004;36(11):1985–96.

43. Kraemer WJ, Ratamess NA. Fundamentals of resistance training: progression and exercise prescription. *Med Sci Sports Exerc*. 2004;36(4):674–88.

44. Kraemer WJ, Ratamess NA. Hormonal responses and adaptations to resistance exercise and training. *Sports Med*. 2005; 35(4):339–61.

45. Krieger J. Single versus multiple sets of resistance exercise: a meta-regression. *J Strength Cond Res*. 2009;23(6):1890–901.

46. Kuroda Y, Sato Y, Ishizaka Y, Yamakado M, Yamaguchi N. Exercise motivation, self-efficacy, and enjoyment as indicators of adult exercise behavior among the transtheoretical model stages. *Glob Health Promot*. 2012;19(1):14–22.

47. Lemmer JT, Hurlbut DE, Martel GF, et al. Age and gender responses to strength training and detraining. *Med Sci Sports Exerc*. 2000;32(8):1505–12.

48. Leong DP, Teo KK, Rangarajan S, et al. Prognostic value of grip strength: findings from the Prospective Urban-Rural Epidemiology (PURE) study. *Lancet*. 2015;386(9990): 266–73.

49. Loustalot F, Carlson SA, Kruger J, Buchner DM, Fulton JE. Muscle-strengthening activities and participation among adults in the United States. *Res Q Exerc Sport*. 2013;84(1):30–8.

50. Lyons T, McLester J, Arnett S, Thoma M. Specificity of training modalities on upper body one repetition maximum performance: free weights vs. hammer strength equipment. *J Strength Cond Res*. 2010;24(11):2984–8.

51. Mangione KK, Miller AH, Naughton IV. Cochrane review: improving physical function and performance with progressive resistance strength training in older adults. *Phys Ther*. 2010;90(12):1711–5.

52. Mason C, Brien S, Craig C, Gauvin L, Katzmarzyk P. Musculoskeletal fitness and weight gain in Canada. *Med Sci Sports Exerc*. 2007;39(1):38–43.

53. Mazzetti S, Kraemer W, Volek J, et al. The influence of direct supervision of resistance training on strength performance. *Med Sci Sports Exerc*. 2000;32(6):1175–84.

54. McPhate L, Simek EM, Haines TP, Hill KD, Finch CF, Day L. "Are your clients having fun?" The implications of respondents' preferences for the delivery of group exercise programs for falls prevention. *J Aging Phys Act*. 2016;24(1):129–38.

55. Molanorouzi K, Khoo S, Morris T. Motives for adult participation in physical activity: type of activity, age, and gender. *BMC Public Health*. 2015;15:66.

56. Morgan F, Battersby A, Weightman A, et al. Adherence to exercise referral schemes by participants — what do providers and commissioners need to know? A systematic review of barriers and facilitators. *BMC Public Health*. 2016;16:227.

57. Newton M, Morgan G, Sacco P, Chapman D, Nosaka K. Comparison of responses to strenuous eccentric exercise of the elbow flexors between resistance-trained and untrained men. *J Strength Cond Res*. 2008;22(2):597–607.

58. Pesce C. Shifting the focus from quantitative to qualitative exercise characteristics in exercise and cognition research. *J Sport Exerc Psych*. 2012;34(6):766–86.

59. Quatman C, Myer G, Khoury J, Wall E, Hewett T. Sex differences in "weightlifting" injuries presenting to United States emergency rooms. *J Strength Cond Res*. 2009;23(7):2061–7.

60. Ramírez-Campillo R, Martínez C, de La Fuente C, et al. High-speed resistance training in older women: the role of supervision. *J Aging Phys Act*. 2016;1–30. http://dx.doi.org /10.1123/japa.2015-0122

61. Ratamess NA. *ACSM's Foundations of Strength Training and Conditioning*. Philadelphia (PA): Lippincott Williams & Wilkins; 2012. 560 p.

62. Ratamess NA, Alvar B, Evetoch T, et al. Progression models in resistance training in healthy adults. *Med Sci Sports Exerc*. 2009;41(3):687–708.

63. Ratamess NA, Faigenbaum AD, Hoffman JR, Kang J. Self-selected resistance training intensity in healthy women: the influence of a personal trainer. *J Strength Cond Res*. 2008; 22(1):103–11.

64. Ratamess NA, Falvo MJ, Mangine GT, Hoffman JR, Faigenbaum AD, Kang J. The effect of rest interval length on metabolic responses to the bench press exercise. *Eur J Appl Physiol*. 2007;100(1):1–17.

65. Reilly T, Morris T, Whyte G. The specificity of training prescription and physiological assessment: a review. *J Sport Sci*. 2009;27:575–89.

66. Rhea M, Alvar B, Burkett L. Single vs multiple sets for strength: a meta-analysis to address the controversy. *Res Q Exerc Sport*. 2002;73:485–8.

67. Rhea M, Alvar B, Burkett LN, Ball S. A meta-analysis to determine the dose response for strength development. *Med Sci Sports Exerc*. 2003;35(3):456–64.

68. Riebe D, Franklin B, Thompson P, et al. Updating ACSM's recommendations for exercise preparticipation health screening. *Med Sci Sports Exerc*. 2015;47(11):2473–9.

69. Sáez-Sáez de Villarreal E, Requena B, Newton R. Does plyometric training improve strength performance? A meta-analysis. *J Sci Med Sport*. 2010;13(5):513–22.

70. Schoenfeld B, Wilson J, Lowery R, Krieger J. Muscular adaptations in low- versus high-load resistance training: a meta-analysis. *Eur J Sport Sci*. 2016;16(1):1–10.

71. Shimano T, Kraemer W, Spiering B, et al. Relationship between the number of repetitions and selected percentages of one

repetition maximum in free weight exercises in trained and untrained men. *J Strength Cond Res.* 2006;20(4):819–23.

72. Sillanpää E, Laaksonen D, Häkkinen A, et al. Body composition, fitness and metabolic health during strength and endurance training and their combination in middle-aged and older women. *Eur J Appl Physiol.* 2009;106(2):285–96.

73. Steib S, Schoene D, Pfeifer K. Dose-response relationship of resistance training in older adults: a meta-analysis. *Med Sci Sports Exerc.* 2009;42(5):902–14.

74. Swank A, Kachelman J, Bibeau W, et al. Prehabilitation before total knee arthroplasty increases strength and function in older adults with severe osteoarthritis. *J Strength Cond Res.* 2011;25(2):318–25.

75. Sylvester B, Standage M, McEwan D, et al. Variety support and exercise adherence behavior: experimental and mediating effects. *J Behav Med.* 2016;39(2):214–24.

76. Thompson W. Worldwide survey of fitness trends for 2015. *ACSM's Health Fitness J.* 2015;18(6):8–17.

77. Valenzuela T, Okubo Y, Woodbury A, Lord SR, Delbaere K. Adherence to technology-based exercise programs in older adults: a systematic review. *J Geriatr Phys Ther.* Epub 2016 Jun 29.

78. Vezina JW, Der Ananian CA, Greenberg E, Kurka J. Sociodemographic correlates of meeting US Department of Health and Human Services muscle strengthening recommendations in middle-aged and older adults. *Prev Chronic Dis.* 2014;11:E162.

79. Viljoen J, Christie C. The change in motivating factors influencing commencement, adherence and retention to a supervised resistance training programme in previously sedentary post-menopausal women: a prospective cohort study. *BMC Public Health.* 2015;15:236.

80. Westcott W. Resistance training is medicine: effects of strength training on health. *Curr Sports Med Rep.* 2012;11(4):209–16.

81. Willardson J. A brief review: factors affecting the length of the rest interval between resistance exercise sets. *J Strength Cond Res.* 2006;20(4):978–84.

82. World Health Organization. *Global Recommendations on Physical Activity for Health.* Geneva (Switzerland): WHO Press; 2010. 60 p.

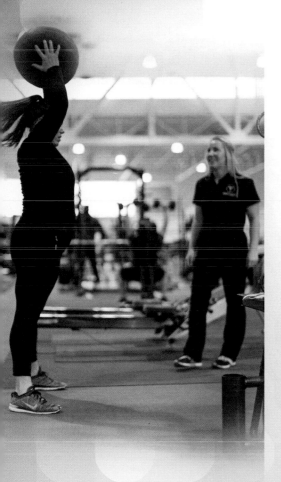

5

Flexibility Assessments and Exercise Programming for Apparently Healthy Participants

OBJECTIVES

- To understand the context of flexibility as it relates to health and wellness.

- To describe the basic anatomy and physiology of the musculoskeletal system related to flexibility.

- To differentiate modes of range of motion exercises and their strengths and weaknesses.

- To select appropriate assessment protocols for flexibility and analyze the results of those assessments.

- To formulate appropriate programs for development of whole body flexibility.

INTRODUCTION

Development and maintenance of flexibility has long been a recommended component of health-related fitness (24). The President's Council on Physical Fitness and Sports was in part prompted by the report of Kraus and Hirschland (56) indicating American children performed poorly compared with European children in a fitness assessment, especially on flexibility. The American College of Sports Medicine (ACSM) released its first position stand on cardiorespiratory and muscular fitness in 1981; however, it didn't include recommendations for flexibility exercises until 1998 (1). Similar to other components of fitness, it is important to maintain an adequate range of motion (ROM) necessary for activities of daily living. However, this increase in ROM through flexibility training does not seem to decrease the incidence of low back pain or muscle soreness (38,82,99), and it has not been shown to improve athletic performance. In some cases, it actually has been shown to decrease performance (7,52,54,55,106). Flexibility requirements are specific to the demands of individual activities, with some activities requiring more than average ROM at particular joints (*e.g.*, gymnastics and ballet) (28,71).

Basic Principles of Flexibility

Visit thePoint to watch video 5.1, which demonstrates dynamic arm circles.

Flexibility is defined as ROM of a joint or group of joints, as per the skeletal muscles and not any external forces (40). The flexibility of any given movable joint includes both static and dynamic components. Static flexibility is the full ROM of a given joint because of external forces. It can be achieved by the use of gravitational force, a partner, or specific exercise equipment (3). In contrast, dynamic flexibility is the full ROM of a given joint achieved by the voluntary use of skeletal muscles in combination with external forces (91). Although it is recognized that dynamic flexibility is greater than static flexibility for a given joint, the two may be independent of each other (43). Each movable joint has its own anatomical structure that helps define the ROM in which that joint can move. Due to this joint specificity, the ROM of one particular joint may not predict the ROM of other joints, although individuals participating in a full-body ROM program or performing activities that move several joints through their full ROM will generally have a greater full-body flexibility (32).

Factors Affecting Flexibility

ROM of a given joint is determined by several factors, including muscle properties, physical activity and exercise, anatomical structure, age, and gender.

Muscle properties: The inherent properties of muscle tissue play a major role in the ROM of a given joint. Skeletal muscles, when stretched, exhibit both viscous and elastic properties (viscoelastic properties), which allow them to extend through the process of creep and stress relaxation (78). In addition, research has suggested that the viscoelastic properties of skeletal muscle may be altered and lead to an increase in ROM by either an external thermal modality (*i.e.*, heat pad) or a physically active warm-up (79,89,90,96). Nevertheless, this finding is not well documented in humans, and therefore, more research is needed to further validate these findings (31,32).

Physical activity and exercise: Both single and multiple bouts of physical activity can lead to greater flexibility of the affected joints, primarily by moving joints through a fuller ROM during exercise

Visit thePoint to watch video 5.2, which demonstrates the soldier walk.

than would normally occur (26,43,86). In addition, resistance training programs that incorporate full ROM exercises may also increase flexibility of the affected joints (59,97), assuming both agonist and antagonist muscles around the joint are being trained (12). For instance, pull-ups or chin-ups move the shoulder through a ROM not normally encountered in day-to-day activities, thereby increasing shoulder ROM. Furthermore, athletes who regularly perform ROM exercise during aerobic, resistance, or flexibility exercise improve performance, at least in part, through an enhanced level of flexibility (44,50,108). Nonetheless, discrepancies exist in the level of flexibility necessary for a variety of activities (28), such as athletes in the same sport but at different competitive levels (collegiate vs. professional) (95) and athletes in the same sport but in a different position (27,80). Additionally, there is also a difference in the level of flexibility between dominant and non-dominant limbs in athletes who participate in sports that involve bilateral asymmetrical motions such as tennis and baseball (21,62).

Anatomical structures: The ROM of a given joint is influenced by its structure and the anatomical structures surrounding it. Freely moveable joints (synovial) may be classified into one of six groups, each with a specific permissible plane or planes of movement (Fig. 5.1) (32,105). Furthermore, joint flexibility is not affected equally by connective tissues around joints. Johns and Wright (48) demonstrated that relative contributions of various soft tissues to joint stiffness are as follows: joint capsule (47%), muscles (41%), tendons (10%), and the skin (2%). In addition, soft tissue bulk including muscle and subcutaneous fat tissues may affect joint flexibility because of potential movement restriction (16,105).

Age and gender: Several studies have examined the relationship between the degree of flexibility within a given joint relative to age and gender. These studies have demonstrated that with aging, there is a reduction in collagen solubility, which may lead to increases in tendon rigidity and therefore reduction in joint ROM (81). This reduction may be further exacerbated by age-related conditions such as past injuries, degenerative joint disease, and decreased levels of physical activity) (42,81). Normative data collected on thousands of men and women at The Cooper Institute show that women consistently have greater ROM across almost all measured joints compared with men (100).

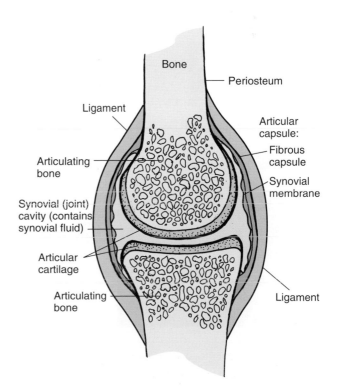

FIGURE 5.1. Classification of synovial joints. (From Bushman B, editor. *ACSM's Resources for the Personal Trainer*. 4th ed. Baltimore [MD]: Lippincott Williams & Wilkins; 2014. 592 p.)

Some of the reasons for increased female flexibility include smaller muscles and wider hips (60) and differences in hormonal levels (83). A study by Park et al. (83) has demonstrated that changes in estradiol and progesterone levels during ovulation led to a greater degree of knee joint laxity. Furthermore, it was also demonstrated that women have a more compliant Achilles tendon, resulting in greater ankle flexibility and lower muscle stiffness (49).

Modes of Flexibility Training

There are four types of flexibility training modes. Three of these modes — static, ballistic, and proprioceptive neuromuscular facilitation (PNF) — are considered "traditional" flexibility training modes (92). Dynamic flexibility training is becoming more common especially as part of the warm-up routine (31,66) to better prepare the body for competition (9). Of all the different modes, static flexibility training is most commonly utilized and can be further subdivided into three categories: (a) slow and constant stretch with a partner (passive), (b) slow and constant stretch without any assistance, or "self-stretching," and (c) slow and constant stretch against a stationary object (isometric) (95).

Static Flexibility

Static stretching is the most commonly used flexibility protocol of all due to the fact that it can be easily administered without assistance (95), and regardless of the type of static stretching, each involves a slow and constant motion that is held in the final position, or point of mild discomfort, for 15–30 seconds (1). To achieve an optimal degree of ROM, it is recommended to repeat each exercise no more than four times, because there are only minimal gains with additional repetitions (98). The advantage of using this method involves both relaxing and concurrent elongation of the stretched muscle without stimulation of the stretch reflex (78). Several studies have demonstrated that static stretching can lead to both short- and long-term gains in flexibility (4,19,67) through a decrease in muscle/tendon stiffness and viscoelastic stress relaxation (63,64). Although many researchers and practitioners view static stretching as effective and beneficial (4,5,19,78) (Fig. 5.2),

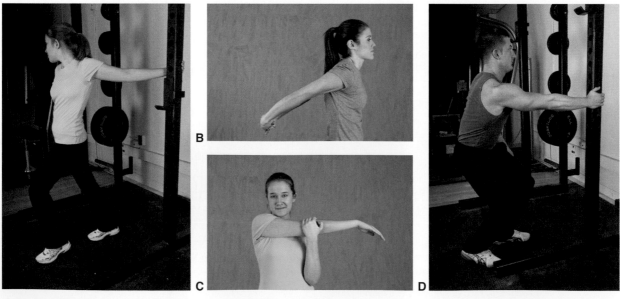

FIGURE 5.2. Examples of static stretches: **(A)** pectoral wall stretch, **(B)** posterior shoulder hyperextension, **(C)** anterior cross-arm stretch, and **(D)** lat stretch. (From Ratamess N. *ACSM's Foundations of Strength Training and Conditioning*. Baltimore [MD]: Lippincott Williams & Wilkins; 2012. 560 p.)

others have raised concerns. Because static stretching is slow and controlled, it does not provide an increase in muscle temperature and blood flow redistribution that is needed before exercise particularly prior to competitive sports performance (69,93,94). In addition, the view that static stretching may improve performance is ambiguous, with several studies reporting an increase (44,50,108), several reporting a decrease (8,17,67), and others reporting no changes (98,109) in performance.

Ballistic Flexibility

Ballistic stretching involves rapid and bouncing-like movements in which the resultant momentum of the body or body segments is used to extend the affected joint through the full ROM (32). This type of stretching technique, as opposed to static stretching and PNF, is no longer advocated as common practice for most individuals (57,102) to improve a joint's ROM. However, ballistic stretching is still used by some athletes and coaches to increase the blood flow to the muscle prior to competition or practice. Current research in this area indicates that properly performed ballistic stretching is equally as effective as static stretching in increasing joint ROM and may be considered for adults who engage in activities that involve ballistic movements such as basketball (25,107). However, given the nature of the movements, this type of stretching produces a rapid and high degree of tension inside the muscle, which may potentially lead to muscle and tendon injuries (78,79,92). The risk of injury may be further exacerbated by stimulating a myotatic reflex (also referred to as the stretch reflex), which is common with this mode of stretching (32). However, the hypothesis that ballistic stretching leads to muscle or connective tissue injury has never been supported by the scientific literature (76,103). In respect of the effectiveness of this technique and when compared with static stretching, ballistic stretching does not provide any added benefit (5,41,61). Thus, it is recommended to use techniques that are viewed as safer and may potentially be more effective such as static stretching, dynamic stretching, and PNF (31).

Proprioceptive Neuromuscular Facilitation

PNF is a collection of stretching techniques combining passive stretch with isometric and concentric muscle actions designed to use the autogenic and reciprocal inhibition responses of the Golgi tendon organs (GTOs) (31,32). It is hypothesized that through the responses of the GTO, the muscle and tendon are able to elongate and achieve greater ROM and increasing neuromuscular efficiency (31,39). PNF stretching (Fig. 5.3) was first developed not only as a stretching technique but also as a strengthening technique through a series of diagonal patterns to help physical therapists treat patients with neuromuscular paralysis (51) and later adopted for use by athletes as a technique to increase ROM (91).

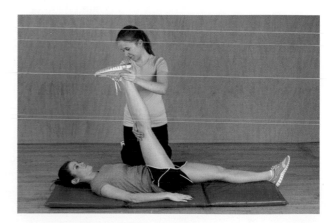

FIGURE 5.3. PNF stretching. (From Ratamess N. *ACSM's Foundations of Strength Training and Conditioning.* Baltimore [MD]: Lippincott Williams & Wilkins; 2012. 560 p.)

Visit thePoint to watch video 5.3, which demonstrates PNF stretching.

There are three types of PNF stretching techniques: (a) hold–relax, (b) hold–relax with antagonist contraction, and (c) agonist contraction (11,14,73,97). Of the three, the hold–relax and the hold–relax with antagonist contraction are most frequently used (39). Each technique comprises three phases: (a) a passive prestretch, (b) passive stretch, and (c) contractions (3). When PNF is compared with other stretching techniques with respect to effectiveness of improving ROM, the data are inconsistent. Some studies have demonstrated that PNF is superior to both static and ballistic stretching techniques (41,88,104), whereas others have found no difference (10,12,29,61). Despite the wide support that the PNF stretching has among researchers and practitioners, there are some limitations with these techniques such as the need for a trained partner and the potential risk for musculature injury (15,37).

EXERCISE IS MEDICINE CONNECTION

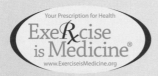

Moonaz S, Bingham C III, Wissow L, Bartlett S. Yoga in sedentary adults with arthritis: effects of a randomized controlled pragmatic trial. *J Rheumatol.* 2015:42(7);1194–202. (72)

Yoga has been used for more than 5,000 years around the world as a means of health improvement, with well-documented studies showing increased in flexibility and ROM, a key aspect of health-related fitness. Yoga's use has increased dramatically as a popular exercise modality in the United States in the recent past. It is estimated that the number of Americans that practice yoga increased by 29% between the years 2008 and 2012.

In addition to the benefits to flexibility, yoga has often been used to ease pain and dysfunction associated with arthritis, a debilitating condition that results in inflammation, stiffness, and pain at and around the joints and affects over 50 million Americans. Recent evidence suggested that yoga training may improve physical activity adherence and physical and psychological health.

Visit thePoint to watch videos 5.4 and 5.5, which demonstrate the kneeling cat and modified cobra positions.

Moonaz, Bingham, Wissow, and Bartlett randomly assigned 75 physically inactive adults with rheumatoid arthritis (RA) or knee osteoarthritis (OA) to an 8-week yoga program group or a control group. Per week, the yoga program group completed two 60-minute classes and one home practice. Outcome measures included physical and mental components representing health-related quality of life (HRQL) domains and disease activity. In the yoga group, the researchers followed the participants for an additional 9 months to examine the long-term effects of the program. The results of this study demonstrated that an 8-week yoga program led to improved physical and mental components, improved walking capacity, and reduced depressive symptoms. It was also demonstrated that most of these benefits were maintained 9 months after the cessation of the program.

In summary, appropriately designed yoga programs can be an effective treatment for improving physical and psychological health and physical abilities in patients with RA and OA.

Dynamic Flexibility

As opposed to the previously mentioned stretching techniques, dynamic flexibility uses slow and controlled, sport-specific movements that are designed to increase core temperature and enhance activity-related flexibility and balance (5,36,66). In view of the fact that these exercises are sport-specific, there is no comprehensive list of dynamic exercises. The design of such exercises is only limited by the knowledge and resourcefulness of the coach/trainer (36). In the past few years, several studies have examined the effectiveness of dynamic flexibility in relation to the degree of flexibility and athletic performance and the effects of preexercise static and dynamic stretches on anaerobic performance in different populations. One study has demonstrated that both static and dynamic stretches improve the ROM of the hamstring muscle; yet, static stretching was more effective (5). Furthermore, whereas some studies have demonstrated that a warm-up that included dynamic stretching was superior for improving sport performance to the one that included static stretching (70,74,101), others have failed to show those differences (13,33,103). Also related to dynamic stretching, eccentric training was recently introduced as a new technique that is designed to reduce the occurrence of injuries and improve flexibility and performance. Using this technique, the participant is instructed to resist a flexion in a given joint by eccentrically contracting the antagonist muscles during the entire ROM (76). Two studies examining this technique have demonstrated some merit when compared with static stretching (76,77). These recent findings emphasize the controversy that surrounds the issue of the usefulness of different stretching techniques.

Muscle and Tendon Proprioceptors

There are two types of sensory organs that provide muscular dynamic and limb movement information to the central nervous system (68). These sensors, muscle spindles (Fig. 5.4), and GTOs (Fig. 5.5) should be considered when discussing stretching and flexibility. Muscle spindles are a collection of 3–10 intrafusal, specialized muscle fibers that are innervated by gamma motor neurons and provide information about the rate of change in muscle length. The intrafusal muscle fibers run parallel to the extrafusal muscle fibers (regular muscle fibers), which are innervated by alpha motor neurons and are responsible for tension development (30,32) (see Fig. 5.4). When muscle

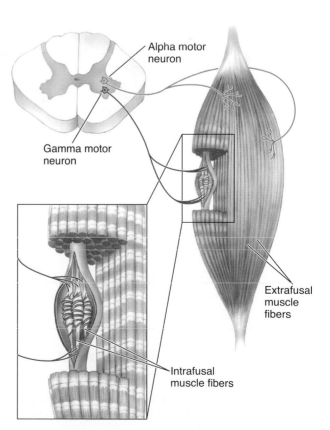

FIGURE 5.4. Structure and location of the muscle spindles. (From Bear MF, Connors BW, Parasido MA. *Neuroscience: Exploring the Brain.* 2nd ed. Philadelphia [PA]: Lippincott Williams & Wilkins; 2001. 855 p.)

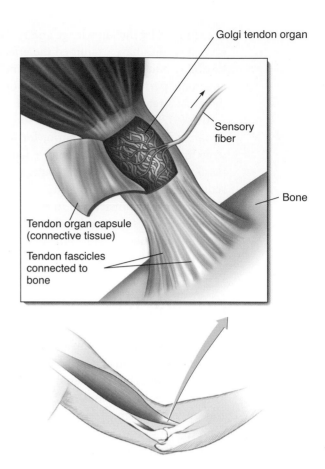

FIGURE 5.5. Structure and location of the GTO. (From Premkumar K. *Anatomy & Physiology: The Massage Connection.* 2nd ed. Baltimore [MD]: Lippincott Williams and Wilkins; 2004.)

spindles are stimulated, there is a dual response in which a rapid tension development is initiated in the stretched muscle and inhibited in the antagonist muscle. The response in the stretched muscle is known as a stretch or myotatic reflex, and the response in the antagonist muscle is known as reciprocal inhibition (12,32,73). These responses serve an important role in both static stretching and PNF. Because the myotatic reflex is less likely to occur in slow and controlled movements, static stretch is viewed as a safer and more effective technique than ballistic stretch (32). During PNF stretching when there is an increase in tension in the antagonist muscle with a concurrent elongation of the agonist muscle, a further lengthening of the stretched muscle is thought to be mediated by reciprocal inhibition (31).

GTOs are located in the musculotendinous junction and respond to changes in muscle tension (see Fig. 5.5). These organs are encapsulated in a series with 10–15 muscle fibers and can identify and provide a response to changes in the amount of tension (static) and the rate of tension (dynamic) development. When the GTOs are stimulated, there is a dual response in which tension development is inhibited in the contracting muscle (autogenic inhibition) and initiated in the antagonist muscles to protect the muscle tissue from damage (30,32). Similar to the muscle spindles' response, the GTO plays an important role in PNF. The active tension development in the muscle prior to a stretch elicits autogenic inhibition, which promotes further lengthening of the affected muscle (12,30,73).

Flexibility Assessment Protocols

Different methods and tools are used to measure ROM and flexibility. Among the most common are the use of goniometers, sit-and-reach tests, and functional movement screenings.

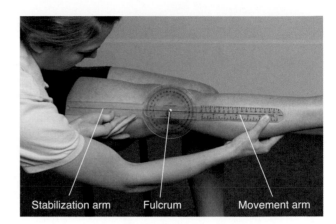

FIGURE 5.6. A goniometer includes the body axis or fulcrum, a stabilization arm, and a movement arm.

Stabilization arm   Fulcrum   Movement arm

Goniometers

Quantitative assessment of ROM is necessary to identify deficiencies resulting from injury or the need for a flexibility training program relative to the individual's needs. Given that ROM is joint-specific, knowing the ROM ranges for the specific joint will help to address any problematic areas that need attention. The most useful method for determining individual joint flexibility is through the use of a goniometer (Fig. 5.6). Once established, an appropriate flexibility prescription with the goal of increasing or maintaining ROM can be implemented.

A goniometer is similar to a protractor and is used to measure a joint's ROM expressed in degrees. Proper procedures followed by a certified exercise physiologist (EP-C), provide both valid and reliable results (58). Proper positioning of the instrument includes first, identifying the specific joint line and placing the axis (pin) of the goniometer at the joint's axis of rotation. Second, line up the arms with the given anatomical reference points on the body. The goniometer consists of two arms: a stabilization arm that is fixed and aligned with specific anatomical reference points on the proximal body segment and a movement arm that aligns with specific anatomical reference points that follow the distal body segment as it is moved through its ROM. Procedures for goniometry assessment of commonly measured joints are listed in Table 5.1. General guidelines for proper goniometry assessment include the following:

- Before assessment, provide the client with an overview of the process.
- Demonstrate proper technique for movement of the joint being assessed.

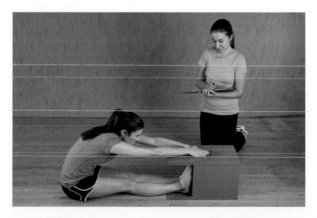

FIGURE 5.7. Sit-and-reach tests. Test using a sit-and-reach box. (From Ratamess N. *ACSM's Foundations of Strength Training and Conditioning.* Baltimore [MD]: Lippincott Williams & Wilkins; 2012. 560 p.)

Table 5.1 Procedures for Goniometry Assessment of Joints Commonly of Concern to Health and Fitness Professionals

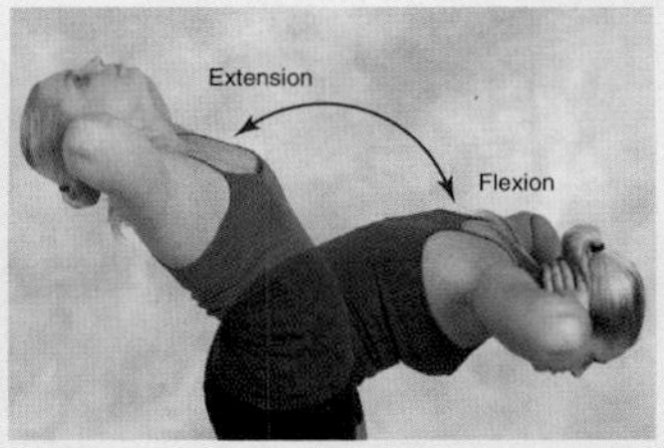

FIGURE 5.8. Lumbar flexion and extension. (From Bushman B, editor. *ACSM's Resources for the Personal Trainer.* 4th ed. Baltimore [MD]: Lippincott Williams & Wilkins; 2014. 592 p.)

Movement	Plane of Motion	Axis of Motion	Average Range	Goniometer Position	Stabilization	Starting/Ending Body Position
Spine						
					Upper Body	
Lumbar flexion	Sagittal	Bilateral	4-in increase	Tape measure position 1. Top point: spinous process C7 2. Bottom point: level to posterior superior iliac spine (PSIS)	Client is seated on floor or table with pelvis stabilized to prevent anterior/posterior tilting with legs extended.	Client is in good posture with a stabilized cervical, thoracic, and lumbar spine in 0° of flexion, extension, rotation, or lateral flexion. Head is in neutral position. Client performs lumbar flexion until first sign of resistance.
Lumbar extension	Sagittal	Bilateral	2-in difference as spine extends	Tape measure position 1. Top point: spinous process C7 2. Bottom point: level to PSIS	Client is seated on floor or table with pelvis stabilized to prevent anterior/posterior tilting with legs extended.	Client is in good posture with a stabilized cervical, thoracic, and lumbar spine in 0° of flexion, extension, rotation, or lateral flexion. Head is in neutral position. Client performs lumbar extension until first sign of resistance.

Continued

FIGURE 5.9. Glenohumeral flexion and extension. (From Bushman B, editor. *ACSM's Resources for the Personal Trainer.* 4th ed. Baltimore [MD]: Lippincott Williams & Wilkins; 2014. 592 p.)

Shoulder

Glenohumeral flexion	Sagittal	Bilateral	0°–180°	1. Axis point: lateral aspect of greater tubercle 2. Stabilization arm: perpendicular to the floor 3. Movement arm: Align with midline of humerus and reference the lateral epicondyle.	Client is in good posture with a stabilized scapula (retracted), thoracic, and lumbar spine. Stabilize scapula to prevent tilting, rotation, or elevation.	Client is seated with glenohumeral in 0° of flexion, extension, abduction, or adduction. Head is in neutral position. Palm of hand should be facing the body. Elbow should be extended completely. Client performs glenohumeral flexion until the first sign of resistance. 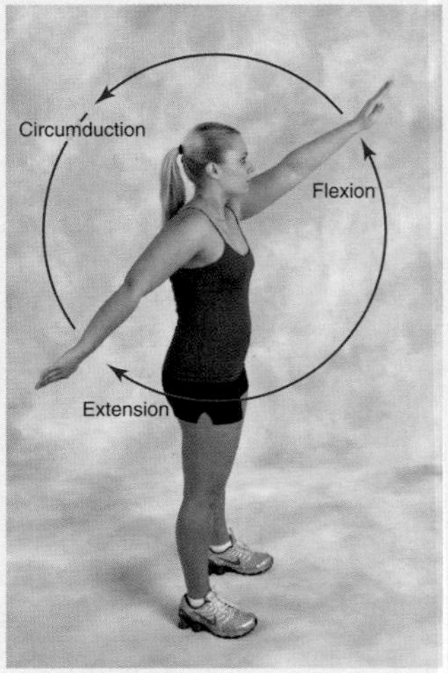
Glenohumeral extension	Sagittal	Bilateral	0°–60°	1. Axis point: lateral aspect of greater tubercle 2. Stabilization arm: perpendicular to the floor 3. Movement arm: Align with midline of humerus and reference the lateral epicondyle.	Client is in good posture with a stabilized scapula (retracted), thoracic, and lumbar spine. Stabilize scapula to prevent tilting, rotation, or elevation. Place towel under humerus to stabilize and align with acromion process.	Client is prone on table with glenohumeral in 0° of flexion, extension, abduction, or adduction. Head is in neutral position. Palm of hand should face the body. Elbow should be extended completely. Client performs glenohumeral extension until the first sign of resistance.

Table 5.1 Procedures for Goniometry Assessment of Joints Commonly of Concern to Health and Fitness Professionals (continued)

Movement	Plane of Motion	Axis of Motion	Average Range	Goniometer Position	Stabilization	Starting/Ending Body Position
Upper Body						
Shoulder						
Glenohumeral internal rotation	Transverse	Longitudinal	0°–70°	1. Axis point: olecranon process of the elbow 2. Stabilization arm: perpendicular to the floor 3. Movement arm: Align with lateral midline of ulna and reference the ulnar styloid.	Client is in good posture with a stabilized scapula (retracted), thoracic, and lumbar spine. Stabilize scapula to prevent tilting, rotation, or elevation. Place towel under humerus to stabilize and align with acromion process.	Client is supine on table with humerus abducted at 90° and elbow is flexed at 90°. Elbow is at 0° of supination and pronation. Client performs glenohumeral internal rotation until the first sign of resistance 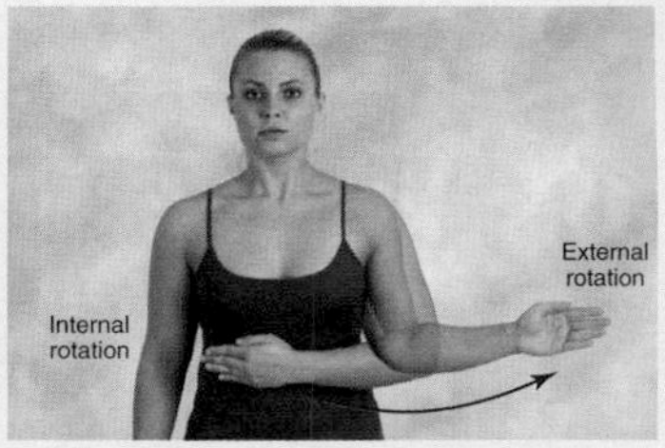
Glenohumeral external rotation	Transverse	Longitudinal	0°–90°	1. Axis point: olecranon process of the elbow 2. Stabilization arm: perpendicular to the floor 3. Movement arm: Align with lateral midline of ulna and reference the ulnar styloid.	Client is in good posture with a stabilized scapula (retracted), thoracic, and lumbar spine. Stabilize scapula to prevent tilting, rotation, or elevation. Place towel under humerus to stabilize and align with acromion process.	Client is supine on table with humerus abducted at 90° and elbow is flexed at 90°. Elbow is at 0° of supination and pronation. Client performs glenohumeral external rotation until the first sign of resistance.

FIGURE 5.10. Glenohumeral internal rotation and external rotation. (From Bushman B, editor. *ACSM's Resources for the Personal Trainer.* 4th ed. Baltimore [MD]: Lippincott Williams & Wilkins; 2014. 592 p.)

Lower Body

Hip

Hip flexion (testing leg fully extended)	Sagittal	Bilateral	0°–90°	1. Axis point: greater trochanter of the lateral thigh 2. Stabilization arm: lateral midline of the pelvis 3. Movement arm: lateral midline of the femur, using the lateral epicondyle as a reference	Client is in good posture with a stabilized scapula, thoracic, lumbar spine, and pelvic area. Pelvis should not rise off table. Opposite leg not being assessed should have knee flexed and foot flat on table for added stability and protection for the back.	Client is supine on table with hip in 0° of flexion, extension, abduction, adduction, and rotation. Testing leg has knee fully extended. Client performs hip flexion until the first sign of resistance or until the pelvis rotates or knee breaks extension. 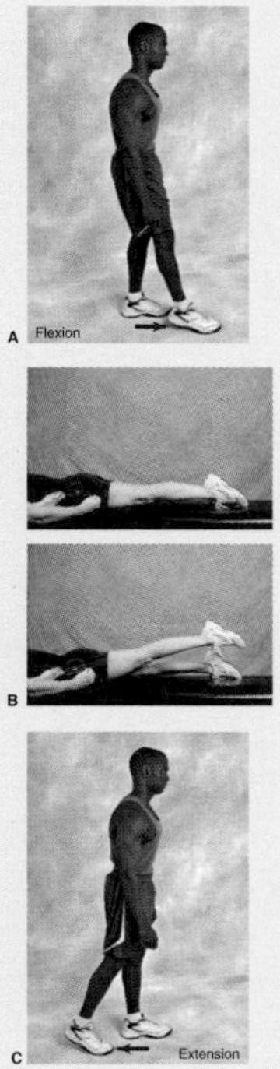
Hip flexion (testing knee flexed 90° and hip flexed 90°)	Sagittal	Bilateral	0°–120°	1. Axis point: greater trochanter of the lateral thigh 2. Stabilization arm: lateral midline of the pelvis 3. Movement arm: lateral midline of the femur, using the lateral epicondyle as a reference	Client is in good posture with a stabilized scapula, thoracic, lumbar spine, and pelvic area. Pelvis should not rise off table. Opposite leg not being assessed should have knee flexed and foot flat on table for added stability and protection for the back.	Client is supine on table with knee flexed at 90° and hip flexed at 90°, and hip is in 0° of abduction, adduction, and rotation. Knee is flexed to reduce contraction of hamstrings. Client performs hip flexion until the first sign of resistance or until the pelvis rotates.

FIGURE 5.11. Hip flexion with the testing leg fully extended **(A)** and with the testing knee and hip both flexed 90° **(B)**; hip extension with the testing leg fully extended **(C)**. (**A** and **C** from Bushman B, editor. *ACSM's Resources for the Personal Trainer.* 4th ed. Baltimore [MD]: Lippincott Williams & Wilkins; 2014. 592 p. **B** from Kaminsky L. *ACSM's Health-Related Physical Fitness Assessment Manual.* 4th ed. Baltimore [MD]: Lippincott Williams & Wilkins; 2014. 192 p.)

Continued

Table 5.1   **Procedures for Goniometry Assessment of Joints Commonly of Concern to Health and Fitness Professionals** *(continued)*

Movement	Plane of Motion	Axis of Motion	Average Range	Goniometer Position	Stabilization	Starting/Ending Body Position
Lower Body						
Hip						
Hip extension (testing leg fully extended)	Sagittal	Bilateral	0°–30°	1. Axis point: greater trochanter of the lateral thigh 2. Stabilization arm: lateral midline of the pelvis 3. Movement arm: lateral midline of the femur, using the lateral epicondyle as a reference	Client is in good posture with a stabilized scapula, thoracic, lumbar spine, and pelvic area. Pelvis should not rise off table. Opposite leg not being assessed should have leg fully extended on table for added stability.	Client is prone on table with hip in 0° of flexion, extension, abduction, adduction, and rotation. Testing leg has knee fully extended. Client performs hip extension until the first sign of resistance or until the pelvis rotates.

FIGURE 5.12. Hip adduction and abduction. (From Bushman B, editor. *ACSM's Resources for the Personal Trainer.* 4th ed. Baltimore [MD]: Lippincott Williams & Wilkins; 2014. 592 p.)

Hip abduction	Frontal	Anterior/ posterior	0°–45°	1. Axis point: locate anterior superior iliac spine (ASIS) 2. Stabilization arm: imaginary line connecting axis point ASIS to other ASIS 3. Movement arm: anterior midline of the femur, using the midline of the patella as a reference	Client is in good posture with a stabilized scapula, thoracic, lumbar spine, and pelvic area. Stabilize for lateral trunk flexion on both sides.	Client is supine on table with hip in 0° of flexion, extension, and rotation. Testing leg has knee fully extended. Client performs hip abduction until the first sign of resistance or lateral trunk flexion occurs on either side. 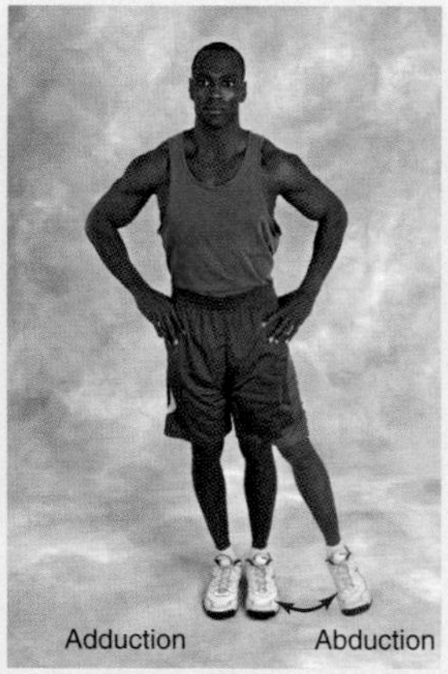
Hip adduction	Frontal	Anterior/ posterior	0°–30°	1. Axis point: located at the ASIS 2. Stabilization arm: imaginary horizontal line connecting axis point ASIS to other ASIS 3. Movement arm: anterior midline of the femur, using the midline of the patella as a reference	Client is in good posture with a stabilized scapula, thoracic, lumbar spine, and pelvic area. Opposite leg not being tested should be abducted fully to allow for testing hip to be assessed.	Client is supine on table with hip in 0° of flexion, extension, and rotation. Testing leg has knee fully extended. Client performs hip adduction until the first sign of resistance or lateral trunk flexion or pelvic rotation occurs.

- Instruct the client to move slowly through the proper ROM.
- Stabilize the stationary portion of the body.
- During movement, ensure that the goniometer maintains proper orientation relative to pre-defined anatomical landmarks (it may be helpful to mark specific body segments to assure consistent placement over time).
- Measure three consecutive trials averaging the values as the final score.
- If average ROM is lesser than 50°, it is recommended that the measures fall within ±5° of the mean. If the average ROM is greater than 50°, the three measures should fall within ±10° of the mean. Measurements should continue until they meet the criteria or are otherwise considered invalid (2,58).

Sit-and-Reach Tests

Whereas goniometry is the most accurate method to assess joint-specific ROM when used properly, the sit-and-reach test is perhaps the most commonly used assessment for flexibility in the lower back and hip joint. Although other joints in the body (including the spine and shoulder girdle) can and should be assessed for flexibility, there is a lack of tests and norms for flexibility assessment of these joints. The sit-and-reach test may be useful to evaluate ROM of the spine and hips for effective completion of activities of daily living, although there has not been evidence demonstrating reduction in low back pain relative to ROM measured by the sit-and-reach (47). It should be noted that sit-and-reach testing may need to be modified for various subpopulations, including the young, the old, and the pregnant, although specific procedures and norms are lacking. Procedures for two different sit-and-reach tests (Fig. 5.7) are described in the box titled "How to Perform the Sit-and-Reach Test." Normative data for these sit-and-reach tests are in Tables 5.2.

Table 5.2	Fitness Categories for Trunk Forward Flexion Using a Sit-and-Reach Box (cm)[a] by Age and Sex								
	Age (year)								
Category	20–29		30–39		40–49		50–59		60–69	
Sex	M	W	M	W	M	W	M	W	M	W
Excellent	≥40	≥41	≥38	≥41	≥35	≥38	≥35	≥39	≥33	≥35
Very good	34–39	37–40	33–37	36–40	29–34	34–37	28–34	33–38	25–32	31–34
Good	30–33	33–36	28–32	32–35	24–28	30–33	24–27	30–32	20–24	27–30
Fair	25–29	28–32	23–27	27–31	18–23	25–29	16–23	25–29	15–19	23–26
Poor	≤24	≤27	≤22	≤26	≤17	≤24	≤15	≤24	≤14	≤22

[a]These norms are based on a sit-and-reach box in which the "zero" point is set at 26 cm. When using a box in which the zero point is set at 23 cm, subtract 3 cm from each value in this table.

M, men; W, women.

Reprinted with permission from the Canadian Society for Exercise Physiology. *Canadian Society for Exercise Physiology — Physical Activity Training for Health (CSEP-PATH®)*; 2013.

Flexibility Program Design

The framework for developing and maintaining whole body ROM is structured around the same underlying principles that all health-related fitness components utilize: progressive overload, specificity of training, individual differences, and reversibility. The components of a health-related fitness program consisting of frequency, intensity, time, and type (FITT) are the foundation for which flexibility programs are developed (1,25).

Assessment of ROM at specific joints helps determine the need for a flexibility program. Healthy individuals with inadequate ROM for particular activities should engage in a program that caters to their specific needs.

Once adequate ROM is achieved, a maintenance program should be prescribed. For individuals with hypermobility in joint ROM, there does not seem to be a benefit of participation in a flexibility training program (28,52,54,55,106).

The principle of progressive overload in the context of flexibility demonstrates that for ROM to improve, it must be stressed beyond its normal range. This may be accomplished by completing the flexibility exercises recommended below or by participating in activities that elicit greater ROM in targeted joints.

The principle of overload for flexibility training may be applied by

- Increasing frequency (sessions per day or week)
- Increasing intensity (point of stretch)
- And/or increasing time for each session.

Individual differences as it relates to neuromuscular function and structure should be taken into consideration in the design of a flexibility program. However and to date, there are no specific guidelines for optimal progression (1,25). The principle of reversibility should also be considered with respect to flexibility training like other modes of exercise. Feland et al. (22) demonstrated that flexibility gains are lost within 4–8 weeks of ceasing flexibility exercises.

After assessment of flexibility, a training program may be necessary to increase or maintain ROM relative to individual goals. See Table 5.3 for an evidence-based flexibility exercise program recommendation. To improve ROM, two to three training sessions per week for at least 3–4 weeks may be required (18,20,22), although daily stretching exercises may be more effective (25). During each of the training sessions, each exercise should include two to four repetitions in which the stretch is held between 10 and 30 seconds, with 30–60 seconds in older individuals, with a goal of accumulating 60 seconds of stretch across two to four repetitions (25,87,102). Increasing the duration of each repetition beyond 30–60 seconds does not seem to lead to improved ROM benefits except perhaps in an elderly population (6,22,25). Generally, joints of the neck, shoulders, upper and lower back, pelvis, hips, and legs will need to be trained as it relates to daily activity and performance (98). Flexibility training should be conducted when a muscle is warm and therefore should be completed after an aerobic warm-up of at least 5 minutes and some general flexibility exercises. Also, testing may occur subsequent to cardiovascular or strength sessions. Since some researchers have demonstrated that acute preexercise flexibility training may have negative effects on ensuing performance, postexercise flexibility training may be more beneficial (52,54,55,106). The intensity of the flexibility training is dependent on the individual, but it is recommended that a given stretch will be held to the point of tightness or slight discomfort (23). The duration of the training session may vary on the basis of the mode of the flexibility exercise. Static ROM training session should be at minimum 10 minutes, and if PNF stretching is being employed, a 20%–75% maximum voluntary contraction should be held for 3- to 6-second contraction followed

Visit thePoint to watch videos 5.7 and 5.8, which demonstrate pendulum leg swings and dynamic hip rotation, respectively.

Table 5.3	Flexibility Exercise Evidence-Based Recommendations
FITT-VP	**Evidence-Based Recommendation**
Frequency	■ $\geq$2–3 d · wk^{-1} with daily being most effective
Intensity	■ Stretch to the point of feeling tightness or slight discomfort.
Time	■ Holding a static stretch for 10–30 s is recommended for most adults. ■ In older individuals, holding a stretch for 30–60 s may confer greater benefit. ■ For proprioceptive neuromuscular facilitation (PNF) stretching, a 3- to 6-s light-to-moderate contraction (*e.g.*, 20%–75% of maximum voluntary contraction) followed by a 10- to 30-s assisted stretch is desirable.
Type	■ A series of flexibility exercises for each of the major muscle-tendon units is recommended. ■ Static flexibility (*i.e.*, active or passive), dynamic flexibility, ballistic flexibility, and PNF are each effective.
Volume	■ A reasonable target is to perform 60 s of total stretching time for each flexibility exercise.
Pattern	■ Repetition of each flexibility exercise two to four times is recommended. ■ Flexibility exercise is most effective when the muscle is warmed through light-to-moderate aerobic activity or passively through external methods such as moist heat packs or hot baths.
Progression	■ Methods for optimal progression are unknown.

Adapted with permission from American College of Sports Medicine. *ACSM's Guidelines for Exercise Testing and Prescription*. 10th ed. Philadelphia (PA): Lippincott Williams & Wilkins; 2018 (Table 6.7).

by a 10- to 30-second assisted stretch is recommended (1,2). The mode of the flexibility program should depend on the individual and available equipment. Generally, increased ROM has been demonstrated in all modes of flexibility training (65,110). Table 5.4 lists some static stretches for the major muscle groups.

Numerous examinations have reported no link between ROM training and prevention of low back pain, injury, or postexercise muscle soreness (38,82,84,85,99). In addition, individuals with ROM imbalances may be at an increased risk for injury during activity (53) and therefore benefit from ROM exercises. This benefit, however, may be limited to those with ROM imbalances and not be effective as a simple means of injury prevention. Furthermore, there has been recent research suggesting a link between antibiotics and musculotendinous injuries. Individuals who are using fluoroquinolone antibiotics are at an increased risk for tendon rupture and joint and muscle damage and therefore should approach flexibility exercises with extreme caution (45,46).

Table 5.4   Static Stretches for the Major Muscle Groups

Stretch	Muscle Involved	Starting Position	Description
Upper Body			
Neck			
Flexion for stretching extensors (Fig. 5.13A)	■ Obliquus capitis superior Rectus capitis superior major Rectus capitis superior minor Obliquus capitis inferior Semispinalis capitis Splenius cervicis Longissimus capitis Levator scapulae	Standing or sitting	Starting with the superior segments, first retract your chin then slowly flex your cervical spine so that your chin moves toward your chest. Maintain your chest and shoulders in a static position.
Lateral bending (Fig. 5.13C)	■ Upper trapezius Anterior, middle, and posterior scalene Sternocleidomastoid Splenius capitis	Standing or sitting	Take your right hand and reach over the top of your head, placing it palm down on your head so that your middle two fingers touch your left ear. Carefully, pull your head directly toward the right side, being careful not to let your head move forward or back. Repeat to the left.
Rotation (Fig. 5.13D)	■ Sternocleidomastoid Longissimus capitis Splenius capitis Obliquus capitis inferior	Standing or sitting	Use your left hand to reach behind your back and pull your right forearm gently inferiorly and toward the left, depressing your right shoulder. Carefully turn your head toward the left. Repeat toward the right.

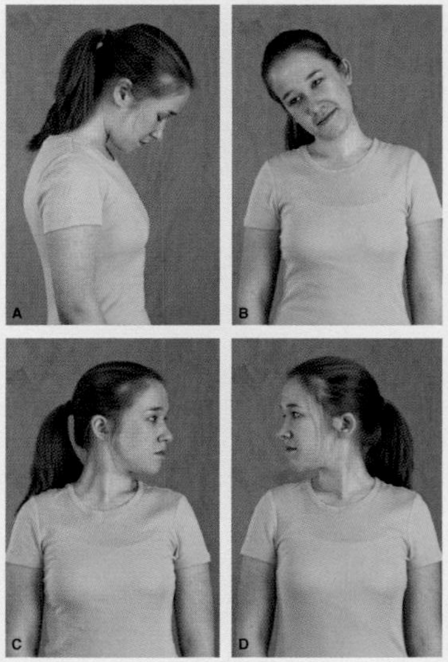

FIGURE 5.13. Neck flexion (**A**), extension (**B**), lateral flexion (**C**), and rotation (**D**). (From Ratamess N. *ACSM's Foundations of Strength Training and Conditioning.* Baltimore [MD]: Lippincott Williams & Wilkins; 2012. 560 p.)

Continued

Table 5.4   Static Stretches for the Major Muscle Groups (continued)

Upper Body

Stretch	Muscle Involved	Starting Position	Description
Shoulder			
Extension for stretching flexors	■ Pectoralis major Anterior deltoid Long head of biceps brachii Coracobrachialis	Standing	Lock your hands together behind back with elbows only slightly flexed. Lift interlocked hands up behind your back, extending your shoulders. No need to bend your back forward.
Flexion for stretching extensors	■ Latissimus dorsi Teres major Posterior deltoid Long head of the triceps brachii Rhomboid major and minor through their action on the scapula	Standing in front of a chair	Place both hands on the back of a chair or object of similar height. Then, carefully bend at the waist until arms are straightened overhead with a roughly 90° angle at the waist. Be careful to keep your lower back straight, allowing the forward bend to come from flexion at the hips.
Adduction for abductors	■ Middle deltoid Supraspinatus Upper trapezius through its action in superiorly rotating the scapula (a necessary and integral motion in abducting the shoulder)	Standing	Reach your right hand behind your back. Grasp your right forearm with your left hand. Adduct your right arm by carefully pulling it toward the left until a gentle stretch is felt at the right shoulder. Then slowly lean your head toward the left, increasing the stretch at both your right shoulder and your upper trapezius. Repeat toward the right.
Abduction for adductors	■ Pectoralis major Latissimus dorsi Teres major Rhomboids major and minor via their action on the scapula	Standing	Extend your right arm overhead, palm facing to the left. Reach your entire arm directly toward the left and continue with left side-bending of your torso. Repeat to the right leading with your left hand.

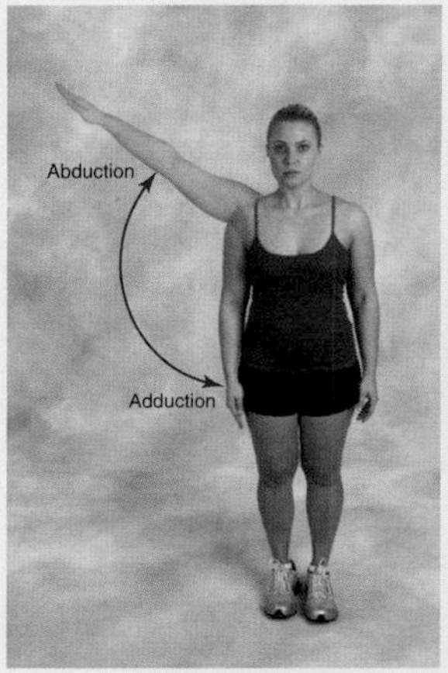

FIGURE 5.14. Shoulder abduction and adduction. (From Bushman B, editor. *ACSM's Resources for the Personal Trainer.* 4th ed. Baltimore [MD]: Lippincott Williams & Wilkins; 2014. 592 p.)

FIGURE 5.15. Shoulder horizontal adduction and horizontal abduction. (From Bushman B, editor. *ACSM's Resources for the Personal Trainer.* 4th ed. Baltimore [MD]: Lippincott Williams & Wilkins; 2014. 592 p.)

Exercise	Muscles	Position	Instructions
Horizontal abduction for horizontal adductors	■ Anterior deltoid Sternal portion of pectoralis major Coracobrachialis	Standing	Adduct arms to shoulder level with palms facing upward. Horizontally abduct both shoulders, keeping them at shoulder level. You may use a doorway to help assist with this movement. Ideally, both sides can be stretched simultaneously (as the tension from one side stabilizes the origin on the other side); however, this is not necessary, and effective stretches can be performed unilaterally. 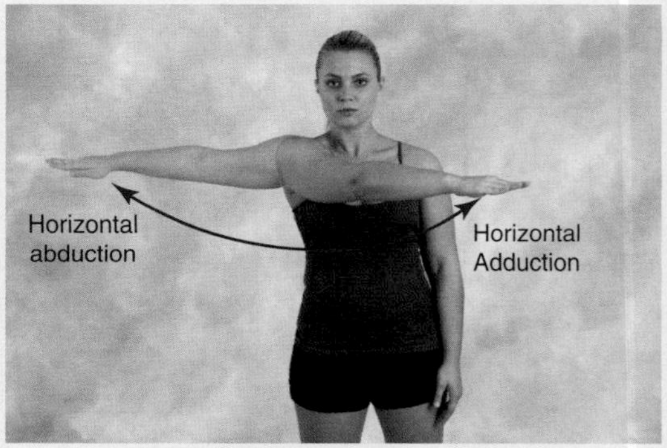
Horizontal adduction for horizontal abductors	■ Posterior deltoid Teres minor Infraspinatus Upper and middle trapezius Rhomboid major and minor via their attachment to the scapula	Standing	To stretch your left shoulder horizontal abductors, grasp the posterior aspect of your left elbow with your right hand. Horizontally adduct your left shoulder by pulling your left elbow horizontally across toward your right shoulder just beneath the chin. Repeat with the right.
External rotation for internal rotators	■ Subscapularis Latissimus dorsi Pectoralis major Teres major Anterior deltoid	Standing in a doorway, right arm at your side, elbow flexed to 90°, and palm facing forward against the doorframe	To stretch your right shoulder internal rotators, keep your right elbow at your side and right hand against the door frame, then carefully turn your body toward the left until you feel a gentle stretch. Repeat for your left shoulder.

Continued

Table 5.4   Static Stretches for the Major Muscle Groups (continued)

Stretch	Muscle Involved	Starting Position	Description
Upper Body			
Shoulder			
Internal rotation for external rotators	Infraspinatus Teres minor Posterior deltoid	Standing	Internally rotate your left shoulder by placing your left hand behind your back with the palm facing posteriorly. Place the palm of your right hand over the anterior aspect of your left shoulder. Back into a doorway with the posterior surface of the left elbow against the door jam. While maintaining firm support of the anterior shoulder with the left palm and hand (do not let the shoulder push forward), carefully move your entire body backward, forcing the elbow forward, until an easy stretch is felt in your left shoulder. Repeat on the opposite side to stretch your right shoulder.
Elbow			
Extension for flexors	Long and short heads of the biceps brachii Brachialis Brachioradialis	Standing	Clasp your hands together behind your lower back, extend your elbows completely, and then externally rotate your arms so that your palms are facing your buttocks. Now extend both shoulders by lifting the hands up and away from your buttocks.

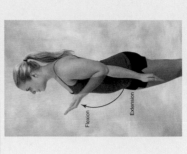

FIGURE 5.16. Elbow flexion and extension. (From Bushman B, editor. *ACSM's Resources for the Personal Trainer.* 4th ed. Baltimore [MD]: Lippincott Williams & Wilkins; 2014. 592 p.)

Continued

FIGURE 5.17. Elbow supination and pronation. (From Bushman B, editor. *ACSM's Resources for the Personal Trainer.* 4th ed. Baltimore [MD]: Lippincott Williams & Wilkins; 2014. 592 p.)

Flexion for extensors	■ Long, medial, and middle heads of the triceps brachii Anconeus	Standing	Extend your right arm overhead and flex your elbow maximally. Place the palm of your left hand against your right forearm just distal to the elbow, with your fingers curving over your right elbow. Squeeze your elbow joint to keep it maximally flexed, and then slowly pull it posteriorly and medially. Repeat with the left arm.
Pronation for supinators	■ Supinator Biceps brachii	Standing with arms relaxed at sides	To stretch the supinators of your right arm, flex your right elbow slightly and pronate your right forearm so that the palm is facing down. Using your left hand, grasp your right forearm just proximal to your wrist. Pronate your right forearm while externally rotating your right humerus. Repeat with the left forearm. 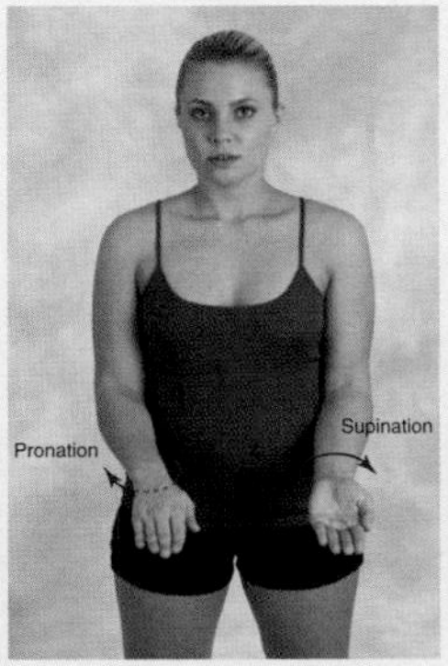
Supination for pronators	■ Pronator teres Pronator quadratus	Standing	To stretch the pronators of your right forearm, extend your right elbow and supinate your right hand. With your left hand, grasp your right forearm just proximal to the wrist. Using your left hand, rotate your right wrist externally, further supinating your right forearm. Be sure to keep your upper arm from externally rotating as well — this may require an active contraction of the shoulder internal rotators. Repeat with the left forearm.

Table 5.4 Static Stretches for the Major Muscle Groups (continued)

Stretch	Muscle Involved	Starting Position	Description
Upper Body			
Wrist and Hand			
Flexion for extensors	▪ Extensor carpi radialis Extensor digitorum Extensor indicis Extensor digiti minimi Extensor carpi radialis Extensor pollicis longus Extensor pollicis brevis	Sitting or standing	To stretch the extensors of your left arm and hand, extend your left arm out in front of you with your elbow extended, forearm pronated. Flex your left wrist and then attempt to flex fingers 2–5 into a fist. Repeat on the right arm. 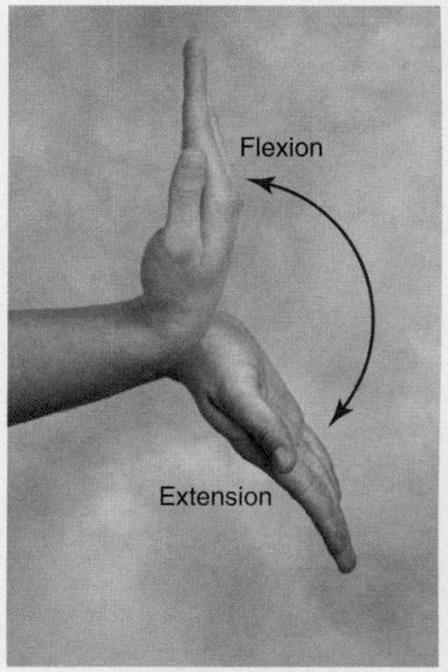
Extension for flexors	▪ Flexor carpi radialis Flexor digitorum profundus Flexor digitorum superficialis Palmaris longus Flexor pollicis longus Flexor carpi ulnaris	Sitting or standing	To stretch the flexors of your left wrist and hand, extend your left arm out in front of you with your elbow extended and palm supinated. Use your right hand to extend the fingers and the wrist of your left hand by carefully pulling the fingers back toward you. Repeat with the right.

FIGURE 5.18. Wrist extension and flexion. (From Bushman B, editor. *ACSM's Resources for the Personal Trainer.* 4th ed. Baltimore [MD]: Lippincott Williams & Wilkins; 2014. 592 p.)

Fingers

Extension and abduction for flexors and adductors	Umbricales Interossei (plantar adductors, dorsal abductors) Flexor pollicis brevis Abductor pollicis brevis Abductor pollicis longus Flexor digiti minimi Opponens pollicis Opponens digiti minimi	Sitting or standing with upper arms at sides, elbows flexed, and palms together	Place your hands together in front of you, matching your palms and fingers as if you are about to pray. With elbows flexed and wrists and fingers extended, elevate both elbows by flexing both shoulders, while lowering both hands extending the wrists. Keep palms together and finger matched. Now maximally abduct all fingers.

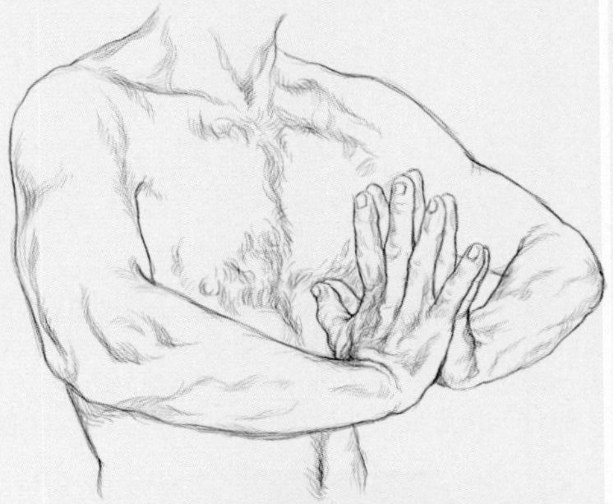

FIGURE 5.19. Finger flexion and adduction. (From Armiger P, Martyn M. *Stretching for Functional Flexibility*. Baltimore [MD]: Lippincott Williams & Wilkins; 2009. 464 p.)

Trunk

Flexion for extensors (Fig. 5.20A)	Multifidus Spinalis thoracis Longissimus thoracis Iliocostalis thoracis Quadratus lumborum Erector spinae	Lying on the floor, supine	Bring both of your knees up to your chest flexing both hips. Using your arms and hands, pull both of your knees closer to your chest. Continue pulling until your buttocks are off the floor, flexing your mid and lower spine. You may carefully flex your cervical and upper thoracic spine by pulling your head up toward your knees. 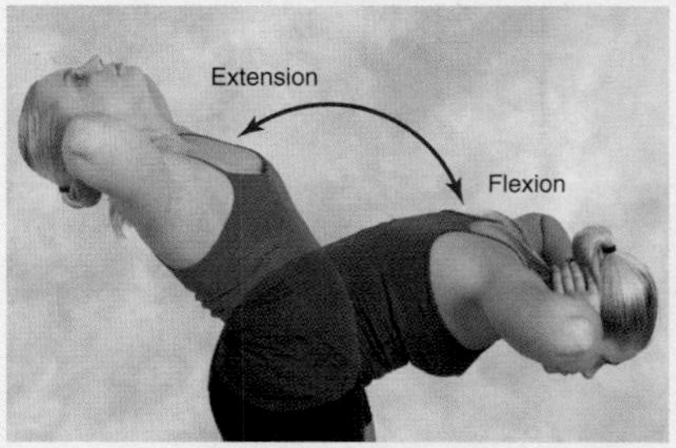
Extension for flexors (Fig. 5.20A)	Rectus abdominis External oblique Internal oblique	Lying on the floor, prone, with elbows flexed and palms on the floor just beneath the shoulders	Slowly attempt to press your chest and shoulders up and forward while taking care not to extend your head and neck. Your hip bones (ASIS) should remain in contact with the floor.

FIGURE 5.20. **A.** Trunk extension and flexion. *(continued)*

Continued

Table 5.4 Static Stretches for the Major Muscle Groups (continued)

Upper Body

Stretch	Muscle Involved	Starting Position	Description
Trunk			
Lateral flexors bending (Fig. 5.20B)	Internal oblique External oblique Iliocostalis lumborum Multifidus Quadratus lumborum	Lying on the floor on your left side	To stretch the lateral flexors on your left side, laterally flex your torso toward the right by pressing up with your left arm and hand. Be sure to bend directly sideways, staying in the frontal plane. Repeat on the right side.
Rotation (Fig. 5.20C)	Internal and external oblique Rotators Semispinalis Multifidus	Sitting on the floor with both legs extended	Straighten your spine and then step your left foot over and place it on the right side of your right knee. Now rotate your upper body and head toward the left, placing your right elbow against the lateral side of your left knee. Continue turning to the left by applying pressure against your left knee with your right elbow. Repeat on the opposite side.

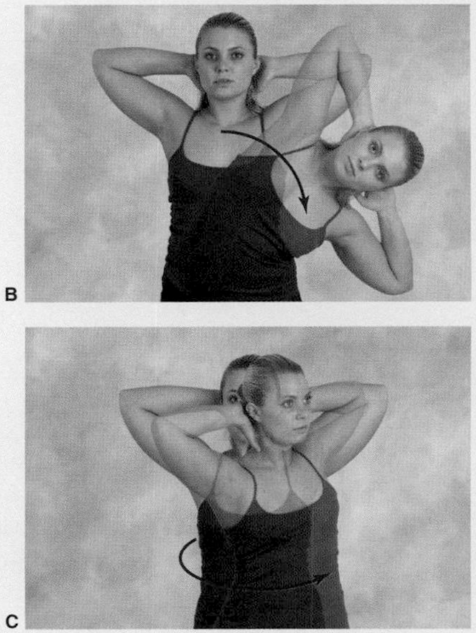

FIGURE 5.20. *(continued)* **B.** Trunk lateral flexion. **C.** Trunk rotation. (From Bushman B, editor. *ACSM's Resources for the Personal Trainer.* 4th ed. Baltimore [MD]: Lippincott Williams & Wilkins; 2014. 592 p.)

Continued

Lower Body

Hip

Flexors	Psoas major and minor Iliacus Rectus femoris Sartorius Tensor fasciae latae	Standing	To stretch the hip flexors on your right side, first step forward about 2 ft with your left foot. While keeping your torso and hips facing forward, move your upper body and hips anteriorly over your left foot by flexing your left knee and allowing a relaxed flexion in your right knee and ankle. You may allow your right heel to come off the floor. Contract your abdominals to keep your lower back from extending. Repeat on your left side.
Extensors	Gluteus maximus Hamstrings Semimembranosus Semitendinosus Long head of biceps femoris	Lying supine	To stretch the hip extensors on your left side, grasp your left knee with your right hand. Using your right arm and hand, pull your left knee up and across your torso toward your right shoulder, flexing and adducting your left hip. While keeping your knee in this position, actively extend your left knee to add stretch to the hamstrings, which also extend the hip. Repeat on the opposite side.
Adductors	Adductor magnus Adductor longus Adductor brevis Pectineus gracilis	Lying on the floor with knees extended and legs abducted	Using the abductors of your hips, abduct your legs to their end range. You may assist this stretch by placing the medial borders of your feet against a wall. As you achieve a stretching sensation, you can scoot your feet slightly farther apart on the wall.
Abductors	Gluteus medius Gluteus minimus Tensor fasciae latae	Standing	To stretch your left hip abductors, step forward and toward the left with your right foot so that your right foot rests just ahead and to the left of your left foot. Using your left hand, reach overhead and toward the right. Continue bending toward the right with your upper body

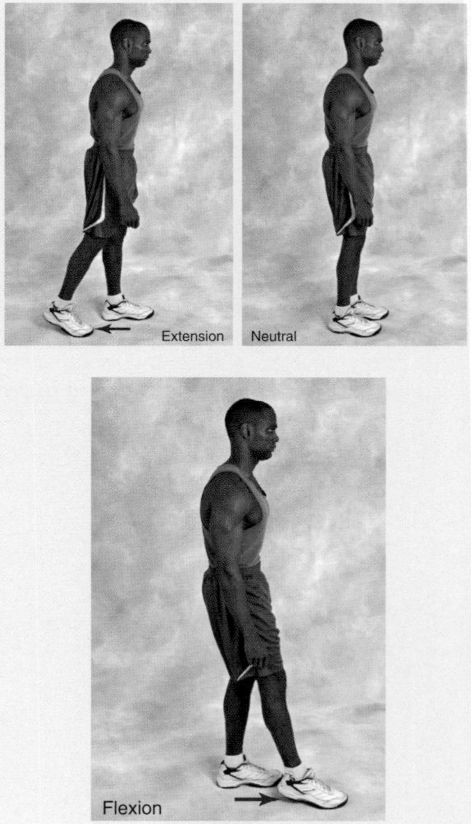

FIGURE 5.21. Hip flexion and extension. (From Bushman B, editor. *ACSM's Resources for the Personal Trainer.* 4th ed. Baltimore [MD]: Lippincott Williams & Wilkins; 2014. 592 p.)

Table 5.4 Static Stretches for the Major Muscle Groups (continued)

Stretch	Muscle Involved	Starting Position	Description
Hip			
Internal rotators	■ Anterior fibers of the gluteus medius Hip adductors and medial hamstrings (semimembranosus and semitendinosus)	Lying supine, with the left knee flexed to 90°	To stretch the internal rotators of your left hip, place the ankle of your left leg on top of and across the right thigh, making sure that the lateral lower left leg is lying on top of the right femur. Now, place your left hand on your left knee and carefully press it toward the floor, taking care not to let your hips twist. Repeat on the right. 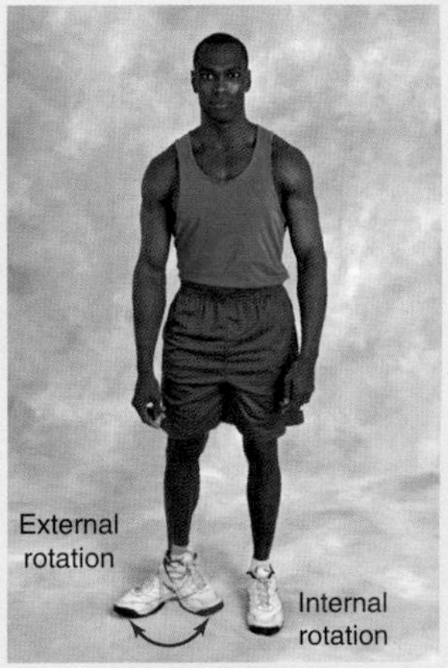
External rotators	■ Piriformis Gluteus maximus Posterior fibers of gluteus medius Inferior and superior gemelli Obturator internus and externus Quadratus femoris	Lying on the floor, supine	To stretch the external rotators of your left hip, flex your left hip to just above 90°. Next, adduct your left hip by pulling your left knee over toward the right by pulling with your right hand. You may allow your left hip/buttock to come slightly off the floor. Repeat for the right hip.

FIGURE 5.22. Hip internal rotation and external rotation. (From Bushman B, editor. *ACSM's Resources for the Personal Trainer.* 4th ed. Baltimore [MD]: Lippincott Williams & Wilkins; 2014. 592 p.)

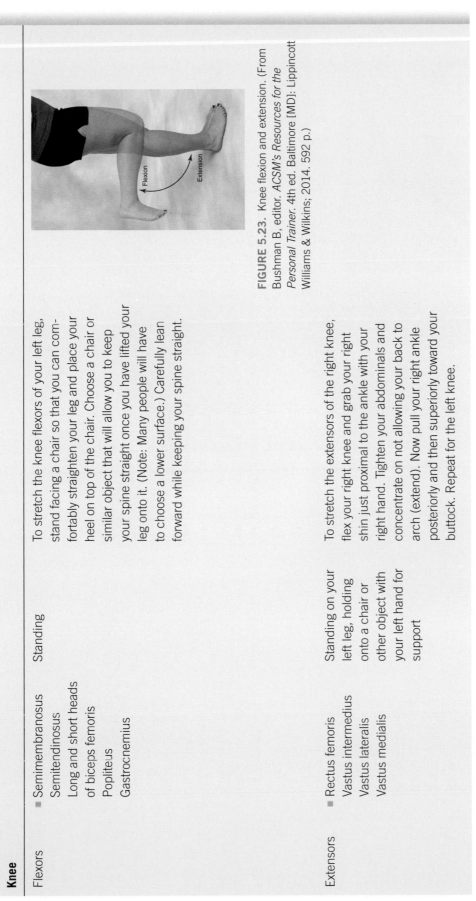

FIGURE 5.23. Knee flexion and extension. (From Bushman B, editor. *ACSM's Resources for the Personal Trainer.* 4th ed. Baltimore [MD]: Lippincott Williams & Wilkins; 2014. 592 p.)

Continued

Knee

Flexors	■ Semimembranosus Semitendinosus Long and short heads of biceps femoris Popliteus Gastrocnemius	Standing	To stretch the knee flexors of your left leg, stand facing a chair so that you can comfortably straighten your leg and place your heel on top of the chair. Choose a chair or similar object that will allow you to keep your spine straight once you have lifted your leg onto it. (Note: Many people will have to choose a lower surface.) Carefully lean forward while keeping your spine straight.
Extensors	■ Rectus femoris Vastus intermedius Vastus lateralis Vastus medialis	Standing on your left leg, holding onto a chair or other object with your left hand for support	To stretch the extensors of the right knee, flex your right knee and grab your right shin just proximal to the ankle with your right hand. Tighten your abdominals and concentrate on not allowing your back to arch (extend). Now pull your right ankle posteriorly and then superiorly toward your buttock. Repeat for the left knee.

Table 5.4 Static Stretches for the Major Muscle Groups (continued)

Stretch	Muscle Involved	Starting Position	Description
Lower Body			
Ankle and Foot			
Extensors (dorsiflexors)	■ Anterior tibialis Extensor digitorum longus Extensor digitorum brevis Extensor hallucis longus Extensor hallucis brevis Peroneus tertius	Standing	To stretch the extensors of the right ankle, foot, and toes, flex the right knee and plantar flex the foot and toes. Place the dorsum of your right foot and toes on the floor about 18 in behind you. Slowly bend your left knee, applying a gentle stretch to your right ankle, foot, and toes, bending them further into plantar flexion. Repeat on the left.
Flexors (plantar flexors)	■ Gastrocnemius Soleus Peroneus brevis Posterior tibialis Flexor digitorum longus Flexor digitorum brevis Flexor hallucis longus Flexor hallucis brevis	Standing	To stretch the flexors of the ankle, foot, and toes of your right leg, step forward about 18 in with your left foot. Flex both knees while keeping your right heel on the ground. Maintain a neutral-to-high right arch (this may require a slight external rotation of your right tibia). You may move slightly forward over your left foot. Repeat to stretch the left ankle, foot, and toes.

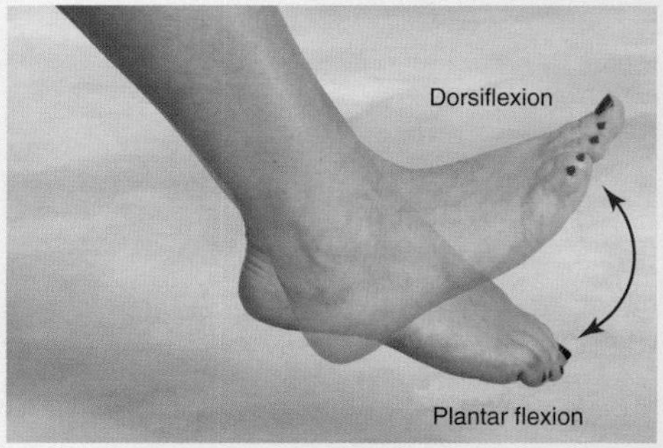

FIGURE 5.24. Ankle dorsiflexion and plantarflexion. (From Bushman B, editor. *ACSM's Resources for the Personal Trainer.* 4th ed. Baltimore [MD]: Lippincott Williams & Wilkins; 2014. 592 p.)

Invertors	Tibialis posterior Tibialis anterior Flexor digitorum longus Flexor hallucis longus	Seated with your left ankle supported across your right knee	To stretch the invertors of the left foot, use your right hand to dorsiflex the toes of your left foot and then continue to push your left forefoot into dorsiflexion and eversion (sole of the foot away from you). Repeat for the right foot.
Evertors	Peroneus longus, brevis, and tertius Extensor digitorum longus	Standing	To stretch the evertors of your right footstep, place your right foot on top of your left foot. Now carefully align your right foot to roll over onto its outside edge. Next, bend carefully bend your right knee, moving it forward. Repeat for the left foot.
Toes			
Extensors	Extensor digitorum longus Extensor digitorum brevis Extensor hallucis longus Extensor hallucis brevis Extensor digiti minimi	Seated with left ankle crossed over your right knee	To stretch the extensors of your left foot and toes, place your right hand over the dorsal surface of the toes of your left foot. Carefully flex all five toes toward dorsal surface of your foot. Repeat for the right foot.

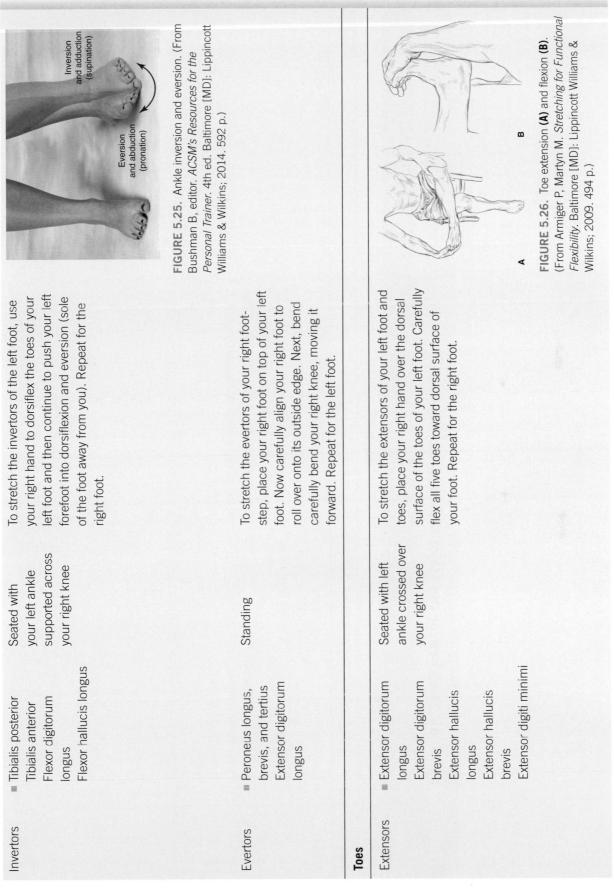

FIGURE 5.25. Ankle inversion and eversion. (From Bushman B, editor. *ACSM's Resources for the Personal Trainer.* 4th ed. Baltimore [MD]: Lippincott Williams & Wilkins; 2014. 592 p.)

FIGURE 5.26. Toe extension **(A)** and flexion **(B)**. (From Armiger P, Martyn M. *Stretching for Functional Flexibility.* Baltimore [MD]: Lippincott Williams & Wilkins; 2009. 494 p.)

Continued

Table 5.4   Static Stretches for the Major Muscle Groups (continued)

Stretch	Muscle Involved	Starting Position	Description
Lower Body			
Toes			
Flexors	■ Flexor digitorum longus Flexor digitorum brevis Flexor hallucis longus Flexor hallucis brevis Flexor digiti minimi brevis	Seated with your left ankle crossed over the right knee	To stretch the toe flexors of your left foot, grasp the toes of your left foot with the fingers and palm of your right hand. Extend all five toes and dorsiflex your ankle by pushing the toes toward the shin and allowing the ankle to dorsiflex. Repeat for your right foot.

> ### HOW TO   Perform the Sit-and-Reach Test
>
> Pretest: Before testing, the participant should remove his or her shoes and perform a short warm-up of approximately 5-minute moderate aerobic activity followed by a few select flexibility exercises. It is also recommended that the participant refrain from fast, jerky movements.
>
> For the Canadian Trunk Forward Flexion test, the client sits without shoes and the soles of the feet flat against the flexometer (sit-and-reach box) at the 26-cm mark. Inner edges of the soles are placed within 2 cm of the measuring scale.
>
> The participant should slowly reach forward with both hands as far as possible, holding this position approximately 2 seconds. Be sure that the participant keeps the hands parallel and does not lead with one hand. Fingertips can be overlapped and should be in contact with the measuring portion of the sit-and-reach box.
>
> The score is the most distant point (in centimeters or inches) reached with the fingertips. The best of two trials should be recorded. To assist with the best attempt, the participant should exhale and drop the head between the arms when reaching (and otherwise breath normally, never holding breath). Testers should ensure that the knees of the participant stay extended; however, the participant's knees should not be pressed down. Norms for the Canadian test are presented in Table 5.2. Note that these norms use a sit-and-reach box in which the zero point is set at the 26-cm mark. If you are using a box in which the zero point is set at 23 cm (*e.g.,* FitnessGram), subtract 3 cm from each value in this table.
>
> Source: Reprinted with permission from Canadian Society for Exercise Physiology. *Canadian Society for Exercise Physiology — Physical Activity Training for Health (CSEP-PATH).* Ottawa (Canada): Canadian Society for Exercise Physiology; 2013. 210 p. and YMCA of the USA. *YMCA Fitness Testing and Assessment Manual.* 4th ed. Champaign (IL): Human Kinetics; 2000. p. 158–60. 250 p.

Overall Range of Motion Recommendations

To determine appropriate program design, one must differentiate between flexibility training with the sole purpose of increasing ROM (often using static stretching) and flexibility exercises with the primary purpose of preparing for fitness training or sport-specific training. The former may be necessary for someone who has limited ROM due to genetics or disuse because of injury or lack of activity. The latter is generally part of a dynamic warm-up prior to more intense or skill-dependent exercise and therefore allows for better preparation (35,99). However, ROM warm-up activities that do not include a dynamic component (and therefore do not tend to increase body temperature, blood flow, etc.) have not shown a benefit to performance or reduction in injury rate during subsequent activity (38,54,55,82,85,99,106).

Acute beneficial effects from static flexibility exercise as it relates to performance are not well supported. Preactivity static flexibility training has been shown to decrease strength, sprint performance, endurance performance, and efficiency because it relates to energy expenditure and power output (52–55,106). With the demonstrated detrimental effects of static stretching, it is therefore recommended that preactivity ROM be dynamic and/or that flexibility programming occur postactivity or during the training session. Dynamic exercise during the warm-up period with the purpose of increasing body temperature and blood flow will naturally increase ROM during the activity. To date, there is not sufficient evidence to advocate against routine flexibility exercises, especially those following, or separate from, other exercise sessions (6), as chronic increases in ROM have yielded conflicting results related to injury prevention and performance. In addition, some research has demonstrated a reduction of overuse injuries among individuals with increased flexibility (34), whereas others demonstrate that typical muscle stretching programs do not produce a reduction in exercise-related injuries (85). Perhaps, the most prudent recommendation to the health professional is to assess individual client needs and requirements and determine the ROM necessary for desired activity. Initial assessment of joint-specific ROM to determine client status would be the first step in the development of a program. If the client is in need of increased ROM, it would be prudent to implement a flexibility training program as previously described. A client with adequate or hyper ROM may be placed on a maintenance program or focus on other areas of health-related fitness until time for reassessment.

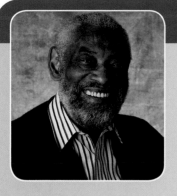

The Case of Allen

Submitted by **Stephanie Marie Otto, PhD, ACSM EP-C, Assistant Professor, Gustavus Adolphus College, St. Peter, MN**

Allen is a retired Navy officer who experienced tightening in his chest and dizziness during a recent walk.

Narrative

Allen retired from the Navy 10 years ago and is currently not working. He spends his days gardening and playing with his four grandchildren. Every morning, he walks along the beach for 20 minutes, and he regularly engages in strength-training activities from his Navy days, but he never has done much flexibility exercise. Allen has played bingo twice a week at the local bingo hall for the past year, but his wife complains because he comes home smelling of smoke. During a recent walk, Allen experienced tightness in his chest and dizziness. He is concerned and not sure what to do. He cannot believe he might be at risk for cardiovascular disease. He comes to you for advice and guidance. After your some preliminary testing and information gathering, you discover that Allen's blood pressure is 160/88 mm Hg, and he also revealed to you that his father passed away from a heart attack at the age of 53 years. His total cholesterol is 190 mg $\cdot$ dL^{-1}, low-density lipoprotein is 149 mg $\cdot$ dL^{-1}, and high-density lipoprotein is 43 mg $\cdot$ dL^{-1}. Allen is 58 years old, and his body mass index is 23. Allen came in a year ago for an assessment, and his results were as follows.

Aerobic fitness ($\dot{V}O_{2max}$): 40.3 mL $\cdot$ kg^{-1} $\cdot$ min^{-1}
(no chest pain reported during this exercise test)
Upper body strength (bench press weight ratio): 0.98
Leg strength (leg press weight ratio): 1.97

Push-ups: 32
Curl-ups: 28
YMCA sit-and-reach: 4 in
Skinfold: 19.1%

Allen is worried about his experience during his last walk and comes to you for advice about his current activity participation and lifestyle. He cannot understand how this could be happening to him since he has been active for most of his life and worked hard to control his weight.

Goals

Goal 1: Improve flexibility.
Goal 2: Understand what may have been causing the chest pain and dizziness during his last walk.
Goal 3: Maintain current weight.

QUESTIONS

- Given the information above, identify the risk factors and determine the risk stratification for Allen.
- How would you proceed after this initial conversation with Allen?
- Assuming Allen is cleared for exercise, how would you plan for his next session with you?
- What other lifestyle factors would you want to discuss with Allen that are contributing to his risk of developing cardiovascular disease?
- Assuming Allen is cleared for exercise, and considering his goals, what would you recommend as an activity plan?

References

1. American College of Sports Medicine. *ACSM's Guidelines for Exercise Testing and Prescription.* 8th ed. Philadelphia (PA): Lippincott Williams & Wilkins; 2010. 400 p.
2. Neiman D. *Exercise Testing and Prescription: A Health Related Approach.* 7th ed. New York (NY): McGraw Hill; 2011. 672 p.
3. Garber CE, Blissmer B, Deschenes MR, et al. Quantity and quality of exercise for developing and maintaining cardiorespiratory, musculoskeletal, and neuromotor fitness in apparently healthy adults: guidance for prescribing exercise. *Med Sci Sports Exerc.* 2011;43(7):1334–59.

SUMMARY

Development and maintenance of flexibility is one of the five components of health-related fitness, and maintaining an adequate ROM is important for activities of daily living. Nevertheless, controversy exists in regard to the overall benefits of flexibility training for injury prevention or sport performance. Because flexibility training involves multiple modes, the EP-C can choose which is best for each client and implement these as part of a dynamic warm-up or during the cool-down phase of exercise. Many different methods and tools are used to assess ROM and flexibility. Among the most common are the use of goniometers for the measurement of ROM and the sit-and-reach tests for the measurement of distance. Overall, flexibility exercise prescription depends on the mode of the exercise and should be set on the basis of established ACSM guidelines.

STUDY QUESTIONS

1. Characterize the various modes of flexibility training, including the advantages and disadvantages of each.
2. Differentiate between the two types of sensory organs that provide muscular dynamic and limb movement information to the central nervous system with respect to location and function.
3. Design a sample static flexibility exercise prescription based on the FITT principle.
4. Assess the controversy that surrounds the need for flexibility training with respect to health and athletic performance.

REFERENCES

1. American College of Sports Medicine. *ACSM's Guidelines for Exercise Testing and Prescription*. 10th ed. Philadelphia (PA): Lippincott Williams & Wilkins; 2018.

2. American College of Sports Medicine Position Stand. The recommended quantity and quality of exercise for developing and maintaining cardiorespiratory and muscular fitness, and flexibility in healthy adults. *Med Sci Sports Exerc*. 1998;30(6):975–91.

3. Baechle TR, Earle RW, editors. *Essentials of Strength Training and Conditioning*. 3rd ed. Champaign (IL): Human Kinetics; 2008. 656 p.

4. Bandy WD, Irion JM. The effect of time on static stretch on the flexibility of the hamstring muscles. *Phys Ther*. 1994;74(9):845–50; discussion 850–2.

5. Bandy WD, Irion JM, Briggler M. The effect of static stretch and dynamic range of motion training on the flexibility of the hamstring muscles. *J Orthop Sports Phys Ther*. 1998;27(4):295–300.

6. Bandy WD, Irion JM, Briggler M. The effect of time and frequency of static stretching on flexibility of the hamstring muscles. *Phys Ther*. 1997;77(10):1090–6.

7. Barroso R, Tricoli V, Dos Santos Gil S, Ugrinowitsch C, Roschel H. Maximal strength, number of repetitions, and total volume are different affected by static-, ballistic-, and proprioceptive neuromuscular facilitation stretching. *J Strength Cond Res*. 2012;26(9):2432–7.

8. Behm DG, Bambury A, Cahill F, Power K. Effect of acute static stretching on force, balance, reaction time, and movement time. *Med Sci Sports Exerc*. 2004;36(8):1397–402.

9. Chatzopoulos D, Galazoulas C, Patikas D, Kotzamanidis C. Acute effects of static and dynamic stretching on balance, agility, reaction time, and movement time. *J Sports Sci Med*. 2014;13(2):403–9.

10. Chen CH, Nosaka K, Chen HL, Lin MJ, Tseng KW, Chen TC. Effects of flexibility training on eccentric exercise-induced muscle damage. *Med Sci Sports Exerc*. 2011;43(3):491–500.

11. Cherry DB. Review of physical therapy alternatives for reducing muscle contracture. *Phys Ther*. 1980;60(7):877–81.

12. Church JB, Wiggins MS, Moode FM, Crist R. Effect of warm-up and flexibility treatments on vertical jump performance. *J Strength Cond Res*. 2001;15(3):332–6.

13. Clark L, O'Leary CB, Hong J, & Lockard M. The acute effects of stretching on presynaptic inhibition and peak power. *J Sports Med Phys Fitness*. 2014;54(5):605–10.

14. Condon SM, Hutton RS. Soleus muscle electromyographic activity and ankle dorsiflexion range of motion during four stretching procedures. *Phys Ther*.1987;67(1):24–30.

15. Cornelius WL. Flexibility exercise: effective practices. *Natl Str Cond Assoc J*. 1989;11(6):61–2.

16. Cornelius WL, Hinson MM. The relationship between isometric contractions of hip extensors and subsequent flexibility in males. *J Sports Med Phys Fitness*. 1980;20(1):75–80.

17. Cramer JT, Housh TJ, Weir JP, Johnson GO, Coburn JW, Beck TW. The acute effects of static stretching on peak torque, mean power output, electromyography, and mechanomyography. *Eur J Appl Physiol*. 2005;93(5–6):530–9.

18. Decoster LC, Cleland J, Altieri C, Russell P. The effects of hamstring stretching on range of motion: a systematic literature review. *J Orthop Sports Phys Ther*. 2005;35(6):377–87.

19. Depino GM, Webright WG, Arnold BL. Duration of maintained hamstring flexibility after cessation of an acute static stretching protocol. *J Athl Train*. 2000;35(1):56–9.

20. de Weijer VC, Gorniak GC, Shamus E. The effect of static stretch and warm-up exercise on hamstring length over the course of 24 hours. *J Orthop Sports Phys Ther*. 2003;33(12):727–33.

21. Ellenbecker TS, Roetert EP, Piorkowski PA, Schulz DA. Glenohumeral joint internal and external rotation range of motion in elite junior tennis players. *J Orthop Sports Phys Ther*. 1996;24(6):336–41.

22. Feland JB, Myrer JW, Schulthies SS, Fellingham GW, Measom GW. The effect of duration of stretching of the hamstring muscle group for increasing range of motion in people aged 65 years or older. *Phys Ther*. 2001;81(5):1110–7.

23. Freitas SR, Vilarinho D, Rocha Vaz J, Bruno PM, Costa PB, Mil-homens P. Responses to static stretching are dependent on stretch intensity and duration. *Clin Physiol Funct Imaging*. 2015;35(6):478–84.

24. Friedrich LJ. *A Treatise on Gymnastics*. Northampton (MA): Simeon and Butler; 1828. 216 p.

25. Garber CE, Blissmer B, Deschenes MR, et al. Quantity and quality of exercise for developing and maintaining cardiorespiratory, musculoskeletal, and neuromotor fitness in apparently healthy adults: guidance for prescribing exercise. *Med Sci Sports Exerc*. 2011;43(7):1334–59.

26. Getchell B. *Physical Fitness: A Way of Life*. 2nd ed. New York (NY): Wiley; 1979. 352 p.

27. Gleim GW. The profiling of professional football players. *Clin Sports Med*. 1984;3(1):185–97.

28. Gleim GW, McHugh MP. Flexibility and its effects on sports injury and performance. *Sports Med*. 1997;24(5):289–99.

29. Godges JJ, Macrae H, Longdon C, Tinberg C, Macrae PG. The effects of two stretching procedures on hip range of motion and gait economy. *J Orthop Sports Phys Ther*. 1989;10(9):350–7.

30. Guyton AC, Hall JE. *Textbook of Medical Physiology*. 11th ed. Philadelphia (PA): Elsevier Saunders; 2006. 1116 p.

31. Haff GG. Roundtable discussion: flexibility training. *Strength Cond*. 2006;28(2):64–85.

32. Hall SJ. *Basic Biomechanics*. 5th ed. Boston (MA): McGraw-Hill; 2007. 544 p.

33. Handrakis JP, Southard VN, Abreu JM, et al. Static stretching does not impair performance in active middle-aged adults. *J Strength Cond Res*. 2010;24(3):825–30.

34. Hartig DE, Henderson JM. Increasing hamstring flexibility decreases lower extremity overuse injuries in military basic trainees. *Am J Sports Med*. 1999;27(2):173–6.

35. Harvey L, Herbert R, Crosbie J. Does stretching induce lasting increases in joint ROM? A systematic review. *Physiother Res Int*. 2002;7(1):1–13.

36. Hedrick A. Dynamic flexibility training. *Strength Cond J*. 2000;22(5):33–8.

37. Hedrick A. Flexibility: flexibility and the conditioning program. *Natl Str Cond Assoc J*. 1993;15(4):62–7.

38. Herbert RD, Gabriel M. Effects of stretching before and after exercising on muscle soreness and risk of injury: systematic review. *BMJ*. 2002;325(7362):468.

39. Hindle KB, Whitcomb TJ, Briggs WO, Hong J. Proprioceptive neuromuscular facilitation (PNF): its mechanism and effects on range of motion and muscular function. *J Hum Kinet*. 2012;31:105–113.

40. Holt J, Holt LE, Pelhan TW. Flexibility redefined. In: Bauer T, editor. *XIIIth International Symposium for Biomechanics in Sport*. Ontario (Canada): Lakehead University; 1996. p. 170–4.

41. Holt LE, Travis TM, Okita T. Comparative study of three stretching techniques. *Percept Mot Skills*. 1970;31(2):611–6.

42. Houck JC, De Hesse C, Jacob R. The effect of ageing upon collagen metabolism. *Symp Soc Exp Biol*. 1967;21:403–25.

43. Hubley CL, Kozey JW, Stanish WD. The effects of static stretching exercises and stationary cycling on range of motion at the hip joint. *J Orthop Sports Phys Ther*. 1984;6(2):104–9.

44. Hunter JP, Marshall RN. Effects of power and flexibility training on vertical jump technique. *Med Sci Sports Exerc*. 2002;34(3):478–86.

45. Huston KA. Achilles tendinitis and tendon rupture due to fluoroquinolone antibiotics. *N Engl J Med*. 1994;331(11):748.

46. Information for Healthcare Professionals: Fluoroquinolone Antimicrobial Drugs [ciprofloxacin (marketed as Cipro and generic ciprofloxacin), ciprofloxacin extended-release (marketed as Cipro XR and Proquin XR), gemifloxacin (marketed as Factive), levofloxacin (marketed as Levaquin), moxifloxacin (marketed as Avelox), norfloxacin (marketed as Noroxin), and ofloxacin (marketed as Floxin)] [Internet]. Silver Spring (MD): U.S. Food and Drug Administration; [cited 2015 September 1]. Available from: http://www.fda.gov

47. Jackson AW, Morrow JR Jr, Brill PA, Kohl HW III, Gordon NF, Blair SN. Relations of sit-up and sit-and-reach tests to low back pain in adults. *J Orthop Sports Phys Ther*. 1998;27(1):22–6.

48. Johns RJ, Wright V. Relative importance of various tissues in joint stiffness. *J Appl Physiol*. 1962;17(5):824–8.

49. Kato E, Toshiaki O, Kentaro C, et al. Musculotendinous factors influencing difference in ankle joint flexibility between men and women. *Int J Sport Health Sci*. 2005;3:218–25.

50. Kerrigan DC, Xenopoulos-Oddsson A, Sullivan MJ, Lelas JJ, Riley PO. Effect of a hip flexor-stretching program on gait in the elderly. *Arch Phys Med Rehabil*. 2003;84(1):1–6.

51. Kisner C, Colby LA. *Therapeutic Exercise: Foundations and Techniques*. 4th ed. Philadelphia (PA): F.A. Davis; 2002. 844 p.

52. Kistler BM, Walsh MS, Horn TS, Cox RH. The acute effects of static stretching on the sprint performance of collegiate men in the 60- and 100-m dash after a dynamic warm-up. *J Strength Cond Res*. 2010;24(9):2280–4.

53. Knapik JJ, Bauman CL, Jones BH, Harris JM, Vaughan L. Preseason strength and flexibility imbalances associated with athletic injuries in female collegiate athletes. *Am J Sports Med*. 1991;19(1):76–81.

54. Knudson D, Noffal G. Time course of stretch-induced isometric strength deficits. *Eur J Appl Physiol*. 2005;94(3):348–51.

55. Knudson DV, Noffal GJ, Bahamonde RE, Bauer JA, Blackwell JR. Stretching has no effect on tennis serve performance. *J Strength Cond Res*. 2004;18(3):654–6.

56. Kraus H, Hirschland R. Minimum muscular fitness tests in school children. *Res Q*. 1954;25:178–88.

57. Lamontagne A, Malouin F, Richards CL. Viscoelastic behavior of plantar flexor muscle-tendon unit at rest. *J Orthop Sports Phys Ther*. 1997;26(5):244–52.

58. Lea RD, Gerhardt JJ. Range-of-motion measurements. *J Bone Joint Surg Am*. 1995;77(5):784–98.

59. Leighton JR. A study of the effect of progressive weight training on flexibility. *J Assoc Phys Ment Rehabil*. 1964;18:101–4.

60. Liguori G, Carroll-Cobb S. *FitWell: Questions and Answers*. New York (NY): McGraw Hill; 2011. 512 p.

61. Lucas RC, Koslow R. Comparative study of static, dynamic, and proprioceptive neuromuscular facilitation stretching techniques on flexibility. *Percept Mot Skills*. 1984;58(2):615–8.

62. Magnusson SP, Gleim GW, Nicholas JA. Shoulder weakness in professional baseball pitchers. *Med Sci Sports Exerc*. 1994;26(1):5–9.

63. Magnusson SP, Simonsen EB, Aagaard P, Sorensen H, Kjaer M. A mechanism for altered flexibility in human skeletal muscle. *J Physiol*. 1996;497(Pt 1):291–8.

64. Magnusson SP, Simonsen EB, Dyhre-Poulsen P, Aagaard P, Mohr T, Kjaer M. Viscoelastic stress relaxation during static stretch in human skeletal muscle in the absence of EMG activity. *Scand J Med Sci Sports*. 1996;6(6):323–8.

65. Mahieu NN, McNair P, De Muynck M, et al. Effect of static and ballistic stretching on the muscle-tendon tissue properties. *Med Sci Sports Exerc*. 2007;39(3):494–501.

66. Mann DP, Jones MT. Guidelines to the implementation of a dynamic stretching program. *Strength Cond J*. 1999;21(6):53–55.

67. Marek SM, Cramer JT, Fincher AL, et al. Acute effects of static and proprioceptive neuromuscular facilitation stretching on muscle strength and power output. *J Athl Train*. 2005;40(2):94–103.

68. McArdle WD, Katch FI, Katch VL. *Exercise Physiology: Energy, Nutrition, and Human Performance*. 6th ed. Philadelphia (PA): Lippincott Williams & Wilkins; 2007. 1068 p.

69. McGlynn GH, Laughlin NT, Rowe V. Effect of electromyographic feedback and static stretching on artificially induced muscle soreness. *Am J Phys Med*. 1979;58(3):139–48.

70. McMillian DJ, Moore JH, Hatler BS, Taylor DC. Dynamic vs. static-stretching warm up: the effect on power and agility performance. *J Strength Cond Res*. 2006;20(3):492–9.

71. McNeal JR, Sands WA. Stretching for performance enhancement. *Curr Sports Med Rep*. 2006;5(3):141–6.

72. Moonaz S, Bingham C III, Wissow L, Bartlett S. Yoga in sedentary adults with arthritis: effects of a randomized controlled pragmatic trial. *J Rheumatol*. 2015;42(7);1194–202.

73. Moore MA, Hutton RS. Electromyographic investigation of muscle stretching techniques. *Med Sci Sports Exerc*. 1980;12(5):322–9.

74. Needham RA, Morse CI, Degens H. The acute effect of different warm-up protocols on anaerobic performance in elite youth soccer players. *J Strength Cond Res*. 2009;23(9):2614–20.

75. Nelson AG, Kokkonen J. Acute ballistic muscle stretching inhibits maximal strength performance. *Res Q Exerc Sport*. 2001;72(4):415–9.

76. Nelson RT. A comparison of the immediate effects of eccentric training vs static stretch on hamstring flexibility in

high school and college athletes. *N Am J Sports Phys Ther.* 2006;1(2):56–61.

77. Nelson RT, Bandy WD. Eccentric training and static stretching improve hamstring flexibility of high school males. *J Athl Train.* 2004;39(3):254–8.

78. Noakes T. *Lore of Running.* 4th ed. Champaign (IL): Human Kinetics; 2003. 931 p.

79. Noonan TJ, Best TM, Seaber AV, Garrett WE Jr. Thermal effects on skeletal muscle tensile behavior. *Am J Sports Med.* 1993;21(4):517–22.

80. Oberg B, Ekstrand J, Moller M, Gillquist J. Muscle strength and flexibility in different positions of soccer players. *Int J Sports Med.* 1984;5(4):213–6.

81. O'Brien M. Functional anatomy and physiology of tendons. *Clin Sports Med.* 1992;11(3):505–20.

82. Park DY, Chou L. Stretching for prevention of Achilles tendon injuries: a review of the literature. *Foot Ankle Int.* 2006;27(12):1086–95.

83. Park SK, Stefanyshyn DJ, Loitz-Ramage B, Hart DA, Ronsky JL. Changing hormone levels during the menstrual cycle affect knee laxity and stiffness in healthy female subjects. *Am J Sports Med.* 2009;37(3):588–98.

84. Pieber K, Herceg M, Quittan M, Csapo R, Müller R, Wiesinger GF. Long-term effects of an outpatient rehabilitation program in patients with chronic recurrent low back pain. *Eur Spine J.* 2014;23(4):779–85.

85. Pope RP, Herbert RD, Kirwan JD, Graham BJ. A randomized trial of preexercise stretching for prevention of lower-limb injury. *Med Sci Sports Exerc.* 2000;32(2):271–7.

86. Raab DM, Agre JC, McAdam M, Smith EL. Light resistance and stretching exercise in elderly women: effect upon flexibility. *Arch Phys Med Rehabil.* 1988;69(4):268–72.

87. Roberts JM, Wilson K. Effect of stretching duration on active and passive range of motion in the lower extremity. *Br J Sports Med.* 1999;33(4):259–63.

88. Sady SP, Wortman M, Blanke D. Flexibility training: ballistic, static or proprioceptive neuromuscular facilitation? *Arch Phys Med Rehabil.* 1982;63(6):261–3.

89. Safran MR, Garrett WE Jr, Seaber AV, Glisson RR, Ribbeck BM. The role of warmup in muscular injury prevention. *Am J Sports Med.* 1988;16(2):123–9.

90. Sawyer PC, Uhl TL, Mattacola CG, Johnson DL, Yates JW. Effects of moist heat on hamstring flexibility and muscle temperature. *J Strength Cond Res.* 2003;17(2):285–90.

91. Shellock FG, Prentice WE. Warming-up and stretching for improved physical performance and prevention of sports-related injuries. *Sports Med.* 1985;2(4):267–78.

92. Shrier I. Does stretching improve performance? A systematic and critical review of the literature. *Clin J Sport Med.* 2004;14(5):267–73.

93. Simic L, Sarabon N, Markovic G. Does pre-exercise static stretching inhibit maximal muscular performance? A meta-analytical review. *Scand J Med Sci Sports.* 2013;23(2):131–48.

94. Smith LL, Brunetz MH, Chenier TC, et al. The effects of static and ballistic stretching on delayed onset muscle soreness and creatine kinase. *Res Q Exerc Sport.* 1993;64(1):103–7.

95. Sprague HA. Relationship of certain physical measurements to swimming speed. *Res Q.* 1976;47(4):810–4.

96. Strickler T, Malone T, Garrett WE. The effects of passive warming on muscle injury. *Am J Sports Med.* 1990;18(2):141–5.

97. Tanigawa MC. Comparison of the hold-relax procedure and passive mobilization on increasing muscle length. *Phys Ther.* 1972;52(7):725–35.

98. Taylor DC, Dalton JD Jr, Seaber AV, Garrett WE Jr. Viscoelastic properties of muscle-tendon units. The biomechanical effects of stretching. *Am J Sports Med.* 1990; 18(3):300–9.

99. Thacker SB, Gilchrist J, Stroup DF, Kimsey CD Jr. The impact of stretching on sports injury risk: a systematic review of the literature. *Med Sci Sports Exerc.* 2004;36(3):371–8.

100. The Cooper Institute. *Physical Fitness Assessments and Norms.* Dallas (TX): The Cooper Institute; 2005. 72 p.

101. Thompsen AG, Kackley T, Palumbo MA, Faigenbaum AD. Acute effects of different warm-up protocols with and without a weighted vest on jumping performance in athletic women. *J Strength Cond Res.* 2007;21(1):52–6.

102. Thompson WR. *ACSM's Guidelines for Exercise Testing and Prescription.* 8th ed. Philadelphia (PA): Lippincott Williams & Wilkins; 2009. 380 p.

103. Unick J, Kieffer HS, Cheesman W, Feeney A. The acute effects of static and ballistic stretching on vertical jump performance in trained women. *J Strength Cond Res.* 2005; 19(1):206–12.

104. Wallin D, Ekblom B, Grahn R, Nordenborg T. Improvement of muscle flexibility. A comparison between two techniques. *Am J Sports Med.* 1985;13(4):263–8.

105. Watkins J. *Structure and Function of the Musculoskeletal System.* 2nd ed. Champaign (IL): Human Kinetics; 2010. 96 p.

106. Wilson JM, Hornbuckle LM, Kim JS, et al. Effects of static stretching on energy cost and running endurance performance. *J Strength Cond Res.* 2010;24(9):2274–9.

107. Woolstenhulme MT, Griffiths CM, Woolstenhulme EM, Parcell AC. Ballistic stretching increases flexibility and acute vertical jump height when combined with basketball activity. *J Strength Cond Res.* 2006;20(4):799–803.

108. Worrell TW, Smith TL, Winegardner J. Effect of hamstring stretching on hamstring muscle performance. *J Orthop Sports Phys Ther.* 1994;20(3):154–9.

109. Young W, Clothier P, Otago L, Bruce L, Liddell D. Acute effects of static stretching on hip flexor and quadriceps flexibility, range of motion and foot speed in kicking a football. *J Sci Med Sport.* 2004;7(1):23–31.

110. Yuktasira B, Kayab F. Investigation into the long-term effects of static and PNF stretching exercises on range of motion and jump performance. *J Body Mov Ther.* 2009;13(1):11–21.

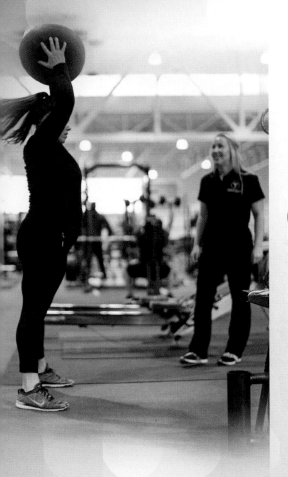

6

Functional Movement Assessments and Exercise Programming for Apparently Healthy Participants

OBJECTIVES

- To understand the integration of the motor system and the sensory system in developing motor patterns.

- To examine the importance of stability, mobility, and proprioception within the context of progressive exercise programing.

- To understand the relevance of optimizing posture for improved neuromuscular function.

- To identify the muscles commonly affected by neuro-muscular imbalances.

- To describe appropriate assessments and exercise prescription and self-myofascial release strategies to improve movement potential.

INTRODUCTION

One of the most salient features of successful strength and conditioning programs is progressively overloading the body to the extent that adaptation occurs. This progression is optimized when three fundamental features are present: sensory acuity, optimal stabilization strategies, and mobility. There are, however, a number of pervasive issues, including obesity and overweight, sedentary lifestyles, poor posture, improper training and aging that are known to compromise these preconditions of progression. With knowledge of biomechanics, motor control, and optimal alignment, the American College of Sports Medicine (ACSM) exercise practitioner is in a position to make the necessary program adjustments and offer lifestyle recommendations to accommodate for these ever-present issues. Ultimately, these accommodations can lay the foundation for optimal gains in functional capacity, strength, and performance.

 ## Sensorimotor Control

Motor Learning

During early phases of motor learning, performance is largely under conscious control, meaning a great deal of focus and concentration is needed in order to successfully perform the movement. Upon repeated practice, control of individual movements becomes integrated into motor patterns. These motor patterns are stored in the central nervous system (CNS), not unlike saving a document on a computer. Once motor patterns are integrated and stored, they become automatic and are fine-tuned by unconscious sensory feedback. The saving of motor patterns makes the neuromuscular system more efficient when the body is exposed to similar demands in the future. For this reason, after sufficient practice, we do not really have to think about riding a bike, hitting a golf ball, or performing a clean and jerk. The problem lies in the saving of faulty motor patterns, as once stored, motor patterns can be challenging to correct.

Proprioception

The sensory system and the motor control system, collectively known as the sensorimotor system, work together to control movement, balance, posture, and joint stability (15,24,31). Essentially, in order for optimal movement to occur, the body requires the brain to process afferent sensory information from multiple sources. Dr. Charles Sherrington (53) was the first to characterize this input as proprioception. Currently, proprioception is understood to be the sense of knowing where one's body is in space and is composed of static (joint position sense) and dynamic (kinesthetic movement sense) (16). Proprioception enables us, with closed eyes, to estimate the size of our feet, describe the width of our pelvis, and scratch our noses. Table 6.1 describes common movements that are derived from proprioceptive acuity. This sensory input is gathered from specialized nerve endings, termed mechanoreceptors, that are located within the skin, muscles, fascia, and joints (49). Information collected from visual and vestibular centers further supports proprioception, and when taken together, the result is precise body awareness and well-adapted motor actions (Fig. 6.1).

Proprioception is an important mediator of joint stability and mobility and ultimately the calibration of movement (18). It follows that this sensory acuity is central to safely perform

Table 6.1	Salient Features of Proprioceptive Acuity
Characteristic	**Example**
Postural control	Maintaining balance during perturbations (a force, such as a gentle tap or vibration, that is applied with the intention of altering balance)
Precise calibration of limb position in space	Threading a needle
Maintenance of steady muscle force production/ movement amplitudes	Unbroken, smooth motion during the eccentric and concentric phases of a dumbbell chest press
Discrimination of object weight	Tailoring the effort required to lift a 5-lb weight and a 25-lb weight
Production of coordinated gait patterns	Biomechanically efficient walking; running
Controlling the timing of muscular contraction for dynamic stabilization and multisegmental movement	Executing a tennis serve or a clean and jerk
Feedback and feed-forward motor control	Reaction time and anticipatory responses in a soccer game

many of the resistance training exercises that are included in conventional exercise programs. If there are disturbances in proprioception, reactive (feedback) and preparatory/anticipatory (feed-forward) motor control and stability will be altered, increasing the risk of injury (48). It is also important to note that problems with stability and/or mobility issues will perpetuate proprioceptive deficits. Figure 6.2 describes the afferent and efferent pathways involved in the sensorimotor system.

Key Point

Motor control is developed through enhancing proprioceptive acuity and grooving proper movement patterns through practice.

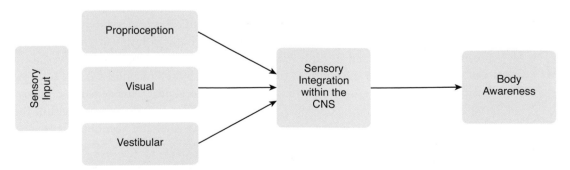

FIGURE 6.1. Sensory input from vestibular, visual, and proprioception are integrated within the central nervous system resulting in relatively keen body awareness.

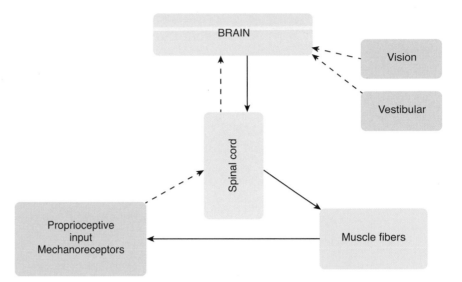

FIGURE 6.2. The sensorimotor system integrates all sensory (afferent) and muscular (efferent) activity. Afferent activity is indicated by the dotted lines, whereas the solid lines indicate efferent activity. (Adapted from Riemann BL, Lephart SM. The sensorimotor system, part I: the physiologic basis of functional joint stability. *J Athl Train*. 2002;37[1]:71–9.)

Stability and Mobility

There is a good reason why we prefer driving a car with aligned tires, lug nuts tightened, and fan belts secured. For example, if the fan belt is secured (stability), it can move at a very high speed (mobility) for many miles without wear and tear. If these requisite features are not present, we can expect to shell out money for repairs far sooner than the manufacturer originally predicted. We might also expect far-reaching changes to the overall structure and function of the car. The factors that contribute to the mechanical efficiency and the long life of our cars are akin to the features needed for optimal function in the body, stability, and mobility.

Stability has been defined as the state of remaining unchanged, even in the presence of forces that would normally change the state or condition (26). Others have defined stability as the state of a joint remaining or promptly returning to proper alignment through an equalization of forces (47). Joint stabilization then occurs through coordinated muscle coactivation, creating a suitable amount of stiffness to maintain joint alignment (35).

Stabilization strategies are managed at the subcortical level, where the generation of stability is somewhat automatic and requires quality proprioceptive input. For example, a tennis player does not consciously consider the use of the rotator cuff muscles (glenohumeral stabilizers) while serving, rather the player is more focused on the voluntary actions of the ball toss and the service motion. Ideally, the muscles of the rotator cuff perform the job of joint centration (keeping the humeral head in an optimal position within the glenoid fossa) in an anticipatory manner, described as glenohumeral stabilization (37). To this end, the sensorimotor system is responsible for providing awareness,

---

Key Point

Optimal stabilization strategies require

1. A stable base from which forces are transferred
2. Adequate muscular capacity (strength and endurance)
3. CNS motor programming (integration of sensory input) that produces synchronous activation of the muscles

Table 6.2	Muscle Classification
Mobilizers	**Stabilizers**
Upper trapezius	Deep cervical flexors
Levator scapulae	Lower trapezius
Pectoralis major and minor	Serratus anterior
Deltoids	Rotator cuff (infraspinatus, supraspinatus, teres minor, subscapularis)
Erector spinae	Middle and lower trapezius
Iliopsoas	Transversus abdominis
Quadriceps	Multifidus
Rectus abdominis	Gluteus medius and maximus

coordination, and feedback to maintain optimal positioning of the shoulder joint, thereby enhancing the quality of movement and reducing the chance of injury (22,59). Conversely, if the stabilizing rotator cuff muscles are not recruited with proper timing and speed and proper muscle patterns, the humeral head is subject to the pulling forces of the deltoid muscles, which can cause the humeral head to shift upward within the socket. The upward translation is problematic in that several musculotendinous structures (*e.g.*, biceps tendon and rotator cuff tendons) that are located in this area can become impinged between the acromion process and the head of the humerus. Other illustrations of the automation of healthy stabilization strategies are the anticipatory bracing that occurs when a dog unexpectedly pulls on the leash, the bracing of the neck and trunk when cyclist rides over a pothole, or the postural adjustments that are made during abrupt change directions on the tennis court.

Some researchers have categorized muscles as two distinct, yet interdependent systems, stabilizers or mobilizers (6,46). Categorization is largely based on their relative contributions to movement and maintaining posture, and position in the body (Table 6.2).

Classifying muscles in this way is beneficial for the exercise practitioner, as stabilizing muscles have unique characteristics (Table 6.3) that require specialized training approaches, which will be

Table 6.3	Mobilizer and Stabilizer Characteristics
Mobilizers	**Stabilizers**
Fast twitch	Slow twitch
Fatigues easily	Resistant to fatigue
Superficial	Deep
Relatively small proprioceptive role	Major contributor to proprioception
High force production	Low force production
Prone to hold excess tension/shorten	Prone to inhibition/weakness
Concentric	Isometric/eccentric
Gross movement	Joint stabilization

What Is the Core?

Perhaps the most common discussion of stabilization relates to core function. This is because the hips and the trunk serve as our center of mass and attempts to centralize the strength and coordination of the core are believed to yield optimal force production through the limbs. The principle of core stability can be illustrated in a simple comparison, shooting a canon off of a canoe versus a stable surface. To date, there is no universally accepted definition of the core, where some researchers describe the core as a muscular cylinder with the abdominals comprising the front, the multifidus and gluteals the back, the diaphragm as the roof, and the pelvic floor as the base of the cylinder (6–8,35). Tse et al. (60) defined the core as all muscles of the trunk and pelvis that contribute to maintaining a stable spine. Other researchers suggest that the core is an integrated system composed of passive structures (*e.g.*, ligaments and bone), the active spinal muscles and thoracolumbar fascia, and the neural control unit (40,41). Precise definition notwithstanding, there is universal agreement that the core is central to all kinetic chains, and that upper and lower extremity movement is optimized in conditions where there is sufficient endurance and neuromuscular control of the core (6–8). Moreover, proper core function improves the spine's ability to withstand the various loads and directional forces that it encounters during daily activities, sport and exercise.

described later in this chapter. Generally speaking, mobilizing muscles are superficially located and responsible for controlling locomotion, alignment, and balancing forces imposed on the spine. Stabilizing muscles are more centrally located and largely function to create stiffness across joints. These muscles are shorter in length and respond to changes in posture and extrinsic loads. Conversely, mobilizers, or global muscles, comprise long lever arms, allowing greater force production, torque and gross multiplanar movements.

Mediators of the Proprioception, Mobility, and Stability

Overweight and Obesity and Physical Inactivity

Overweight and obesity is a worldwide epidemic and is associated with elevated risk for a number of chronic diseases such as diabetes, hypertension, and the metabolic syndrome. Among adult men and women, obesity and overweight has been shown to be associated with alterations in motor function and postural control, possibly due to reductions in muscular strength and endurance, postural distortion, discomfort with movement, and the perception of stiffness (29,54). Unfortunately, associations of poor motor control and elevated BMI have also been reported in children and adolescents (11,13,14). Moreover, obesity and overweight in growth and developmental stages is believed to contribute to aberrant motor patterning, which extends to adulthood (54).

Propensity for Inhibition of Stabilizing Muscles

Dr. Vladimir Janda, a key figure in 20th century rehabilitation and one of the first to characterize the sensorimotor system, suggested that certain muscles had an inherent propensity for weakening or inhibition, while other muscles were prone to hypertonicity (24). Ultimately, the tendencies of certain muscles to weaken or tighten may lead to postural distortion and alterations in motor control (24). This altered regulation of the sensorimotor system may occur due to participation in sports involving repetitive actions, overtraining, poor ergonomics, sedentary lifestyle, trauma, or disease.

Previous Injury and Pain

Disturbances in the motor control system often follow injury and leave residual effects (45,56). In other words, although the client is pain-free, mobility and stability problems and sensory deficits remain. This sets the stage for a perpetuating cycle of motor control impairment and mobility and stability limitations. Specifically, these alterations lead to inappropriate magnitudes of muscle forces and stiffness across joints, allowing for a joint to buckle or undergo shear translation (as described in the rotator cuff example earlier) (35). The loss of stability may be due to damage incurred to the passive structures of the joint (*e.g.*, tendons, ligaments) where they can no longer support joint integrity. Additionally, sensory receptors within the joints may be compromised, which will result in the delayed action of stabilizing muscles (56). The delay in action changes the order of muscle activation that is necessary for joint centration (20,46).

Everyday Posture and Limited Variety of Movement

Sahrmann (33) proposes that movement impairment stems from a biomechanical cause. In which case, repeated movements in one direction or sustained postures result in the remodeling of sarcomeres, whereby muscle lengths adaptively shorten or lengthen. The adaptive shortening represents a loss of sarcomeres, whereas muscle lengthening represents the addition of sarcomeres in series, taken together results in overall muscle imbalance (33). In effect, we stray from a neutral position and begin to adopt the posture that we are in most of the time (51). The muscle length adaptations then influence length tension and force-coupling relationships, motor control, and ultimately how we are able, or in many cases unable, to move (51). This set of circumstances is often seen in individuals that are sedentary, where the muscles of the anterior torso, and internal rotators of the shoulder tend to shorten. Athletes are also susceptible to development of faulty stabilization strategies and mobility, particularly those who perform repeated unvaried or unidirectional movement patterns (*e.g.*, cyclists, runners, golfers, overhead athletes).

From a performance standpoint, a tight and shortened agonist (prime mover) has a lowered activation threshold and is described as hypertonic. This simply means that it will not take much stimulus to activate the muscle. In which case, hypertonic muscles suppress (decrease neural activity via reciprocal inhibition) the activity of lengthened antagonists and cause further weakening of that muscle (61). For example, hypertonic iliopsoas muscles often result from repeated hip flexion as seen in long distance cycling or running, or from prolonged seated postures. The hypertonicity of the hip flexors then contributes to the progressive weakening of the gluteus maximus via reciprocal inhibition. The gluteus maximus is an important hip extensor; thus, when forceful hip extension is necessary, the hamstrings (a synergist of the gluteus maximus) will compensate for the weakened gluteus maximus. This compensatory pattern is problematic for two main reasons. First, the pattern overworks the synergists (in the example, the hamstrings), which increases the risk for injury. Second, this compensatory pattern becomes etched within the sensorimotor system and will alter quality proprioception, mobility and stability. These alterations then tend to perpetuate further postural distortion. For example, when the hamstrings become hypertonic (also due to sedentary posture), they exert a downward force upon the proximal attachment site at the ischial tuberosity of the pelvis. This force rotates the pelvis posteriorly, which reduces the neutral curvature of the lumbar spine (flattens the low back) (51).

Joint Structure

Mobility and stability are partly derived from the articular geometry, or the shape and depth of joints. It is important to realize that some clients will present with structural anomalies that will prohibit full range of motion (ROM) on certain exercises. For example, an individual's hip joint may have a capsular structure that prevents performing a deep squat with the feet pointed in a neutral alignment. In such cases, the ACSM professional should encourage movement that is most comfortable for the client and not attempt to stretch through this nonmodifiable limitation.

Age

The adverse effects of aging on proprioception, stability and mobility are well established (18,62). This is particularly relevant for the exercise professional, as the percentage of individuals over the age of 60 years continues to increase and the risk of falls, due to diminished kinesthesia and postural control, increases with age. These factors highlight the functional significance of balance and stability training in older populations. The reasons behind proprioceptive decline in the elderly include a reduction in the number of joint mechanoreceptors, changes to the structure and sensitivity of mechanoreceptors, inadequate processing of proprioceptive input within the CNS (1,2,17,23).

Key Points

Alterations in movement quality can stem from multiple factors including obesity and overweight, sedentary behavior, poor postures, unvaried movement, joint structure, propensity for certain muscles to become inhibited, and age. It follows that fitness practitioners must consider each of these omnipresent factors when designing exercise programs.

What Is Neutral Position and Why Is It so Important?

Panjabi (41) describes neutral position as "the posture of the spine in which the overall internal stresses in the spinal column and muscular effort to hold the posture are minimal." A nice illustration of mechanical importance of neutral can be seen in a tent that has supporting wires equally tight around the structure. Conversely, if one set of support wires is tighter in comparison to the

Implications for Exercise Practitioners

Context for the Principles of Overload, Specificity, and Other Training Variables
The principle of overload is a fundamental construct of resistance training design (30). The overload principle suggests that in order to enhance muscular fitness, the body must exercise at an intensity that exceeds what it is normally accustomed to. It is important to recognize that overload represents a specific threshold that must be met in order for adaptation to occur. The way in which we introduce overload, however, must consider a superseding principle, which is quality movement should not be compromised, as flawed motor patterns can be easily ingrained and are difficult to correct once they take hold. To put it another way, overload should not outpace the client's sensory awareness, capacity to stabilize, and ability to move through a full ROM without compensation.

The principle of specificity suggests that specific adaptations occur upon application of specific demands. Accordingly, to improve proprioceptive acuity, sensory-specific training is necessary. More to the point, strength training is not the most effective way to improve sensory deficits.

In summary, fundamental principles of exercise prescription must be taken within context of quality movement. This means the adjustment of resistance training variables, including exercise selection, velocity of movement, and the number of repetitions and sets, should all be based on the client's sensorimotor capacity.

other side, the tent will likely collapse. In humans, maintaining neutral is important because it organizes the body into its most biomechanically efficient posture (40,41). More specifically, neutral position (a) optimizes ideal muscle length-tension and force-coupling relationships, (b) minimizes compressive and shear forces imposed on the joint, and (c) optimizes the timing and speed of contraction of stabilizing muscles.

Assessment and Prescription

Establishing a Movement Baseline

A widely held belief is that simple bodyweight movement is an appropriate place to begin a strength and conditioning program. This logic is based on the assumption that the client already has sufficient proprioceptive acuity, mobility, and appropriate command of the stabilizing muscles to maintain optimal alignment. Given the pervasive contributors of muscle imbalance described earlier, this assumption is a chancy supposition, whereby further exploration into the client's true movement baseline is likely needed (51).

Considering the majority of fitness assessments will take place in fitness centers, gyms, and studios, without the use of sophisticated laboratory equipment, the most pragmatic strategies for the exercise professional are left to observation of static and dynamic postures and symmetry of movement. It is important to note that if pain is present during any of the following assessments or exercises, the ACSM practitioner should recommend a medical exam by a qualified medical professional.

Assessment of Static Neutral Posture

Although static posture does not necessarily capture how an individual moves, it does provide the exercise practitioner some insight regarding specific muscle imbalances. This information can then be used in the selection of stabilization exercises and stretching and self-myofascial release (SMR) strategies. Static postural assessments also help clients develop an awareness of neutral posture, which holds great relevance when clients are performing dynamic movements that require maintenance of neutral while under load (*e.g.*, squat, lunge, deadlift, farmer's carries).

PLUMB LINE ASSESSMENT

Use of a plumb line or a static posture app is useful in identifying deviations from a neutral position. Clients should be barefoot, wear form-fitting clothing that enables the assessor to identify bony landmarks, and be encouraged to assume their everyday, relaxed posture during the assessment. Table 6.4 describes a basic plumb line postural assessment.

WALL TEST

In addition to the plumb line assessment, a wall assessment of normal lumbar curvature and forward head posture is helpful. Instruct the client to stand with his or her back against a wall and feet approximately 6 in from the wall. Ideally, the back of the head should be positioned against the wall and the assessors hand should be able to fit snuggly in between the wall of the client's lumbar spine and the wall. Taken together, these static postural assessments expose areas of tightness and/or weakness. There are occasions where simply drawing the client's attention to the postural distortion and offering verbal cues will prove helpful (Table 6.5). Additionally, Table 6.5 offers specific stretching targets that correspond to the listed postural deviations.

PROGRESSIVE APPROACH TO DEVELOPING POSTURAL AWARENESS

Unfortunately, due to various sensory, mobility, and stability limitations, the ability to distinguish neutral spine may be challenged. To begin, the ACSM practitioner should cue the client,

Table 6.4	Basic Plumb Line Static Postural Assessment	
View	**Setup for Assessment**	**Alignment Checkpoints (the plumb line should pass through these anatomical landmarks)**
Sagittal	Client should stand sideways to the plumb line, with the line positioned slightly anterior to the client's ankle (lateral malleolus)	External auditory meatus (ear canal) Acromioclavicular joint Greater trochanter of the femur Tibial tuberosity
Anterior	Client should stand facing the plumb line, with feet equidistant from the line. Align the plumb line with the pubis.	Navel Sternum Chin Nose Eyes are equidistant from the line. Additionally, the shoulder girdle should be level.

Adapted from Kendall FP. *Muscles: Testing and Function with Posture and Pain.* 5th ed. Baltimore (MD): Lippincott Williams & Wilkins; 2005. 560 p.

both manually and verbally, to arch the low back and then flatten the low back (see Table 6.6 for progressive postural staging of this process). This should be repeated several times, upon which the client should be asked to find the middle of the two extremes. Once neutral alignment is found, the client should be instructed to hold this posture for several seconds and then lose neutral by arching or flattening the low back, only to regain neutral position again. The client should begin performing each stage with eyes open and then eyes closed. When more dynamic movements, such as hip hinging and squatting, are introduced a dowel placed along the spine provides valuable tactile feedback for the client. The client should be encouraged to maintain three points of contact with the dowel: the back of the head, the upper thoracic spine, and the pelvis.

Table 6.5	Postural Corrective Suggestions	
Postural Deviation	**Suggestive Verbal Cues**	**Stretching Target**
Forward head posture	"Tuck the chin."	Pectoralis major and minor; latissimus dorsi; abdominals
Increased thoracic curvature	"While tucking your chin, stand or sit as tall as possible."	Pectoralis major and minor; latissimus dorsi; abdominals
Internal rotation of the shoulders	"Create as much width between your shoulders."	Pectoralis major and minor; latissimus dorsi
Posterior pelvic tilt	"Align your rib cage over your pelvis."	Hamstrings; abdominals
Hyperextension of lumbar spine	"Gently contract your glute muscles." "Lock your ribcage on top of your pelvis."	Erector spinae; quadratus lumborum; quadriceps; iliopsoas

Table 6.6	Progressive Stages for Neutral Posture

Stage 1 Lying on the ground

Stage 2 Seated

Stage 3 Standing

Stage 4 Standing and adding in hip hinging

Stage 5 Farmer carries with bilateral loading

Stage 6 Farmer carries with unilateral loading

Integrative Assessments and Corrections

As muscles rarely work in isolation, assessments that consider the body as an integrated system, involving various segments of the body responding to movements in a synchronous coordinated fashion, are quite valuable (60). Although the following patterns may seem rudimentary, keep in mind that poor posture, fatigue, repeated asymmetrical movements, stress, and poor exercise practices have the potential to corrupt even the most primal motor patterns (24,28,32,35,51). Reclaiming these basic patterns then feeds the reflexive and intentional stabilization strategies needed for more functional movements such as the deadlift, squat, lunges etc. (9,38).

WALL PLANK-AND-ROLL

The wall plank-and-roll (WPR) is not only an assessment of lumbar stability but can also serve as an exercise to enhance lumbar torsional (anti-rotational) control (63). The client should be instructed to face a wall, with feet positioned approximately 2 ft from the wall. The client's elbows should be positioned on the wall, with forearms lying one on top of the other. The client should then be instructed to "brace" or stiffen the trunk (35), and pivot on the balls of their feet while pulling one elbow off the wall ending in a side plank position. The client should be encouraged to rotate the entire body as a single unit. No lumbar or pelvic motion should be observed while pivoting from side to side. Once the client demonstrates sufficient stability for the wall roll, progressions include side planks on the floor, initially performed on the knees and ultimately performed in a full body side plank position. Of practical relevance, in order to optimize the effectiveness of isometric endurance exercises such as the side plank (also called the side bridge), Dr. Stuart McGill recommends performing repeated sets of short-duration holds (8–10 s) rather than having the client perform one set of a prolonged (>30 s) (35).

TEACHING HOW TO BRACE

With respect to teaching clients how to brace, a few concepts are important to emphasize. First, the client should be instructed to precontract, or brace, the abdominal wall prior to performing isometric exercises such as a plank or isotonic movements such as squatting movements. Stuart McGill (35) suggests the use of the simple cue of "pretend you are about to be hit in the stomach." It is worth mentioning that the "hit" is not necessarily a full force strike to the stomach, rather only intended to create the image of creating sufficient stability to maintain neutral alignment but not too much stiffness where motion is prevented (35). In other words, *the intensity of the brace should be tailored to the **relative intensity** of the exercise*, where the resultant coactivation of the trunk muscles is ample to protect the spine during lifting tasks but does not encumber proper mobility. For example, a client performing a bodyweight squat may require a low level of bracing intensity; however, when performing a one repetition maximum (1-RM) squat, the client should be encouraged to brace with closer to a maximal effort to maintain spinal integrity.

DIAPHRAGMATIC BREATHING ASSESSMENT AND CORRECTIVE METHODS

Evaluation of diaphragmatic control is important for several reasons. First, the diaphragm muscles are not only the prime muscles of respiration but they are also a vital muscle of core stabilization. To this end, if proper diaphragmatic control is not present, the generation of intra-abdominal pressure required to stabilize the spine during lifting tasks can be compromised (27,38). Second, breathing pattern problems have been shown to result in muscular imbalance, motor control alterations, and chronic low back pain (12,35,38). Third, as with proper conditioning of any muscle in the body, improving the endurance of the respiratory muscles enables these muscles to perform at higher capacities, ultimately leading to improved work capacity and prolonged time to fatigue (34). Fourth, those who tend to breathe at quicker rates, described as hyperventilation, exceed the gas exchange needs of metabolism. To this end, over-breathing has the potential to drastically lower carbon dioxide (CO_2) levels, which can raise pH levels (34). Not only is this a performance limiting issue, if hyperventilation is severe enough, light-headedness and possibly unconsciousness can result. Finally, alterations in breathing mechanics have been correlated with low scores on the Functional Movement Screen (9), an evaluation of movement quality that explores seven different movement patterns.

Healthy breathing patterns, or diaphragmatic breathing, involve the expansion of the rib cage and abdomen and involves proper recruitment and endurance of the diaphragm muscles (43). Conversely, altered breathing involves breathing from the upper chest, as shown by rib cage elevation, and often involves shallow and quick breathing rates (12). The Hi-Lo Assessment is a simple assessment of proper diaphragmatic control during breathing and is detailed in Table 6.7.

Ideally, the hand on the upper abdomen should rise before the hand on the chest. Additionally, the hand on the chest should move slightly forward and not upward toward the chin (12). Conveniently, this simple assessment also serves as a means to correct the breathing pattern problem. The basic approach, detailed in Table 6.8, involves the client practicing a diaphragmatic breathing pattern while progressing through more challenging postures and movements. Clients demonstrating improper breathing habits should be encouraged to regularly practice breathing (using the same hand positions) that is focused on expansion of the rib cage and upper abdomen prior to any chest movement and to increase the length of each breath, in particular the client should be encouraged to fully exhale. Routine follow-up breathing pattern assessment should be performed to monitor for changes and to emphasize the relevance of diaphragmatic breathing patterns in optimizing core stability and overall health.

Table 6.7	Hi-Lo Assessment
Client places one hand on his or her sternum and one hand on his or her upper abdomen.	
The client is then instructed to perform 10 breathing cycles.	
The client reports which hand moved first at the beginning of the inhalation phase during the majority of the assessment. In addition, the practitioner should observe the hand movements of the client.	

Adapted from Chaitow L. Breathing pattern disorders, motor control, and low back pain. *J Osteopath Med.* 2004;7(1):33–40.

Table 6.8	Diaphragmatic Breathing Pattern Progression	
Stage	Description	Postural Progression
Static	Maintenance of postural stability while breathing diaphragmatically	Supine on stable surface Seated Standing
Dynamic	Simultaneous limb movement while maintaining postural stability and diaphragmatic breathing patterns	Supine on floor with arm or leg movement Supine on foam roller with arm or leg movement Seated with arm or leg movement Standing with arm or leg movement
Advanced	Increase ventilation by performing any type of aerobic exercise	Immediately stop the aerobic exercise and perform an isometric exercise (*e.g.*, side-plank, bird dog, curl-up). This will assist in improve the coordination of the diaphragm during tasks of core stabilization. Note: For these low loading challenges, abdominal bracing should occur in concert with diaphragmatic breathing.

Adapted from Nelson N. Diaphragmatic breathing: the foundation of core stability. *Strength Cond J.* 2012;34(5):34–40; McGill SM. *Low Back Disorders: Evidence-Based Prevention and Rehabilitation.* 2nd ed. Champaign (IL): Human Kinetics; 2007. 328 p.

ROLLING PATTERNS: ASSESSMENT AND CORRECTION

Although infants can roll with relative efficiency by 6–8 months of age, the pattern may become altered later in life due to mobility deficits or insufficient core stabilization patterning (21). More specifically, demonstration of efficient rolling patterns reveals proper recruitment sequencing of the core stabilizing muscles (*i.e.*, initiated with the deeper trunk stabilizers, including the transversus abdominis, multifidus, diaphragm and pelvic floor, and followed by recruitment of the more superficial or global muscles including the internal and external obliques, rectus abdominis, quadratus lumborum, erector spinae). However, given the lack of variety of daily movement among many individuals (including athletes performing motions in one direction), symmetrical rotational efficiency may be altered. The objective of the assessment is to observe the rolling strategy of the client in eight different patterns, leading from all four quadrants of the body. Ideally, the client should be able to roll with equal ease in all directions. When first performing the rolling assessments, use limited cues (Table 6.9), as the goal is to observe their movement plan and "cheating" methods.

There are times where clients will have difficulty completing rolling patterns. In which case, Table 6.10 and the following figures provide some of the common associated mobility and stability limitations and corresponding corrections. The rolling pattern itself can also be modified by placing a foam roller under one side of the trunk (just lateral to the spine); this will assist the client in rolling away from the bolstered side.

The client should be encouraged to practice each of the patterns (particularly the patterns where coordination and symmetry of movement was poor) while keeping the cues offered in Table 6.11 in mind.

Addressing Alignment Issues

It is essential for the ACSM exercise professional to be able to critically appraise the quality of movement during an exercise session. In the fitness center setting, this evaluation will often

Table 6.9	Assessment of Rolling Patterns	
Rolling Direction[a]	**Beginning Position**	**Cues**
Supine to prone leading with the right or left arm	Supine, legs straight, and slightly abducted; arms overhead and slightly abducted; when looking down at the client, they should resemble an "X."	"With no help from the legs, roll onto your belly."
Supine to prone leading with the right or left leg	Supine, legs straight, and slightly abducted; arms overhead and slightly abducted	"With no help from your arms, roll onto your belly."
Prone to supine leading with the right or left arm	Prone, legs straight, and slightly abducted; arms overhead and slightly abducted	"With no help from your legs, roll onto your back."
Supine to prone leading with the right or left leg	Prone, legs straight, and slightly abducted; arms overhead and slightly abducted	"With no help from your arms, roll onto your back."

[a]Each pattern should be performed right to left and left to right, totaling eight patterns.

Table 6.10	Correctives for Those Who are Initially Unable to Perform Rolling Patterns
Exercise Progression for Rolling Patterns	
Strength or mobility limitation	**Corrective stretch or exercise**
Thoracic spine mobility	Modified cobra stretch (Fig. 6.3); doorway pectoralis major stretch
Gluteus maximus weakness	Bird dog (Fig. 6.4) or quadruped exercises; glute bridges (Fig. 6.5)
Gluteus medius weakness	Lateral band walks (Fig. 6.6); clam shell exercises (Fig. 6.7)
Core endurance	Wall plank-and-roll; side plank performed on knees (Fig. 6.8)

Table 6.11	Verbal Cues for Rolling Patterns
Rolling Direction[a]	**Verbal Cues**
Supine to prone leading with the right arm	"Begin by looking to the left, lead with the eyes and head; lift the right arm; look into the left shoulder and roll over like a rag doll."
Supine to prone leading with the right leg	"Flex the hip and then cross the right leg over the left and roll."
Prone to supine leading with the right arm	"Lift the right arm, look up and over the opposite shoulder and roll."
Prone to supine leading with the right leg	"Bend the right knee, lift the foot toward the ceiling, cross the right leg over the left and roll."

[a]These sample cues are for rolling from right to left. Simply reverse the cuing when rolling from left to right.

Adapted from Hoogenboom BJ, Voight ML, Cook G, Gill L. Using rolling to develop neuromuscular control and coordination of the core and extremities of athletes. *N Am J Sports Phys Ther.* 2009;4(2):70–82.

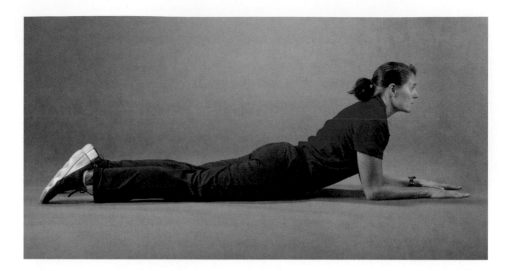

FIGURE 6.3. Modified cobra stretch.

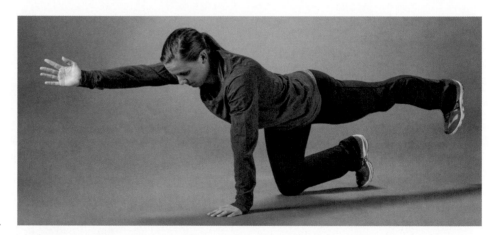

FIGURE 6.4. Bird dog.

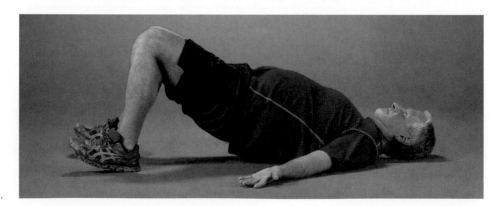

FIGURE 6.5. Glute bridge.

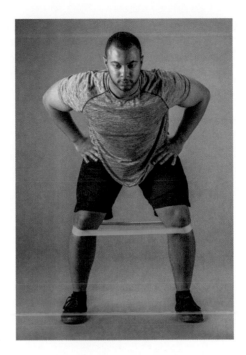

FIGURE 6.6. Lateral band walks.

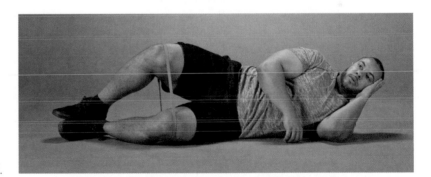

FIGURE 6.7. Clam shell.

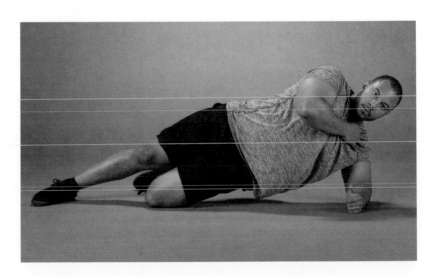

FIGURE 6.8. Side plank performed on the knees.

Table 6.12	Alignment Fault Checklist

Loss of cervical neutral — head positioned in front of the body or tilting up or down

Loss of thoracic extension — rounding of the thoracic spine

Internal rotation of the shoulders

Posterior pelvic tilt — loss of neutral lordosis in the lumbar spine or flattening of lumbar spine

Anterior pelvic tilt — excessive arching of low back

Knee valgus — knees collapsing inward

rely on observing any alignment faults that may present during the performance of an exercise (Table 6.12). Many times, verbal and manual cuing can correct the problem; however, there are occasions where alignment faults are the result of low endurance, timing issues of the stabilizing muscles, and/or tightness in the mobilizing muscles that were outlined earlier in this chapter (Table 6.13).

The training goal is to improve the endurance and functional stabilization capacity of these muscles. In which case, a good place to start is incorporating isometric exercises applied at various joint specific angles for the weakened or inhibited muscles (3), with short duration hold and relax cycles (5–8 s). For example, if weakness is noted in the rhomboid muscles (demonstrated by excessive thoracic kyphosis), an effective approach might involve the following:

■ Instruct the client to maintain a tall neutral posture while retracting and depressing the scapula, holding this position for 5–8 seconds and then relaxing.
■ Progression 1: Have the client perform multiple sets of this exercise, still using 5- to 8-second holds.

Table 6.13	Common Alignment Faults Along with Corresponding Inhibited or Weak Stabilizing Muscles	
Alignment Fault	**Associated Weak or Inhibited Muscles**	**Suggested Corrective Exercises**
Loss of cervical neutral	Deep cervical flexors (longus colli, capitis)	Chin tucks (Fig. 6.9); isometric cervical exercise (*e.g.*, using hands on forehead resisting neck flexion effort)
Loss of thoracic extension	Middle and lower trapezius	Scapular retraction with no weight (Fig. 6.10); progressing to seated rows
Internal rotation of the shoulders	External rotators of the shoulder (infraspinatus)	Band or dumbbell shoulder external rotation (Fig. 6.11)
Posterior pelvic tilt	Gluteus medius and maximus; multifidus	Glute bridges; quadruped or bird dog
Anterior pelvic tilt	Gluteus medius and maximus; transversus abdominis	Curl-up; side plank/bridge
Knee valgus	Gluteus medius and maximus	Lateral band walks; clam shells; glute bridges; bird dog

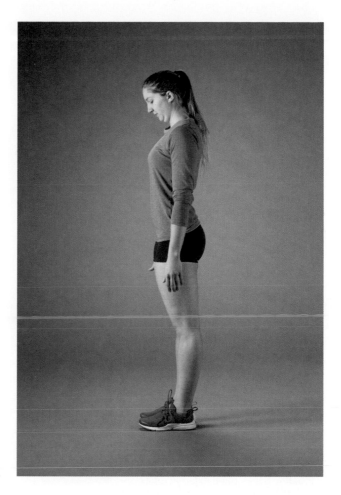

FIGURE 6.9. Chin tucks.

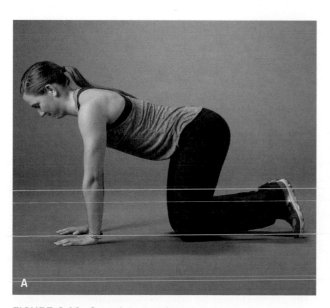

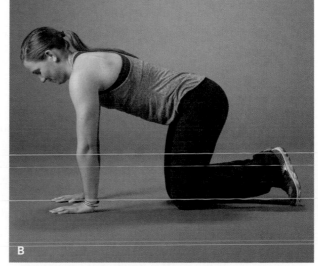

FIGURE 6.10. Scapular retraction.

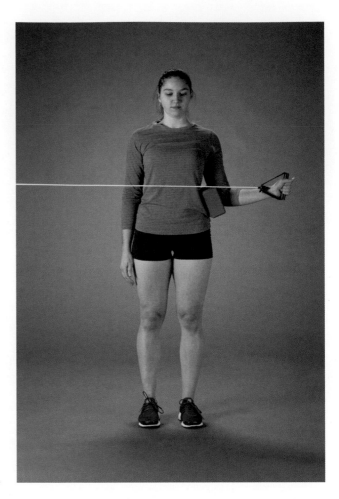

FIGURE 6.11. Band external rotation.

- Progression 2: Have the client perform the same isometric hold against light resistance tubing.
- Progression 3: As the client develops endurance and greater recruitment efficiency of the rhomboids, introduce more dynamic movements, such as a seated row or single arm dumbbell row. In this case, repetitions schemes should be focused on enhancing muscular endurance (12–15 repetitions).

INSTABILITY TRAINING

Instability training is a method of training that challenges a client's ability to maintain balance while challenging the client's center of gravity. This is often accomplished by narrowing the client's base of support (*e.g.*, by moving the legs closer together, maintaining single leg postures, or performing exercises on unstable surfaces). By challenging posture in this way, instability training is thought to improve feed-forward and feedback mechanisms, ultimately improving stability and proprioception. It is worth noting that the goal of instability training is to improve stability and sensory acuity, not necessarily to improve strength in the extremities, thus should involve low load tasks. When planning instability training, it is essential to tailor the difficulty of the exercise to the client's relative functional capacity. In effect, the client should be able to demonstrate some level of postural control, but at the same time, the exercise should require a great deal of concentration. Once the client has mastered one level, the client should progress to the next level of difficulty. Table 6.14 illustrates a systematic approach to instability training. Once the client can adequately perform the exercise on the floor, the next stage would involve having the client perform the same

Table 6.14	Instability Training Progression Example	
Exercise	Position	Demonstration of Mastery
A1. Wide staggered stance on the floor Eyes open (Fig. 6.12)	Client stands on the floor with one foot in front of the other, wide stance to increase the base of support.	Maintains optimal alignment without significant swaying for 30 s
A2. Wide staggered stance on the floor Eyes closed	Client stands on the floor with one foot in front of the other, wide stance to increase the base of support.	Maintains optimal alignment without significant swaying for 30 s
A3. Wide staggered stance on the floor with weight shift Eyes closed	Client stands on the floor with one foot in front of the other, wide stance to increase the base of support. Instruct client to shift majority of weight onto front foot then to back foot.	Maintains optimal alignment without significant swaying for 30 s
B1. Narrow staggered stance Eyes open	Client stands on the floor with one foot directly in front of the other as if standing on a balance beam.	Maintains optimal alignment without significant swaying for 30 s
B2. Narrow staggered stance Eyes closed	Client stands on the floor with one foot directly in front of the other as if standing on a balance beam.	Maintains optimal alignment without significant swaying for 30 s
B3. Narrow staggered stance Eyes closed with weight shift	Client stands on the floor with one foot directly in front of the other as if standing on a balance beam. Instruct client to shift majority of weight onto front foot then to back foot.	Maintains optimal alignment without significant swaying for 30 s
C1. Single-leg stance Eyes open	Client stands on one foot on the floor.	Maintains optimal alignment without significant swaying for 30 s
C2. Single-leg stance Eyes closed (Fig. 6.13)	Client stands on one foot on the floor.	Maintains optimal alignment without significant swaying for 30 s
C3. Single-leg stance with reach	Client stands on one foot on floor and reaches with opposite hand to a specific target.	Able to perform several reaches without losing balance

sequence of exercises, only on an unstable surface, such as a cushioned surface or an Airex pad. The next stage might incorporate the use of a wobble board or Bosu trainer, as the client performs functional challenges such as medicine ball tosses or sport specific tasks (Figs. 6.14 and 6.15).

Self-Myofascial Release and Stretching

Another important component of a well-rounded exercise prescription is managing hypertonic muscles and soft tissue restriction that compromise mobility. Although stretching approaches such as proprioceptive neuromuscular facilitation (PNF), and static stretching are known to improve ROM, several reviews have reported significant deleterious effects on neuromuscular performance when done prior to activity (5,25). Conversely, several recent investigations have shown that SMR elicits improvements in ROM without concomitant performance decrements when done prior to activity (19,42,55).

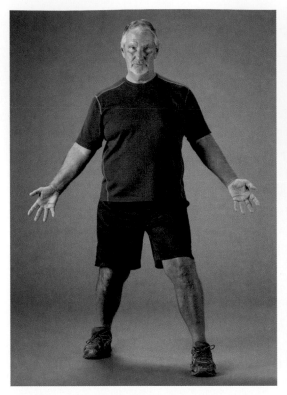

FIGURE 6.12. Wide staggered stance, eyes open.

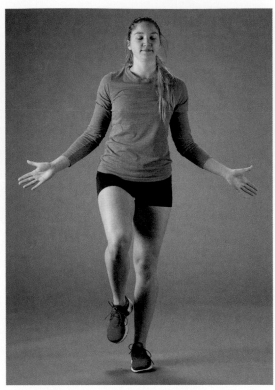

FIGURE 6.13. Single-leg stance, eyes closed.

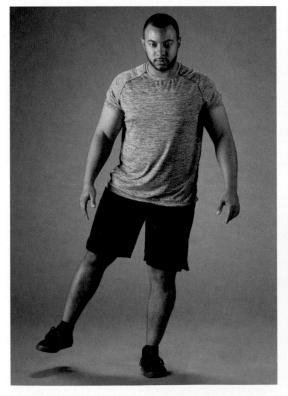

FIGURE 6.14. Progression option: one leg on floor.

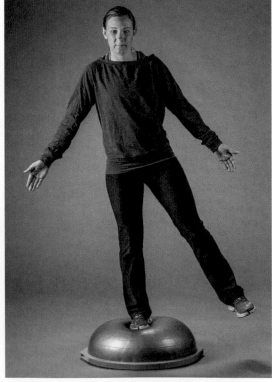

FIGURE 6.15. Progression option: one leg on Bosu.

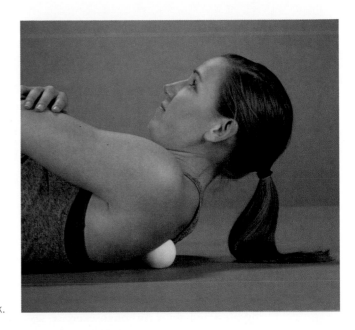

FIGURE 6.16. Lacrosse ball on upper back.

SMR is based on a form of manual therapy believed to alleviate the discomfort associated with tender spots within the myofascia, known as trigger points (10,58), and relax hypertonic areas within soft tissue (36). SMR involves the compression of soft tissue using tools such as foam rollers, roller massagers, or tennis balls and is performed by the individual rather than by a therapist (Figs. 6.16 and 6.17). Currently, the mechanisms behind SMR are unclear, although prevailing theories suggest that the compressive forces imposed on the myofascia stimulate various mechanoreceptors that reduce muscle-firing rates (50,52,57). Additionally, mechanical pressure induced by SMR may improve the viscous and fluid qualities of fascia, described as thixotropism (52). Other theories have proposed that the myofascia becomes restricted due to local inflammation (4). Although it is unclear how SMR might reduce inflammation, there is evidence indicating that SMR transiently increases local blood flow (39,44). To this end, the increased blood flow may aid in the reduction of inflammation. Table 6.15 includes a few suggested SMR and stretching targets for common alignment issues.

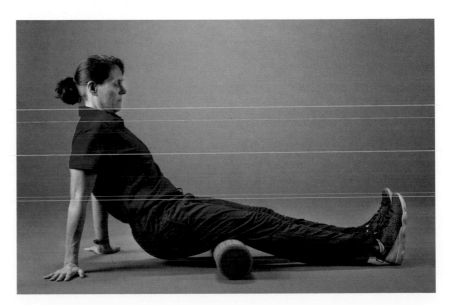

FIGURE 6.17. Foam rolling hamstrings.

Table 6.15	Alignment Issues and Soft Tissue Targets
Alignment Fault	**Self-Myofascial Release and Stretching Targets**
Excessive kyphosis of the thoracic spine	Pectoralis major and minor; latissimus dorsi; abdominals
Internal rotation of the shoulders	Pectoralis major and minor; latissimus dorsi
Posterior pelvic tilt	Hamstrings (see Fig. 6.17); abdominals
Hyperextension of the lumbar spine	Quadratus lumborum; quadriceps; iliopsoas

Lifestyle Recommendations

Stability, mobility, and sensory issues develop over long periods of time and are often mediated by lifestyle habits. Although exercise sessions are a critical piece of the repatterning process, the ACSM exercise professional should also offer recommendations that address lifestyle issues known to perpetuate muscle imbalance. Suggestions might include improving the ergonomics of the work environment, setting a recurring alarm to serve as a reminder to stand and walk around the office, practice of diaphragmatic breathing, and foam rolling while watching television.

SUMMARY

Although progressive overload is essential for improvements in strength and endurance outcomes, it should not come at the expense of proper movement patterning. To this end, it is critical for the ACSM practitioner to recognize that stability, mobility, and proprioception are requisite features of motor patterning and collectively serve as the foundation for strength and functional development. Unfortunately, pervasive issues such as sedentary behavior, obesity and overweight, and limited variety in movement impair these foundational components of fitness. If insufficient stabilizing strategies, lack of mobility, and low proprioceptive acuity are observed, practitioners must incorporate a systematic, progressive approach to improve baseline function prior to advancing the client into more conventional exercise prescription.

REFERENCES

1. Adamo D, Martin B, Brown S. Age-related differences in upper limb proprioceptive acuity. *Percept Mot Skills*. 2007; 104(3 Pt 2):1297–309.

2. Aydog S, Korkusuz P, Doral M, Tetick O, Demirel H. Decrease in the numbers of mechanoreceptors in rabbit ACL: the effects of aging. *Knee Surg*. 2006;14(4):325–9.

3. Baechle TR, Earle RW. *Essentials of Strength Training and Conditioning*. 2nd ed. Champaign (IL): Human Kinetics; 2000. 672 p.

4. Bednar DA, Orr FW, Simon GT. Observations on the pathomorphology of the thoracolumbar fascia in chronic mechanical back pain: a microscopic study. *Spine*. 1995;20(10): 1161–4.

5. Behm DG, Chaouachi A. A review of the acute effects of static and dynamic stretching on performance. *Eur J Appl Physiol*. 2011;111(11):2633–51.

6. Bergmark A. Stability of the lumbar spine: a study in mechanical engineering. *Acta Orthop Scand*. 1989;230(Suppl):20–4.

7. Bliss L, Teeple P. Core stability: the centerpiece of any training program. *Cur Sports Med Rep*. 2005;4(3):179–83.

8. Borghuis J, Hof A, Lemmink K. The importance of sensory-motor control in providing core stability. *Sports Med*. 2008;38(11):893–916.

9. Bradley H, Esformes J. Breathing pattern disorders and functional movement. *Int J Sports Phys Ther*. 2014;9(1):28–39.

10. Bron C, Dommerholt JD. Etiology of myofascial trigger points. *Curr Pain Headache Rep*. 2012;16(5):439–44.

11. Cattuzzo MT, dos Santos H, Ré A, et al. Motor competence and health related physical fitness in youth: a systematic review. *J Sci Med Sport*. 2016;19(2):123–9.

12. Chaitow L. Breathing pattern disorders, motor control, and low back pain. *J Osteopath Med*. 2004;7(1):33–40.

13. Ðokic Z. Relationship between overweight, obesity and the motor abilities of 9-12 year old school children. *Phys Cult*. 2013;67(2):91–102.

14. Duncan MJ, Stanley M, Wright SL. The association between functional movement and overweight and obesity in British primary school children. *BMC Sports Sci Med Rehabil*. 2013; 5(1):1–8.

15. Franklin DW, Wolpert DM. Computational mechanisms of sensorimotor control. *Neuron*. 2011;72(3):425–42.

16. Gandevia SC, Refshauge KM, Collins DF. Proprioception: peripheral inputs and perceptual interactions. *Adv Exp Med Biol*. 2002;508:61–8.

17. Goble DJ, Brown SH. Task-dependent asymmetries in the utilization of proprioceptive feedback for goal-directed movement. *Exp Brain Res*. 2007;180(4):693–704.

18. Goble DJ, Coxon JP, Wenderoth N, Van Impe A, Swinnen SP. Proprioceptive sensibility in the elderly: degeneration, functional consequences and plastic-adaptive processes. *Neurosci Biobehav Rev*. 2009;33(3):271–8.

19. Healey KC, Hatfield DL, Blanpied P, Dofrman LR, Riebe D. The effects of myofascial release with foam rolling on performance. *J Strength Cond Res*. 2014;28(1):61–8.

20. Hodges PW, Richardson CA. Altered trunk muscle recruitment in people with low back pain with upper limb movement at different speeds. *Arch Phys Med Rehabil*. 1999;80(9): 1005–12.

21. Hoogenboom BJ, Voight ML, Cook G, Gill L. Using rolling to develop neuromuscular control and coordination of the core and extremities of athletes. *N Am J Sports Phys Ther*. 2009;4(2):70–82.

22. Ionta S, Heydrich L, Lenggenhager B, et al. Multi-sensory mechanisms in temporo-parietal cortex support self-location and first-person perspective. *Neuron*. 2011;70(2):363–74.

23. Iwasaki T, Goto N, Goto J, Ezure H, Moriyama H. The aging of human Meissner's corpuscles as evidenced by parallel sectioning. *Okajimas Folia Anat*. 2003;79(6):185–9.

24. Jull GA, Janda V. Muscles and motor control in low back pain: assessment and management. In: Twomey LT, Taylor JR, editors. *Physical Therapy of the Low Back*. New York (NY): Churchill Livingstone; 1987. p. 253–78.

25. Kay AD, Blazevich AJ. Effect of acute static stretch on maximal muscle performance: a systematic review. *Med Sci Sports Exerc*. 2012;44(1):154–64.

26. Kersey R. Taber's Cyclopedic Medical Dictionary, 20th ed. *Athl Ther Today*. 2006;11(3):47.

27. Key J. 'The core': understanding it, and retraining its dysfunction. *J Bodywork Movement Ther*. 2013;17(4):541–59.

28. Kibler WB, Press J, Sciascia A. The role of core stability in athletic function. *Sports Med*. 2006;36(3):189–98.

29. Kováčiková Z, Svoboda Z, Neumannová K, Bizovská L, Cuberek R, Janura M. Assessment of postural stability in overweight and obese middle-aged women. *Acta Gymnica*. 2014;44(3):149–53.

30. Kraemer WJ, Ratamess NA. Fundamentals of resistance training: progression and exercise prescription. *Med Sci Sports Exerc*. 2004;36(4):674–88.

31. Lephart S, Riemann F, Fu F. *Proprioception and Neuromuscular Control in Joint Stability*. Champaign (IL): Human Kinetics; 2000. 439 p.

32. Lin YH, Li CW, Tsai LY, Liing R. The effects of muscle fatigue and proprioceptive deficits on the passive joint senses of ankle inversion and eversion. *Isokinet Exerc Sci*. 2008;16(2):101–5.

33. MacIntosh BR, Gardiner P, McComal AJ. *Skeletal Muscle: Form and Function*. 2nd ed. Champaign (IL): Human Kinetics; 2006. 432 p.

34. McArdle WD, Katch FI, Katch VL. *Exercise Physiology: Nutrition, Energy, and Human Performance*. 8th ed. Baltimore, MD: Wolters Kluwer; 2015. 1088 p.

35. McGill SM. *Low Back Disorders: Evidence-Based Prevention and Rehabilitation*. 2nd ed. Champaign (IL): Human Kinetics; 2007. 328 p.

36. McKenney K, Elder AS, Elder C, Hutchins A. Myofascial release as a treatment for orthopaedic conditions: a systematic review. *J Athl Train*. 2013;48(4):522–7.

37. Myers J, Wassinger C, Lephart S. Sensorimotor contribution to shoulder stability: effect of injury and rehabilitation. *Man Ther*. 2006;11(3):197–201.

38. Nelson N. Diaphragmatic breathing: the foundation of core stability. *Strength Condition J*. 2012;34(5):34–40.

39. Okamoto T, Masuhara M, Ikuta K. Acute effects of self-myofascial release using a foam roller on arterial function. *J Strength Cond Res*. 2014;28(1):69–73.

40. Panjabi MM. The stabilizing system of the spine. Part I. Function, dysfunction, adaptation, and enhancement. *J Spinal Disord*. 1992;5(4):383–9.

41. Panjabi MM. The stabilizing system of the spine. Part II. Neutral zone and instability hypothesis. *J Spinal Disord*. 1992; 5(4):390–7.

42. Peacock CA, Krein DD, Silver TA, Sanders GJ, Carlowitz KA. An acute bout of self-myofascial release in the form of foam rolling improves performance testing. *Int J Exerc Sci*. 2014;7(3):202–11.

43. Pryor JA, Prasad SA. *Physiotherapy for Respiratory and Cardiac Problems*. Edinburgh (United Kingdom): Churchill Livingstone; 2002. 618 p.

44. Quere N, Noel E, Lieutaud A, d'Alessio P. Fasciatherapy combined with pulsology touch induces changes in blood turbulence potentially beneficial for vascular endothelium. *J Bodywork Movement Ther*. 2009;13(13):239–45.

45. Richardson C, Jull G, Hodges P, Hides J. *Therapeutic Exercise for Spinal Segmental Stabilisation in Low Back Pain*. Edinburgh (United Kingdom): Churchill Livingstone; 1999. 192 p.

46. Richardson C, Hodges PW, Hides J. *Therapeutic Exercise for Lumbopelvic Stabilization : A Motor Control Approach for the Treatment and Prevention of Low Back Pain*. 2nd ed. Edinburgh (United Kingdom): Churchill Livingstone; 2004. 271 p.

47. Riemann BL, Lephart SM. The sensorimotor system, part I: the physiologic basis of functional joint stability. *J Athl Train*. 2002;37(1):71–9.

48. Röijezon U, Clark NC, Treleaven J. Proprioception in musculoskeletal rehabilitation. Part 1: basic science and principles of assessment and clinical interventions. *Man Ther*. 2015;20(3):368–77.

49. Rothwell J. *Control of Human Voluntary Movement*. London (United Kingdom): Chapman and Hall; 1994. 325 p.

50. Roylance DS, George JD, Hammer AM, et al. Evaluating acute changes in joint range-of-motion using self-myofascial release, postural alignment exercises, and static stretches. *Int J Exerc Sci*. 2013;6(4):310–319.

51. Sahrmann S. *Diagnosis and Treatment of Movement Impairment Syndromes*. St. Louis (MO): Mosby; 2002. 384 p.

52. Schleip R. Fascial plasticity — a new neurobiological explanation: part 1. *J Bodywork Movement Ther*. 2003;7(1):11–9.

53. Sherrington C. *The Integrative Action of the Nervous System*. New Haven (CT): Yale University Press; 1906. 128 p.

54. Shultz S, Byrne N, Hills A. Musculoskeletal function and obesity: implications for physical activity. *Curr Obes Rep*. 2014;3(3):355.

55. Sullivan KM, Silvey D, Button DC, Behm DG. Roller-massager application to the hamstrings increases sit-and-reach range of motion within five to ten seconds without performance impairments. *Int J Sports Phys Ther*. 2013;8(3): 228–36.

56. Switlick T, Kernozek TW, Meardon S. Differences in joint-position sense and vibratory threshold in runners with and without a history of overuse injury. *J Sport Rehab*. 2015; 24(1):6–12.

57. Tozzi P. Selected fascial aspects of osteopathic practice. *J Bodyw Mov Ther*. 2012;16(4):503–19.

58. Travell JG, Simons DG, Simons DG. *Myofascial Pain and Dysfunction: The Trigger Point Manual*. Baltimore (MD): Williams & Wilkins; 1983. 628 p.

59. Tripp B, Yochem E, Uhl T. Functional fatigue and upper extremity sensorimotor system acuity in baseball athletes. *J Athl Train*. 2007;42(1):90–8.

60. Tse MA, McManus AM, Masters RSW. Development and validation of a core endurance intervention program: implications for performance in college-age rowers. *J Strength Cond Res*. 2005;19(3):547–55.

61. Whittle MW. *Gait Analysis: An Introduction*. 4th ed. Edinburgh (Scotland): Butterworth Heineman Elsevier; 2007. 255 p.

62. Wingert JR, Welder C, Foo P. Age-related hip proprioception declines: effects on postural sway and dynamic balance. *Arch Phys Med Rehabil*. 2014;95(2):253–61.

63. Yoon C, Lee J, Kim K, Chan Kim H, Chung SG. Original research: quantification of lumbar stability during wall plank-and-roll activity. *PM R*. 2015;7(8):803–13.

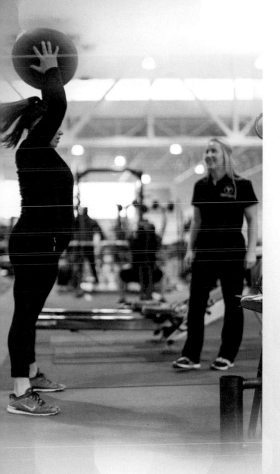

7

Body Composition and Weight Management

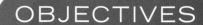

OBJECTIVES

- To understand and apply the various methods for assessing body composition.

- To evaluate body composition assessment as related to patient population and body mass index (BMI) status.

- To understand the key nutrition messages as described by the 2015 U.S. Department of Agriculture (USDA) Dietary Guidelines.

- To understand and apply the American College of Sports Medicine's (ACSM) metabolic calculations.

INTRODUCTION

The prevalence of overweight and obesity has been increasing in the United States and in developed countries around the world. Recent estimates indicate that approximately 68% of the US population are classified as overweight or obese (body mass index [BMI] $\geq$25 kg $\cdot$ m^{-2}), with approximately 34% classified as obese (BMI $\geq$30 kg $\cdot$ m^{-2}) and 6% as severely obese (BMI $\geq$40 kg $\cdot$ m^{-2}) (17). Population studies suggest that obesity rates have been relatively stable since 2003, but the prevalence of extreme obesity continues to increase (17,48,51). Obesity rates among children and adolescents have tripled since the 1980s and are now at 18% and 21%, respectively (50). The prevalence of obesity varies by racial and ethnic groups, with higher rates found in African American, Hispanic, and Mexican American populations compared with non-Hispanic Whites (17,51).

Overweight and obesity are characterized by high amounts of body fat in relation to overall lean body mass and are linked to numerous chronic diseases, including hypertension, cardiorespiratory disease, dyslipidemia, Type 2 diabetes, some cancers, sleep apnea, arthritis, and other musculoskeletal problems (62). It is estimated that obesity-related conditions account for more than 7% of total health care costs in the United States (9). Several medical conditions exist that promote weight gain (*e.g.*, Cushing syndrome); however, these conditions are uncommon. In most individuals, overweight and obesity are the result of excess caloric consumption and/or inadequate energy expenditure.

Obesity is associated with premature mortality from cardiorespiratory disease and other diseases such as cancer (62). Central (abdominal) obesity is associated with the metabolic syndrome, a clustering of metabolic factors that increase the risk of cardiovascular disease (CVD) (46). Other comorbidities associated with obesity such as Type 2 diabetes, dyslipidemia, and hypertension, as well as poor dietary habits and a sedentary lifestyle, also increase the risk of cardiorespiratory disease.

Body composition is an important component of health-related physical fitness. It is important for the certified exercise physiologist (EP-C) to understand how to properly measure body composition, make sound weight loss goals, and formulate exercise and nutritional recommendations for weight loss and weight management. Due to the high prevalence of obesity, the percentage of body fat is often emphasized. However, it is equally important to consider the changes in body composition that accompany aging. Sarcopenia is the age-related loss of muscle mass that is accompanied by a decrease in strength. The body composition assessments completed in most health fitness settings do not provide a precise measurement of muscle mass, but muscle mass is a major component of the fat-free mass that is estimated and should be discussed with the client.

This chapter discusses the different methods for measuring body composition, reviews American College of Sports Medicine (ACSM) exercise guidelines for weight loss, and provides sound physical activity (PA) and nutritional information regarding weight management.

Measuring Body Composition

Anthropometric Methods

Anthropometrics are a set of noninvasive, quantitative techniques for determining body size by measuring, recording, and analyzing specific dimensions of the body, such as height, weight, and body circumference.

Height and Weight

Height is measured using a wall-mounted stadiometer (a vertical ruler mounted on a wall with a wide horizontal headboard). The clients should remove their shoes and hair ornaments, stand straight with their heels together, and look straight ahead. Before taking the measurement, ask that the clients take a deep breath and hold it. Height is recorded in either inches or centimeters.

Weight is measured using a calibrated balance beam or electronic scale. The clients should wear only light clothing, remove their shoes, empty their pockets, void if necessary, and stand in the center of the platform with weight distributed evenly on both feet. Weight is recorded in either pounds or kilograms.

Body Mass Index

BMI is a measure of weight in relation to a person's height. It is calculated by dividing body weight in kilograms by height in meters squared (refer to the "How to Calculate BMI" box) or can be determined with a BMI table (Table 7.1).

Body Mass Index is used to classify individuals as underweight (<18.5 kg · m^{-2}), normal weight (18.5–24.9 kg · m^{-2}), overweight (25.0–29.9 kg · m^{-2}), or obese (≥ 30 kg · m^{-2}) (17) and to identify individuals at risk for obesity-related diseases (Table 7.2). For most individuals, obesity-related health problems increase with a BMI ≥ 25.0 kg · m^{-2}. A BMI ≥ 30.0 kg · m^{-2} is associated with hypertension, dyslipidemia, coronary heart disease, and mortality (63). A BMI of <18.5 kg · m^{-2} also increases mortality risk (18). BMI can be used to classify children and adolescents as overweight or obese using the standard BMI formula along with a BMI for age growth chart provided

HOW TO   Calculate Body Mass Index

The following example can be used to learn how to calculate BMI. An individual weighing 150 lb (or 68.18 kg [divide weight in pounds by 2.2]), standing 66 in tall (or 1.68 m tall [multiply height in inches by 0.0254]) has a BMI of:

BMI = weight (kg) / height (m^2)
    = 68.18 kg / (1.68 m)^2
    = 68.18 / 2.82
    = 24.2 kg · m^{-2}

Another formula eliminates the need to convert pounds and inches to kilograms and meters. Using the same example:

BMI = (weight [lb] / height [in^2]) × 704.5
    = (150 lb / 66 in^2) × 704.5
    = (0.0344352) × 704.5
    = 24.2 kg · m^{-2}

Table 7.1	Body Mass Index Chart													
BMI (kg · m⁻²)	19	20	21	22	23	24	25	26	27	28	29	30	35	40
Height (in)	Weight (lb)													
58	91	96	100	105	110	115	119	124	129	134	138	143	167	191
59	94	99	104	109	114	119	124	128	133	138	143	148	173	198
60	97	102	107	112	118	123	128	133	138	143	148	153	179	204
61	100	106	111	116	122	127	132	137	143	148	153	158	185	211
62	104	109	115	120	126	131	136	142	147	153	158	164	191	218
63	107	113	118	124	130	135	141	146	152	158	163	169	197	225
64	110	116	122	128	134	140	145	151	157	163	169	174	204	232
65	114	120	126	132	138	144	150	156	162	168	174	180	210	240
66	118	124	130	136	142	148	155	161	167	173	179	186	216	247
67	121	127	134	140	146	153	159	166	172	178	185	191	223	255
68	125	131	138	144	151	158	164	171	177	184	190	197	230	262
69	128	135	142	149	155	162	169	176	182	189	196	203	236	270
70	132	139	146	153	160	167	174	181	188	195	202	207	243	278
71	136	143	150	157	165	172	179	186	193	200	208	215	250	286
72	140	147	154	162	169	177	184	191	199	206	213	221	258	294
73	144	151	159	166	174	182	189	197	204	212	219	227	265	302
74	148	155	163	171	179	186	194	202	210	218	225	233	272	311
75	152	160	168	176	184	192	200	208	216	224	232	240	279	319
76	156	164	172	180	189	197	205	213	221	230	238	246	287	328

Adapted from U.S. Department of Health and Human Services, National Health, Lung, and Blood Institute, People Science Health. Body Mass Index Table 1 [Internet]. [cited 2017 Feb 23]. Available from: http://www.nhlbi.nih.gov/guidelines/obesity/bmi_tbl.htm

by the Centers for Disease Control and Prevention (10). In children and adolescents, overweight is defined as the ≥85th to <95th percentile of BMI for age and sex, whereas obesity is defined as ≥95th percentile for age and sex.

BMI does not differentiate between fat and fat-free mass, so it is not a true measure of body fatness. Limitations of using BMI to classify individuals as normal, overweight, or obese must be recognized. Individuals with high levels of muscle mass can be misclassified as overweight or, in extreme cases, obese (*e.g.*, elite body builder). BMI can underestimate body fat in persons who have lost muscle mass (*e.g.*, older adults). High BMI in very short individuals (under 5 ft) may not reflect fatness. Despite these limitations, BMI is a very useful measurement, particularly when assessing large groups of people, because of its convenience and low cost. When possible, the EP-C should use clinical judgment when assessing individual clients and use BMI with other measures of body composition for a more complete profile of an individual. It is possible to predict percentage body fat from BMI, but this is not recommended because of the high margin of error associated with this technique (±5% fat) (16).

Table 7.2	Classification of Disease Risk Based on BMI and Waist Circumference (62)		
		Disease Risk[a] Relative to Normal	
		Waist Circumference	
		Men ≤102 cm	**Men >102 cm**
Weight	**BMI**	**Women ≤88 cm**	**Women >88 cm**
Underweight	<18.5	—	—
Normal	18.5–24.9	—	—
Overweight	25.0–29.9	Increased	High
Obesity			
Class I	30.0–34.9	High	Very high
Class II	35.0–39.9	Very high	Very high
Class III	≥40	Extremely high	Extremely high

[a]Disease risk for Type 2 diabetes, hypertension, and cardiovascular disease. Dashes (—) indicate that no additional risk at these levels of BMI was assigned. Increased waist circumference can also be a marker for increased risk even in persons of normal weight.

Circumference Measures

Circumference measures are a beneficial adjunct to other anthropometric measures. They are easily understood by clients and can be used with severely obese individuals, particularly when skinfold thicknesses are too large for standard skinfold calipers. Circumference measures can be used to determine body fat distribution, an important predictor of the health risks of obesity. Central obesity (also referred to as abdominal or android obesity) is associated with a higher risk of hypertension, metabolic syndrome, Type 2 diabetes mellitus, dyslipidemia, CVD, and premature death compared with gynoid obesity, which is characterized by a greater proportion of fat distributed on hips and thighs (54). The standard circumference sites are described in Table 7.3 and shown in Fig. 7.1.

Body fat distribution can be determined using the waist-to-hip ratio (WHR). This assessment helps the EP-C identify individuals with higher amounts of abdominal fat. To determine the WHR, divide the circumference of the waist by the circumference of the hips (buttocks/hips; Table 7.3). If a female client has a waist circumference of 31 in and a hip circumference of 42 in, her WHR is 35/42 = 0.83. Health risks increase as WHR increases, and standards for risk vary with age and sex (see Table 7.4).

Waist circumference alone can be used as an indicator of health risk because it reflects the level of abdominal obesity (8). Health risks are high when the waist circumference is ≥35 in (88 cm) for women and ≥40 in (102 cm) for men. Furthermore, waist circumference can be used with BMI to more precisely classify disease risk (see Table 7.2). It is important to note that these risk criteria are based on data derived from white men and women. African American men and women may have different BMI and waist circumference cut points (7,35). One study found that BMI and WHR correlated with mortality in whites, but not in African Americans; however, the risk of mortality associated with waist circumference was almost identical between races (35).

Circumference measurements should be taken using a flexible yet inelastic tape measure with a spring loaded handle (*e.g.*, Gulick tape measure) standardizes the tension of the tape on the skin. Each site should be measured twice in a rotational order and an average of the two measures is used to represent the circumference value. The EP-C should retest if duplicate measures are not within 5 mm (or 0.5 cm).

Visit thePoint to watch videos 6.1 and 6.2, which explain how to measure waist circumference for men and women.

Table 7.3	Standardized Description of Circumference Sites (1,2)
Site	**Location Description**
Abdomen	With the subject standing upright and relaxed, a horizontal measure taken at the greatest anterior extension of the abdomen, usually at the level of the umbilicus
Arm	With the subject standing erect and arms hanging freely at the sides with hands facing the thigh, a horizontal measure is taken midway between the acromion and the olecranon processes.
Buttocks/hips	With the subject standing erect and feet together, a horizontal measure is taken at the maximal circumference of buttocks. This measure is used for the hip measure in a waist/hip measure.
Calf	With the subject standing erect (feet apart ~20 cm), a horizontal measure taken at the level of the maximum circumference between the knee and the ankle, perpendicular to the long axis
Forearm	With the subject standing, arms hanging downward but slightly away from the trunk and palms facing anteriorly, a measure is taken perpendicular to the long axis at the maximal circumference.
Hips/thigh	With the subject standing, legs slightly apart (~10 cm), a horizontal measure is taken at the maximal circumference of the hip/proximal thigh, just below the gluteal fold.
Mid-thigh	With the subject standing and one foot on a bench so the knee is flexed at 90°, a measure is taken midway between the inguinal crease and the proximal border of the patella, perpendicular to the long axis.
Waist	With the subject standing, arms at the sides, feet together, and abdomen relaxed, a horizontal measure is taken at the narrowest part of the torso (above the umbilicus and below the xiphoid process). The National Obesity Task Force (NOTF) suggests obtaining a horizontal measure directly above the iliac crest as a method to enhance standardization. Unfortunately, current formulae are not predicated on the NOTF suggested site.

Percentage Body Fat Methods

Anthropometric measurements provide important information about the relationship between obesity and health but do not provide precise estimates of body composition. Body composition is the relative proportion of fat and fat-free tissue in the body. Determining body composition, or percentage body fat, helps the EP-C (a) identify individuals with high and low levels of body fat that are associated with increased health risks, (b) design appropriate exercise prescriptions, (c) formulate dietary recommendations, (d) assess the progress of a client in response to a weight management program, and (e) estimate weight loss goals. Body composition can be measured using various techniques that vary in terms of accuracy, cost, and complexity. The more common body composition measurements that are used in health/fitness settings include skinfolds and bioelectrical impedance. Laboratory measures include underwater weighing, plethysmography, and dual-energy X-ray absorptiometry (DEXA).

Tables 7.5 and 7.6 provide percentile values for percentage body fat in men and women, respectively. Experts have not agreed on an exact percentage body fat value associated with optimal health risk; however, a range of 10%–22% for men and 20%–32% for women is considered satisfactory for health (40).

Skinfold Measurements

Skinfold measurements are used to determine the amount of subcutaneous fat, that is, the fat located directly below the skin. Skinfold measures can be used to determine body composition

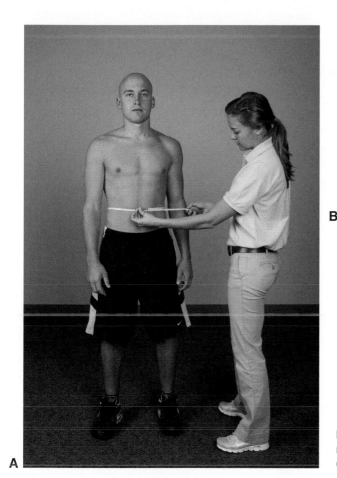

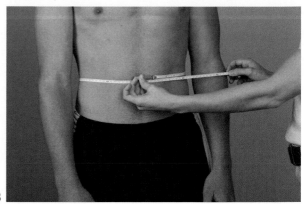

FIGURE 7.1. Measuring waist circumference. The waist is measured at the smallest circumference above the umbilicus (usually 1–2 in).

Table 7.4	Waist-to-Hip Ratio Norms for Men and Women (4)		
Age	Low Risk	Moderate Risk	High Risk
Men (yr)			
20–29	<0.83	0.83–0.88	>0.88
30–39	<0.84	0.84–0.91	>0.91
40–49	<0.88	0.88–0.95	>0.95
50–59	<0.90	0.90–0.96	>0.96
60–69	<0.91	0.91–0.98	>0.98
Women (yr)			
20–29	<0.71	0.71–0.77	>0.77
30–39	<0.72	0.72–0.78	>0.78
40–49	<0.73	0.73–0.79	>0.79
50–59	<0.74	0.74–0.81	>0.81
60–69	<0.76	0.76–0.83	>0.83

Table 7.5	Body Composition (% Body Fat) for Men						
	Age (yr)						
% Body Fat	20–29	30–39	40–49	50–59	60–69	70–79	
99	4.2	7.3	9.5	11.1	12.0	13.6	VL[a]
95	6.4	10.3	13.0	14.9	16.1	15.5	
90	7.9	12.5	15.0	17.0	18.1	17.5	E
85	9.1	13.8	16.4	18.3	19.2	19.0	
80	10.5	14.9	17.5	19.4	20.2	20.2	
75	11.5	15.9	18.5	20.2	21.0	21.1	G
70	12.6	16.8	19.3	21.0	21.7	21.6	
65	13.8	17.7	20.1	21.7	22.4	22.3	
60	14.8	18.4	20.8	22.3	23.0	22.9	
55	15.8	19.2	21.4	23.0	23.6	23.6	F
50	16.7	20.0	22.1	23.6	24.2	24.1	
45	17.5	20.7	22.8	24.2	24.9	24.5	
40	18.6	21.6	23.5	24.9	25.6	25.2	
35	19.8	22.4	24.2	25.6	26.4	25.7	P
30	20.7	23.2	24.9	26.3	27.0	26.3	
25	22.1	24.1	25.7	27.1	27.9	27.1	
20	23.3	25.1	26.6	28.1	28.8	28.0	
15	25.1	26.4	27.7	29.2	29.8	29.3	VP
10	26.6	27.8	29.1	30.6	31.2	30.6	
5	29.3	30.2	31.2	32.7	33.5	32.9	
1	33.7	34.4	35.2	36.4	37.2	37.3	
n =	1,938	10,457	16,032	9,976	3,097	571	

Total n = 42,071. Norms are based on Cooper Clinic patients. VL, very lean; E, excellent; G, good; F, fair; P, poor; VP, very poor.

[a]Very lean — No less than 3% body fat is recommended for males.

Reprinted with permission from The Cooper Institute, Dallas, Texas. Updated 2013. For more information: www.cooper institute.org

and correlate well with body composition determined by underwater weighing and DEXA. This technique is based on the assumptions that (a) approximately one-third of total body fat is located subcutaneously (41) and (b) the amount of subcutaneous fat is proportional to total body fat (2). However, these assumptions vary with sex, age, and ethnicity, which introduce some error into the prediction of percentage body fat from skinfold measurements. Other factors that may contribute to measurement error include poor technique and/or an inexperienced evaluator, a severely obese or extremely lean client, and an improperly calibrated caliper. In severely obese individuals, the skinfold thickness may exceed the maximum aperture of the caliper. To avoid embarrassing the client, the EP-C can use circumference measures only or use a different technique for measuring

Table 7.6	Fitness Categories for Body Composition (% Body Fat) for Women by Age						
	Age (yr)						
% Body Fat	20–29	30–39	40–49	50–59	60–69	70–79	
99	11.4	11.0	11.7	13.5	13.8	13.7	VL[a]
95	14.1	13.8	15.2	16.9	17.7	16.4	
90	15.2	15.5	16.8	19.1	20.1	18.8	E
85	16.1	16.5	18.2	20.8	22.0	21.2	
80	16.8	17.5	19.5	22.3	23.2	22.6	
75	17.7	18.3	20.5	23.5	24.5	23.7	G
70	18.6	19.2	21.6	24.7	25.5	24.5	
65	19.2	20.1	22.6	25.7	26.6	25.4	
60	20.0	21.0	23.6	26.6	27.5	26.3	
55	20.7	22.0	24.6	27.4	28.3	27.1	F
50	21.8	22.9	25.5	28.3	29.2	27.8	
45	22.6	23.7	26.4	29.2	30.1	28.6	
40	23.5	24.8	27.4	30.0	30.8	30.0	
35	24.4	25.8	28.3	30.7	31.5	30.9	P
30	25.7	26.9	29.5	31.7	32.5	31.6	
25	26.9	28.1	30.7	32.8	33.3	32.6	
20	28.6	29.6	31.9	33.8	34.4	33.6	
15	30.9	31.4	33.4	34.9	35.4	35.0	VP
10	33.8	33.6	35.0	36.0	36.6	36.1	
5	36.6	36.2	37.0	37.4	38.1	37.5	
1	38.4	39.0	39.0	39.8	40.3	40.0	
n =	1,342	4,376	6,392	4,496	1,576	325	

Total *n* = 18,507. Norms are based on Cooper Clinic patients. VL, very lean; E, excellent; G, good; F, fair; P, poor; VP, very poor.
[a]Very lean, no less than 10–13% body fat is recommended for women.

Reprinted with permission from The Cooper Institute, Dallas, Texas. Updated 2013. For more information: www.cooperinstitute.org

body composition, if available, the accuracy of predicting the percentage body fat from skinfolds is ±3.5%, assuming that proper technique is used when taking measures and that an appropriate regression equation is used to estimate percentage body fat (25).

Various regression equations have been developed to predict body density or percentage body fat from skinfold measurements. Table 7.8 lists generalized equations that allow calculation of body density for a wide range of individuals. Other population-specific equations that are sex-, age-, ethnicity-, fatness-, and sport-specific are available and may provide a more accurate estimate of body composition. Most regression equations use two or three skinfolds to predict body density,

HOW TO — Measure Skinfolds

Skinfolds are measured at standardized sites, described in Table 7.7 and shown in Figure 7.2. The skinfold sites must be precisely located using anatomical landmarks, and the following procedures must be followed for the accurate determination of body composition (1,6):

- Take all measurements on the right side of the client's body with the client standing upright. The client's skin should be dry and lotion-free. Do not take skinfold measurement immediately after exercise.
- Identify and mark all sites before measuring.
- Firmly grasp the skinfold (two layers of skin and subcutaneous fat) between the thumb and the index finger of your left hand, 1 cm above the site to be measured. To grasp the skinfold, place the thumb and index finger about 3 in apart on a line that is perpendicular to the long axis of the skinfold. Pull the skinfold up and away from the body.
- Keep the fold elevated while the measurement is being taken. Keep pinching the fold with your left hand throughout the entire measurement.
- Hold the caliper in the right hand with the dial facing up. Place the jaws of the calibers perpendicular to the fold 1 cm below the fingers and halfway between the crest and the base of the fold and release all pressure on the scissor grip while keeping the caliper perpendicular to the skinfold.
- Record the skinfold measurement to the nearest 0.5 mm, 1–2 seconds after releasing the scissor grip.
- Take skinfold measures in rotational order to allow time for the skinfold to regain its normal thickness.
- Take a minimum of two measurements at each site. If duplicate measurements are not within 1 or 2 mm (or 10%), retest this site.
- Calculate the average for each skinfold site. Using the client's measurements and validated skinfold equations, percentage body fat can be estimated.

which can then be converted to percentage body fat. The following are two of the most commonly used body density regression equations (5,58):

Brozek equation: % body fat = (495 / body density) − 450
Siri equation: % body fat = (457 / body density) − 414.2

Population-specific formulas for estimating percentage body fat from body density that are sex-, age-, ethnicity- and fatness-specific are also available (25).

Bioelectrical Impedance

Bioelectrical impedance analysis (BIA) is a rapid, noninvasive body composition assessment tool. In this method, a harmless electrical current is passed through the body and the impedance to that current is measured. Electrical impedance is related to the percentage of water contained in various body tissues. Lean tissue, which is composed of mostly water and electrolytes, is a good electrical conductor, whereas fat tissue, which contains much less water, acts as an impedance to the electrical current. BIA estimates total body water and relies on regression equations to estimate percentage body fat.

Table 7.7	Standardized Descriptions of Skinfold Sites (1,2)
Site	**Location Description**
Abdominal	Vertical fold; 2 cm to the right side of the umbilicus
Triceps	Vertical fold; on the posterior midline of the upper arm, halfway between the acromion and the olecranon processes, with the arm held freely to the side of the body
Biceps	Vertical fold; on the anterior aspect of the arm over the belly of the biceps muscle, 1 cm above the level used to mark the triceps site
Chest/ pectoral	Diagonal fold; one-half the distance between the anterior axillary line and the nipple (men), or one-third of the distance between the anterior axillary line and the nipple (women)
Medial calf	Vertical fold; at the maximum circumference of the calf on the midline of its medial border
Midaxillary	Vertical fold; on the midaxillary line at the level of the xiphoid process of the sternum. An alternate method is a horizontal fold taken at the level of the xiphoid/sternal border in the midaxillary line.
Subscapular	Diagonal fold (at a 45° angle); 1–2 cm below the inferior angle of the scapula
Suprailiac	Diagonal fold; in line with the natural angle of the iliac crest taken in the anterior axillary line immediately superior to the iliac crest
Thigh	Vertical fold; on the anterior midline of the thigh, midway between the proximal border of the patella and the inguinal crease (hip)

The accuracy of predicting the percentage body fat from BIA ranges between ±2.7% and 6.3% (23). Selecting an appropriate regression equation and controlling potential sources of measurement error help keep measurement error in the lower end of this range. Factors that alter hydration status are a major source of error; therefore, it is essential for client to follow pretesting guidelines. These guidelines will assist in attaining an accurate prediction of percentage body fat using BIA (24):

- No eating or drinking within 4 hours of the test
- No exercise within 12 hours of the test
- Completely void the bladder within 30 minutes of the test
- No alcohol consumption within 48 hours of the test
- No diuretic medication within 7 days of the test (clients should not discontinue use of prescribed diuretic medication unless approved by their personal physician)
- Avoid taking measurements prior to menstruation to avoid the possible effects of water retention in women
- Use the same BIA analyzer when measuring change in a client's body composition over time
- Complete measurements in a thermoneutral environment

Laboratory Methods for Measuring Body Composition

There are a number of sophisticated methods that you can use to determine percentage body fat. These methods tend to be more precise than the methods described in the preceding text but require expensive specialized equipment that is not available in most health/fitness settings. However, the EP-C should have knowledge of these advanced techniques, as they are often used as the reference that the simpler measures are compared with.

Hydrostatic (underwater) weighing (HW) is a widely used technique for determining body composition. This technique calculates body density from body volume, based on Archimedes principle, which states that the weight under water is directly proportional to the volume of water displaced by the body volume. The protocol requires that a person be weighed on land and underwater.

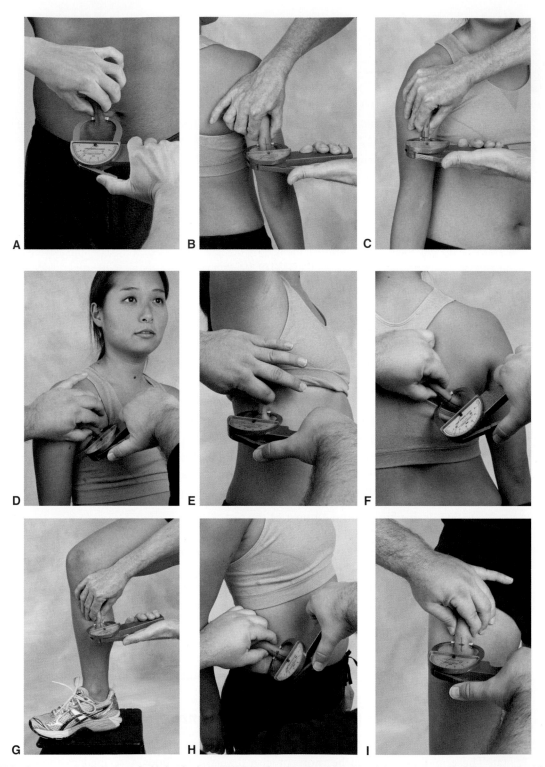

FIGURE 7.2. Common skinfold sites. **A.** Abdominal: vertical fold, 2 cm to the right side of the umbilicus. **B.** Triceps: vertical fold on the posterior midline of the upper arm, halfway between the acromion and the olecranon processes, with the arm held freely to the side of the body. **C.** Biceps: vertical fold on the anterior aspect of the arm over the belly of the biceps muscle, 1 cm above the level used to mark the triceps site. **D.** Chest: diagonal fold, one-half the distance between the anterior axillary line and the nipple (men) or one-third of the distance between the axillary line and the nipple (women). **E.** Midaxillary: vertical fold on the midaxillary line at the level of the xiphoid process of the sternum. **F.** Subscapular: diagonal fold (at a 45° angle), 1–2 cm below the inferior angle of the scapula. **G.** Medial calf: vertical fold at the maximum circumference of the calf on the midline of its medial border. **H.** Suprailium: diagonal fold in line with the natural angle of the iliac crest taken in the anterior axillary line immediately superior to the iliac crest. **I.** Thigh: vertical fold, on the anterior midline of the thigh, midway between the proximal border of the patella and the inguinal crease (hip). (From Bushman B, editor. *ACSM's Resources for the Personal Trainer.* 4th ed. Baltimore [MD]: Lippincott Williams & Wilkins; 2014.)

Table 7.8	Generalized Skinfold Equations to Determine Body Density (28,55)	
	Men	**Women**
Seven-site formula (chest, midaxillary, triceps, subscapular, abdomen, suprailiac, and thigh)	BD = 1.112 − 0.00043499 (sum of seven skinfolds) + 0.00000055 (sum of seven skinfolds)^2 − 0.00028826 (age) [See 0.008 or ~3.5% fat]	BD = 1.097 − 0.00046971 (sum of seven skinfolds) + 0.00000056 (sum of seven skinfolds)^2 − 0.00012828 (age) [See 0.008 or ~3.8% fat]
Three-Site Formula		
Chest, abdomen, and thigh	BD = 1.10938 − 0.0008267 (sum of three skinfolds) + 0.0000016 (sum of three skinfolds)^2 − 0.0002574 (age) [See 0.008 or ~3.4% fat]	NA
Chest, triceps, and subscapular	BD = 1.1125025 − 0.0013125 (sum of three skinfolds) + 0.0000055 (sum of three skinfolds)^2 − 0.000244 (age) [See 0.008 or ~3.6% fat]	NA
Triceps, suprailiac, and thigh	NA	BD = 1.099421 − 0.0009929 (sum of three skinfolds) + 0.0000023 (sum of three skinfolds)^2 − 0.0001392 (age) [See 0.009 or ~3.9% fat]
Triceps, suprailiac, and abdominal	NA	BD = 1.089733 − 0.0009245 (sum of three skinfolds) + 0.0000025 (sum of three skinfolds)^2 − 0.0000979 (age) [See 0.009 or ~3.9% fat]

BD, body density; NA, not applicable.

The densities of muscle and bone are higher than the density of water, whereas fat is less dense than water. A person with high levels of muscle and bone will be heavier in water compared with a person with higher levels of fat. HW has a standard error of the estimate of ±2.7% body fat (39).

Air displacement plethysmography (ADP) also measures body volume and is an alternative to HW for determining body composition. ADP has many advantages over HW, in that it is quick and noninvasive, does not require submersion in water, and accommodates children, adults, and older adults as well as individuals who are obese or disabled. There is one commercial system currently available (BOD POD, Life Measurement Instruments, Concord, CA). The accuracy of ADP is similar to that of HW (2).

DEXA uses very low current X-rays at two energy levels to measure bone mineral content, body fat, and lean soft tissue mass. This method requires an individual to lie supine on a table while being scanned from head to toe. DEXA is safe and easy to use, but the instrumentation can be very expensive. With appropriate standards and methodology, the reproducibility of DEXA is 1.7% for percentage body fat (3).

Weight Management

The causes of obesity are complex and multifactorial and are a mixture of genetic, behavioral, physiological, geographical, economic, and social factors. The *F as in Fat* report (38) noted that the states with the highest levels of physical inactivity and the lowest levels of fruit and vegetable consumption had the highest rankings of obesity. Although many other factors contribute to an individual's body weight, a healthy diet and regular PA are critical for attaining and/or maintaining a healthy weight.

Weight Loss Goals

Developing realistic weight loss goals is important when working with those who are trying to lose weight. The National Heart, Lung, and Blood Institute recommends that a 5%–10% weight reduction results in improved overall health (63). New guidelines indicate that a 3%–5% reduction in body weight produces health benefits (32).

Safe and effective weight loss should occur at a rate of 1–2 lb · week^{-1} (63). For example, an EP-C may work with a person who weighs 213 lb and has a percentage body fat of 31% and who has a goal weight of 196 lb and a target body fat of 25%. It would take 8.5–17 weeks or 2.5–4.25 months for the person to reach his or her desired weight. Although people can lose 2 lb · week^{-1}, it is difficult to maintain this amount of weight loss consistently over time, and the time frame of 8.5 weeks or 2.5 months is most likely unrealistic for most people. Thus, it is possible to reduce a person's percentage body fat 3%–6% in 3–4 months; however, it may take longer depending on the person. Depending on the weight loss goal, multiple (*i.e.*, three to four) goals may need to be created until the person reaches the desired percentage body fat and weight, especially if the goal is more than a 10% weight reduction.

Measuring body weight is a good method to use for weekly tracking because depending on which percentage body fat method is used, there could be a 3%–6% error in the estimated value. Therefore, if percentage body fat was measured each week, it would be difficult to determine either whether a change has actually occurred or whether it is a reflection of measurement error. This problem does not exist with absolute weight, although it is best to measure weight at a consistent time of day. Also, a person can weigh himself or herself each week without having to see a specialist to be measured (36).

Energy Balance

The management of body weight is dependent on energy balance: energy intake (the amount of calories consumed) and energy expenditure (the amount of calories expended). To reduce body weight, energy expenditure must exceed energy intake, referred to as a negative energy balance. Conversely, an individual gains weight when in a positive energy balance, that is, when energy intake exceeds energy expenditure. Body weight is maintained when an individual is in energy balance — expending the same number of calories as they are consuming.

Total energy expenditure (TEE) is the total number of calories expended each day and reflects the amount of energy required to carry out all metabolic processes within the body. Examples of these metabolic processes include growth of new cells, maintaining the functions of body tissues, and providing fuel for movement of the body, including exercise. There are three components to determining TEE:

- Resting energy expenditure (REE *or* resting metabolic rate [RMR] *or* basal metabolic rate [BMR]): 60%–70% TEE
- Thermic effect of food: 10% TEE
- PA expenditure: 20%–30% TEE

REE is the largest component of TEE and is the energy required to maintain normal regulatory balance and body functions at rest. In the simplest terms, REE (sometimes referred to as BEE or basal energy expenditure) is the amount of calories a person uses if he or she was to do no activity throughout the day. There are several factors that influence REE. To some degree, everyone's "metabolism" is determined by their genes; however, there are several other factors within the individual that contribute to a person's REE, including the body composition. Lean body mass, such as skeletal muscle, has a major influence on REE. Body tissues, such as the brain, the liver, and other organs, and even fat mass contribute to one's metabolism, although fat mass is much less metabolically active than other body tissues. A person's age, gender, and ethnicity also influence REE, primarily because of the impact on lean body mass.

Another component that contributes to a person's TEE is the thermic effect of food. Although this may account for a small percentage of a person's total metabolism, it is important to note that

HOW TO	Estimate Desired Body Weight and Percentage Body Fat

Knowing a person's percentage body fat and current body weight is needed to develop weight loss goals. Below is an equation that can be used to develop a desired body weight once the person's percentage body fat is known and a desired percentage body fat has been determined.

1. Estimate percentage body fat (using one of the methods discussed earlier in this chapter)
2. Fat mass = Total body mass × (Percentage body fat / 100)
3. Fat-free mass = Total body mass − Fat mass
4. Desired weight = Fat-free mass / [1 − (Desired percentage body fat / 100)]

Example:

1. Percentage body fat = 31%; Total body mass = 213 lb; Desired percentage body fat = 25%
2. Fat mass = Total body mass × (Percentage body fat / 100)

$$= 213 \times 0.31$$
$$= 66.03 \text{ lb}$$

3. Fat-free mass = Total body mass − Fat mass

$$= 213 - 66.03$$
$$= 146.97 \text{ lb}$$

4. Desired weight = Fat-free mass / [1 − (Desired percentage body fat / 100)]

$$= 146.97 / [1 - 0.25]$$
$$= 146.97 / 0.75$$
$$= 195.96 \; (\sim 196 \text{ lb})$$

the act of eating and digestion of foods require energy. The most controllable of all the influences on a person's total metabolism, however, is how active he or she is. The more physically active an individual is, the greater his or her TEE.

To calculate an individual's total energy needs, REE must first be measured or calculated using predictive equations. Next, an activity factor is used to calculate TEE for that individual. REE can be measured using indirect calorimetry, which measures an individual's oxygen consumption, although is not widely available. Predictive equations can also be used to estimate REE; however, predictive equations that incorporate fat-free mass provide the most accurate prediction of REE. Predictive equations take into account an individual's age, gender, height, and weight or fat-free mass (21). Table 7.9 provides examples of commonly used predictive equations for adults.

In determining an individual's daily energy needs, there are two approaches. One may use a predictive equations for REE (such as the Mifflin–St. Jeor equation) and then multiply this by a PA factor to give TEE (20).

Another method is to use the Institute of Medicine (IOM) TEE equations which factor in a physical activity level (PAL) based on gender (22):

For men:
Sedentary: PA = 1.0, when $1.0 \leq$ PAL <1.4
Low active: PA = 1.12, when $1.4 \leq$ PAL <1.6
Active: PA = 1.27, when $1.6 \leq$ PAL <1.9
Very active: PA = 1.54, when $1.9 \leq$ PAL <2.5

Table 7.9	Common Resting Energy Expenditure (kcal · day⁻¹) Predictive Equations for Adults	
	Men	**Women**
Harris–Benedict (for adults)	66.47 + 13.75 (weight in kg) + 5 (height in cm) − 6.8 (age in yr)	665 + 9.6 (weight in kg) + 1.8 (height in cm) − 4.7 (age in yr)
Mifflin–St. Jeor (for obese adults)	10 (weight in kg) + 6.3 (height in cm) − 5 × age + 5	10 (weight in kg) + 6.3 (height in cm) − 5 × age − 161

For women:

Sedentary: PA = 1.0, when $1.0 \leq$ PAL <1.4

Low active: PA = 1.14, when $1.4 \leq$ PAL <1.6

Active: PA = 1.27, when $1.6 \leq$ PAL <1.9

Very active: PA = 1.45, when $1.9 \leq$ PAL <2.5

Thus, PA is entered into the TEE equation in the following text to give total daily energy requirements for an individual:

For men:

TEE = 864 − 9.72 × age (yr) + PA × [(14.2 × weight (kg) + 503 × height (m)]

For women:

TEE = 387 − 7.31 × age (yr) + PA × [(10.9 × weight (kg) + 660.7 × height (m)]

Table 7.10	Estimated Calorie Needs per Day by Age, Gender, and Physical Activity Level (60,61)		
		Physical Activity Level		
Gender	**Age (yr)**	**Sedentary**	**Moderately Active**	**Active**
Female	2–3	1,000	1,000–1,200	1,000–1,400
	4–8	1,200–1,400	1,400–1,600	1,400–1,800
	9–13	1,400–1,600	1,600–2,000	1,800–2,200
	14–18	1,800	2,000	2,400
	19–30	1,800–2,000	2,000–2,200	2,400
	31–50	1,800	2,000	2,200
	51+	1,600	1,800	2,000–2,200
Male	2–3	1,000	1,000–1,400	1,000–1,400
	4–8	1,200–1,400	1,400–1,600	1,600–2,000
	9–13	1,600–2,000	1,800–2,200	2,000–2,600
	14–18	2,000–2,400	2,400–2,800	2,800–3,200
	19–30	2,400–2,600	2,600–2,800	3,000
	31–50	2,200–2,400	2,400–2,600	2,800–3,000
	51+	2,000–2,200	2,200–2,400	2,400–2,800

Table 7.11	Common Activity Factors Used with Resting Energy Expenditure to Calculate Total Daily Calorie Needs for Weight Maintenance in Adults (42)	
Level of Physical Activity	**Common Activity Factor**	
Sedentary (little to no activity)	1.2	
Light activity	1.375	
Moderate activity	1.55	
Very active	1.725	
Exceedingly active	1.9	

It is important to consider that using either method of determining an individual's energy needs gives total calories for weight maintenance. When calculating for weight loss, the recommended rate in adults is 1–2 lb · week^{-1}, which is equal to a daily caloric deficit of 500–1,000 calories.

When calculating energy needs for weight loss, first determine REE with either indirect calorimetry or the appropriate predictive equation. Then, multiply this by the appropriate activity factor. Table 7.10 shows daily energy needs for various population groups.

Following is an example for determining TEE prediction for a 35-year-old man, who is 6 ft 0 in, weighs 180 lb, and is lightly active. Using the Mifflin–St. Jeor equation, the calculated REE would be:

$$1{,}781 \text{ kcal (REE)} \times 1.375 \text{ (lightly active)} = 2{,}448 \text{ kcal} \cdot \text{day}^{-1}$$

In the earlier example, the individual needs about 2,500 cal · day^{-1} to maintain his weight at a low activity level (Table 7.11). To achieve 1 lb of weight loss per week, this person's caloric requirements would be approximately 2,100 cal · day^{-1}, or a 500-calorie daily deficit. It should be noted that it is not recommended for an individual to consume less than 1,200 cal · day^{-1} unless medically indicated, as this low-calorie intake is not likely to meet basic nutrient needs.

Treatment of Obesity through Exercise

ACSM Position Stand

In 2009, ACSM developed a position stand on appropriate PA interventions for weight loss and prevention of weight gain in adults (14). Regarding weight loss, the combination of diet and moderate-to-vigorous physical activity (MVPA) (≥150 min · wk^{-1}) produces the largest weight loss compared with diet or PA only.

Although the exact amount of PA necessary for weight maintenance after weight loss is currently unknown, it is well established that regular MVPA is necessary to prevent weight regain after weight loss has occurred. Furthermore, to prevent general weight gain, engaging in MVPA for at least 150 minutes a week is typically sufficient; however, the ACSM position stand indicates that engaging in more than 250 minutes a week of MVPA would result in better weight maintenance. Thus, it can be concluded that MVPA has a greater role in the prevention of weight regain and weight maintenance after weight loss has occurred rather than as a stand-alone weight loss method (14).

Weight Loss Using the FITT Principle

Exercise is defined as a PA that is structured and repetitive, uses large muscle groups, and has the intent of changing one or more fitness components. Exercise promotes increased levels of energy expenditure and should be done at a moderate to vigorous intensity. Types of exercise activities that work well for the overweight and obese include walking, swimming, water aerobics, jogging/walking in water, biking, and elliptical and rowing machines (12). All these activities can be done at an appropriate intensity and for a long duration without negatively impacting the knee and hip joints. Resistance training is also important to include after an aerobic activity has been incorporated into a person's routine, as it will not only improve muscular strength and endurance but also provide other health benefits, such as improvements in blood glucose levels and insulin sensitivity and increased bone mass.

Depending on the amount of excess body weight and the aerobic fitness of the client, the FITT principle can be adjusted to meet the needs of the client. There have been numerous studies examining the amount and type of PA that is needed to promote and maintain weight loss (29–31). Often, the person who is trying either to lose weight or to maintain weight loss will be working with a nutritionist for dietary advice. This is important as a reduction in energy consumption and an increase in energy expenditure will result in more weight loss than either method used alone. If an EP-C is working with a client who has not exercised in a long time, has never exercised, or is severely obese, initially doing exercise in 10-minute bouts at least three times a day may be necessary. The client may exercise for longer durations as their fitness level increases. This is also a good strategy to use if the client has a very busy schedule and cannot fit in one 30-minute bout.

Another strategy when working with an overweight or obese client is to have them decrease their time spent in sedentary behaviors. Sedentary behaviors involve activities that are no more than 1.5 metabolic equivalents (METs) (52). Examples of sedentary behaviors would be items that are completed while sitting, reclining or lying down, such as watching television, playing video games, non–work-related computer use, or using a tablet or smart phone. Sedentary behavior is not be confused with physical inactivity which is often used to describe people who may engage in some PA but not enough to meet recommended PALs.

The FITT principle for weight loss following ACSM guidelines is as follows:

Frequency: $\geq$5 days · week^{-1} to maximize caloric expenditure
Intensity: Moderate- to vigorous-intensity aerobic activity should be encouraged. Initial exercise training intensity should be moderate (*i.e.*, $\geq$40%–<60% $\dot{V}O_2R$ or HRR). Eventual progression to more vigorous exercise intensity (*i.e.*, $\geq$60% $\dot{V}O_2R$ or HRR) may result in further health and physical fitness benefits.
Time: A minimum of 30 minutes · day^{-1} (*i.e.*, 150 min · wk^{-1}) progressing to 60 minutes · day^{-1} (*i.e.*, 300 min · wk^{-1}) or more of moderate-intensity aerobic activity. Incorporating more vigorous-intensity exercise into the total volume of exercise may provide additional health benefits. However, vigorous-intensity exercise should be encouraged in individuals who are both capable and willing to exercise at higher than moderate-intensity levels with recognition that vigorous-intensity exercise is associated with the potential for greater injuries (53). Accumulation of intermittent exercise of at least 10 minutes is an effective alternative to continuous exercise and may be a particularly useful way to initiate exercise (29).
Type: The primary mode of exercise should be aerobic physical activities that involve the large muscle groups. As part of a balanced exercise program, resistance training and flexibility exercise should be incorporated.

Demonstrating Exercises

Demonstrating exercises to clients is a critical element to program implementation. Exercise demonstration allows the client to see what has been verbally explained and also allows key aspects of the exercise to be highlighted. This is especially true with either an overweight or an obese client. Depending on the severity of obesity, it may also be necessary to identify suitable equipment. Keep in mind that some equipment has a maximum weight limit or the person may not fit or be comfortable while exercising on the equipment. Furthermore, certain basic activities may be difficult, such as going down and getting up from the floor or bending over. Thus, specific exercises in a person's exercise program may need to be either modified or removed. All these aspects should be considered when designing an exercise program for an overweight and obese client.

General Training Principles

When designing a training program for overweight and obese clients, it may be of considerable value for the EP-C to become familiar with the 2009 ACSM position stand (14). Because each person will be at a different starting point and will have different goals regarding weight loss, the 2009 position stand combined with the *2015 Dietary Guidelines for Americans* will help the EP-C to individualize specific weight loss plans (12).

Although there are numerous approaches to planning exercise for weight loss, the basic principles of exercise prescription are outlined in Chapter 3. In addition, Chapter 8 provides detailed information about exercise prescription in people with cardiovascular, metabolic, and pulmonary disease, many of which are often present in the overweight and obese. Most importantly, if someone is overweight, obese, and currently sedentary, the EP-C needs to use caution and empathy in the early stages of an exercise program. The sedentary overweight and obese person is likely to find exercise initially uncomfortable and accompanied by soreness the following day or two (delayed onset muscle soreness or DOMS). These feelings may also bring about lower levels of self-efficacy and a lower desire to achieve the intended weight loss goals. Therefore, prescribing exercise becomes just as much art as science when working with this population.

Metabolic Equations

The ACSM metabolic equations can be used to estimate the amount of calories that will be expended during a workout or to estimate the length of time an individual has to exercise to expend a certain amount of calories. A calorie, also known as a kilocalorie (kcal), is an expression of energy intake and expenditure. It takes approximately 3,500 calories to make and store 1 lb of body weight. The following is an example of using metabolic equations to determine caloric expenditure. Either of these yields a reasonable estimate of calories expended and can be useful in setting exercise and dietary goals with a client.

These metabolic calculations yield a range of caloric expenditures that can be expected while performing the exercise. Keep in mind also that this value of $kcal \cdot min^{-1}$ includes the calories that would have been expended at rest, so this is the "gross" caloric expenditure for the 30 minutes. Refer to Chapters 3 and 8 to determine "net" caloric expenditure, or the calories strictly from the exercise.

Weight Management Myths

When working with someone who is trying to lose weight, they may ask about some common myths.

Myth 1: Fat Turns into Muscle or Vice Versa

Fat and muscle are two separate tissues in the body. It is impossible to change one type into the other. During weight loss, fat mass in the body typically decreases while the amount of muscle mass may increase if exercise is of sufficient intensity (overload principle).

EXERCISE IS MEDICINE CONNECTION

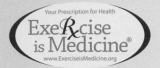

The Look AHEAD Research Group. Long-term effects of a lifestyle intervention on weight and CVD risk factors in individuals with Type 2 diabetes mellitus: four-year results of the look AHEAD trial. *Arch Intern Med.* 2010;170:1566–75.

The Look AHEAD (Action for Health in Diabetes) group conducted a 4-year randomized clinical trial that compared the effects of a lifestyle intervention with diabetes support and education (DSE) standard care. The purpose of this study was to examine the effects the Look AHEAD trial had on weight loss and CVD risk factors. The lifestyle intervention consisted of diet modification, PA, and behavior modification and was designed to produce at least a 7% weight loss at 1 year. The diet consisted of a 1,200–1,800 kcal $\cdot$ day^{-1} goal based on initial weight, with less than 30% of total calories from fat and at least 15% of total calories from protein. The exercise goal was to obtain at least 175 minutes of PA a week through walking. The behavioral strategies stressed included self-monitoring, goal setting, and problem solving. The lifestyle intervention group met with counselors weekly for the first 6 months and three times a week for the next 6 months. For years 2–4, they met with the counselors at least once a month. The DSE group was invited to attend three group sessions each year where diet, PA, or social support was discussed. Weight, aerobic fitness, blood draw, and blood pressure were measured annually, and the participants received an honorarium. Although the paper presents results for all CVD risk factors, only the results for the weight loss and maintenance are going to be discussed. At the end of the first year, the lifestyle group lost more weight (8.6% change) than did the DSE group (1% change). Furthermore, the lifestyle group was able to maintain the weight loss better than the DSE group over the 4-year period (4.7% vs. 1.1%, respectively; $p < .001$). When the weight loss was averaged over the 4 years, the lifestyle group lost more weight (mean change: 6.15% from initial weight) than the DSE group (mean change: 0.88% from initial weight). This is the first study to track weight loss and weight loss maintenance for such a long period. The results are very encouraging given the fact weight loss among that patients with Type 2 diabetes is very challenging. The participants in this study had an average BMI of 36.0 ± 5.6 kg $\cdot$ m^{-2}, so they were considered obese. This study shows that the combination of diet, PA, and behavioral modification is necessary not only to promote weight loss but also to maintain the weight loss over a long period.

Myth 2: Spot Reducing Works

It is not possible to reduce fat in a chosen region of the body. Fat reduction occurs in a somewhat random fashion and is not likely to be the same for any two persons. What will happen, however, is that if a client wants to lose fat around his or her waist and does an excessive number of core exercises, he or she will increase his or her core muscle mass but not necessarily reduce the fat located around the core.

Myth 3: Gaining Weight at the Start of an Exercise Program Is from Increased Muscle

Muscle hypertrophy occurs only after 6–8 weeks of higher intensity resistance training, and therefore, it is highly unlikely to see any muscle gain in the first 2 months of exercise. Even beyond that point, most people will not exercise at an intensity to produce significant increases in muscle mass. Instead, what is more likely, and discouraging, is that those new to exercise may overcompensate their calorie intake, thinking their newfound exercise "allows" them to eat more, thereby increasing their overall body weight.

> ### HOW TO   Calculate Metabolic Equations (Weight Management)
>
> Here is an example calculating caloric expenditure using metabolic equations.
>
> Female — height: 63 in, weight: 68 kg, BMI: 26.6 kg · m⁻²
>
> Client walks on a treadmill at 3.5 mph and a 5% grade for 30 minutes.
>
> What is the client's total caloric expenditure?
>
> $$\text{mph} \times (26.8 \text{ m} \cdot \text{min}^{-1}) = \text{m} \cdot \text{min}^{-1}$$
> $$(3.5 \text{ mph}) \times (26.8 \text{ m} \cdot \text{min}^{-1}) = 93.8 \text{ m} \cdot \text{min}^{-1}$$
> $$5\% \text{ grade} = 0.05$$
> $$\dot{V}O_2 \, (\text{mL} \cdot \text{kg}^{-1} \cdot \text{min}^{-1}) = (0.1 \times \text{m} \cdot \text{min}^{-1}) + (1.8 \times \text{m} \cdot \text{min}^{-1} \times \text{grade}) + 3.5$$
> $$\dot{V}O_2 \, (\text{mL} \cdot \text{kg}^{-1} \cdot \text{min}^{-1}) = (0.1 \times 93.8) + (1.8 \times 93.8 \times 0.05) + 3.5$$
> $$\dot{V}O_2 \, (\text{mL} \cdot \text{kg}^{-1} \cdot \text{min}^{-1}) = 9.38 + 8.44 + 3.5$$
> $$\dot{V}O_2 = 21.32 \text{ mL} \cdot \text{kg}^{-1} \cdot \text{min}^{-1}$$
> $$(\text{mL} \cdot \text{kg}^{-1} \cdot \text{min}^{-1}) \times 1,000 \, / \, \text{kg} = \dot{V}O_2 \, \text{L} \cdot \text{min}^{-1}$$
> $$(21.32 \times 1,000)/58 = 1.24 \text{ L} \cdot \text{min}^{-1}$$
> $$\text{L} \cdot \text{min}^{-1} \times 5 = \text{kcal} \cdot \text{min}^{-1}$$
>
> Note: Approximately 5 kcal are consumed for every liter of oxygen.
>
> $$1.24 \times 5 = 6.2 \text{ kcal} \cdot \text{min}^{-1}$$
> $$6.2 \text{ kcal} \cdot \text{min}^{-1} \times 30 \text{ min} = 186 \text{ kcal}$$
>
> Total caloric expenditure on treadmill = 186 kcal for 30 min
>
> This information can then be used to determine how many minutes, over how many days, the client will need to exercise to achieve her weight loss goals.

Treatment of Obesity through Nutrition

Every 5 years, a new edition of the *Dietary Guidelines for Americans* is available to the public. It is intended to help Americans aged 2 years to older adults improve overall health through evidence-based recommendations for healthy food choices (Table 7.12). The most current recommendations, the *2015-2020 Dietary Guidelines for Americans*, builds upon the 2010 Dietary Guidelines and provides five Guidelines with associated Key Recommendations. A key expansion of the Dietary Guidelines is that the focus is now more related to healthy eating patterns rather than individual food groups or nutrients. As stated in the *2015 Dietary*

Table 7.12	Recommended Macronutrient Proportions by Age (26)		
	Carbohydrate (%)	Protein (%)	Fat (%)
Young children (1–3 yr)	45–65	5–20	30–40
Older children and adolescents (4–18 yr)	45–65	10–30	25–35
Adults (≥19 yr)	45–65	10–35	20–35

Guidelines Executive Summary: "These Guidelines also embody the idea that a healthy eating pattern is not a rigid prescription, but rather, an adaptable framework in which individuals can enjoy foods that meet their personal, cultural, and traditional preferences and fit within their budget" (12).

The Guidelines for the *2015 Dietary Guidelines for Americans* are as follows (http://health.gov /dietaryguidelines/2015/guidelines/executive-summary/) (12):

1. **Follow a healthy eating pattern across the lifespan.** All food and beverage choices matter. Choose a healthy eating pattern at an appropriate calorie level to help achieve and maintain a healthy body weight, support nutrient adequacy, and reduce the risk of chronic disease.
2. **Focus on variety, nutrient density, and amount.** To meet nutrient needs within calorie limits, choose a variety of nutrient-dense foods across and within all the food groups in recommended amounts.
3. **Limit calories from added sugars and saturated fats and reduce sodium intake**. Consume an eating pattern low in added sugars, saturated fats, and sodium. Cut back on foods and beverages higher in these components that fit within a healthy eating pattern.
4. **Shift to healthier food and beverage choices.** Choose nutrient-dense foods and beverages across and within all food groups in place of less healthy choices.
5. **Support healthy eating patterns for all.** Everyone has a role in helping to create and support healthy eating patterns in multiple settings nationwide, from home to school to work to communities.

The Key Recommendations provide individuals with more guidance on how to follow the mentioned Guidelines:

Consume a healthy eating pattern that accounts for all foods and beverages within an appropriate calorie level.

A healthy eating pattern includes

- A variety of vegetables from all of the subgroups — dark green, red and orange, legumes (beans and peas), starchy and other
- Fruits, especially whole fruits
- Grains, at least half of which are whole grains
- Fat-free or low-fat dairy, including milk, yogurt, cheese, and/or fortified soy beverages
- A variety of proteins, including seafood, lean meats and poultry, eggs, legumes (beans and peas), and nuts, seeds, and soy products
- Oils

A healthy eating pattern limits

- Saturated fats and *trans* fats, added sugars, and sodium

Specifically,

- Consume less than 10% of cal $\cdot$ day^{-1} from added sugars
- Consume less than 10% of cal $\cdot$ day^{-1} from saturated fats
- Consume less than 2,300 mg $\cdot$ day^{-1} of sodium
- If alcohol is consumed, it should be consumed in moderation — up to one drink per day for women and up to two drinks per day for men — and only by adults of legal drinking age.

The MyPlate concept is still a very useful way to visualize a healthy eating pattern and is in accordance with the updated *Dietary Guidelines* (Fig. 7.3). The MyPlate website can be an evidence-based resource for all health, nutrition, and exercise professionals: http://www.choosemyplate.gov /dietary-guidelines (11).

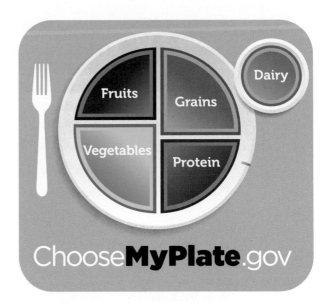

FIGURE 7.3. MyPlate: the new healthy eating guide.

The *2015 Dietary Guidelines* also recommend that individuals of all ages — children, adolescents, adults, and older adults — should meet the *Physical Activity Guidelines for Americans*.

Another key message of the *2015 Dietary Guidelines for Americans* is that there are relationships among individual food choices and the context and settings within which these choices are made to include the family environment, social and work settings, living situations, and communities. Thus, this edition of the *Dietary Guidelines* encourages efforts among health professionals, communities, businesses and industries, organizations, governments, and other areas of society to help support individuals in making healthy food choices and in meeting PA recommendations that are recommended in the *Dietary Guidelines*. It is the responsibility of the EP-C to keep abreast of changes that occur with the *Dietary Guidelines*.

Treatment of Obesity through Other Methods

Different strategies exist for modifying a person's body composition and promoting weight loss. Although many of these strategies are effective, some are considered unsafe and should not be used by individuals trying to lose weight. Inappropriate weight loss methods include saunas, electric stimulators, sweat suits, vibrating belts, body wraps, overexercising, very low calorie diets, fad diets, and dietary supplements (Table 7.13).

Appropriate weight loss methods include exercise, dietary changes, behavioral strategies, and bariatric surgery. Bariatric surgery rates have increased from 7.0 to 38.6 per 100,000 adults between 1998 and 2002 (59), and current rates are estimated to be almost double that of 2002. Although this surgery is very effective at producing weight loss (57), the effects of exercise in combination with this surgery are currently unknown. Moreover, it is unknown whether the exercise prescription should be different from those who chose not to undergo the surgery (1). For many people, though, bariatric surgery is medically indicated because of severe obesity and/or comorbidities threatening their health. The EP-C should recognize that weight loss is not easy, and for some people, the health risk of being overweight or obese is such that medical care should be sought. However, for those not interested or indicated for surgery, adding a behavioral component to their exercise and diet plan may aid them in achieving their weight loss goals.

Table 7.13	Inappropriate Weight Loss Methods and Consequences (13,15,33,56,66)
Method	**Negative Consequences**
Saunas	Dehydration, only lose water weight, low amount of weight loss, temporary weight loss
Vibrating belts	No weight loss
Body wraps	Small weight loss, temporary weight loss, skin irritation
Overexercising	Overuse injury, unhealthy amount of weight loss
Electric muscle stimulators	No change in body composition, bruising, and skin irritation
Sweat suits	Dehydration, only lose water weight, low amount of weight loss, temporary weight loss
Dietary supplements	Not regulated by FDA, so dosage may not be known; may have nutrient drug interactions, drug–drug interactions, and other side effects such as nausea, dizziness, and racing heart
Very low calorie diets	May not meet nutrient needs of the individual promoting deficiencies in specific nutrients (*e.g.*, calcium deficiency leads to brittle, broken bones, hip fractures); could lead to dehydration, constipation, or fatigue
Fad diets	Often "cut out" a food group, which leads to specific nutrient, vitamin, and mineral deficiencies; not sustainable for long periods; could lead to "yo-yo" dieting (*i.e.*, intervals of weight loss followed by weight gain); low carbohydrate diets do not meet body's requirement for a minimum of 130 g of carbohydrates a day; could lead to fatigue and lack of energy; could lead to dehydration and/or constipation; not recommended

Behavioral Strategies

Interventions that combine diet, PA, and behavior therapy are the most effective programs for weight loss and weight maintenance (62). Behavioral weight loss programs not only target dietary intake and PA but also provide clients with strategies to help them make the necessary lifestyle changes. Key strategies used in behavioral weight loss programs include the following:

- Self-monitoring — keeping food or PA logs or monitoring body weight on a regular basis
- Goal setting — setting realistic goals for the number of minutes of exercise one will accomplish during the next week or month
- Stimulus control — modifying one's environment to enhance successful behavior change such as removing "risky" foods from the refrigerator or hanging an exercise adherence calendar in a prominent spot
- Problem solving — identifying situations that pose a problem for overeating (such as holidays) and developing a solution to eat healthy and avoid excess caloric intake

There are many additional behavioral strategies that clients can use to enhance a weight management program. See Chapter 12 for more information on behavioral strategies that can assist with weight loss goals.

Weight Loss Supplements

The EP-C has a responsibility to encourage healthy weight loss, when indicated, by eating a balanced diet including adequate fruit and vegetables, limiting sugary beverages and energy-dense foods, and including regular exercise and activity. Taking this approach is considered safe and reasonable and should provide sufficient nutrition to meet daily needs. However, despite this, many different weight loss products and supplements are available to the public, often with little or no evidence to support their value. One of the most reputable resources for information on vitamins, minerals, supplements, and herbal products is the Office of Dietary Supplement (49). Although medications and drugs prescribed by a doctor are regulated by the U.S. Food and Drug Administration (FDA), supplements and herbal products are not regulated by the government in terms of efficacy, safety, dosing, and purity of the product. The FDA Web site does list updates and warnings related to supplements (both dietary and herbal) and is an important resource for EP-Cs and their clients (64).

The rating on effectiveness is based on available research (44). Some advertised physiological mechanisms for dietary supplements include increased energy expenditure, modified carbohydrate metabolism, decreased fat production, and blocked absorption of dietary fat. However, numerous safety concerns have been raised with some supplements (*e.g.*, ephedra, bitter orange, and chitosan), occasionally resulting in their removal from the consumer market.

People of all ages experiment with weight loss products, including caffeine and energy drinks. Although a safe upper limit has been established for adults and caffeine ($250–300$ mg $\cdot$ d^{-1}), there is no recommendation for adolescents. Therefore, as a general rule, caffeine and energy drinks should be consumed with caution, particularly in the younger/adolescent population. Many energy drinks are also high in sugar and calories, so regardless of age, the consumption of these drinks may be a source of excess calories and not "cost-effective" in terms of the benefits outweighing the risks. Side effects of energy drinks and caffeine depend on the individual's sensitivity but may include sleeplessness, nervousness, irritability, and anxiety. Resources for additional information on supplements and herbal products can be found at the end of this chapter.

Dieting

Although many people may also experiment with "dieting" for weight loss, in general, most popular diets are to be approached with caution. Ideally, individuals interested in the current popular diet fads should first seek the advice of a registered dietitian or other health care professional trained in nutrition to determine the safety and effectiveness of the diet. Diets to be cautious of include those promoting low carbohydrates, excessive protein intake, or any meal pattern that eliminates or emphasizes any one particular food group. For instance, the IOM recommends at least 130 g of carbohydrate each day for all age groups (28). Thus, diets prescribing low carbohydrate intake may fall short of this requirement and likely lead to cravings. Individuals need a variety of foods from each food group to meet their needs for growth, development, and maintenance throughout the lifespan. Any client who wishes to "go on a diet" should first consider his or her optimal health/ dietary needs. A more prudent approach may be to consider permanent dietary changes (such as eating more fruits and vegetables) as opposed to "going on a diet."

Medications

Table 7.14 shows the effect of common medications on weight management and their physiological action (15,19,34,37,43,45). Many of these medications, taken for high blood pressure, seizure disorders, allergies, and so on, can actually promote weight gain. Therefore, it is important to know all the medications your client is taking, as they may inhibit your client's weight loss attempts.

Table 7.14	Effect of Medication on Weight Management and the Action on the Body (16,19,37,43,45,65)	
Medication	**Effect**	**Action**
Corticosteroid		
Prednisone	Weight gain	Increased appetite/decreased ability to absorb blood glucose
Antidepressant		
Paxil	Weight gain	
Zoloft	Weight gain	
Wellbutrin	Weight loss	
Prozac	Weight loss	
Antihypertensive		
Cardura and Inderal	Weight gain	Fatigue/shortness of breath/water retention
Hormone replacement therapy/oral contraceptives	Weight gain	
Antiseizure		
Depakote	Weight gain	
Zonegran	Weight loss	
Topamax	Weight loss	
Diabetes Medication		
Insulin	Weight gain	Weight gain: decreases resting RMR; stimulates insulin secretion; increases number of fat cells
Sulfonylureas	Weight gain	
Thiazolidinediones	Weight gain	
Glucophage	No change	
Precose	No change	
Byetta	Weight loss	
Symlin	Weight loss	
Heartburn		
Nexium	Weight gain	
Prevacid		
Antihistamine	Weight gain	Increase food intake via hypothalamic receptors and leptin regulative system
Other		
α-Blockers	Weight gain	Unknown
β-Blockers	Weight gain	Decreased RMR; increased fatigue and causes reduction in physical activity
Migraine medication	Weight gain	Increased appetite; stimulated insulin secretion
Nicotine	Weight loss (?)	Reducing appetite; increasing RMR
Caffeine	Weight loss (?)	Reducing appetite; stimulate thermogenesis; promote water loss

RMR, resting metabolic rate.

Nutrition through the Lifespan

Along with regular exercise, it is important to incorporate proper daily nutrition habits to achieve and successfully maintain weight loss. However, this should not be considered a "one-time" diet but instead a lifelong strategy of healthy eating. Specific needs for pregnant women, children, and older adults are discussed in the following sections.

Pregnancy

During pregnancy, there are increased energy and nutrient needs to support the growth of the developing fetus. The pregnant woman needs an additional 300 calories each day to ensure that enough essential nutrients are available for both mother and baby. Although pregnant women are strongly encouraged to eat a well-rounded diet, it is also important for the pregnant women to take a vitamin specifically designed for prenatal purposes.

In addition to the increased daily need for protein, there is also an increased dietary need for folic acid and iron that is provided in a prenatal vitamin. Folic acid (a B vitamin) is important in the prevention of serious birth defects such as neural tube defect and congenital heart disease. Extra iron is needed to help support the increased blood supply needed to carry extra oxygen throughout the pregnancy. It is usually recommended that pregnant women take a prenatal vitamin as directed by her doctor because taking higher or lower doses of a given vitamin or mineral could be harmful to the developing baby. It is also recommended that pregnant women do not take herbal or botanical supplements because they are not FDA regulated in terms of dosage, purity, and testing. Harmful effects of herbal supplements are not yet fully known, and therefore, it is best for woman to avoid these altogether while pregnant. In addition, given that the demand for other nutrients such as calcium, protein, and carbohydrate increase during pregnancy, this is certainly not an appropriate time for a woman to go on any type of self-prescribed "diet," especially one intended for weight loss.

Children and Older Adults

The EP-C should also have sufficient knowledge of the unique dietary needs of children and older adults. Vitamin D recommendations for children and adolescents ages 1–18 years is 600 IU, and recommendations for adults older than 71 years is 800 IU. Also in the older adult, vitamin D is particularly important in its role of promoting the absorption of calcium and in maintaining serum calcium levels, which in turn protects bone strength (48). Although sunlight is a natural source of vitamin D, it is also fortified into many foods, including dairy, breads, and cereals and can therefore be obtained rather easily in most diets.

Calcium is an important nutrient during childhood and adolescence. Current recommendations are 1,000 mg $\cdot$ day^{-1} for 4- to 8-year-olds, with an increase of calcium for 9- to 18-year-olds to 1,300 mg $\cdot$ day^{-1} (27).

It is crucial for bone and teeth health at this life stage and is also important in the prevention of osteoporosis later in life. Adults aged 19–50 years need 1,000 mg calcium $\cdot$ day^{-1}. Calcium absorption declines with age, thus increasing the need of this nutrient in the older adult population. Postmenopausal women (51 yr and older) tend to experience greater bone loss and decreased absorption of calcium, which increases the need in this population to 1,200 mg $\cdot$ day^{-1}. Older men aged 70 years and older also have increased needs at 1,200 mg $\cdot$ day^{-1}. Calcium supplements are best absorbed when doses are 500 mg or less.

In older adults, vitamin B$_{12}$ supplementation can be important, as 10%–30% of older individuals develop atrophic gastritis, a condition that decreases secretion of hydrochloric acid in the stomach, which in turn decreases the absorption of naturally occurring vitamin B$_{12}$ (47). Thus, it is recommended that adults 50 years and older either take a vitamin B$_{12}$ supplement or consume sufficient amounts of fortified foods such as breakfast cereals.

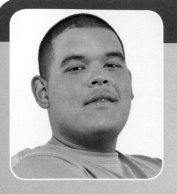

The Case of Ryan

Submitted by **Linda Vaughn, MS, MBA, ACSM EP-C, YMCA of Metropolitan Atlanta, Atlanta, GA**

Ryan, a 22-year-old, 425-lb man, presented at his local YMCA to seek help in losing weight, specifically stating, "I'm 22 years old and weigh less than the rest of my family. I've never had a date and I don't want any more male 'boobies.'"

Narrative

The EP-C coach informed Ryan that his goals would require at least a 2-year commitment to healthy eating and regular exercise, to which Ryan agreed. Ryan stated that he had recently lost 50 lb. He said that he lived with his grandmother while he was in college and that she consistently served Southern home–style (fried) meals, and it was hard to say "no" to her cooking; he was afraid of offending her. His affect was somewhat flat at presentation. The EP-C coach used calibrated scales to verify that his body weight was 425 lb. The EP-C coach then administered the Resources for Exercise Maintenance Survey (1) to determine what type of support Ryan needed. It was determined that Ryan needed specific support in his inability to tolerate discomfort, his lack of self-management skills, and his lack of social support among family members. On investigating Ryan's preferred activities, the EP-C coach advised Ryan to begin walking on a treadmill for at least 20 minutes, three times a week, at an intensity of 64%–70% of his maximum heart rate; to begin a strength training program (no more than two sets of 8–10 repetitions of at least eight different muscle groups); and to begin tracking his food intake. Within 3 weeks, Ryan reported a weight loss of 27 lb to his coach and revealed to his coach that he was "working out" three times a day every day and eating Clif bars and salads for his meals (approximately 1,000 cal · day^{-1}). The coach verified Ryan's workouts via the FitLinxx system to reflect that he was swimming at least 20–30 minutes a day, attending group cycling classes, step aerobics classes, Taekwondo classes, or yoga classes daily (55 min), as well as running outdoors (33–40 min). In addition, he reported to his coach that he was weight training everyday with no off-days between workouts; this was reflected in the FitLinxx system as calisthenics at an intensity of level 9 out of 10 for, on average, 45–60 minutes, however, not always daily. The coach advised Ryan that he needed to eat more to sustain himself at rest at his present body weight and even more to support 3 hours of workouts a day. After calculating Ryan's caloric needs for REE and his TEE, the EP-C coach advised Ryan that he needed to eat more food or exercise less to avoid muscle degradation in his efforts. Ryan was resistant, stating "No one has ever told me I had to eat more, and I feel good!"

QUESTIONS

- What is the TEE for Ryan based on his current body weight and his current exercise regimen?
- What modifications should occur in Ryan's self-imposed fitness prescription?
- How can Ryan effectively deal with his grandmother's cooking?
- How can Ryan deal with his lack of familial support in his efforts to be become healthier?

References

1. Annesi JJ. *The Coach Approach: An Exercise Support Process Implementation Handbook*. 3rd ed. Atlanta, GA: YMCA of Metropolitan Atlanta; 2007. 51 p.

Additional Resources

1. Donnelly JE, Blair SN, Jakicic JM, Manore MM, Rankin JW, Smith BK. Appropriate physical activity intervention strategies for weight loss and prevention of weight regain for adults. *Med Sci Sports Exerc*. 2009;41(2):459–71.
2. Fitness Education Network. *American College of Sports Medicine Certified Personal Trainer Workshop Course Workbook*. Atlanta (GA): Fitness Education Network; 2009. 53 p.

SUMMARY

Obesity has reached epidemic levels in the United States, and determining a person's obesity status is a key part of the EP-C job duties. Each EP-C should be experienced in a variety of methods to measure obesity status, as different methods may be better for different individuals. Although some methods are quite precise (*e.g.*, HW and DEXA), they are not very practical. Therefore, regular practice with BMI, skinfolds, circumferences, and so on, is important for the EP-C. Once a person's obesity status is determined, realistic weight loss or weight maintenance goals can be created. Through the 2009 ACSM position stand, the EP-C has a guideline for developing exercise programs that address weight management with regard to frequency, intensity, time, and type of exercise and goals for caloric intake.

A person's nutritional needs change over time because of medical conditions, aging, pregnancy, and so on. Although working with a registered dietitian is ideal, the EP-C should be aware of the different nutritional needs for pregnant women, children, and older adults. The 2010 dietary guidelines are a good resource for the EP-C when discussing client nutritional needs. The information highlighted in this chapter will enable the EP-C to fully support a client with weight management by appropriately incorporating nutrition, PA, and behavior modification in individual client goal setting.

STUDY QUESTIONS

1. Discuss the pros and cons of percentage body fat measurement methods in individuals with a BMI >35 kg $\cdot$ m^{-2}.
2. Compare and contrast the difference between the Food Guide Pyramid and the MyPlate campaign.
3. Robert walked on a treadmill at a speed 2.5 mph and a grade of 10% for 40 minutes. How many kilocalories did he expend?

REFERENCES

1. American College of Sports Medicine. *ACSM's Guidelines for Exercise Testing and Prescription*. 8th ed. Baltimore (MD): Lippincott Williams & Wilkins; 2010. 400 p.

2. American College of Sports Medicine. *ACSM's Guidelines for Exercise Testing and Prescription*. 9th ed. Philadelphia (PA): Lippincott Williams & Wilkins; 2014. 456 p.

3. Bray GA. *A Guide to Obesity and the Metabolic Syndrome*. Boca Raton (FL): CRC Press; 2011. 412 p.

4. Bray GA, Gray DS. Obesity. Part I — pathogenesis. *West J Med*. 1988;149(4):429–41.

5. Brozek J, Grande F, Anderson JT, Keys A. Densitometric analysis of body composition: revision of some quantitative assumptions. *Ann N Y Acad Sci*. 1963;110:113–40.

6. Callaway CW, Chumlea WC, Bouchard C. Circumferences. In: Lohman TG, Roche AF, Martorell R, editors. *Anthropometric Standardization Reference Manual*. Champaign (IL): Human Kinetics; 1988. p. 39–54.

7. Camhi SM, Bray GA, Bouchard C, et al. The relationship of waist circumference and BMI to visceral, subcutaneous, and total body fat: sex and race differences. *Obesity*. 2011;19(2):402–8.

8. Canoy D. Distribution of body fat and risk of coronary heart disease in men and women. *Curr Opin Cardiol*. 2008;23(6): 591–8.

9. Cawley J, Meyerhoefer C. The medical care costs of obesity: an instrumental variables approach. *J Health Econ*. 2012; 31(1):219–30. doi:10.1016/j.jhealeco.2011.10.003.

10. Centers for Disease Control and Prevention. About child & teen BMI [Internet]. Atlanta (GA): Centers for Disease Control and Prevention; [cited 2011 Jul 20]. Available from: http://www.cdc.gov/healthyweight/assessing/bmi/childrens_bmi/about_childrens_bmi.html

11. ChooseMyPlate Web site [Internet]. Alexandria (VA): U.S. Department of Agriculture; [cited 2011 Jul 20]. Available from: http://www.choosemyplate.gov

12. Compendium of Physical Activities [Internet]. [cited 2011 Nov 11]. Available from: https://sites.google.com/site/compendiumofphysicalactivities/

13. Doheny K. Body wraps: what to expect [Internet]. Atlanta (GA): WebMD; [cited 2011 Aug 2]. Available from: http://www.webmd.com/healthy-beauty/features/body-wraps-what-to-expect

14. Donnelly JE, Blair SN, Jakicic JM, Manore MM, Rankin JW, Smith BK. Appropriate physical activity intervention strategies for weight loss and prevention of weight regain for adults. *Med Sci Sports Exerc*. 2009;41(2):459–71.

15. Do vibration exercise machines work? [Internet]. [cited 2011 Aug 2]. Available from: http://www.weighttraining.com/faq/do-vibration-exercise-machines-work

16. Duren DL, RJ Sherwood, SA Czerwinski, et al. Body composition methods: comparisons and interpretation. *J Diabetes Sci Technol*. 2008;2(6):1139–46.

17. Flegal KM, Carroll MD, Odgen CL, Curtin LR. Prevalence and trends in obesity among US adults. *JAMA*. 2010;303(3):235–41.

18. Flegal KM, Graubard BI, Williamson DF, Gail MH. Excess deaths associated with underweight, overweight, and obesity. *JAMA*. 2005;293(15):1861–7.

19. http://www.fitwoman.com/blog/medications-weight-gain-2/. Accessed Feb 23, 2017.

20. Frankenfield D. Bias and accuracy of resting metabolic rate equations in non-obese and obese adult. *Clin Nutr*. 2013; 32(6):976–82.

21. Frankenfield D, Roth-Yousey L, Compher C. Comparison of predictive equations for resting metabolic rate in healthy non-obese and obese adults: a systematic review. *J Am Diet Assoc*. 2005;105(5):775–89.

22. Gerrior S, Juan W, Basiotis P. An easy approach to calculating estimated energy requirements. *Prev Chronic Dis*. 2006; 3(4):A129.

23. Graves JE, Kanaley JA, Garzareooa L, Pollock ML. Anthropometry and body composition assessment. In: Maud PJ, Foster C, editors. *Physiological Assessment of Human Fitness*. 2nd ed. Champaign (IL): Human Kinetics; 2006. p. 185–225.

24. Heyward VH. *Advanced Fitness Assessment and Exercise Prescription*. 6th ed. Champaign (IL): Human Kinetics; 2010. 480 p.

25. Heyward VH, Wagner DR. *Applied Body Composition Assessment*. 2nd ed. Champaign (IL): Human Kinetics; 2004. 280 p.

26. Institute of Medicine. *Dietary Reference Intakes (DRIs): Acceptable Macronutrient Distribution Ranges* [Internet]. Washington (DC): National Academies Press; [cited 2016 Jan 15]. Available from: http://fnic.nal.usda.gov/sites/fnic.nal.usda.gov/files/uploads/recommended_intakes_individuals.pdf

27. Institute of Medicine. *Dietary Reference Intakes (DRIs): Recommended Dietary Allowances and Adequate Intakes, Elements* [Internet]. Washington (DC): National Academies Press; [cited 2016 Jan 15]. Available from: http://fnic.nal.usda.gov/sites/fnic.nal.usda.gov/files/uploads/recommended_intakes_individuals.pdf

28. Jackson AS, Pollock ML. Practical assessment of body composition. *Physician Sportsmed*. 1985;13(5):76–90.

29. Jakicic JM, Marcus BH, Gallagher KL, Napolitano M, Lang W. Effect of exercise duration and intensity on weight loss in overweight, sedentary women: a randomized trial. *JAMA*. 2003;290(10):1323–30.

30. Jakicic JM, Winters C, Lang W, Wing RR. Effect of intermittent exercise and use of home exercise equipment on adherence, weight loss, and fitness in overweight women: a randomized trial. *JAMA*. 1999;282(16):1554–60.

31. Jeffery RW, Wing RR, Sherwood NE, Tate DF. Physical activity and weight loss: does prescribing higher physical activity goals improve outcome? *Am J Clin Nutr*. 2003;78(4):684–9.

32. Jensen MD, Ryan DH, Apovian CM, et al. 2013 ASA/ACC/TOS guideline for the management of overweight and obesity in adults: a report of the American College of Cardiology/American Heart Association Task Force on Practice Guidelines and The Obesity Society. *Circulation*. 2014;129(25 Suppl 2):S102–38.

33. Johannes L. Cinching your belt without a crunch [Internet]. *The Wall Street Journal*. [cited 2011 Aug 2]. Available from: http://online.wsj.com/article/SB10001424052748704779704574553790579199098.html

34. Johns Hopkins Health Alert. Prescription drugs that cause weight gain [Internet]. [cited 2011 Jul 5]. Available from: http://www.johnshopkinshealthalerts.com/alerts/prescription_drugs/JohnsHopkinsPrescriptionsDrugsHealthAlert_656-1.html.

35. Katzmarzyk PT, Mire E, Bray GA, Greenway FL, Heymsfield SB, Bouchard C. Anthropometric markers of obesity and mortality in white and African American adults: the Pennington Longitudinal Study. *Obesity*. 2013;21(5):1070–5.

36. Klem ML, Wing RR, McGuire MT, Seagle HM, Hill JO. A descriptive study of individuals successful at long-term maintenance of substantial weight loss. *Am J Clin Nutr*. 1997; 66(2):239–46.

37. Laino C. Is your medicine cabinet making you fat? [Internet]. [cited 2011 Jul 5]. Available from: http://www.medicinenet.com/script/main/art.asp?articlekey=56339&page=1

38. Levi J, Vinter S, St. Larent R, Segal LM. *F as in Fat: How Obesity Threatens American's Future*. Washington (DC): Trust for American's Health, Robert Wood Johnson Foundation; 2010. 115 p.

39. Lohman TG. *Advances in Body Composition Assessment*. Champaign (IL): Human Kinetics; 1992. 150 p.

40. Lohman TG. Body composition methodology in sports medicine. *Physician Sports Med*. 1982;10(12):46–7.

41. Lohman TG. Skinfolds and body density and their relations to body fatness: a review. *Hum Biol*. 1981;53(2):181–225.

42. Lutz C, Mazur E, Litch N. *Nutrition and Diet Therapy*. 6th ed. Philadelphia (PA): F.A. Davis; 2015. 523 p.

43. Mayo Clinic. *Does Caffeine Help with Weight Loss?* [Internet]. Scottsdale (AZ): Mayo Clinic; [cited 2011 Jul 5]. Available from: http://www.mayoclinic.com/health/caffeine/HQ00369

44. Mayo Clinic. *Over-the-Counter Weight-Loss Pills* [Internet]. Scottsdale (AZ): Mayo Clinic; [cited 2011 Jul 21]. Available from: http://www.mayoclinic.com/health/weight-loss/HQ01160

45. MedicineNet. *Prescription Drugs Causing Weight Gain?* [Internet]. San Clemente (CA): MedicineNet; [cited 2011 Jul 5]. Available from: http://www.medicinenet.com/script/main/art.asp?articlekey=56339&page=2

46. National Cholesterol Education Program. *Third Report of the National Cholesterol Education Program (NCEP) Expert Panel on Detection, Evaluation, and Treatment of High Blood Cholesterol in Adults (Adult Treatment Panel III): Final Report*. Washington (DC): National Institutes of Health; 2002. 284 p.

47. National Institutes of Health Office of Dietary Supplements. Vitamin B$_{12}$ [Internet]. Bethesda (MD): U.S. Department of Health and Human Services; [cited 2011 Jul 21]. Available from: http://ods.od.nih.gov/factsheets/vitaminb12/

48. National Institutes of Health Office of Dietary Supplements. Vitamin D [Internet]. Bethesda (MD): U.S. Department of Health and Human Services; [cited 2011 Jul 21]. Available from: http://ods.od.nih.gov/factsheets/vitamind/

49. National Institutes of Health Office of Dietary Supplements Web site [Internet]. Bethesda (MD): U.S. Department of Health and Human Services; [cited 2011 Jul 21]. Available from: http://ods.od.nih.gov

50. Ogden CL, Carroll MD, Curtin LR, Lamb MM, Flegal KM. Prevalence of high body mass index in US children and adolescents, 2007–2008. *JAMA*. 2010;303(3):242–9.

51. Ogden CL, Carroll MD, Kit BK, Flegal KM. Prevalence of childhood and adult obesity in the United States, 2011-2012. *JAMA*. 2014;311(8):806–14.

52. Owen N, Leslie E, Salmon J, Fotheringham MJ. Environmental determinations of physical activity and sedentary behavior. *Exer Sport Scie Rev*. 2000;28(4):153–8.

53. Perri MG, Anton SD, During PE, et al. Adherence to exercise prescriptions: effect of prescribing moderate versus high levels of intensity and frequency. *Health Psychol*. 2002;21(5):452–8.

54. Pi-Sunyer FX. The epidemiology of central fat distribution in relation to disease. *Nutr Rev*. 2004;62(7 Pt 2):S120–6.

55. Pollack ML, Schmidt DH, Jackson AS. Measurement of cardiorespiratory fitness and body composition in the clinical setting. *Compr Ther*. 1980;6(9):12–27.

56. Porcari JP, McLean KP, Foster C, Kernozek T, Crenshaw B, Swensen C. Effects of electrical muscle stimulation on body composition, muscle strength, and physical appearance. *J Strength Cond Res*. 2002;16(2):165–72.

57. Schauer PR, Burgera B, Ikramuddin S, et al. Effect of laparoscropic Roux-en Y gastric bypass on type 2 diabetes mellitus. *Ann Surg*. 2003;238(4):467–84.

58. Siri WE. Body composition from fluid spaces and density: analysis of methods. 1961. *Nutrition*. 1993;9(5):480–91; discussion 480,492.

59. Smoot TM, Xu P, Hilsenrath P, Kuppersmith NC, Singh KP. Gastric bypass surgery in the United States, 1998–2002. *Am J Public Health*. 2006;96(7):1187–9.

60. U.S. Department of Agriculture. Appendix 2. Estimated calorie needs per day, by age, sex, physical activity level [Internet]. [cited 2016 Jan 15]. Available from: http://health.gov/dietaryguidelines/2015/guidelines/appendix-2/

61. U.S. Department of Agriculture. Executive summary [Internet]. [cited 2016 Jan 15]. Available from: http://health.gov/dietaryguidelines/2015/guidelines/executive-summary/.

62. U.S. Department of Health and Human Services. Public Health Service, National Institutes of Health. National Heart, Lung, and Blood Institute. *Clinical Guidelines on the Identification, Evaluation, and Treatment of Overweight and Obesity in Adults: The Evidence Report* (NIH Publication No 98-4083). Bethesda (MD): National Heart, Lung, and Blood Institute; 1998. 262 p.

63. U.S. Department of Health and Human Services. Public Health Service, National Institutes of Health. National Heart, Lung, and Blood Institute. *The Practical Guide: Identification, Evaluation, and Treatment of Overweight and Obesity in Adults* (NIH Publication No. 00-4084). Bethesda (MD): National Heart, Lung, and Blood Institute; 2000. 94 p.

64. U.S. Food and Drug Association Web site [Internet]. Silver Spring (MD): U.S. Food and Drug Association; [cited 2012 Oct 12]. Available from: http://www.fda.gov/

65. Wikipedia. Nicotine [Internet]. [cited 2011 Jul 5]. Available from: http://en.wikipedia.org/wiki/Nicotine

66. wiseGeek. Will a sauna help me lose weight? [Internet]. Sparks (NV): Conjecture Corporation; [cited 2011 Aug 2]. Available from: http://www.wisegeek.com/will-a-sauna-help-me-lose-weight.htm

Additional Resources for Information about Supplements and Herbal Products

http://www.consumerlab.com — This site reports results of an independent testing lab to measure active ingredients in popular supplements. Products must have within 20% of what is on the label. Some information is free. Detailed lists of products require payment.

http://www.iherb.com — The Natural Pharmacist is a trusted reference for 500 dietary supplements.

http://www.herbmed.org HerbMd information on herbals with evidence and warnings — Short research summaries. Promotes alternative medical treatments but does not support outlandish claims.

http://www.uspverified.org — Has information about products that have passed the USP test. Brochures to use for a class or health fair may be available.

http://www.herbalgram.org — This site is maintained by the American Botanical Council.

American Association of Clinical Endocrinologists medical guidelines for the clinical use of dietary supplements and nutraceuticals. 2003. http://guidelines.gov

http://dietary-supplements.info.nih.gov/databases/ibids.html

The National Center for Complementary and Alternative Medicine. http://nccam.nih.gov

Fact sheets at http://ods.od.nih.gov

Center for Food Safety and Applied Nutrition, U.S. Food and Drug Administration. Dietary Supplements. http://www.cfsan.fda.gov/~dms/ds-prod.html

Food and Nutrition Information Center. National Agricultural Library/U.S. Department of Agriculture, 10301 Baltimore Ave, Room 105, Beltsville MD 2005-2351. Dietary Supplements Resource List. See http://www.nal.usda.gov/fnic/etext/000015.html

PART III

Exercise Programming for Special Populations

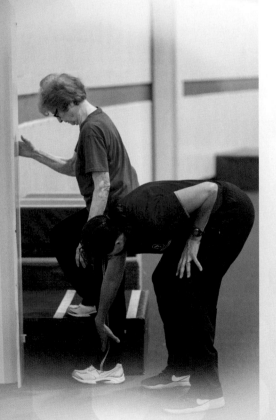

Exercise for Individuals with Controlled Cardiovascular, Pulmonary, and Metabolic Diseases

OBJECTIVES

- To describe the pathophysiology of common cardiovascular, metabolic, and pulmonary conditions.

- To describe the role medications play in altering the exercise response in various chronic diseases.

- To explain the nuances of exercise prescription in various chronic diseases compared with apparently healthy individuals.

INTRODUCTION

The certified exercise physiologist (EP-C) is responsible for developing exercise prescriptions for healthy clients and those with medically controlled diseases who are cleared by their physician for independent exercise. The role of physical activity and exercise training in primary and secondary disease prevention is well established (6,10,62,113). Developed guidelines provide recommendations regarding the amount of physical activity and exercise that offers significant health fitness benefits. Individuals with chronic diseases often present unique and challenging exercise limitations, but physical activity and exercise should not be avoided. Instead, exercise should become part of their medical management plan. Individuals with a chronic condition can experience health fitness benefits such as reduced disease symptoms, reduced medication reliance, and restoration of mental well-being (62). Because diseases usually impose exercise limitations and restrictions, the EP-C must know these limitations to ensure a safe and effective exercise prescription and just as importantly must recognize when to refer someone back to his or her physician or to more specialized exercise training with a clinical exercise physiologist or registered clinical exercise physiologist. This chapter reviews disease pathology, exercise considerations and contraindications, and the process for developing a proper FITT (frequency, intensity, time, and type) plan to allow optimal physical activity and exercise programming for the client with a cardiovascular, metabolic, and pulmonary disease who has been cleared by his or her physician for independent exercise training.

Pathophysiology of Common Cardiovascular, Metabolic, and Pulmonary Diseases

Cardiovascular Disease

Cardiovascular diseases (CVDs) account for more American deaths than any other disease, with nearly 650,000 total deaths annually (35). The financial cost and prevalence, along with the associated morbidity and mortality, make it important for the EP-C to understand the cardiovascular pathology and exercise measures for working with this population. A strong understanding of the disease pathology and specific exercise nuances will allow the EP-C to effectively design an exercise prescription to lessen the effects of CVD and improve the client's health fitness status and quality of life.

Coronary Heart Disease

Coronary artery disease (CAD) is one of the most prevalent types of CVD and also accounts for the most cardiovascular deaths (35). CAD is characterized by any one of several factors, including a buildup of atherosclerotic plaques, vascular remodeling resulting in luminal stenosis, and inflammation, brought on by numerous factors, including dyslipidemia and hypertension (HTN). Central to CAD is the formation of atherosclerotic plaque in the elastic and smooth lining inside

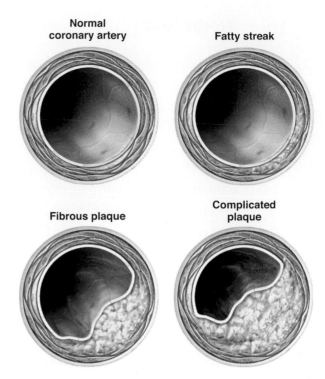

FIGURE 8.1. Depiction of the typical progression for plaque buildup in a coronary artery. The disease process begins with a normal coronary artery and the progression to fatty streak to an artery with complicated plaque. (Asset provided by Anatomical Chart Co.)

of arteries (Fig. 8.1). Plaque formations in the coronary arteries will obstruct blood flow to cardiac muscle tissue downstream of the obstruction resulting in reduced cardiac function and/or tissue death (necrosis) (58,95). Atherosclerosis is a process where fatty streaks develop causing the artery wall to thicken while reducing luminal diameter. This arterial narrowing is a progressive and dangerous arterial buildup of fat and fibrous plaques. The atherosclerotic process begins with a focal injury to the lining of the artery that eventually causes damage to the endothelium. The endothelium then becomes more permeable to lipids, allowing low-density lipoprotein cholesterol (LDL-C) to easily move through the damaged endothelium and into the arterial intima layer. Once inside the intima, macrophages oxidize LDL-C and begin the formation of arterial foam cells. As these foam cells evolve and begin to release cholesterol into the surrounding areas of the cell, fatty streaks start to form around the initial injury site and the plaque formation process begins (97). Fatty streak formation starts a repeating cycle of repair and remodeling in the artery during which the luminal diameter is progressively reduced until either a partial or complete reduction of luminal diameter occurs (67). A partial impairment of coronary artery blood flow and thus oxygen delivery to cardiac tissue is referred to as myocardial ischemia, whereas the complete obstruction of blood flow to the cardiac myocardial tissue is referred to as a myocardial infarction (MI) or a heart attack and results in tissue death or necrosis (58).

Myocardial ischemia is an imbalance between myocardial oxygen demand and supply. Two common types of myocardial ischemia are stable and unstable ischemia. Stable ischemia is often a result of increased oxygen demand of the heart, as seen with exercise. The impaired ability to deliver blood to the cardiac tissue during exercise starves the tissue from needed oxygen and results in chest pain known as angina and decreased exercise capacity (128). The symptoms of stable ischemia lessen as the oxygen demands of the heart decrease, or when exercise eases or ceases, allowing the coronary arteries to effectively supply the cardiac tissue with an adequate supply of blood flow and oxygen. Unstable ischemia is a more severe condition often seen with symptoms at rest and during a time of little exertional stress. Individuals with unstable ischemia need to seek medical treatment immediately, as unstable ischemia may be a warning sign that a heart attack is imminent (128). In no case should this person perform exercise or an exercise test.

Hypertension

HTN is common among patients with CAD. HTN is considered the "silent killer" because this condition's signs and symptoms often go unnoticed. The severity of HTN, however, cannot be overlooked because if left untreated is a major risk factor for developing multiple complications such as atherosclerosis, stroke, heart attack, chronic heart failure, kidney failure, and blindness (22).

HTN is characterized as a persistent elevation in either systolic blood pressure (SBP) (>140 mm Hg) or diastolic blood pressure (DBP) (>90 mm Hg) (116) and is categorized as either primary or secondary in its etiology. Primary HTN accounts for 90%–95% of all cases, has no established pathology, and is thus considered idiopathic (arising spontaneously or from an obscure or unknown cause) (67,127). Secondary HTN, which accounts for very few cases, is associated with identifiable causes such as renal disease, stress, drug-induced side effects, sleep apnea, neurologic disorders, and many others (67).

Blood pressure is regulated by two factors: cardiac output, or $\dot{Q}$ (a function of heart rate [HR] and stroke volume [SV]), and total peripheral vascular resistance. Increased peripheral resistance is the most common characteristic of primary and secondary HTN and is caused by chronic vasoconstriction, or narrowing of the peripheral arterioles, or by vascular plaque buildup. When HTN is present, arterioles lose elasticity because of the increased presence of fibrous collagen tissue. Collagen buildup decreases proper arteriole constriction and relaxation, which is important in normal blood flow regulation. In time, this condition leads to increased vascular resistance, increased blood pressure, and eventually increased atherosclerosis development (67).

Current guidelines for the management of HTN provide specific instructions on the implementation of pharmacologic therapies in addition to emphasizing lifestyle modifications that include habitual physical activity as initial therapy to lower blood pressure (BP) and to prevent or attenuate progression to HTN in individuals with pre-HTN (80).

Peripheral Artery Disease

The pathologic development of peripheral artery disease (PAD) mimics CAD with the primary difference being the location of the affected blood vessels. Specifically, PAD is characterized by occlusion or narrowing of peripheral arteries or vessels of the upper and lower limbs as a result of the buildup of atherosclerotic plaques (117). Although blood vessels of the upper and lower limbs may be affected, most cases of PAD are observed in the arterial network of the lower limbs (14). As a result of this vascular remodeling and subsequent dysfunction, blood flow is reduced to the vasculature distal to the area of occlusion. This reduced blood flow often leads to a mismatch between oxygen supply and demand leading to the development of ischemia that often manifests as pain and easy fatigability (73).

The most common symptom of PAD is intermittent claudication that is characterized by a repeatable aching, cramping sensation, or fatigue affecting the muscles of the calf in one or both legs. These sensations are often triggered by weight-bearing exercises and normally dissipate with the cessation of activity (14). The severity of PAD is based on the extent of claudication and is quantified by the use of ankle/brachial systolic pressure index (ABI) (74). PAD severity is rated on a 4-point scale in which grade 0 = asymptomatic, grade 1 = intermittent claudication, grade 2 = ischemic rest pain, and grade 4 = minor/major tissue loss in the limbs. ABI is a ratio of SBP measurements taken in a supine position at rest at the level of the ankle and brachial artery and is calculated with the equation: ABI = ankle SBP / brachial SBP (1). Values of >0.90 are considered normal, whereas ≤0.90 is the threshold for PAD confirmation. Although there are limitations in the use of ABI as a diagnostic criteria for PAD (117,125), ABI is generally accepted as an effective predictive measurement (124).

Metabolic Diseases/Disorders

Metabolic diseases/disorders have varying genetic or environmental causes that alter metabolic processes. The most common of these causes are diabetes mellitus (DM), hyperlipidemia, and obesity, each of which responds well to exercise therapy. If not treated properly, each can lead to various metabolic problems including CAD.

Diabetes

Type 1 and Type 2 DM are defined by a decrease in the production, release and/or effectiveness, and action of insulin. Either form of DM results in increased blood glucose levels, a condition referred to as hyperglycemia (20). In addition, diabetes can cause vasculature damage and starves cells of needed glucose.

Type 1 diabetes is quite uncommon found in only 5%–10% of all patients with diabetes and is characterized by an absolute deficiency in blood insulin release because of the destruction of pancreatic insulin secreting beta cells (44). Patients with Type 1 diabetes should be referred to exercise professionals with more specialized training to prescribe and monitor exercise.

The patient with Type 2 diabetes has elevated glucose levels which is typically a result of increasing insulin resistance. Excessive abdominal fat is a leading cause of Type 2 diabetes. The disease responds well to exercise therapy and drugs that either increase insulin sensitivity or decrease blood glucose levels.

Hyperlipidemia

Hyperlipidemia, defined as elevated blood cholesterol and triglyceride levels, is caused by a combination of genetic and/or environmental factors (77). Lipids are packaged with protein and travel through the blood as lipoproteins. Lipoproteins are classified by their density: chylomicrons, very low density lipoproteins (VLDLs), low-density lipoproteins (LDLs), and high-density lipoproteins (HDLs) (104). HDL is responsible for aiding in the removal of lipids from the circulation, through reverse cholesterol transport. Hence, HDL cholesterol (HDL-C) is referred to as the "good" cholesterol. Also, if HDL-C levels are less than 40 mg $\cdot$ dL^{-1}, very little reverse cholesterol transport occurs, leading to further vascular lipid accumulation and accelerated atherosclerosis rates. Excessive amounts of total blood cholesterol (>200 mg $\cdot$ dL^{-1}) and LDL-C, or "bad" cholesterol (>130 mg $\cdot$ dL^{-1}), is associated with increased risk of atherosclerosis and CAD. Within these four lipoprotein classifications exist associated subfractions, including intermediate-density lipoprotein (IDL; an intermediate step in VLDL catabolism), lipoprotein(a) (Lp[a]), an LDL subfraction that is highly related to CAD, small and large LDL subfractions, and two HDL subfractions: HDL$_2$ and the more dense HDL$_3$. Both the small and large LDL particles are associated with increased risk for CAD. Nonetheless, the current belief is that the small LDL particles are more atherogenic than the large particles because of their greater oxidation potential and the relationship of the small particles to other metabolic abnormalities principally high levels of triglyceride-rich lipoproteins such as VLDL and low serum HDL-C concentrations (89).

Obesity

Obesity is defined as an excessive accumulation of body fat and is associated with a body mass index (BMI) ≥30 kg $\cdot$ m^{-2} (118). Although the causes of obesity are complex and multifaceted, the combination of increased caloric consumption and decreased daily physical activity are the primary contributors (34). Regardless of its genesis, obesity is associated with a multitude of comorbidities, including insulin resistance, decreased growth hormone, increased cholesterol synthesis and excretion (29), and an increased incidence of all-cause mortality (27).

Metabolic Syndrome

Metabolic syndrome involves a clustering of metabolic risk factors including hyperglycemia (or current blood glucose medication use), elevated blood pressure (or current HTN medication use), dyslipidemia (or current lipid lowering medication use), and central adiposity based on waist circumference (3,23). Causes for the metabolic syndrome are multifactorial where genetics and health behavior are critical components. Mortality rates caused by CVD are substantially higher in those having the metabolic syndrome (88).

Pulmonary Diseases

Most pulmonary diseases are grouped into two categories: chronic obstructive pulmonary diseases (COPDs) and chronic restrictive pulmonary diseases (CRPDs). However, patients with pulmonary disease can present a multitude of unique challenges for exercise therapy and therefore are typically referred for more specialized care.

Chronic Obstructive Pulmonary Disease

COPD is an umbrella term for a collection of pulmonary diseases, including chronic bronchitis, emphysema, and asthma (Fig. 8.2) (110). COPD is characterized by progressive airflow limitation associated with an abnormal inflammatory lung response that limits the lung's ability to move air during inhalation and exhalation (110). Chronic bronchitis is characterized by a cough lasting for at least 3 months (77), resulting in chronic pulmonary inflammation which leads to damage of the bronchial lining and impeded lung function and airflow obstruction (18). Emphysema is the permanent enlargement of airspaces along with necrosis of alveolar walls (91), causing an accumulation of air in the lung tissue (67).

Asthma consists of both inflammation and increased smooth muscle constriction in the lungs in response to various stimuli (91). Triggers for asthma include environmental, biochemical, autonomic, immunologic, infectious, endocrine, and psychological factors (67). During an asthmatic episode, inflammatory mediators are released causing bronchial smooth muscle spasm, edema formation, and the production of mucous resulting in vascular congestion.

Chronic Restrictive Pulmonary Disease

CRPD, also known as interstitial lung disease, is made up of a small group of diseases that cause inflammation resulting in lung tissue necrosis and decreased lung volume (91). Both clients with

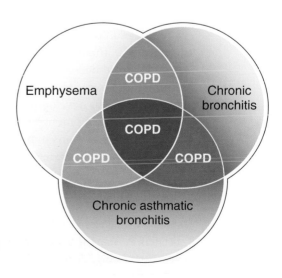

FIGURE 8.2. The relationships among emphysema, chronic bronchitis, chronic asthmatic bronchitis, and COPD. Most clients with COPD have a combination of these diseases. (From McConnell TH. *The Nature of Disease: Pathology for the Health Professions.* Philadelphia [PA]: Lippincott Williams & Wilkins; 2007. 739 p.)

COPD and CRPD have limited gas exchange within the lungs, frequent shortness of breath, and difficulty breathing. The EP-C's scope of practice does not include most aspects of pulmonary disease, given the disease's unique physiological challenges. Therefore, other than exercise-induced asthma, and particularly in emphysema and CRPD, individuals suffering from pulmonary disease should be referred to more specialized care.

Role of Exercise Training in Mediating Common Cardiovascular, Metabolic, and Pulmonary Diseases

Exercise has been shown to have positive effects on both primary and secondary disease prevention (71). An estimated 90 million Americans are currently living with a chronic health condition, and this number is expected to rise with a rapid expansion of the older population. Even in light of the increased prevalence of disease, many people are unaware of the potential disease-altering benefits that exercise can provide (70). Therefore, the EP-C is in a unique position to use this knowledge for the individual and collective improvement of health through appropriately applied exercise prescriptions.

Cardiovascular

Exercise training is beneficial for individuals with a history of or at high risk for an MI (62). Exercise has been shown to decrease coronary inflammatory markers (*e.g.*, C-reactive protein [CRP] and lipoprotein-associated phospholipase A2 [PLAC or Lp-PLA2]) (84), decrease stress and damage on the coronary arteries, and increase new blood vessel growth (angiogenesis) and vascular regeneration which are all likely to promote faster recovery from an MI (112). Regular exercise can also decrease blood platelet adhesiveness, fibrinogen levels, and blood viscosity, all of which reduce the risk of clotting and the likelihood for a second MI (134). In addition, regular exercise can improve self-efficacy and psychosocial well-being (62). Patients who engage in exercise after an MI can restore their health to near or above pre-MI fitness status and are able to return their lives to a pre-MI state (62). For clients suffering from ischemia and thus at high MI risk, the effect of exercise can help reduce the risk of an initial MI while also raising the overall quality of life (60). Exercise has also been shown to prevent, slow, and even reverse vasculature atherosclerotic plaque development, allowing for an increase in the ischemic threshold during daily activities or exercise (24).

For individuals with PAD, regular exercise training has been shown to have a profound impact on alleviating claudication by increasing the ischemic threshold allowing affected persons to work longer and at higher work intensities before exhibiting symptoms. This observation is supported by increases in pain-free walking time (48), pain-free walking distance (49), and maximal walking distance (92). In addition, regular exercise in patients with PAD has been shown to improve ABI scores (33) and decrease mortality risk (79).

Endurance exercise does lower resting SBP and DBP values by 5–7 mm Hg (68), and for individuals at risk for developing HTN, endurance exercise is thought to slow blood pressure rise and delay HTN development (116). Although not fully understood, possible mechanisms for exercise-induced reductions in blood pressure include an alteration in renal functioning, a decrease in plasma norepinephrine levels, and an increase in circulating vasodilator substances (135).

Metabolic

Patients with Type 2 diabetes gain health fitness benefits rather quickly once an exercise program is initiated. Perhaps, the most beneficial aspect is the improved insulin sensitivity that is reported with exercise training (20,123) which may result in a lower medication requirement and greater control

EXERCISE IS MEDICINE CONNECTION

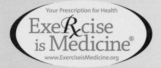

Milani RV, Lavie CJ, Mehra MR. Reduction in C-reactive protein through cardiac rehabilitation and exercise training. *J Am Coll Cardiol.* 2004;43(6):1056–61.

Milani and colleagues (2004) studied the effects of a 3-month formal phase II cardiac rehabilitation and exercise training program on CRP levels. The study consisted of two groups with the populations of both groups having diagnosed CAD. The exercise group underwent a 3-month phase II cardiac rehabilitation program, and the control group did not. Patients in the exercise group received formalized exercise instruction, met three times a week for a duration of an hour each session, and were encouraged to exercise on their own (one to three times a week) in between sessions. Patients also received individual and group counseling from a registered dietitian who stressed dietary management as recommended by the Adult Treatment Panel III guidelines and also placed special emphasis on the Mediterranean diet. Results showed people who engaged in the cardiac rehabilitation program had significant decreases in the levels of CRP and blood triglycerides and a significant increase in HDL-C. Because many of the patients in the exercise group were also taking medications, the data were analyzed to determine whether the medications or the exercise (or a combination) caused reduced CRP levels. Also found was that patients taking a statin medication had significant decrease in CRP levels over the course of the rehabilitation program. Also, exercising patients who were not taking a statin medication showed the same decreases in CRP levels as the statin users. The authors reported the favorable effects of exercise training on CRP levels independent of statin therapy. This study demonstrates that therapeutic lifestyle modifications, promoted by a 3-month cardiac rehabilitation and dietary management can produce significant improvements in CRP levels and other cardiac risk factors, such as blood lipids and can increase exercise capacity which in turn can promote health and overall well-being.

of blood glucose levels (123). In addition, if body fat is reduced, as may occur from the indirect effect of exercise, further increases in insulin sensitivity are found (20,123).

Dyslipidemic clients engaging in physical activity and exercise reduce postprandial lipidemia or the amount of cholesterol in their blood after a meal (59). Exercise also provides a positive benefit on other blood lipid values by lowering blood concentrations of LDL-C and increasing concentrations of HDL-C (20,55,129).

The role of exercise in treating obesity is most effective when used in combination with caloric restriction (61,131). As expected, increased exercise in an obese client can promote regional fat loss, especially abdominal fat deposits (29,133) which can also result in improved psychological well-being (29). With noticeable reductions in body weight and fat, clients have a tangible result that can increase self-image and self-esteem. However, even when reductions in body fat or weight do not occur, exercise participation will still produce other positive health fitness benefits (52).

Risk factors associated with the metabolic syndrome are improved by engaging in physical activity and modifying dietary behaviors (57). Exercise is shown effective for lowering blood pressure, blood glucose, and body mass while improving cholesterol levels. Treating individuals with the metabolic syndrome is consistent with guidelines for healthy adults where both aerobic and resistance exercises are recommended as part of the exercise prescription. However, each cardiovascular risk factor must be taken into account by the EP-C as each risk factor needs to be accounted for individually when designing the exercise prescription.

Ultimately, regular exercise yields improvement in many obesity comorbidities, including decreased fasting blood glucose levels, increased insulin sensitivity, decreased triglyceride levels, and decreased CAD risk factors (75). The EP-C is expected to have an understanding of the basic mechanisms involved in these positive changes to better prescribe exercise that is meaningful to each individual client.

Pulmonary

The scientific literature is mixed regarding the extent that exercise plays a role in reducing the pathologies of pulmonary diseases (114). Although exercise does not cure pulmonary diseases, exercise does bring a noticeable increase in quality of life in the pulmonary client (47). In fact, the overall benefit of exercise allows the pulmonary client to exercise longer at higher exercise intensities (77).

The Art and Science of Exercise Prescription and Programming in Controlled Disease Populations

A "one size fits all" approach may not be the most effective method to creating individualized exercise prescriptions or programs. Rather, the successful EP-C should create specific and individualized programs to meet the client's needs and health goals (10). The American College of Sports Medicine (ACSM) metabolic equations are useful mathematical tools as they help tailor caloric expenditure and exercise intensity to meet the needs of each client (5) (see Chapters 3 and 7 for more exercise prescription details); however, these calculations are specific to apparently healthy individuals and may not be as reliable when used in individuals with certain chronic conditions (5).

The body of scientific information regarding exercise prescription for individuals with chronic disease has increased significantly in the past 20 years (8,20). Nonetheless, the application of these principles should not be completed in an exceedingly rigid and precise fashion. Rather, the procedures presented in this chapter are in fact principles and accordingly should be utilized with flexibility and careful attention to the contraindications, limitations, and goals of the individual. Because the physiological responses vary considerably across individuals regarding exercise responses and adaptations, and particularly in those with chronic conditions, the EP-C must be prepared to modify exercise prescriptions accordingly. The EP-C uses the basic scientific process, knows the individual client's needs, and develops and implements an appropriate exercise prescription with an overriding goal of promoting a more physically active lifestyle.

Chronic diseases present unique and challenging limitations for the EP-C in developing an appropriate exercise program. The role of the EP-C is to be aware of such limitations and use scientifically developed principles in conjunction with his or her own experiences to adapt and implement a properly designed exercise prescription that is effective in optimizing health fitness benefits and ensures safety. Thus, the EP-C must recognize that the process of making an exercise prescription is an art as well as a science.

Special FITT Considerations for Persons with Chronic Diseases

Clients with cardiovascular, metabolic, or pulmonary systems need to include physical activity and exercise as part of their lifestyle. The ACSM endorses the use of the FITT-VP (V = volume; P = progression) principle in developing an exercise prescription (8); however, when considering chronic disease populations presented in this chapter, the focus is on the "FITT" components only with each disease discussed more thoroughly. The EP-C needs to be diligent in using the FITT principle carefully to develop an individualized exercise program that ensures patient safety while maximizing functional capacity and developing optimal health fitness benefits. Tables 8.1 and 8.2 present general aerobic and resistance exercise guidelines for patients diagnosed with chronic diseases, respectively.

Table 8.1	General Aerobic Training Guidelines to Be Applied in the Effective Development of Exercise Prescriptions for the Treatment of a Population with Chronic Disease
Frequency (d · wk^{-1})	CVD: 3–7 (3 days if all are vigorous) PAD: 3–5 DM: 3–7 Pulmonary: 3–5
Intensity	CVD: moderate 40%–59% HRR or RPE <11–14 (6–20 scale); vigorous 60%–89% HRR; or deconditioned 30%–39% HRR PAD: 40%–59% $\dot{V}O_2$ reserve or to the exercise intensity in which the patient experiences moderate pain (*e.g.*, 3–4 out of 5 points on the claudication pain scale) DM: 50%–79% HRR or RPE = 12–16 (6–20 scale) Pulmonary: prescribed on an individual basis, based on GXT with scale for dyspnea
Time	CVD: achieve 1,500–2,000 kcal of energy expenditure each week or 20–60 min per session PAD: 30–50 min per session (excluding rest periods) DM: 20–60 min per session At least 150 min · wk^{-1} at moderate intensity (*e.g.*, 600 METs · min · wk^{-1}) or 90 min · wk^{-1} at vigorous intensity (*e.g.*, 540 METs · min · wk^{-1}) Pulmonary: 20–60 min a session
Type	CVD: large dynamic muscle group exercises PAD: weight bearing: walking or treadmill DM: walk, bicycle, jogging, water aerobics activities Pulmonary: Walking and cycling are most strongly recommended.

Information taken with permission from Cooper CB. Exercise in chronic pulmonary disease: aerobic exercise prescription. *Med Sci Sports Exerc.* 2001;33(7 suppl):S671–9; American College of Sports Medicine. Exercise prescription for patients with cardiac, peripheral, cerebrovascular, and pulmonary disease. In: Riebe D, editor. *ACSM's Guidelines for Exercise Testing and Prescription.* 10th ed. Philadelphia (PA): Wolters Kluwer; 2018. p. 226–67; Hirsch AT, Haskal ZJ, Hertzer NR, et al. ACC/AHA 2005 practice guidelines for the management of patients with peripheral arterial disease (lower extremity, renal, mesenteric, and abdominal aortic): a collaborative report from the American Association for Vascular Surgery/Society for Vascular Surgery, Society for Cardiovascular Angiography and Interventions, Society for Vascular Medicine and Biology, Society of Interventional Radiology, and the ACC/AHA Task Force on Practice Guidelines (Writing Committee to Develop Guidelines for the Management of Patients With Peripheral Arterial Disease): endorsed by the American Association of Cardiovascular and Pulmonary Rehabilitation; National Heart, Lung, and Blood Institute; Society for Vascular Nursing; TransAtlantic Inter-Society Consensus; and Vascular Disease Foundation. *Circulation.* 2006;113(11):e463–654; American College of Sports Medicine. Exercise prescription for individuals with metabolic disease and cardiovascular disease risk factors. In: Riebe D, editor. *ACSM's Guidelines for Exercise Testing and Prescription.* 10th ed. Philadelphia (PA): Wolters Kluwer; 2018. p. 268–96; Schairer JR. Exercise prescription in patients with cardiovascular disease. In: Swain DP, editor. *ACSM's Resource Manual for Guidelines for Exercise Testing and Prescription.* 7th ed. Philadelphia (PA): Lippincott Williams & Wilkins; 2014. p. 624; Verity L. Exercise prescription in patients with diabetes. In: Ehrman J, editor. *ACSM's Resource Manual for Guidelines for Exercise Testing and Prescription.* 6th ed. Philadelphia (PA): Lippincott Williams & Wilkins; 2010. p. 600–17.

High-Intensity Interval Training

High-intensity interval training (HIIT) is an exercise training protocol consisting of alternating high- and low-intensity exercise intervals with an underlying premise that HIIT participants are able to complete greater exercise volumes at higher intensity levels than during a sustained, continuous effort (25,65,90). HIIT principles are flexible and allow for the adjustment of duration and intensity of both the high- and low-intensity exercise intervals to alter accordingly to meet individual fitness levels and goals. HIIT is an effective exercise training method producing beneficial changes in various physiological, performance, and health-related factors, which are similar or superior to those improvements reported for steady-state moderate-intensity continuous exercise training (25,65,90). The use of HIIT can also provide functional benefits for clients with chronic

Table 8.2	General Resistance Training Guidelines to Be Applied in the Effective Development of Exercise Prescriptions for the Treatment of a Chronic Diseased Population
Frequency (d · wk^{-1})	CVD: 2–3 PAD: 2–4, performed on nonconsecutive days DM: 2–3 Pulmonary: 2–3 (4–5 d · wk^{-1} for respiratory muscles)
Intensity	CVD: 60%–80% 1-RM low to moderate PAD: 60%–80% 1-RM low to moderate RPE ~14–16 (6–20 scale) DM: 60%–80% 1-RM low to moderate RPE ~14–16 (6–20 scale) Pulmonary: 50%–80% 1-RM low to moderate RPE ~12–15 (6–20 scale) (possibly lower depending on severity of COPD)
Time	CVD: 8–12 exercises 1–4 sets per exercise PAD: 8–12 exercise 2–3 sets per exercise, 8–12 repetitions DM: 8–12 exercises 2–3 sets per exercise Pulmonary: 8–12 exercises 2–3 sets per exercise
Type	CVD: elastic bands, light (1–5 lb) hand weights, light free weights with wall pulleys, and machines PAD: all major muscle groups, emphasis on lower limbs if time is limited DM: all major muscle groups Upper body: 4–5 exercises Lower body: 4–5 exercises Pulmonary: free weights, elastic bands, body weight exercises, and machine exercises

Information taken with permission from Cooper CB. Exercise in chronic pulmonary disease: aerobic exercise prescription. *Med Sci Sports Exerc.* 2001;33(7 suppl):S671–9; American College of Sports Medicine. Exercise prescription for patients with cardiac, peripheral, cerebrovascular, and pulmonary disease. In: Riebe D, editor. *ACSM's Guidelines for Exercise Testing and Prescription.* 10th ed. Philadelphia (PA): Wolters Kluwer; 2018. p. 226–67; Hirsch AT, Haskal ZJ, Hertzer NR, et al. ACC/AHA 2005 practice guidelines for the management of patients with peripheral arterial disease (lower extremity, renal, mesenteric, and abdominal aortic): a collaborative report from the American Association for Vascular Surgery/Society for Vascular Surgery, Society for Cardiovascular Angiography and Interventions, Society for Vascular Medicine and Biology, Society of Interventional Radiology, and the ACC/AHA Task Force on Practice Guidelines (Writing Committee to Develop Guidelines for the Management of Patients With Peripheral Arterial Disease): endorsed by the American Association of Cardiovascular and Pulmonary Rehabilitation; National Heart, Lung, and Blood Institute; Society for Vascular Nursing; TransAtlantic Inter-Society Consensus; and Vascular Disease Foundation. *Circulation.* 2006;113(11):e463–654; American College of Sports Medicine. Exercise prescription for individuals with metabolic disease and cardiovascular disease risk factors. In: Riebe D, editor. *ACSM's Guidelines for Exercise Testing and Prescription.* 10th ed. Philadelphia (PA): Wolters Kluwer; 2018. p. 268–96; Schairer JR. Exercise prescription in patients with cardiovascular disease. In: Swain DP, editor. *ACSM's Resource Manual for Guidelines for Exercise Testing and Prescription.* 7th ed. Philadelphia (PA): Lippincott Williams & Wilkins; 2014. p. 624; Verity L. Exercise prescription in patients with diabetes. In: Ehrman J, editor. *ACSM's Resource Manual for Guidelines for Exercise Testing and Prescription.* 6th ed. Philadelphia (PA): Lippincott Williams & Wilkins; 2010. p. 600–17.

diseases and is a valuable tool that can be part of every comprehensive medical management plan (4,51). HIIT can improve health-related factors such as exercise capacity and quality of life for CVD (46,69), pulmonary disease (21,87), and clients with diabetes (26). The use of HIIT protocols or any exercise programming does always afford medical concern for client safety. Existing scientific evidence supports that HIIT presents little risk for stable clients with a chronic health condition when the prescribed exercise protocols are followed (21,26,46,69,85).

Cardiovascular Disease

CVD pathology is associated with reduced functional capacity and exercise tolerance, and in general, patients with CVD have higher sedentary rates than most other individuals (71). In addition, other factors such as medications (*e.g.*, β-blockers, β-adrenergic blocking agents, central α_2-agonists, nitrates, nitroglycerin, calcium channel blockers [CCBs], cardiac glycosides, and angiotensin-converting enzyme [ACE] inhibitors), myocardial ischemia, intermittent claudication, and angina all impact the application of the FITT principle when developing an exercise prescription for clients with CVD.

Some clients with CVD may choose to enroll in a cardiac rehabilitation program to initiate an exercise program. Cardiac rehabilitation programming has been shown to reduce disease symptoms and reduce risk of a second cardiovascular event (15). Regardless of the exercise setting, the EP-C can safely prescribe exercise in a stable client with CVD. Exercise frequency is usually prescribed as 5 or more days each week (9), and in the very low fit person, multiple daily exercise episodes lasting as little as 10 minutes and totaling at least 30 minutes could provide numerous health benefits (9). Clients with CVD usually have limited functional capacities; therefore, shorter exercise episodes of 10–15 minutes performed two or three times each day may be useful and often result in exercise being better tolerated. In addition, intermittent work (alternating higher and lower intensity exercise) can also be useful (71). Clients with CVD making lifestyle modifications to include physical activity and exercise may experience concerns with program adherence and motivation. The EP-C has a significant role in helping facilitate the motivation and support the adherence of clients making lifestyle modifications.

Typically, exercise intensity is measured as a percentage of volume of oxygen consumed per unit time ($\dot{V}O_2$) reserve, or HR reserve (HRR) (10); however, using these variables may be difficult in many cases of cardiac disease because of the effect of HR-modifying medications and/or HR-altering medical conditions (17). In these cases, rating of perceived exertion (RPE) as an alternative measurement of exercise intensity is useful (9). Exercise intensity is always prescribed below the myocardial ischemic threshold; however, any client experiencing ischemia should exercise in the presence of someone with more specific training than the EP-C.

Exercise time or duration varies with the disease severity. The overall exercise goal for clients with CVD is to progress to 60 minutes of aerobic conditioning a day. However, starting with shorter exercise time is appropriate (10- to 15-min periods), and increasing exercise duration from 1 to 5 minutes per session depending on individual exercise tolerance is suggested (10,71).

Resistance training also offers health fitness benefits beyond that of aerobic conditioning alone. The FITT for resistance training is no different than in the general population; however, most cardiac patients will likely start at a low work rate level. Therefore, potential exercise equipment for completing these exercises includes elastic bands, light (1–5 lb) hand weights, light free weights with wall pulleys, and exercise machines.

Metabolic Disease

Clients with Type 2 diabetes should incorporate physical activity and exercise as part of their management plan (11,12). The EP-C can safely work with clients with well-controlled Type 2 diabetes. If a person with Type 2 diabetes experiences frequent swings in blood glucose levels, he or she should be referred to a health care professional and encouraged to exercise under the supervision of more skilled personnel. When developing an exercise prescription for the client with diabetes, an important consideration is the need to reduce overall body fat. This goal, however, can be complicated if the client is taking a glycemic lowering agent, as the potential exists for the combination of exercise and medication to lower blood glucose beyond a safe level (6,132). The EP-C must therefore balance the appropriate exercise prescription with the effect of the medication to avoid any potential diabetes-related complications (130).

Being physically active and exercising 5–7 days $\cdot$ week^{-1} is recommended for the patient with Type 2 diabetes (6). Because weight loss is so important, special consideration is given to physical activity and exercise volume and frequency to maximize weight loss (30). Exercise intensity usually ranges between 50% and 80% HRR and $\dot{V}O_2$ reserve and corresponds to an RPE of 12–16 (6). Exercise duration begins with a daily accumulation of 20 minutes and should progress to 60 minutes of daily aerobic conditioning. The time for a client to reach 60 minutes of daily accumulated exercise is variable and may take many weeks or months. Some clients may never achieve this goal. As with clients with CVD, multiple daily physically activity or exercise episodes of 10 minutes or more may be used as well as the use of intermittent work (lower exercise intensity mixed with higher exercise intensity). The overall goal is to obtain the health fitness benefits associated with 150 minutes of total physical activity and exercise each week. Also additional health fitness benefits are obtained when a goal of 300 minutes of physical activity and exercise is reached (31). Aerobic exercise that emphasizes large muscle groups using rhythmic motion is recommended, although the type of exercise chosen should reflect the individual's interest and goals.

Resistance training for clients with diabetes is recommended as long as there is an absence of contraindications such as retinopathy and recent laser treatment (6). Exercise frequency and intensity recommendations are not different from those used for healthy sedentary individuals. Exercise intensity is set at 60%–80% of one repetition maximum (1-RM) with two to three sets of 8–12 repetitions. Exercise duration is usually set at 8–10 multiple-joint exercises involving most if not all major muscle groups and is often performed in one whole-body session or split into multiple sessions (6). Exercise type or mode is based on the presence of exercise limitations and includes free weights, elastic bands, body weight exercises, and any of a variety of machines.

In addition, clients with diabetes must always wear medical identification, and because diabetes slows the healing process, maintaining proper foot care to reduce foot sores and blisters is vital. With longer healing times, foot sores and blisters are more likely to become infected and result in more serious complications. Most importantly, exercising clients with diabetes must have an available source of carbohydrates. Exercising with a partner is often recommended for individuals with diabetes. Finally, exercise in the early evening should be completed with caution because exercising at this time could cause hypoglycemic conditions later in the night, possibly during sleep and could cause dire consequences (132).

Pulmonary Disease

Clients with advanced stages of COPD or CRPD are especially unique among the chronic diseases presented in this chapter (105,109). In most cases, these clients are unlikely to ever fully vanquish their symptoms, and their functional capacity and exercise tolerance will progressively become more restricted (105). The scope of practice for the EP-C does not warrant working with this population and instead encourages referral to the appropriate health care personnel.

The EP-C is prepared to work with clients with well-controlled asthma and should encourage them to perform aerobic exercise at least 3–5 days $\cdot$ week^{-1}. Unfortunately, there is not a true consensus regarding the optimal intensity for aerobic training in the client with asthma, and therefore, guidelines for older adults are often used (see Chapter 10). Another guiding technique used in developing appropriate exercise intensity is the use of the dyspnea scale rating which focuses on a value in the range of 3–5 on a scale of 0–10 (76). Exercise duration recommendations for the client with pulmonary disease are to obtain at least 20 minutes each session and, in the long term, move progressively toward 60 minutes of continuous or intermittent physical activity and aerobic conditioning.

Effects of Myocardial Ischemia, Myocardial Infarction, and Hypertension on Cardiorespiratory Responses during Exercise

CVD continues to be the leading cause of death in the United States for men and women alike (139). The prevalence of CVD continues to rise even as medical technology finds new ways to improve overall survival rates (36–40,41–43). An individual who suffers an MI has likely had a significant level of myocardial ischemia as one key predisposing factor. Being an MI survivor, this individual still has ischemia and limited exercise tolerance and functional capacity.

In addition to CVD, HTN is a common disorder with a prevalence of about 1 in 4 adults reported in the United States (68). Although HTN can go undetected for many years, this disease possesses medical considerations when physical activity and exercise are performed. Therefore, because of the high prevalence of CVD and HTN, the EP-C must be keenly aware of these conditions, their etiology, and their likely impact on an individual's exercise and functional performance.

Myocardial Ischemia

Myocardial ischemia, or simply ischemia, indicates a shortage of oxygenated blood flow to the heart myocardium. The prevalence of ischemia in the United States is approximately 7%, although the proportion of individuals suffering ischemia increases with age. Ischemia is an imbalance of oxygen supply and demand. Impaired blood supply is a result of several mechanisms, the most common being atherosclerosis, congestive heart failure (CHF), or both. Oxygen demand is elevated dramatically during physical or emotional exertion. If oxygen supply fails to match an increased demand, even briefly, then ischemia is present. If ischemia is prolonged, then viable myocardium becomes at risk for necrosis and infarction. Oftentimes, ischemia is associated with chest pain, or angina.

In a typical exercise session, myocardial oxygen demand is increased, which is met by an increased frequency and vigor of the heart pumping action. This linear relationship between oxygen demand and HR continues until an individual reaches maximum exercise capacity. However, in the client with ischemia, maximum exercise capacity is limited by insufficient myocardial oxygen supply. If the heart is deficient such as in the case of CHF or because the arteries are partially blocked as in atherosclerosis, oxygen delivery to target muscle is impaired and exercise capacity is limited and the client has reached the "ischemic threshold." Avoiding this ischemic threshold is a critical concern in prescribing exercise. However, as was previously stated, any client experiencing ischemia should exercise in the presence of someone with more specific training than the EP-C.

Myocardial Infarction

An MI occurs when there is prolonged ischemia and can result in heart tissue death or necrosis (95). The ischemia duration necessary to produce an infarct varies; therefore, the EP-C must design exercise prescriptions that safely avoid the ischemic threshold or the HR at which angina symptoms develop. Also, because necrosis results in the loss of heart tissue, any necrosis will negatively impact the movement of an action potential throughout the heart as well as the contractile state of the heart as a pump, lowering ejection fraction and limiting exercise capacity and tolerance (78).

Initiating exercise in the patient with post-MI is approached with caution. Because access to graded exercise test (GXT) results is less common (58,120), the "art" of exercise prescription takes on greater importance. Known benefits for clients after an MI include reducing the likelihood for a second infarct, decreasing return to work time, increasing overall functional capacity, and improving self-efficacy (64).

Although post-MI exercise is relatively safe (93), including vigorous exercise (50,93), the EP-C must understand each client's exercise limitations and myocardial oxygen supply. Therefore, only after gaining medical clearance and physician approval for independent exercise is the initiation of exercise programming appropriate. The EP-C likely will work with this type of patient after the patient has completed a supervised round of cardiac rehabilitation under the guidance of the medical community.

Hypertension

Daily physical activity and exercise is part of the treatment for HTN, although such programming should be implemented with caution (68,107). Normally, a single exercise session causes a linear increase in SBP while a steady constant DBP is maintained (82,100). In the hypertensive person, SBP changes with exercise are often curvilinear and reach excessively high levels (<250 mm Hg). This dramatic increase in arterial pressure puts undue pressure on the arterial intima increasing the likelihood of dislodging atherosclerotic plaques and/or thrombi precipitating an MI or stroke. In addition, repeated periods of high-intensity exercise could further exacerbate endothelial damage (99,137).

Given the potential concerns associated with exercise and HTN, the EP-C must be aware of and follow guidelines for initiating and terminating exercise in the client with hypertension. By adhering to these standards, the client with hypertension with the guidance from the EP-C can safely use regular physical activity and exercise as an important adjunct to any pharmaceutical therapy in managing blood pressure.

Exercise Concerns, Precautions, and Contraindications Related to Cardiovascular, Metabolic, and Pulmonary Diseases

The information found in Table 8.3 presents the clinical indications and contraindications for patients in cardiac rehabilitation (inpatient and outpatient). This information and the following summarized points are meant to help the EP-C develop and implement a safe exercise prescription as discussed in this chapter.

- As with any chronic disease, the EP-C must foster a safe environment that facilitates clients' understanding of their disease and exercise limitations.
- Before starting exercise, clients must have the knowledge to define angina and its treatment, identify CVD symptoms and provoking factors, and understand their exercise tolerance limits (15). By knowing this information, clients can better understand their disease, their exercise limits, and health implications while fostering safe exercise.
- A primary exercise programming goal is for the CVD client to reduce disease risk and increase the ease in completing activities of daily living. Exercise training will increase functional capacity and exercise tolerance and reduce the chance of experiencing another cardiovascular event (15).
- The early stages of the exercise prescription usually begin with the use of lower, more conservative exercise intensities, usually 10–15 heartbeats per minute below the ischemic threshold (81). Although less than optimal for maximizing cardiorespiratory fitness and optimizing health fitness benefits, this lower exercise intensity level will still increase functional capacity and reduce CVD risk (58).

Table 8.3	Clinical Indications and Contraindications for Inpatient and Outpatient Cardiac Rehabilitation
Indications	**Contraindications**
■ Medically stable after MI ■ Stable angina ■ Coronary artery bypass graft surgery ■ Percutaneous transluminal coronary angioplasty or other transcatheter procedure ■ Stable heart failure ■ Cardiomyopathy ■ Heart or other organ transplantation ■ Other cardiac surgery, including valvular and pacemaker insertion (including implantable cardioverter defibrillator) ■ Peripheral arterial disease ■ At risk for CAD with diagnoses of DM, dyslipidemia, HTN, obesity, or other diseases and conditions ■ Other patients who may benefit from structured exercise and/or patient education based on physician referral and consensus of the rehabilitation team	■ Unstable angina ■ Uncontrolled HTN (resting SBP >180 mm Hg and/or resting DBP >110 mm Hg) ■ Orthostatic BP drop of >20 mm Hg with symptoms ■ Significant aortic stenosis (aortic valve orifice area of <1.0 cm^2 in an average-sized adult) ■ Acute systemic illness or fever ■ Uncontrolled atrial or ventricular dysrhythmias ■ Uncontrolled sinus tachycardia (>120 bpm) ■ Uncompensated CHF ■ Third-degree atrioventricular block without pacemaker ■ Active pericarditis or myocarditis ■ Recent embolism ■ Thrombophlebitis ■ Aortic dissection ■ Resting ST-segment depression or elevation (>2 mm) ■ Uncontrolled DM ■ Severe orthopedic conditions that would prohibit exercise ■ Other metabolic conditions, such as acute thyroiditis, hypokalemia, hyperkalemia, or hypovolemia

■ As fitness levels and exercise tolerance increase, the ischemic threshold is also increased and exercise intensity can therefore also be increased.

■ The client with hypertension can exercise once HTN is controlled (107). In the presence of uncontrolled HTN (>180/110 mm Hg), exercise is only engaged after initiating drug therapy (111). For resting SBP greater than 180 mm Hg or resting DBP greater than 110 mm Hg, even if blood pressure medications are being taken, exercise is contraindicated and is not engaged until blood pressure is under control (107).

■ During exercise, if SBP becomes greater than 220 mm Hg or DBP greater than 105 mm Hg, exercise is stopped, and blood pressure is allowed to return toward resting values (136). The next exercise period is completed at lower exercise intensity to ensure blood pressure stays less than 220/105 mm Hg (136).

■ Also, many HTN medications present unique challenges for the EP-C in prescribing proper exercise. For example, β-blockers can attenuate HR response by as much as 30 bpm (137), and this attenuated HR response may result in the need for using an RPE scale or "beats above resting" as alternative methods for prescribing exercise intensity. Clients taking these medications are advised to have longer cool-down periods, where blood pressure is monitored after exercise to ensure that blood pressure does not fall to unsafe levels (107).

■ The use of a claudication pain perception scale is useful when working with the PAD population. A typical 0–4 scale of 0 = no pain, 1 = onset of pain, 2 = moderate pain, 3 = intense pain, and 4 = maximal pain is commonly employed. Along with the severity of claudication experienced, the time and distance to the onset of symptoms to maximal pain should also be recorded (7).

HOW TO	**Initiate Exercise in a Patient with Coronary Artery Disease in Lieu of a Graded Exercise Test**

Equipment Needed

1. Blood pressure monitoring equipment: stethoscope and blood pressure cuff (sphygmomanometer)

2. Electrocardiogram (ECG) monitoring unit (3- or 12-lead)

3. RPE chart

4. Exercise equipment (*i.e.*, treadmill, recumbent cycle, elliptical)

Important Information and Tips

1. The results of a GXT can be a valuable tool in the initiation of an exercise prescription (1). However, in certain cases, a GXT may not have been previously administered. Yet even without the GXT results, a safe and effective exercise prescription can be developed.

2. Reasons for not performing a GXT before starting an exercise prescription include extreme deconditioning, orthopedic limitations, recent successful percutaneous intervention, or uncomplicated or stable MI (3).

3. Because the client's response to exercise is not documented, client safety is of utmost concern, and the exercise prescription should reflect this. Initiation of exercise at a low intensity, slow exercise intensity progression, and constant monitoring of physiologic symptoms help ensure client safety.

Example of an Exercise Prescription

FITT framework for a patient with CAD without a GXT (3,4,8).

1. Frequency: minimum 3 d $\cdot$ wk^{-1} with additional walking on the days off

2. Intensity: 2–3 metabolic equivalents (METs)

   a. HR: 20–30 bpm above resting value

   b. RPE: 11–14

3. Time: Begin with 3- to 5-min intervals. Allow for adequate rest and recovery between intervals. Aim for an overall exercise duration of 30–45 min.

4. Type: low-intensity modes of exercise

   a. Treadmill (0% grade, low speed)

   b. Cycle ergometer

   c. Arm ergometer

   d. Elliptical

5. Progression: 1–2 METs as tolerated by the client

6. Monitoring: ECG, BP, RPE, and signs or symptoms of ischemia

References

1. American College of Sports Medicine. *ACSM's Guidelines for Exercise Testing and Prescription*. 10th ed. Philadelphia (PA): Wolters Kluwer; 2018.
2. McConnell TR. Exercise prescription when the guidelines do not work. *J Cardiopulm Rehabil*. 1996;16(1):34–7.
3. McConnell TR, Klinger TA, Gardner JK, Laubach CA, Herman CE, Hauck CA. Cardiac rehabilitation without exercise tests for post-myocardial infarction and post-bypass surgery patients. *J Cardiopulm Rehabil*. 1998;18(6):458–63.
4. Visich PS. The value of graded exercise testing in today's world. *Am J Lifestyle Med*. 2009;3(1):57–62.

Suggested Readings

ACSM's Exercise Management for Persons with Chronic Diseases and Disabilities — provides detailed overview on the approach on the proper development of an exercise prescription for persons in a diseased state.

Pollack's Textbook of Cardiovascular Disease and Rehabilitation — provides comprehensive and detailed descriptions of the pathologic effects of CAD and effects on the exercise response.

■ In more severe cases of PAD, some clients may need to begin exercising for only a total of 15 minutes · day^{-1} with gradual increases of 5 minutes · day^{-1} every 2–4 weeks depending on individual progression (138).

■ In persons with PAD, the client may need repeated breaks after the onset of severe claudication symptoms. A specific rest-to-work ratio will need to be tailored and continually modified for every client (7).

■ Non–weight-bearing exercises, such as cycling, may be used as a warm-up modality but should not be the primary type of activity that is prescribed to this population (7).

■ A long warm-up may be needed for persons with PAD as a cold environment may aggravate symptoms of intermittent claudication (32).

Metabolic

Under normal conditions, blood glucose homeostasis is maintained by a precise coordination of hormones and metabolic events. Diabetes interrupts this delicate balance, and individuals with this disease do not respond normally to exercise. Nonetheless, patients with diabetes are able to exercise but with precaution. Because diabetes involves multiple body systems resulting in a multitude of complications, the EP-C must give careful consideration to the presence and severity of diabetes and associated complications, medication regimens, and the schedule for these medications to ensure client safety.

■ Patients with diabetes need constant blood glucose monitoring and the ability to measure before, during, and after exercise (132).

■ A readily available source of carbohydrate, such as fruit juice or hard candy, should be available if needed to increase blood glucose levels (122,123).

■ If preexercise or during exercise blood glucose measurements are less than 70 mg · dL^{-1}, a carbohydrate snack (15 g) is administered, and a blood glucose reading of greater than 100 mg · dL^{-1} is obtained before starting or continuing exercise (122,123).

■ When preexercise blood glucose values are greater than 250 mg · dL^{-1} with the presence of blood ketones or are greater than 300 mg · dL^{-1} with either presence or absence of ketones, blood glucose should be lowered prior to initiating exercise (77). However, provided the client feels well and is adequately hydrated and ketones are not present, postponing exercise is not compulsory based solely on hyperglycemia (128).

■ When an active retinal hemorrhage is present or recent laser corrective surgery for retinopathy is completed, exercise is avoided (132). Postponing exercise will limit the risk of triggering vitreous hemorrhage and retinal detachment (122,123).

■ Because clients with diabetes experience greater time for proper healing process, they should practice good foot care by inspection of feet before and after exercise and by wearing proper shoes and cotton socks to avoid foot sores and blisters.

■ Exercise with a partner or under the supervision of an EP-C to reduce the risk of problems associated with hypoglycemic events (132).

■ Consideration is always given to exercise timing and the taking of insulin or hypoglycemic agents. Exercise is not recommended during peak insulin action because hypoglycemia may result. Because delayed postexercise hypoglycemia is a known risk, late evening exercising is not recommended.

■ Always carry medical identification.

■ The EP-C must use conservative practices according to each CVD and DM risk factor present in individuals with the metabolic syndrome. Refer to the other bullet points regarding each CVD and DM risk factors to help guide the exercise prescription.

Dyslipidemia presents few, if any, exercise limitations, and individuals with elevated blood lipid levels are encouraged to engage in regular physical activity and exercise. To optimize blood lipid concentrations, clients with dyslipidemia are encouraged to exercise for longer durations (55). Presently, clients with dyslipidemia are recommended to set a short-term goal of 150 minutes · week^{-1} and a long-term goal of greater than 300 minutes · week^{-1} and to expend more than 2,000 kcal of expenditure a week (62,63). Both short- and long-term goals are best achieved by exercising 5 or more days · week^{-1} and, in some cases, by incorporating physical activity and exercise in multiple daily episodes. In general, most lipid-lowering drugs have no impact on exercise responses.

Obesity continues as a growing global health concern (16,133). Both reducing energy intake by dietary restriction and increasing energy expenditure by exercise are targeted interventions for treating obesity (133).

- Individuals who are obese are often at risk for other chronic diseases, and these individuals can need additional medical screening and appropriate supervision for exercise testing and programming.
- Individuals who are obese are recommended to engage in moderate physical activity at least 5, if not all, days of the week and progress to accumulating more than 2,000 kcal a week of energy expenditure (16).
- Because clients who are obese are at an increased risk for orthopedic injury and are usually in a deconditioned state, the exercise prescription should emphasize the use of low-impact or non–weight-bearing exercises such as the water-based, elliptical, and/or recumbent cycling. These types of exercises are recommended because of the reduced joint stress and the potential for less musculoskeletal injury.
- Because of likely low fitness level, an exercise prescription that has a slower intensity and duration progression will likely have fewer injuries.
- Clients who are obese may have a propensity for low motivation and drive for making lifestyle change, and thus, additional motivational strategies are often required to help make these changes (133). Incorporating lifestyle strategies such as realistic goal setting and balance sheets is an effective way to provide positive reinforcement and helps develop motivation to start and adhere to lifestyle change.
- Additional considerations for clients who are obese include adequate flexibility, warm-up and cool-down periods, exercising in cool temperatures with low humidity, adequate hydration, and wearing loose-fitting clothing to allow for heat dissipation.

EXERCISE IS MEDICINE CONNECTION

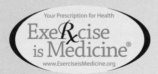

National Institute of Health, National Institute of Diabetes and Digestive and Kidney diseases. Diabetes prevention program [Internet]. Available from: http://diabetes.niddk.nih.gov/dm/pubs/preventionprogram/

The U.S. Diabetes Prevention Program (DPP) was a multicenter trial that compared lifestyle modification with medication in the reduction in incidence of Type 2 DM. All participants ($N = 3,234$) at the start of the study were overweight and had either impaired glucose tolerance (IGT) or impaired fasting glucose (IFG). The main outcome measure was the development of Type 2 diabetes. Participants were randomly assigned to one of three groups: control, medication (metformin), or lifestyle modification. The lifestyle group included intensive dietary and physical activity modifications with a weight loss goal (5%–7% of current body weight) and 150 minutes of weekly aerobic activity. The lifestyle modification group reduced Type 2 diabetes incidence by 58%, and this reduction was true across all participating ethnic groups and for both men and women. The metformin group realized a 31% reduction in diabetes incidence and was effective for both men and women, but it was least effective in people aged 45 years and older.

The DPP study provide results indicating weight loss and physical activity lower the risk of Type 2 diabetes by improving the body's ability to use insulin and process glucose.

Pulmonary

The primary goal when developing an exercise prescription for clients with COPD is to reduce barriers for activities of daily living and to help increase quality of life (114).

- Present scientific information is mixed whether exercise training has an impact on lessening the COPD disease state (45), but because exercise training improves muscle functionality, overall exercise tolerance is improved (114).
- Another exercise training goal for the client with COPD is desensitization to dyspnea — a condition characterized by shortness of breath that often limits exercise. The EP-C must educate the client with COPD to push past this feeling. Once learned, exercise can continue even when dyspnea is increasing, and thus, greater exercise intensities and durations can be completed resulting in greater heath-fitness benefits (77,114).
- Early in the exercise program, the client with COPD will need constant monitoring until they are able to learn pulmonary triggering symptoms (45).
- To ensure safety, many clients with COPD will need constant oxyhemoglobin saturation monitoring. Blood oxygen saturation should be maintained at greater than 90% (114). However, those patients needing this type of monitoring should exercise with closer medical supervision which the EP-C is not trained to provide.
- Fast-acting inhalers are kept available at all times especially while exercising (45).
- A client with CRPD is treated in a similar fashion as a client with COPD, because they have similar exercise limitations and considerations (77).
- Additional considerations for patients with COPD include optimal exercise training time being mid- to late morning and avoiding extreme temperatures and high humidity as they can trigger symptoms and potentiate a medical incident (114).

Effect of Common Medications on Exercise with Cardiovascular, Metabolic, and Pulmonary Diseases

The vast majority of individuals with any form of CVD, metabolic disease, or pulmonary disease are likely to take one or more medications (Table 8.4). Whether medications are over-the-counter (OTC) or prescription, many may have an impact on exercise response or exercise capacity. The expectation for the EP-C is to have at least a cursory knowledge of the most common medications while keeping an updated drug reference guide handy. This preparation will allow the EP-C to make appropriate and necessary adjustments in the exercise prescription while avoiding ischemic and/or other dangerous thresholds while providing a safe and effective exercise experience.

Over-the-Counter Drugs

OTC drug use is limited in treating individuals with a chronic condition. Aspirin, most commonly used for individuals with CVD (72), does not pose any concerns when prescribing exercise (115). The same is true with most herbs, natural remedies, and minerals prescribed for CVD, metabolic, or pulmonary conditions. Nonetheless, these preparations are not regulated by the U.S. Food and Drug Administration (FDA) and should be used with extreme caution. The greater risk of OTC medications is drug interaction, and the interactive effect these drugs can have on many chronic conditions. OTC cold and flu medications often contain some form of ephedrine that has been shown to increase systemic blood pressure. These medications should be avoided or used cautiously in clients with CVD or HTN. When taken, consider postponing exercise for the day or adjusting exercise intensity and duration accordingly to avoid excessive blood pressure increases.

Table 8.4 — Common Medications

Drug Name	Mechanism	Rest/Exercise Response	Special Notes
OTC cold and flu medication	Vary by class of medication	May effect resting and exercise BP and HR but varies by medication type. No significant effect on exercise capacity	Often contain some form of ephedrine that has been shown to increase systemic blood pressure. These medications should be avoided or used cautiously in clients with CVD or HTN. When taken, consider postponing exercise for the day or adjusting exercise intensity and duration accordingly to avoid excessive blood pressure increases.
β-Blockers	Block beta receptors. May alter myocardial contractility depending on chronic condition	Increases exercise capacity with chronic use. Decreased rest and exercise HR and BP	β-Blockers make setting initial exercise intensity difficult, may limit functional capacity, inhibit using HR as an exercise intensity target, and require more rigorous patient self-monitoring. β-Blockers may also block symptoms of hypoglycemia and increase the risk of undetected hypoglycemia during and after exercise.
CCBs and ACE inhibitors	Increase arterial diameter	Decreased rest and exercise BP. No significant effect on exercise capacity	ACE inhibitors may produce an irritating dry cough. In these cases, refer client to physician.
Fibrates and statins	Vary by drug class	No significant effect on exercise capacity	Muscle soreness is an indication that a condition referred to as rhabdomyolysis might be evolving. When symptoms of this condition appear, the client should be referred to his or her physician. Clients taking this drug regimen and showing signs of this condition may need increased recovery time or lower exercise intensities.
Digitalis	Increases myocardial contractility	Increases exercise capacity. May decrease resting HR. Mediates arrhythmias	Can cause ST-segment depression at rest or during exercise
Diuretics	Increase renal water excretion	May increase resting HR. May cause premature ventricular contractions (PVCs). May decrease exercise capacity	Individuals taking diuretics should monitor body weight daily. If weight changes considerably on a given day, physician should be advised prior to exercising.
Oral medications for treating diabetes	Increase hepatic insulin output. Lower insulin resistance. Decrease absorption of carbohydrates	Minimal effect	The exerciser with diabetes needs to monitor blood glucose closely before, during, and after each exercise session.

Ford ES, Giles WH, Dietz WH. Prevalence of the metabolic syndrome among us adults: findings from the third national health and nutrition examination survey. *JAMA.* 2002;287(3):356–9. doi:10.1001/jama.287.3.356.

The patient with diabetes should avoid any OTC drugs that contain alcohol or sugar because they are likely to affect blood glucose levels. In addition, two common nonsteroidal anti-inflammatory drugs (NSAIDs) — ibuprofen and naproxen — are used cautiously in patients with diabetes because both may increase the risk of hypoglycemia (116). Conflicting evidence exists regarding the effect of NSAIDs on blood pressure; therefore, clients with HTN who are taking NSAIDs are monitored closely (102,108,121). OTC cough suppressants can impede "productive cough" and are used cautiously in certain patients with pulmonary disease, although the effect on exercise response is negligible (66).

Prescription Drugs

An abundance of prescription drugs is available to treat CVD, metabolic, and pulmonary disorders/diseases, and many of these drugs impact exercise capacity. The most common class of CVD drugs includes β-blockers, CCBs, ACE inhibitors, digitalis, diuretics, and cholesterol-lowering medications. These drug classes are especially common in treating persons with a history of MI, ischemia, and HTN (94,116).

β-Blockers are well known for decreasing mortality (60,96,119) and risk of a second MI (53,56,83) but also have a profound effect on exercise response. Although β-blockers lower HR and myocardial contractility, these medications also increase exercise capacity by decreasing coronary ischemia (60). This effect makes initial exercise intensity determination difficult, may limit functional capacity, can reduce the use of HR as an exercise intensity target, and requires more rigorous patient self-monitoring. β-Blockers may also block symptoms of hypoglycemia and increase the risk of undetected hypoglycemia during and after exercise (123).

CCBs (used for treating HTN and angina) and ACE inhibitors (used for treating HTN) both increase arterial diameter, thereby lessening blood pressure and decreasing the work by the heart. CCB's effect is central, whereas ACE inhibitors have a peripheral effect. Although CCBs have some effect on HR and contractility, the extent of this effect is not as great as that found for β-blockers. Therefore, CCBs and ACE inhibitors pose less concern regarding exercise responses, but the EP-C must be aware of unusual changes in blood pressure or HR both before and during exercise. ACE inhibitors do work in the lungs and can produce an irritating dry cough; if this occurs, the EP-C should refer the client to his or her physician.

Niacin and other cholesterol-lowering drugs tend to have very little effect on HR and contractility and thus no direct impact on exercise response and exercise capacity or the exercise prescription. Because the liver is the site of action of these drugs, liver function should be checked regularly. Statins alone or in combination with fibric acid are often associated with unusual muscle soreness (101). Muscle soreness is an indication that a condition referred to as rhabdomyolysis might be evolving. When symptoms of this condition appear, the client should be referred to his or her physician. Clients taking this drug regimen and showing signs of this condition may need increased recovery time or lower exercise intensities.

Digitalis, commonly used in CHF and for certain persistent arrhythmias, increases contractility, slows HR, and mediates arrhythmias (126). In the patient with CHF, digitalis typically increases exercise capacity. On the other hand, digitalis can cause ST-segment depression at rest or during exercise, so this medication use should be noted at all times (55).

Diuretics are used to control HTN and edema by triggering the kidney to excrete water (103). This increased water excretion may result in an increased resting and submaximal HR. Increased resting HR may be due to decreased blood volume and decreased blood pressure which could have a slight negative impact on exercise capacity (103) as well as thermoregulation. Individuals using diuretics to control edema should check their body weight regularly.

In pulmonary disease, β_2-agonists are commonly used as a bronchodilator for both short-term (13) and long-term (19) relief and management of asthmatic symptoms. Strong evidence exists for using inhaled corticosteroids for managing asthmatic exacerbations and for long-term treatment. However, steroid-based drugs carry long-term complications and are used cautiously.

A variety of oral medications are available to treat diabetes. Mechanisms of action include increasing pancreatic insulin output, lowering insulin resistance, and decreasing absorption of carbohydrates. These drugs may affect exercise capacity as some claim slight improvements in oxygen consumption (111), whereas others report no changes (98). Regardless, the exerciser with diabetes needs to monitor blood glucose closely before, during, and after each exercise session.

Prescribing exercise for clients with CVD, metabolic disease, or pulmonary disease requires some knowledge of common medications, particularly their effect on exercise response, exercise capacity, and hemodynamics. The EP-C is expected to be familiar with the most commonly prescribed medications and understand how to modify an exercise prescription accordingly. It is outside the scope of practice of the EP-C to suggest medication changes; rather, the EP-C should refer patients back to their attending physician for medication concerns.

Teaching and Demonstrating Safe and Effective Exercises for Individuals with Controlled Cardiovascular, Metabolic, and Pulmonary Diseases

When developing a physical activity and exercise prescription for a medically cleared client, the EP-C must complete a thorough review of the client's medical record to gain a full understanding of specific health conditions and possible exercise limitations and to develop an exercise plan. An orientation session is then scheduled to review this plan, discuss the importance of plan adherence to gain optimal health benefits as well as maintain safety, and demonstrate proper execution of all exercises.

Individuals having incurred a recent medical event are encouraged to seek involvement in an organized rehabilitation setting when starting an exercise program (87). The EP-C reviews the medical history, notes, medication history, and any client limitations. This review provides the EP-C with the background information needed to better understand the special health problems and needs surrounding the client's disease, to determine exercise contraindications and limitations, and to develop areas of emphasis in the exercise plan that will help optimize health fitness benefits and maintain safety.

After a complete review of the client's file, the EP-C is ready to meet and discuss all aspects of the plan. Individuals recently diagnosed with a chronic health condition and just starting an exercise program are probably concerned with safety and are often overwhelmed with making numerous lifestyle changes. The EP-C is never to assume client's knowledge of any part of the plan, goals, and specific exercise executions. Assumptions concerning client's exercise knowledge may lead to calamitous consequences, and for this reason, every aspect of the plan is reviewed and all exercises are carefully explained and demonstrated with active client participation. Because making lifestyle change is difficult, a thorough explanation of the plan is critical in helping to overcome potential barriers and increase the client's chance for success in making change (2). On the other hand, if clients do not understand the goals of the program or are confused by incomplete information regarding proper exercise techniques, their likelihood of exercising outside their physical limitations is greatly increased and could result in muscle skeletal injury and excessive fatigue and/or incur an undesirable medical event. Injuries and extreme fatigue can lead to frustration and possible lead to program discontinuation. In addition, because many chronic diseases pose adverse health effects, these individuals have unique limitations putting them at higher risk for injury and unwanted medical events.

Aerobic conditioning is an important component of the exercise program and is relatively easy to describe. Educational sessions provide a vital means for developing patient understanding while enhancing the likelihood in optimizing the FITT principle application. Careful explanation of exercise frequency regarding the number of days each week that exercise is performed and providing information describing various ways to meet exercise frequency goals are essential. For example, suggesting multiple short exercise episodes per day versus one longer continuous exercise session is often appropriate. Exercise intensity is a measure of exercise difficulty or how hard exercise is being performed. Although several ways to measure intensity exist, HR measurement is most commonly used, although less quantitative means of measuring exercise intensity include the RPE scale (28) or the "Talk Test" (106). Once the exercise type or mode is selected, the EP-C gives detailed exercise instructions using demonstrations and provides safety information regarding all exercises and the use of all exercise equipment. For best results, the client performs the exercise while the EP-C observes, and adjustments to the client's program are made. In the early phase of any exercise program, the client is closely monitored for correct exercise movement and appropriate exercise responses. Client records for exercise frequency, intensity, time, and type are developed and kept on file.

Resistance exercise training requires more demonstration than aerobic conditioning because of different exercises used for the various muscle groups and types of resistance equipment. Clients with a chronic disease can have numerous exercise resistance contraindications, and the EP-C must have a strong understanding and/or access of all various diseases and exercise contraindications to ensure client safety while optimizing health fitness benefits (10). As in aerobic conditioning, the FITT principle is also used for developing the resistance exercise prescription (86). A detailed description of how 1-RM is used for determining the exercise intensity for resistance exercise may be provided. The RPE scale is also an effective indicator of resistance exercise intensity (86). The number of exercise repetitions and sets completed is a measure of the exercise time or duration. Unlike aerobic conditioning, a set of resistance conditioning exercises is developed for each major muscle group. Each exercise is described and completely demonstrated to show the appropriate range of motion with proper technique, number of repetitions performed, number of sets completed, and proper description of the concentric and eccentric portions of the motion (54). In conjunction with each exercise being demonstrated, an explanation regarding why each muscle group is exercised, how a particular exercise movement is beneficial, and what if any potential risks or dangers exist when improper technique is used or the client exercises outside the prescribed recommendations is warranted. In addition to the aforementioned exercises, all clients should also be engaged in regular flexibility training, which is covered in greater detail in Chapter 5.

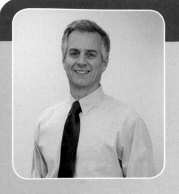

The Case of Frank

Submitted by **Benjamin Gordon, MS, ACSM-CES, and J. Larry Durstine, PhD, FACSM, Department of Exercise Science, University of South Carolina, Columbia, SC**

Frank is an unmotivated, physically inactive, middle-aged accountant. He has several risk factors for CVD but has not been clinically diagnosed with a particular disease.

Narrative

From all outward appearances, Frank seems to be an average middle-aged man. He has been an executive accountant for the past 28 years, and since starting this position as an accountant, Frank has consistently been physically inactive. Often, he will enthusiastically start an exercise program but is very unpredictable and inconsistent with exercising regularly and quits soon after starting. His eating choices and habits are poor and not consistent for good health. He consumes almost no vegetables but lots of saturated fat while consuming several beers with most meals. His most recent endeavor into exercising was spurred on by his daughter, who recommended that he needed to see someone qualified to help him start a program and stay faithful to that exercise program. On this recommendation, Frank went to his college's wellness center to see one of the EP-Cs on staff. During the initial meeting, a comprehensive assessment was carried out to determine Frank's initial fitness level and his readiness to participate in a program.

Physical Information

Age: 49 years old
Height: 5 ft 10 in
Weight: 203 lb
BMI: 29.19 kg $\cdot$ m^{-2}
Body fat percentage (DEXA scan): 29.22
Resting blood pressure: 138/92 mm Hg
Resting HR: 64 bpm

ACSM Guidelines Risk Factors

Age: He is a man, 45 years or older.
Family history: His father had a heart attack at the age of 47 years.
Cigarette smoking: Does not smoke
Physical Activity: Sedentary
Obesity: None (but is considered overweight borderline obese by both his body fat and BMI)
Hypertension: DBP is within hypertensive levels, 138/92 mm Hg.
Dyslipidemia: Total cholesterol: 238 mg $\cdot$ dL^{-1}; LDL-C: 161 mg $\cdot$ dL^{-1}; HDL-C: 39 mg $\cdot$ dL^{-1}
Prediabetes: None (resting blood glucose, 88 mg $\cdot$ dL^{-1})

The following results were from exercise testing:
Aerobic fitness ($\dot{V}O_{2max}$) (Balke protocol): approximately 19.8 mL $\cdot$ kg^{-1} $\cdot$ min^{-1}
Bench press weight ratio for 1-RM: 0.77
Leg press weight ratio for 1-RM: 1.55
YMCA bench press test (total lifts): 15
Partial curl-up test (total repetitions): 12
Forward flexion using a sit-and-reach box: 29 cm

Frank's lifestyle is riddled with long periods of inactivity and no sustained exercise. His low fitness level is affecting his quality of life. He loses his breath and is easily fatigued from menial physical tasks. Unfortunately, Frank isn't really too worried about his health, but his daughter is. He only wants to exercise enough to stop his daughter from nagging him.

QUESTIONS

- What is the biggest problem concerning Frank's health right now?
- What sort of disease is Frank setting himself up for, and does he already have symptoms of the disease?
- Do you think that Frank's workouts should be supervised?
- Should Frank have his aerobic exercise broken up into intermittent exercise sessions or one longer continuous exercise session?

References

1. American College of Sport's Medicine. *ACSM's Exercise Management for Persons with Chronic Diseases and Disabilities*. 4th ed. Champaign (IL): Human Kinetics; 2016. 416 p.
2. American College of Sports Medicine. *ACSM's Guidelines for Exercise Testing and Prescription*. 10th ed. Philadelphia (PA): Wolters Kluwer; 2018.
3. American College of Sports Medicine. *ACSM's Resources for Clinical Exercise Physiology*. 2nd ed. Philadelphia (PA): Lippincott Williams & Wilkins; 2010. 368 p.
4. American College of Sports Medicine. *ACSM's Resource Manual for Guidelines for Exercise Testing and Prescription*. 7th ed. Philadelphia (PA): Wolters Kluwer/Lippincott Williams & Wilkins; 2014. 896 p.

SUMMARY

Regular physical activity and exercise participation can provide primary and secondary prevention health fitness benefits. Medications, specialized diets, and surgeries are generally viewed as first options before exercise is considered as an intervention. Nonetheless, daily physical activity and exercise training are effective tools in developing health fitness benefits for persons with chronic diseases. Although exercise is beneficial, the challenges and limitations presented by diseases must be addressed to properly design the most effective and safest physical activity and exercise program. By adapting the ACSM (62) and U.S. physical activity recommendations (31) for prescribing physical activity and exercise programs, the EP-C is better able to meet the needs of the cardiovascular, metabolic, and pulmonary clients while ensuring program safety. The EP-C must know the limitations and challenges these diseases present for the exercising client and how to adapt the physical activity and exercise programs accordingly.

STUDY QUESTIONS

1. Explain the pathophysiology of atherosclerosis, including the role of the major risk factors.
2. Explain why the patient with asthma may have difficulty breathing, particularly during exercise.
3. Explain the major pathologic differences between Type 1 and Type 2 diabetes, within the context of exercise.
4. Briefly describe the effect of OTC medications on exercise in CAD and pulmonary disease.
5. Describe key differences in prescribing exercise for specific clinical populations.

REFERENCES

1. Aboyans V, Criqui MH, Abraham P, et al. Measurement and interpretation of the ankle-brachial index: a scientific statement from the American Heart Association. *Circulation*. 2012; 126(24):2890–909.

2. Ajzen I. *Attitudes, Personality and Behavior*. Chicago (IL): Dorsey Press; 1988. 116–27 p.

3. Alberti KG, Eckel RH, Grundy SM, et al. Harmonizing the metabolic syndrome: a joint interim statement of the International Diabetes Federation Task Force on Epidemiology and Prevention; National Heart, Lung, and Blood Institute; American Heart Association; World Heart Federation; International Atherosclerosis Society; and International Association for the Study of Obesity. *Circulation*. 2009;120(16):1640–5.

4. American College of Sports Medicine. *ACSM's Exercise Management for Persons with Chronic Diseases and Disabilities*. 4th ed. Champaign (IL): Human Kinetics; 2016. 416 p.

5. American College of Sports Medicine. *ACSM's Metabolic Calculations Handbook*. Baltimore (MD): Lippincott Williams & Wilkins; 2007. 128 p.

6. American College of Sports Medicine. Exercise prescription for individuals with metabolic disease and cardiovascular disease risk factors. In: Riebe D, editor. *ACSM's Guidelines for Exercise Testing and Prescription*. 10th ed. Philadelphia (PA): Wolters Kluwer; 2018. p. 268–96.

7. American College of Sports Medicine. Exercise prescription for patients with cardiac, peripheral, cerebrovascular, and pulmonary disease. In: Riebe D, editor. *ACSM's Guidelines for Exercise Testing and Prescription*. 10th ed. Philadelphia (PA): Wolters Kluwer; 2018. p. 226–67.

8. American College of Sports Medicine. General principles of exercise prescription. In: Riebe D, editor. *ACSM's Guidelines for Exercise Testing and Prescription*. 10th ed. Philadelphia (PA): Wolters Kluwer; 2018. p. 143–79.

9. American College of Sports Medicine. Position stand on exercise for patients with coronary artery disease. *Med Sci Sports Exerc*. 1994;26(3):i–v.

10. American College of Sports Medicine. Position stand on the recommended quantity and quality of exercise for developing and maintaining cardiorespiratory and muscular fitness, and flexibility in healthy adults. *Med Sci Sports Exerc*. 1998;30(6):975–91.

11. American Diabetes Association. Diagnosis and classification of diabetes mellitus. *Diabetes Care*. 2007;30(1):S42–7.

12. American Diabetes Association. Implications of the diabetes control and complications trial. *Diabetes Care*. 2003; 26(1):S25–7.

13. American Pharmaceutical Association. A sample protocol for chronic management of asthma from the American Pharmaceutical Association Respiratory Disease Panelists and Reviewers. *Am Pharm*. 1995;NS35(11):30–5.

14. Askew CD, Parmenter B, Leicht AS, Walker PJ, Golledge J. Exercise & Sports Science Australia (ESSA) position statement on exercise prescription for patients with peripheral artery disease and intermittent claudication. *J Sci Med Sport*. 2014;17(6):623–9.

15. Balady GJ, Williams MA, Ades PA, et al. Core components of cardiac rehabilitation/secondary prevention programs: 2007 update: A scientific statement from the American Heart Association Exercise, Cardiac Rehabilitation, and Prevention Committee, the Council on Clinical Cardiology; the Councils on Cardiovascular Nursing, Epidemiology and Prevention, and Nutrition, Physical Activity, and Metabolism; and the American Association of Cardiovascular and Pulmonary Rehabilitation. *Circulation*. 2007;115(20):2675–82.

16. Barlow CE, Kohl HW III, Gibbons LW, et al. Physical fitness, mortality and obesity. *Int J Obes Relat Metab Disord*. 1995;19(suppl 4):S41–4.

17. Barnard RJ, Gardner GW, Diaco NV, et al. Cardiovascular responses to sudden strenuous exercise — heart rate, blood pressure, and ECG. *J Appl Physiol*. 1973;34(6):833–7.

18. Barnes P. Asthma management: can we further improve compliance and outcomes. *Respir Med*. 2008;98:S8–9.

19. Barnes PJ. Immunology of asthma and chronic obstructive pulmonary disease. *Nat Rev Immunol*. 2008;8(3):183–92.

20. Bayles CM, Chan S, Robare J. Frailty. In: Durstine JL, Moore GE, Painter PL, Roberts SO, editors. *ACSM's Exercise Management for Persons with Chronic Diseases and Disabilities*. 3rd ed. Champaign (IL): Human Kinetics; 2009. p. 206–12.

21. Beauchamp MK, Nonoyama M, Goldstein RS, et al. Interval versus continuous training in individuals with chronic obstructive pulmonary disease — a systematic review. *Thorax*. 2010;65(2):157–64.

22. Beevers G, Lip GY, O'Brien E. ABC of hypertension: the pathophysiology of hypertension. *BMJ*. 2001;322(7291):912–6.

23. Beilby J. Definition of metabolic syndrome: report of the National Heart, Lung, and Blood Institute/American Heart Association Conference on Scientific Issues Related to Definition. *Clin Biochem Rev*. 2004;25(3):195–8.

24. Belardinelli R, Georgiou D, Cianci G, Purcaro A. Randomized, controlled trial of long-term moderate exercise training in chronic heart failure: effects on functional capacity, quality of life, and clinical outcome. *Circulation*. 1999;99(9):1173–82.

25. Billat LV. Interval training for performance: a scientific and empirical practice. Special recommendations for middle- and long-distance running. Part I: aerobic interval training. *Sports Med*. 2001;31:13–31.

26. Bird SR, Hawley JA. Exercise and type 2 diabetes: new prescription for an old problem. *Maturitas*. 2012;72:311–6.

27. Blair SN, Kohl HW III, Barlow CE, Paffenbarger RS Jr, Gibbons LW, Macera CA. Changes in physical fitness and all-cause mortality. A prospective study of healthy and unhealthy men. *JAMA*. 1995;273(14):1093–8.

28. Borg GA. Perceived exertion. *Exerc Sport Sci Rev*. 1974;2(1): 131–53.

29. Bouldin MJ, Ross LA, Sumrall CD, Loustalot FV, Low AK, Land KK. The effect of obesity surgery on obesity comorbidity. *Am J Med Sci*. 2006;331(4):183–93.

30. Boulé NG, Haddad E, Kenny GP, Wells GA, Sigal RJ. Effects of exercise on glycemic control and body mass in type 2 diabetes mellitus: a meta-analysis of controlled clinical trials. *JAMA*. 2001;286(10):1218–27.

31. Buchner D. *2008 Physical Activity Guidelines for Americans*. Washington (DC): U.S. Department of Health and Human Services; 2008. 76 p.

32. Castellani JW, Young AJ, Ducharme MB, et al. American College of Sports Medicine position stand: prevention

of cold injuries during exercise. *Med Sci Sports Exerc.* 2006;38(11):2012–29.

33. Castro-Sánchez AM, Matarán-Peñarrocha GA, Feriche-Fernández-Castanys B, Fernández-Sola C, Sánchez-Labraca N, Moreno-Lorenzo C. A program of 3 physical therapy modalities improves peripheral arterial disease in diabetes type 2 patients: a randomized controlled trial. *J Cardiovasc Nurs.* 2013;28(1):74–82.

34. Centers for Disease Control and Prevention. [Internet]. Atlanta (GA): Centers for Disease Control and Prevention; [cited 2016 Jan]. Available from: https://www.cdc.gov/obesity/adult/defining.html. Accessed January 2017.

35. Centers for Disease Control and Prevention. *Heart Disease Facts* [Internet]. Atlanta (GA): Centers for Disease Control and Prevention; [cited 2016 Jan]. Available from: http://www.cdc.gov/heartdisease/facts.htm

36. Centers for Disease Control and Prevention. *Summary Health Statistics for U.S. Adults: National Health Interview Survey, 2000* [Internet]. Atlanta (GA): Centers for Disease Control and Prevention; [cited 2016 Jan]. Available from: http://www.cdc.gov/nchs/data/series/sr_10/sr10_215.pdf

37. Centers for Disease Control and Prevention. *Summary Health Statistics for U.S. Adults: National Health Interview Survey, 2001* [Internet]. Atlanta (GA): Centers for Disease Control and Prevention; [cited 2016 Jan]. Available from: http://www.cdc.gov/nchs/data/series/sr_10/sr10_218.pdf

38. Centers for Disease Control and Prevention. *Summary Health Statistics for U.S. Adults: National Health Interview Survey, 2002* [Internet]. Atlanta (GA): Centers for Disease Control and Prevention; [cited 2016 Jan]. Available from: http://www.cdc.gov/nchs/data/series/sr_10/sr10_222.pdf

39. Centers for Disease Control and Prevention. *Summary Health Statistics for U.S. Adults: National Health Interview Survey, 2004* [Internet]. Atlanta (GA): Centers for Disease Control and Prevention; [cited 2016 Jan]. Available from: http://www.cdc.gov/nchs/data/series/sr_10/sr10_228.pdf

40. Centers for Disease Control and Prevention. *Summary Health Statistics for U.S. Adults: National Health Interview Survey, 2005* [Internet]. Atlanta (GA): Centers for Disease Control and Prevention; [cited 2016 Jan]. Available from: http://www.cdc.gov/nchs/data/series/sr_10/sr10_232.pdf

41. Centers for Disease Control and Prevention. *Summary Health Statistics for U.S. Adults: National Health Interview Survey, 2007* [Internet]. Atlanta (GA): Centers for Disease Control and Prevention; [cited 2016 Jan]. Available from: http://www.cdc.gov/nchs/data/series/sr_10/sr10_240.pdf

42. Centers for Disease Control and Prevention. *Summary Health Statistics for U.S. Adults: National Health Interview Survey, 2008* [Internet]. Atlanta (GA): Centers for Disease Control and Prevention; [cited 2016 Jan]. Available from: http://www.cdc.gov/nchs/data/series/sr_10/sr10_242.pdf

43. Centers for Disease Control and Prevention. *Summary Health Statistics for U.S. Adults: National Health Interview Survey, 1999* [Internet]. Atlanta (GA): Centers for Disease Control and Prevention; [cited 2016 Jan]. Available from: http://www.cdc.gov/nchs/data/series/sr_10/sr10_210.pdf

44. Cnop M, Welsh N, Jonas JC, Jörns A, Lenzen S, Eizirik DL. Mechanisms of pancreatic beta-cell death in type 1 and type 2 diabetes: many differences, few similarities. *Diabetes.* 2005;(54):S97–107.

45. Cooper CB. Exercise in chronic pulmonary disease: Aerobic exercise prescription. *Med Sci Sports Exerc.* 2001;33 (7 suppl):S671–9.

46. Cornish AK, Broadbent S, Cheema BS. Interval training for patients with coronary artery disease: a systematic review. *Eur J Appl Physiol.* 2011;111(4):579–89.

47. Courser JI, Guthmann R, Hamadeh MA, Kane CS. Pulmonary rehabilitation improves exercise capacity in older elderly patients with COPD. *Chest.* 1995;107(3)730–4.

48. Crowther RG, Leicht AS, Spinks WL, Sangla K, Quigley F, Golledge J. Effects of a 6-month exercise program pilot study on walking economy, peak physiological characteristics, and walking performance in patients with peripheral arterial disease. *Vasc Health Risk Manag.* 2012;8:225–32.

49. Cucato GG, Chehuen Mda R, Costa LA, et al. Exercise prescription using the heart of claudication pain onset in patients with intermittent claudication. *Clinics (Sao Paulo).* 2013;68(7):974–8.

50. DeBusk RF, Haskell W. Symptom-limited vs heart-rate-limited exercise testing soon after myocardial infarction. *Circulation.* 1980;61(4):738–43.

51. Durstine JL, Gordon BT, Wang Z, Luo X. Chronic disease and the link to physical activity. *J Sport Health Sci.* 2013;2(1):3–11.

52. Edmunds J, Ntoumanis N, Duda JL. Adherence and well-being in overweight and obese patients referred to an exercise on prescription program. *Psychol Sport Exerc.* 2007;5(1):722–40.

53. Everly MJ, Heaton PC, Cluxton RJ Jr. Beta-blocker underuse in secondary prevention of myocardial infarction. *Ann Pharmacother.* 2004;38(2):286–93.

54. Fleck SJ, Kraemer WJ. *Designing Resistance Training Programs.* Champaign (IL): Human Kinetics; 2004. 392 p.

55. Fletcher GF, Balady GJ, Amsterdam EA, et al. Exercise standards for testing and training: a statement for healthcare professionals from the American Heart Association. *Circulation.* 2001;104(14):1694–740.

56. Fonarow GC. Beta-blockers for the post-myocardial infarction patient: current clinical evidence and practical considerations. *Rev Cardiovasc Med.* 2006;7(1):1–9.

57. Ford ES, Giles WH, Dietz WH. Prevalence of the metabolic syndrome among US adults: findings from the third National Health and Nutrition Examination Survey. *JAMA.* 2002;287(3):356–9.

58. Franklin BA. Myocardial infarction. In: Durstine LJ, Moore GE, Painter PL, Roberts SO, editors. *ACSM's Exercise Management for Person with Chronic Diseases and Disabilities.* Champaign (IL): Human Kinetics; 2009. p. 49–57.

59. Freese EC, Levine AS, Chapman DP, Hausman DB, Cureton KJ. Effects of acute sprint interval cycling and energy replacement on postprandial lipemia. *J Appl Physiol.* 2011;111(6):1584–9.

60. Friedman D, Roberts SO. Angina and silent ischemia. In: Durstine LJ, Moore GE, Painter PL, Roberts SO, editors. *ACSM's Exercise Management for Person with Chronic Diseases and Disabilities.* Champaign (IL): Human Kinetics; 2009. p. 66–72.

61. Gaesser GA, Angadi SS, Sawyer BJ. Exercise and diet, independent of weight loss, improve cardiometabolic risk profile in overweight and obese individuals. *Phys Sportsmed.* 2011;39(2):87–97.

62. Garber CE, Blissmer B, Deschenes MR, et al. American College of Sports Medicine position stand. Quantity and quality of exercise for developing and maintaining cardiore-

spiratory, musculoskeletal, and neuromotor fitness in apparently healthy adults: guidance for prescribing exercise. *Med Sci Sports Exerc*. 2011;43(7):1334–59.

63. Genest J, McPherson R, Frohlich J, et al. 2009 Canadian Cardiovascular Society/Canadian guidelines for the diagnosis and treatment of dyslipidemia and prevention of cardiovascular disease in the adult — 2009 recommendations. *Can J Cardiol*. 2009;25(10):567–79.

64. Giannuzzi P, Saner H, Björnstad H, et al. Secondary prevention through cardiac rehabilitation: position paper of the Working Group on Cardiac Rehabilitation and Exercise Physiology of the European Society of Cardiology. *Eur Heart J*. 2003;24(13):1273–8.

65. Gibala MJ, Little JP, Macdonald MJ, Hawley JA. Physiological adaptations to low-volume, high-intensity interval training in health and disease. *J Physiol*. 2012;590(5):1077–84.

66. Giron AE, Stansbury DW, Fischer CE, Light RW. Lack of effect of dextromethorphan on breathlessness and exercise performance in patients with chronic obstructive pulmonary disease (COPD). *Eur Respir J*. 1991;4(5):532–5.

67. Goodman CC, Fuller K. *Pathology: Implications for the Physical Therapist*. 3rd ed. St. Louis (MO): Saunders Elsevier; 2009. 1760 p.

68. Gordon NF, Scott CB, Wilkinson WJ, Duncan JJ, Blair SN. Exercise and mild essential hypertension. Recommendations for adults. *Sports Med*. 1990;10(6):390–404.

69. Guiraud T, Nigam A, Gremeaux V, Meyer P, Juneau M, Bosquet L. High-intensity interval training in cardiac rehabilitation. *Sports Med*. 2012;42(7):587–605.

70. Hansen D, Eijnde BO, Roelants M, et al. Clinical benefits of the addition of lower extremity low-intensity resistance muscle training to early aerobic endurance training intervention in patients with coronary artery disease: a randomized controlled trial. *J Rehabil Med*. 2011;43(9):800–7.

71. Haskell WL, Lee IM, Pate RR, et al. Physical activity and public health: updated recommendation for adults from the American College of Sports Medicine and the American Heart Association. *Med Sci Sports Exerc*. 2007;39(8):1423–34.

72. Hennekens CH, Dyken ML, Fuster V. Aspirin as a therapeutic agent in cardiovascular disease: a statement for healthcare professionals from the American Heart Association. *Circulation*. 1997;96(8):2751–3.

73. Hiatt WR, Armstrong EJ, Larson CJ, Brass EP. Pathogenesis of the limb manifestations and exercise limitations in peripheral artery disease. *Circ Res*. 2015;116(9):1527–39.

74. Hirsch AT, Haskal ZJ, Hertzer NR, et al. ACC/AHA 2005 practice guidelines for the management of patients with peripheral arterial disease (lower extremity, renal, mesenteric, and abdominal aortic). *Circulation*. 2006;113(11):e463–654.

75. Hornsby WG, Albright AL. Diabetes. In: Durstine JL, Moore GE, Painter PL, Roberts SO, editors. *ACSM's Exercise Management for Persons with Chronic Diseases and Disabilities*. 3rd ed. Champaign (IL): Human Kinetics; 2009. p. 186–9.

76. Horowitz MB, Littenberg B, Mahler DA. Dyspnea ratings for prescribing exercise intensity in patients with COPD. *Chest*. 1996;109(5):1169–75.

77. Hsia C. Chronic restrictive pulmonary disease. In: Durstine JL, Moore GE, Painter PL, Roberts SO, editors. *ACSM's Exercise Management for Persons with Chronic Diseases and Disabilities*. 3rd ed. Champaign (IL): Human Kinetics; 2009. p. 167–74.

78. Hunt SA. ACC/AHA 2005 guideline update for the diagnosis and management of chronic heart failure in the adult: a report of the American College of Cardiology/American Heart Association Task Force on Practice Guidelines (Writing Committee to Update the 2001 Guidelines for the Evaluation and Management of Heart Failure). *J Am Coll Cardiol*. 2005;46(6):e1–82.

79. Jain A, Liu K, Ferrucci L, et al. Declining walking impairment questionnaire scores are associated with subsequent increased mortality in peripheral artery disease. *J Am Coll Cardiol*. 2013;61(17):1820–9.

80. James PA, Oparil S, Carter BL, et al. 2014 evidence-based guideline for the management of high blood pressure in adults: report from the panel members appointed to the Eighth Joint National Committee (JNC 8). *JAMA*. 2014;311 (5):507–20.

81. Juneau M, Roy N, Nigam A, et al. Exercise above the ischemic threshold and serum markers of myocardial injury. *Can J Cardiol*. 2009;25(10):e338–41.

82. Keteyian SJ. Exercise rehabilitation in chronic heart failure. *Coron Artery Dis*. 2006;17(3):233–7.

83. Kleiner SA, Vogt WB, Gladowski P, et al. Beta-blocker compliance, mortality, and reinfarction: validation of clinical trial association using insurer claims data. *Am J Med Qual*. 2009;24(6):512–9.

84. Kohut ML, McCann DA, Russell DW, et al. Aerobic exercise, but not flexibility/resistance exercise, reduces serum IL-18, CRP, and IL-6 independent of beta-blockers, BMI, and psychosocial factors in older adults. *Brain Behav Immun*. 2006;20(3):201–9.

85. Kortianou EA, Nasis IG, Spetsioti ST, Daskalakis AM, Vogiatzis I. Effectiveness of interval exercise training in patients with COPD. *Cardiopulm Phys Ther J*. 2010;21(3):12–9.

86. Kraemer WJ, Ratamess NA. Fundamentals of resistance training: progression and exercise prescription. *Med Sci Sports Exerc*. 2004;36(4):674–88.

87. Kraus WE. *Physical Activity Status and Chronic Diseases*. 6th ed. Philadelphia (PA): Lippincott Williams & Wilkins; 2009. p. 166–80.

88. Lakka H, Laaksonen DE, Lakka TA, et al. The metabolic syndrome and total and cardiovascular disease mortality in middle-aged men. *JAMA*. 2002;288(21):2709–16.

89. Lamarche B, Moorjani S, Cantin B, et al. Small, dense low-density lipoprotein particles as a predictor of the risk of ischemic heart disease in men. Prospective results from the Québec Cardiovascular Study. *Circulation*. 1997;95(1):69–75.

90. Laursen PB, Jenkins DG. The scientific basis for high-intensity interval training: optimising training programmes and maximising performance in highly trained endurance athletes. *Sports Med*. 2002;32(1):53–73.

91. Leach RJ. Chronic obstructive airways disease. *Respir Dis Manag*. 2009;10:29–40.

92. Leicht AS, Crowther RG, Golledge J. Influence of peripheral arterial disease and supervised walking on heart rate variability. *J Vasc Surg*. 2011;54(5):1352–9.

93. Leon AS. Exercise following myocardial infarction. Current recommendations. *Sports Med*. 2000;29(5):301–11.

94. Li J, Zhang N, Ye B, et al. Non-steroidal anti-inflammatory drugs increase insulin release from beta cells by inhibiting ATP-sensitive potassium channels. *Br J Pharmacol.* 2007; 151(4):483–93.

95. Libby P, Ridker PM. Inflammation and atherothrombosis: from population biology and bench research to clinical practice. *J Am Coll Cardiol.* 2006;48(9):A33–46.

96. Lindenauer PK, Pekow P, Wang K, Mamidi DK, Gutierrez B, Benjamin EM. Perioperative beta-blocker therapy and mortality after major noncardiac surgery. *N Engl J Med.* 2005;353(4):349–61.

97. Mallika V, Goswami B, Rajappa M. Atherosclerosis pathophysiology and the role of novel risk factors: a clinicobiochemical perspective. *Angiology.* 2007;58(5):513–22.

98. McGuire DK, Abdullah SM, See R, et al. Randomized comparison of the effects of rosiglitazone vs. placebo on peak integrated cardiovascular performance, cardiac structure, and function. *Eur Heart J.* 2010;31(18):2262–70.

99. Mittleman MA, Maclure M, Tofler GH, Sherwood JB, Goldberg RJ, Muller JE. Triggering of acute myocardial infarction by heavy physical exertion. Protection against triggering by regular exertion. Determinants of myocardial infarction onset study investigators. *N Engl J Med.* 1993;329(23):1677–83.

100. Naughton J, Raider R. Methods of exercise testing. In: Naughton JP, Hellerstein HK, Mohler IC, editors. *Exercise Testing and Exercise Training in Coronary Heart Disease.* New York (NY): Academic Press; 1973. p. 79–89.

101. Omar MA, Wilson JP, Cox TS. Rhabdomyolysis and HMG-CoA reductase inhibitors. *Ann Pharmacother.* 2001;35(9): 1096–107.

102. Palmer R, Weiss R, Zusman RM, Haig A, Flavin S, MacDonald B. Effects of nabumetone, celecoxib, and ibuprofen on blood pressure control in hypertensive patients on angiotensin converting enzyme inhibitors. *Am J Hypertens.* 2003;16(2):135–9.

103. Parker JD, Parker AB, Farrell B, Parker JO. Effects of diuretic therapy on the development of tolerance to nitroglycerin and exercise capacity in patients with chronic stable angina. *Circulation.* 1996;93(4):691–6.

104. Patsch JR, Sailer S, Kostner G, Sandhofer F, Holasek A, Braunsteiner H. Separation of the main lipoprotein density classes from human plasma by rate-zonal ultracentrifugation. *J Lipid Res.* 1974;15(4):356–66.

105. Pauwels RA, Buist AS, Calverley PM, Jenkins CR, Hurd SS. Global strategy for the diagnosis, management, and prevention of chronic obstructive pulmonary disease. NHLBI/WHO Global Initiative for Chronic Obstructive Lung Disease (GOLD) workshop summary. *Am J Respir Crit Care Med.* 2001;163(5):1256–76.

106. Persinger R, Foster C, Gibson M, Fater DC, Porcari JP. Consistency of the talk test for exercise prescription. *Med Sci Sports Exerc.* 2004;36(9):1632–6.

107. Pescatello LS, Franklin BA, Fagard R, Farquhar WB, Kelley GA, Ray CA. American College of Sports Medicine position stand. Exercise and hypertension. *Med Sci Sports Exerc.* 2004;36(3):533–53.

108. Pope JE, Anderson JJ, Felson DT. A meta-analysis of the effects of nonsteroidal anti-inflammatory drugs on blood pressure. *Arch Intern Med.* 1993;153(4):477–84.

109. Rabe KF, Beghe B, Luppi F, Fabbri LM. Update in chronic obstructive pulmonary disease 2006. *Am J Respir Crit Care Med.* 2007;175(12):1222–32.

110. Rabe KF, Hurd S, Anzueto A, et al. Global strategy for the diagnosis, management, and prevention of chronic obstructive pulmonary disease: GOLD executive summary. *Am J Respir Crit Care Med.* 2007;176(6):532–55.

111. Regensteiner JG, Bauer TA, Reusch JE. Rosiglitazone improves exercise capacity in individuals with type 2 diabetes. *Diabetes Care.* 2005;28(12):2877–83.

112. Rehman J, Li J, Parvathaneni L, et al. Exercise acutely increases circulating endothelial progenitor cells and monocyte-/macrophage-derived angiogenic cells. *J Am Coll Cardiol.* 2004;43(12):2314–8.

113. Riebe D, Franklin BA, Thompson PD, et al. Updating ACSM's recommendations for exercise preparticipation health screening. *Med Sci Sports Exerc.* 2015;47(11):2473–9.

114. Ries AL, Bauldoff GS, Carlin BW, et al. Pulmonary rehabilitation: joint ACCP/AACVPR evidence-based clinical practice guidelines. *Chest.* 2007;131(5 suppl):4S–42S.

115. Romer L. Pathophysiology and treatment of pulmonary disease. In: Ehrman JK, editor. *ACSM's Resource Manual for Guidelines for Exercise Testing and Prescription.* Philadelphia (PA): Lippincott Williams & Wilkins; 2010. p. 20–32.

116. Rosendorff C. Hypertension and coronary artery disease: a summary of the American Heart Association scientific statement. *J Clin Hypertens (Greenwich).* 2007;9(10):790–5.

117. Serrano Hernando FJ, Martin Conejero A. Peripheral artery disease: pathophysiology, diagnosis and treatment. *Rev Esp Cardiol.* 2007;60(9):969–82.

118. Shah K, Villareal DT. Combination treatment to CONQUER obesity? *Lancet.* 2011;377(9774):1295–7.

119. Shekelle PG, Rich MW, Morton SC, et al. Efficacy of angiotensin-converting enzyme inhibitors and beta-blockers in the management of left ventricular systolic dysfunction according to race, gender, and diabetic status: a meta-analysis of major clinical trials. *J Am Coll Cardiol.* 2003;41(9):1529–38.

120. Shephard RJ, Balady GJ. Exercise as cardiovascular therapy. *Circulation.* 1999;99(7):963–72.

121. Sheridan R, Montgomery AA, Fahey T. NSAID use and BP in treated hypertensives: a retrospective controlled observational study. *J Hum Hypertens.* 2005;19(6):445–50.

122. Sigal RJ, Kenny GP, Wasserman DH, Castaneda-Sceppa C. Physical activity/exercise and type 2 diabetes. *Diabetes Care.* 2004;27(10):2518–39.

123. Sigal RJ, Purdon C, Bilinski D, Vranic M, Halter JB, Marliss EB. Glucoregulation during and after intense exercise: effects of beta-blockade. *J Clin Endocrinol Metab.* 1994;78(2): 359–66.

124. Sorensen J, Wilks SA, Jacob AD, Huynh TT. Screening for peripheral artery disease. *Semin Roentgenol.* 2015;50(2): 139–47.

125. Stein R, Hriljac I, Halperin JL, et al. Limitation of the resting ankle-brachial index in symptomatic patients with peripheral arterial disease. *Vasc Med.* 2006;11(1):29–33.

126. Sullivan M, Atwood JE, Myers J, Gustavson SM, Teodorescu V, Olin JW. Increased exercise capacity after digoxin administration in patients with heart failure. *J Am Coll Cardiol.* 1989;13(5):1138–43.

127. Susic D. Hypertension, aging, and atherosclerosis. The endothelial interface. *Med Clin N Am*. 1997;81(5):1231–40.

128. Thompson PD. Exercise and physical activity in the prevention and treatment of atherosclerotic cardiovascular disease. *Arterioscler Thromb Vasc Biol*. 2003;23(8): 1319–21.

129. Thompson PD, Crouse SF, Goodpaster B, Kelley D, Moyna N, Pescatello L. The acute versus the chronic response to exercise. *Med Sci Sports Exerc*. 2001;33(6 suppl):S438–45; discussion S52–3.

130. Verity L. Exercise prescription in patients with diabetes. In: Ehrman J, editor. *ACSM's Resource Manual for Guidelines for Exercise Testing and Prescription*. Philadelphia (PA): Lippincott Williams & Wilkins; 2010. p. 600–17.

131. Villareal DT, Chode S, Parimi N, et al. Weight loss, exercise, or both and physical function in obese older adults. *N Engl J Med*. 2011;364(13):1218–29.

132. Wallace JP, Ray S. Obesity. In: Durstine JL, Moore GE, Painter PL, Roberts SO, editors. *ACSM's Exercise Management for Persons with Chronic Diseases and Disabilities*. 3rd ed. Champaign (IL): Human Kinetics; 2009. p. 192–4.

133. Wallace JP, Shala R. Obesity. In: Durstine JL, Moore GE, Painter PL, Roberts SO, editors. *ACSM's Exercise Management for Persons with Chronic Diseases and Disabilities*. 3rd ed. Champaign (IL): Human Kinetics; 2009. p. 192–9.

134. Wang JS, Jen CJ, Chen HI. Effects of exercise training and deconditioning on platelet function in men. *Arterioscler Thromb Vasc Biol*. 1995;15(10):1668–74.

135. Whelton SP, Chin A, Xin X, He J. Effects of aerobic exercise on blood pressure: a meta-analysis of randomized, controlled trials. *Ann Intern Med*. 2002;136(7):493–503.

136. Williams B, Poulter NR, Brown MJ, et al. British Hypertension Society guidelines for hypertension management 2004 (BHS-IV): summary. *BMJ*. 2004;328(7440):634–40.

137. Willich SN, Lewis M, Lowel H, Arntz HR, Schubert F, Schroder R. Physical exertion as a trigger of acute myocardial infarction. Triggers and Mechanisms of Myocardial Infarction Study Group. *N Engl J Med*. 1993;329(23):1684–90.

138. Womack L, Peters D, Barrett EJ, Kaul S, Price W, Lindner JR. Abnormal skeletal muscle capillary recruitment during exercise in patients with type 2 diabetes mellitus and microvascular complications. *J Am Coll Cardiol*. 2009;53(23):2175–83.

139. Xu JQ, Kochanek KD, Murphy SL, Tejada-Vera B. Deaths: final data for 2007. *Natl Vital Stat Rep* [Internet]. 2010;58(19). Hyattsville (MD): National Center for Health Statistics; [cited 2010 Sep 16]. Available from: http://www.cdc.gov/nchs/

Exercise Programming for Individuals with Musculoskeletal Limitations

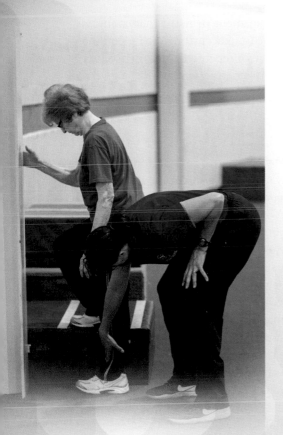

OBJECTIVES

- To understand the causes of, effects of exercise on, and reduction of risks for traumatic injuries, overuse injuries, and selected musculoskeletal diseases.

- To apply appropriate exercise guidelines for traumatic injuries, overuse injuries, and selected musculoskeletal diseases.

- To modify exercise prescription appropriately for traumatic injuries, overuse injuries, and selected musculoskeletal diseases.

INTRODUCTION

In previous chapters, you read about exercise prescription for individuals without limitations. In this chapter, we review selected musculoskeletal injuries and pathologies and discuss causes of, effects of exercise on, and strategies to reduce risks associated with these conditions. This chapter builds on the basic principles of exercise prescription discussed in Part II. This chapter is divided into three sections: traumatic injuries, overuse injuries, and chronic conditions. As you read through these sections, be reminded that safety is first and foremost for your clients. Therefore, it is important to work closely with qualified health care professionals as you develop and implement exercise programs for clients with musculoskeletal limitations.

 ## Traumatic Movement–Related Injuries

Injury to a muscle or tendon is called a *strain*, whereas injury to a ligament, or tissue that connects bones, is called a *sprain*. Both strains and sprains occur in response to unaccustomed stress on the tissue or in response to repeated lower level stress over time because of repetitive motion. In either case, an acute strain or sprain occurs most often during an eccentric contraction and/or when tissue is in an excessively stretched state (1).

Strains

The muscle-tendon unit (MTU) serves to generate force either by concentric contraction to create movement or by eccentric contraction to resist a load (36). Injury to the MTU can occur at any point along the MTU continuum, and the location of injury usually depends on the nature of the rate and magnitude of the applied force and type (intrinsic or extrinsic) of stress. Acute pain generally accompanies a muscle strain; however, muscle pain and dysfunction usually becomes more apparent 1–2 days after the injury because of delayed onset muscle soreness (DOMS). DOMS-related pain may be due to muscle fiber damage and inflammation that accompanies unaccustomed high-intensity eccentric contractions. In sport, the most common injury is a direct impact to the muscle that often causes a *contusion*. A contusion is a soft-tissue hemorrhage and/or hematoma that occurs after disruption of the muscle fibers, with subsequent inflammation and edema. Although muscle strains can occur in any MTU, they are most common in muscles of the calf (gastrocnemius, soleus) and thigh (quadriceps femoris, biceps femoris, semimembranosus, semitendinosus) (36). Contusions are graded by degree. A first-degree contusion is characterized by superficial tissue damage, no weakness or muscle spasm, and mild loss of function, ecchymosis (discoloration) and swelling, and presents no restriction on range of motion (ROM). A second-degree contusion is characterized by superficial and some deep tissue damage, mild to moderate weakness with no muscle spasm, moderate loss of function, and ecchymosis and swelling. This level of damage presents with decreased ROM. Finally, a third-degree contusion is severe and characterized by deep tissue damage, moderate to severe weakness with possible muscle spasm, severe loss of function, and ecchymosis and swelling. Substantial loss of ROM occurs due to swelling (1).

The degree of MTU strain is also classified from first to third (complete rupture) and described in Table 9.1. Assessment of strain severity should be done by a trained health care professional to ascertain the degree of strain and appropriate treatment. In the case of a severe strain, imaging technology (magnetic resonance imaging [MRI] or X-ray) may be required to determine the degree of MTU damage and for follow-up assessment of tissue repair and joint function.

Table 9.1	Grading and Characteristics of MTU Strains		
Classification	**Symptoms**	**Imaging Evidence**	**Treatment**
1st degree: **few torn fibers**	Inflammation, edema, and/or hemorrhage usually near **muscle-tendon junction, painful on contraction** but strong muscle activity	MRI of muscle damage, although not required for diagnosis	**PRICE** (**P**rotect, **R**estrict activity, **I**ce, **C**ompression, **E**levation) followed by therapeutic exercise for strength/ROM
2nd degree: **almost ½ of fibers torn**	Moderate-severe muscle pain on contraction and loss of ROM and strength, edema, and/or hemorrhage	MRI of partial tear of MTU; may not be required for diagnosis	**PRICE** and possibly immobilization followed by therapeutic exercise for strength/ROM
3rd degree: **all fibers torn (rupture)**	Painless, joint instability; moderate-severe edema	**MRI** or X-ray image of malalignment	**PRICE**, immobilization, and/or surgical repair-referral

Adapted from Herzog R. Radiologic imaging in rehabilitation. In: Kibler W, Herring S, Press J, editors. *Functional Rehabilitation of Sports and Musculoskeletal Injuries*. Gaithersburg (MD): Aspen Publishers; 1998. p. 20–70; Booher J, Thibodeau G. Athletic injuries and related skin conditions. In: Booher J, Thibodeau G, editors. *Athletic Injury Assessment*. 4th ed. Boston (MA): McGraw-Hill; 2000. p. 77–106; Anderson MK, Parr GP, Hall SJ. Tissue healing and wound care. In: Anderson MK, Parr GP, Hall SJ, editors. *Foundations of Athletic Training: Prevention, Assessment, and Management*. 4th ed. Philadelphia (PA): Lippincott Williams & Wilkins; 2009. p. 128–59.

Sprains

Ligaments are collagenous fibrous structures that connect bone to bone and provide passive soft-tissue restraint of bone-to-bone contact. Like muscle strains, ligament sprains are graded according to severity as shown in Table 9.2. The most common site of a sprain is the ankle, and the most common mechanism for causing a sprain is inversion (foot falls inward) versus eversion. An inversion sprain typically occurs, for example, when a basketball player lands from a jump on another player's foot, causing the lateral ankle to roll outward while the foot falls inward. Diagnosis of a suspected moderate to serious ligament injury should be left to a trained health care professional who will obtain a detailed history, complete a physical examination, and perform special tests to assess joint stability.

If a client experiences a suspected strain or sprain, provide immediate care by protecting the injured joint/area, having the injured person rest or restrict activity, apply ice with compression, and elevate the injured joint (PRICE) (1). Support and maintain the joint in a position that presents no or minimum discomfort, thus protecting from further injury. Following the acronym "PRICE" will serve to remind you of all steps for immediate care. Also, assist the client, as needed, in seeking medical attention.

Understanding the process of tissue healing is essential to providing safe and effective exercise guidance to an injured client. Although all types of tissue progress through the same phases of healing, the rate and length of each phase varies depending on the type of tissue and degree of tissue damage following injury/surgery. The initial *inflammatory* phase is about 2–3 days or longer. Inflammation occurs in response to acute tissue damage and is mediated chemically (*e.g.*, histamine and bradykinin) to increase blood flow and capillary permeability, causing edema. *Edema* is an accumulation of fluid in surrounding tissues that act as a brace or immobilizer and protects the damaged tissue. It does so by inhibiting contractile tissue activity and stimulating sensory nerves that cause pain to further inhibit activity. The inflammatory phase is important to prepare for the subsequent phase of tissue repair, and therefore, this phase should be accompanied by relative rest

Table 9.2	Grading and Characteristics of Ligament Sprains		
Classification	**Symptoms**	**Imaging Evidence**	**Treatment**
1st degree: **few torn ligamentous fibers**	Pain with stretching, mild instability, decreased ROM	MRI of microscopic fiber disruption, although not required for diagnosis	PRICE, followed by therapeutic exercise for strength/ROM
2nd degree: **almost ½ of ligamentous fibers torn**	Pain with stretching, mild to moderate instability, moderate swelling, decreased ROM	MRI of partial macroscopic tear of ligament; may not be required for diagnosis	PRICE and immobilization to ensure correct healing of torn fibers, followed by therapeutic exercise for strength/ROM
3rd degree: **all ligamentous fibers torn (rupture)**	Joint instability; moderate to severe swelling, severe loss of function	MRI/X-ray image of malalignment and detect possible avulsion of bone	PRICE, immobilization, and/or surgical repair-referral

Adapted from Herzog R. Radiologic imaging in rehabilitation. In: Kibler W, Herring S, Press J, editors. *Functional Rehabilitation of Sports and Musculoskeletal Injuries.* Gaithersburg (MD): Aspen Publishers; 1998. p. 20–70; Booher J, Thibodeau G. Athletic injuries and related skin conditions. In: Booher J, Thibodeau G, editors. *Athletic Injury Assessment.* 4th ed. Boston (MA): McGraw-Hill; 2000. p. 77–106; Anderson MK, Parr GP, Hall SJ. Tissue healing and wound care. In: Anderson MK, Parr GP, Hall SJ, editors. *Foundations of Athletic Training: Prevention, Assessment, and Management.* 4th ed. Philadelphia (PA): Lippincott Williams & Wilkins; 2009. p. 128–59.

and passive modalities or PRICE. Exercise during this phase could interfere with and prolong tissue repair and therefore is not recommended at this time.

The *repair* phase begins within 3–5 days after injury and varies in length depending on the type of tissue and extent of damage but could last up to 2 months. During this phase, damaged tissue is replaced with scar tissue. The quality of scar tissue development relies on proper management of the injury during this phase. As the scar tissue develops, exercise should be designed to prevent muscle atrophy and maintain joint integrity at the site of injury, and promote synthesis and optimum organization of new collagen fibers. Exercise should include gradual progression of low-load stress with no or minimal ROM, such as isometric contractions. Exercise should be administered under the direction of a rehabilitative health care professional (*e.g.*, physical therapist, certified/licensed athletic trainer, or physician).

The final *remodeling* phase is characterized by weakened, repaired tissue. Exercise during this phase is to promote hypertrophy and strength of the newly repaired tissue. Tissue remodeling can take up to 2–4 months, and exercise should be progressive and gradually work toward activity-specific exercises. Early stage progressive loading of tissue is important for collagen fiber alignment and muscle fiber hypertrophy, whereas later stage exercise should transition to activity-specific to prepare for return to activity (85). The three phases of tissue healing are summarized in Table 9.3.

Medications for Strains and Sprains

The goal of medical therapy is to reduce pain during the acute phase of recovery. Medications commonly used to manage pain and inflammation after acute injury are listed in Table 9.4. Be advised that all medications are accompanied by a risk of toxicity and side effects, and knowledge of such risks should be fully understood prior to use. Recommendation of over-the-counter medications is best made by qualified health care providers, including medical doctors, physical therapists, nurse practitioners, physician assistants, and the like.

Table 9.3	Phases and Goals of Tissue Repair			
Phase	**Duration**	**Characteristics**	**Exercise Goals**	
Inflammation	2–3+ d	Pain, edema, redness, ↑ inflammatory cell activity	PRICE for 20 min, 3–4 times a day	
Repair	Up to 2 mo	Collagen fiber production, ↓ collagen fiber organization, ↓ inflammatory cell number	Progressive low-load stress isometric to ↓ muscle atrophy, ↑ joint integrity. Low-level stretching to recover ROM and heat to ↑ blood flow to damaged tissue	
Remodeling	2–4 mo	Optimum collagen fiber alignment, ↑ tissue strength	Initial progressive loading exercises followed by transition to activity-specific exercises for return to activity	

Adapted with permission from Potach D, Ellenbecker T. Clients with orthopedic, injury, and rehabilitation concerns. In: Earle R, Baechle T, editors. *NSCA's Essentials of Personal Training.* Champaign (IL): Human Kinetics; 2004. p. 533–56.

Exercise to Reduce Risk of Strains and Sprains

Appropriate exercises can mitigate the risks of strains and sprains. With regard to connective tissue, physiologic adaptations to resistance training increase ligament and tendon strength, and collagen content, to enhance the overall integrity of connective tissue (53). Similarly, muscle fiber size, fast twitch fibers, and rate of force production increase with resistance training as well, for an overall increase in muscle and connective tissue durability. To reduce the risk of muscle strain, encourage the client to practice the following preventative strategies:

1. Warm up 5–7 minutes prior to vigorous exercise using large muscle group activities such as walking, jogging, cycling, or rowing ergometry.
2. Stretch tight muscles after the general warm-up, holding each stretch for 15–30 seconds. However, some suggest that static stretching may decrease performance in power and strength events. Therefore, dynamic stretching may be performed just prior to a competition or event.
3. Balance regular physical activities/sports with resistance exercises.
4. If possible, avoid exercise/sport when fatigued and increase training volume gradually. Fatigue can increase the risk of injury (1). Balance this with the reality that at certain phases in an athlete's training program, fatigue due to overload is a desired outcome to induce specific adaptations.

Table 9.4	Common Medications for Treatment of Musculoskeletal Injuries		
Class	**Generic Name**	**Brand Name**	**Effect**
NSAIDs	Ibuprofen	Motrin, Advil	Analgesic, anti-inflammatory, antipyretic
	Naproxen	Naprosyn, Aleve, Naprelan	
Analgesic	Acetaminophen	Tylenol, FeverAll, Tempra	Pain control
	Hydrocodone + acetaminophen	Vicodin, Lorcet-HD, Lortab	Pain control with sedating properties
	Acetaminophen + codeine	Tylenol with Codeine	

NSAIDs, nonsteroidal anti-inflammatory drugs.

Adapted from American College of Sports Medicine. *ACSM's Guidelines for Exercise Testing and Prescription.* 10th ed. Philadelphia (PA): Wolters Kluwer; 2018. p. 424–5.

Overuse Injuries

Injuries are generally categorized as acute or overuse. Acute injuries typically occur with a single traumatic event such as joint sprains and muscle strains, joint dislocation, or fracture. Joint sprains and strains were discussed previously. This section focuses on overuse injuries that result from repetitive microtrauma and occur over time. Examples of overuse injury include tendinopathies, plantar fasciitis (PF), and low back pain (LBP).

Tendinopathy

Tendinopathy is a pathological change in the tendon resulting from repeated stress or microtraumas. The most common tendinopathies include tendinitis and tendinosis. *Tendinitis* is an acute inflammatory tendinopathy (98). *Tendinosis* describes a tendon with significant degenerative changes in the absence of an inflammatory response. Tendinosis is the more common of the two as most individuals seek treatment only after the acute inflammatory process has resolved (82,98). Common sites for tendinopathies include rotator cuff, common wrist flexor and extensor tendons, patellar tendon, and Achilles tendon (82).

Clinical Presentation/Assessment

Tendinopathies often result from overload injuries that disrupt the MTU. This overload usually occurs with an acute increase in activity or load. For example, increased mileage in the case of runners or increased repetitive motions in the case of those engaged in racquet sports (32,52). These specific examples of overload are some of the most common mechanisms for tendinopathies. Other causes include premature return to occupational and/or sport and leisure activities after an injury. Individuals with tendinopathies often present with swelling (if acute) and pain, particularly with contraction or stretch of the involved muscle (32,35). Assessment of tendinopathy includes evaluating strength and extensibility of the muscle and palpation of the involved tendon to determine tenderness (100).

Safe and Effective Exercise

For exercises that do not involve the affected joint/extremity, refer to Chapter 4 for exercise guidelines. For the affected area, the following considerations are important. Until pain has subsided, individuals should reduce activity of the affected muscle to decrease repetitive loading of the damaged tendon. Most individuals improve with conservative treatment that includes PRICE (1), stretching, and/or use of analgesics (98). It should be noted that it might take up to 6 months for symptoms to subside. Once symptoms have decreased, strengthening of the affected area is appropriate. There is considerable evidence that supports the use of appropriately graded eccentric exercise as a safe and effective means for strengthening the MTU across the affected joint (57,82,98). Examples of exercises for tendinopathies can be found later in this section.

Exercise Considerations for Tendinopathies

The frequency, intensity, time, and type of eccentric exercise (FITT) is somewhat variable in the literature. However, a review of multiple studies reported a decrease in pain and return to activity with eccentric exercise (96). Refer to Table 9.5 for specific guidelines.

Table 9.5	Exercise Guidelines for Tendinopathies and Plantar Fasciitis	
Condition	**Type**	
	Resistance	**Flexibility/Stretching**
Tendinosis		
Type	Eccentric until pain free; then add concentric and plyometrics as tolerated	Passive elongation of the muscle/tendon
Frequency	3–4 sessions · wk^{-1}	Daily
Intensity	6–15 repetitions (reps)	3 reps
	3–4 sets — use body weight with progressive loading as tolerated	▪ Gradual force to provide gentle stretch
Time	Completion of reps/sets or until pain level reaches threshold to stop exercise	Hold each rep 30 s
Special considerations	Concentric exercise should be avoided early in the healing process until nonsport activities are pain free (57)	
Plantar Fasciitis		
Type		▪ Gentle stretch of the fascia to the point of tension ▪ Stretching: great toe flexors and gastroc soleus
Frequency		3 times a day
Intensity		10 reps (hold 10 s)
Time		To completion of reps
Special considerations	Pain determines exercise intensity and duration.	

Bursitis

Bursitis is an inflammation of a small fluid-filled sac called the bursa. The bursa acts as a cushion to reduce friction between muscles, tendons, and joints. Common areas for bursitis are the shoulders, hips, knees, and elbows (3).

Clinical Presentation/Assessment

Classic symptoms include sharp pain, tenderness, and swelling at the site of the bursa. Assessment of bursitis includes a thorough examination via palpation, mobility, and strength measures. Imaging techniques are usually not needed as part of the assessment but may be necessary in some cases to rule out different diagnoses. Bursitis is best managed conservatively with rest, thermal modalities, and NSAIDs.

Safe and Effective Exercise

Stretching and strengthening exercises can be done within a pain-free ROM.

Plantar Fasciitis

PF is relatively common, affecting upward of 10% of the population of the United States (14). It occurs most commonly with repeated trauma to the origin of the plantar fascia on the medial calcaneal tubercle. This is a common injury in athletes where running is involved. The pathology results from repeated stretching of the fascia during weight-bearing exercise (97).

Clinical Presentation/Assessment

Classic symptoms for PF include pain with first weight-bearing steps in the morning or during the first few minutes of running. Barefoot walking may exacerbate pain as well (13). Pain usually subsides with activity and increases after prolonged rest. Tight plantarflexor muscles along with either pes planus (flat foot) or pes cavus (high arch) may predispose an individual to PF (13,33,97).

Assessment of PF includes palpation along the plantar fascia, evaluating extensibility of the gastrocnemius, and a thorough client history. At the acute stage, PF is best managed with control of pain and minimal exercise. Pain management is often accomplished with ice massage, minimizing excess stress on the fascia (*i.e.*, avoiding barefoot walking) and NSAIDs (97). It should be noted that there is a lack of evidence supporting NSAID use for PF although they may work for some individuals (14).

Safe and Effective Exercise

As the acute phase subsides, it is important to introduce stretching of the plantar fascia as well as the plantarflexors and toe flexors (20,66). Functional weight-bearing exercises may relieve stress on the plantar fascia by supporting the medial longitudinal arch. This is accomplished by strengthening the extrinsic (anterior and posterior tibialis and the peroneus longus) and the intrinsic (abductor hallucis, flexor hallucis brevis, flexor digitorum brevis, abductor digiti minimi, and dorsal interossei) musculature (28,33). Examples of appropriate functional weight-bearing exercises include toe and heel raises (extrinsics) and short foot exercises (intrinsics) (46,47). Qualified professionals may provide orthotic intervention, or taping may be beneficial in supporting the involved structures during weight-bearing exercises (66).

EXAMPLES OF SAFE AND EFFECTIVE EXERCISES FOR OVERUSE INJURIES

As previously noted, exercises to address tendinopathies and PF should focus initially on eccentric loading and stretching. Examples of these exercises are shown for calf, wrist, and foot in Figures 9.1 through 9.4.

Table 9.5 includes exercise guidelines for tendinopathies and PF. As indicated at the bottom of the table, pain should be the limiting factor in the intensity and duration of exercise and the degree of stretch.

Low Back Pain

LBP can be traumatic, acute, or chronic. It is estimated that LBP affects 60%–80% of the adult population at some point in their lives, with an 80% recovery rate within 4–6 weeks, regardless of treatment (65). Unfortunately, unless the underlying cause of the pain is treated, the recurrence of LBP is quite high. There are many causes of LBP, including disc compression, degenerative changes in the lumbar

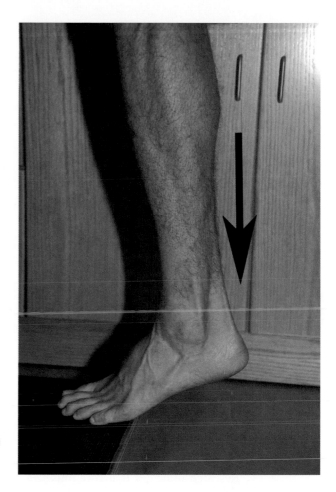

FIGURE 9.1. Eccentric loading of the gastrocnemius. Stand on the edge of a step. Using the uninvolved leg, raise up on toes (plantarflexed position), shift weight to involved leg, and slowly lower to start position. To avoid concentric contractions during the painful stage of healing, ensure that uninvolved limb is used to lift body weight.

spine, various joint and bone pathologies, and muscle imbalances (51). This discussion centers on general LBP resulting from issues of muscle imbalance.

Muscles important to the function of the spine are commonly referred to as the core, consisting of multiple layers of muscles that act to stabilize the spine, pelvis, and kinetic chain during functional movements (25). Core muscles are thought to provide a stable base of support to allow for optimal performance of the spine and extremities and help prevent injury. Also, endurance of core musculature is more critical to overall low back health than strength (Table 9.6) (64).

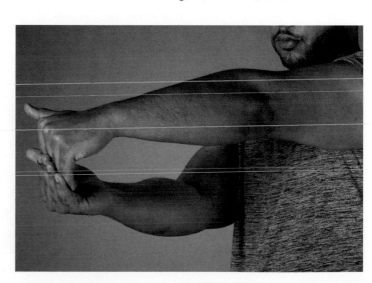

FIGURE 9.2. Stretching exercise for lateral epicondylitis. While sitting or standing, flex the wrist with opposite hand while elbow is extended. Apply pressure until a gentle stretch is felt at the elbow or forearm (wrist extensor) muscles.

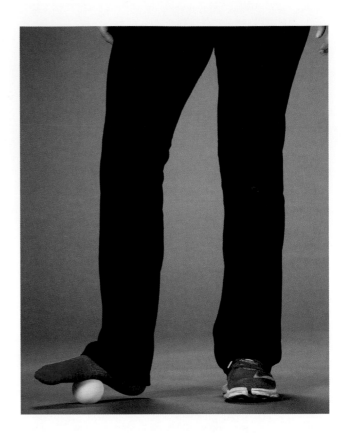

FIGURE 9.3. Stretching exercise for plantar fasciitis (PF). Sitting with involved foot resting on opposite knee, apply stretch by extending great toe and massage arch with opposite hand. Or utilize a tennis or other ball by placing the ball on a flat surface and use the pressure of the ball to massage the tight arch.

Clinical Presentation/Assessment

Research indicates that core muscle activity is different in clients with LBP. The inability of core muscles to adequately stabilize the spine can lead to pain, usually intensified with movement especially toward end of the range and with prolonged postures. Pain questionnaires and other outcome measures are often used to subjectively quantify pain and functional impairment. Examples are the Oswestry Low Back Pain Scale (24) and the McGill Pain Scale (68).

Safe and Effective Exercise

Core stabilization exercises do not fit the normal FITT template but should be incorporated into daily activities and any general exercise program (89). Core stabilization programs progress

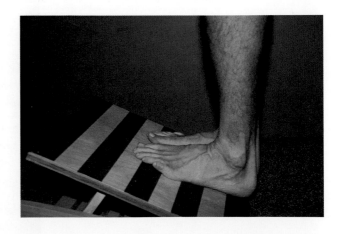

FIGURE 9.4. Stretching exercise for gastrocnemius and soleus. Stand on slanted surface, lean body forward keeping heels in contact with surface until a gentle stretch is felt in the posterior calf. Bend knees slightly to isolate the soleus muscle.

Table 9.6	Core Musculature	
Classification	**Muscle**	**Action**
Global stabilizers	Erector spinae	Extension of vertebral column
	External obliques	Flexion of vertebral column with bilateral contraction, same side lateral flexion and opposite side rotation of vertebral column with unilateral contraction
	Quadratus lumborum	Assists with extension, lateral flexion of lumbar vertebral column
	Rectus abdominis	Flexes vertebral column
Local stabilizers	Internal obliques	Flexion of vertebral column with bilateral contraction, same side lateral flexion, and same side rotation of vertebral column with unilateral contraction
	Multifidus	Extension of vertebral column with bilateral contraction and rotation of vertebral column with unilateral contraction
	Transversus abdominis	Draw abdominal wall toward spine; helps maintain abdominal pressure

Adapted with permission from Kolber M, Beekhuizen K. Lumbar stabilization: an evidence-based approach for the athlete with low back pain. *Strength Cond J.* 2007;29(2):26–37.

through various stages of increasing difficulty or intensity. Stage I, which McGill (62) refers to as abdominal bracing, involves learning to engage the small, deep stabilizing muscles that include the transverse abdominis and multifidi muscles, primarily in a supine position. In stage II, co-contraction of these deep muscles of the core is required while in more challenging positions (*i.e.*, quadruped). Movement of the extremities is also added in this stage. Stage III focuses on maintaining co-contraction of the deep stabilizing muscles while performing exercises designed to recruit larger stabilizers in more functional positions. Regardless of the stage, it is critical for the client to maintain co-contraction of the deep stabilizers. When stabilization can no longer be maintained, the exercise should be stopped. Kolber and Beekhuizen (51) discuss safe and effective lumbar stabilization exercises for LBP (see Table 9.6), and progressions of core exercises are illustrated elsewhere (25).

Examples of selected core exercises are shown in Figures 9.5 through 9.7. In stage I (Fig. 9.5), it is important to develop the abdominal drawing-in maneuver (51). This is referred to as "connecting your abdominals" and is a critical component of all core stabilization exercises.

Position: Lie on back with knees bent and arms relaxed.
Action: Tighten pelvic floor muscles (as if you were stopping the flow of urine); then, draw in lower abdomen as if pulling belly button away from waistband. Think about pulling "up and in" like a zipper zipping up from your pelvis to your ribs (rather than down toward the mat). Hold for a count of six; repeat four times. Avoid holding breath and flattening back (posterior pelvic tilt).

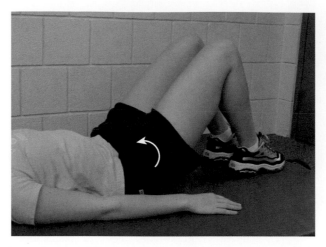

FIGURE 9.5. Example of stage I core stabilization exercise: isolating the transverse abdominis (TA).

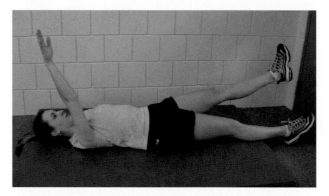

FIGURE 9.6. Example of stage II core stabilization exercise: opposing arm and leg.

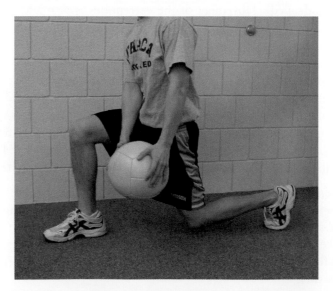

FIGURE 9.7. Example of stage III core stabilization exercise: lunge with medicine ball.

Table 9.7	Exercise Guidelines for Low Back Pain		
	Type		
	Weight-Bearing Aerobic	**Resistance**	**Flexibility/Stretching**
	Fast walking	Bridging, bird dog, curl ups	Limit exercises to unloaded spinal flexion/extension.
Frequency	Daily	2–3 times a week	Daily
Intensity	**Prescribed % of maximum as tolerated below pain threshold**	High reps and low loads	Stretch within pain-free range of motion.
Time	Build up to 30 min · d^{-1}.		Hold for 30+ s. Repeat for 2–3 reps.
Special considerations	Exercise during the first or second hour after rising from bed should be avoided because of disc hydration and subsequent loading. Any exercise that increases the intensity or frequency of pain should be discontinued, and the client should be referred for further evaluation. Exercises resulting in high-impact loading should be avoided.		

Adapted with permission from McGill S. *Ultimate Back Fitness and Performance*. 6th ed. Waterloo (ON): Backfitpro Inc.; 2017.

A stage II exercise shown in Figure 9.6 requires first a contraction of the transverse abdominis followed by simultaneously raising the diagonal arm and leg. Raise the arm to vertical and raise the leg to 45°. Return to starting position and repeat with the other diagonal pair, alternating in a rhythmic fashion. Maintain contact between the lumbar spine and the floor while moving arms and legs. The stage III exercise shown in Figure 9.7 requires connection of the abdominals followed by a lunge forward while maintaining pelvis and spine in a neutral (vertical) position. Return to starting position and repeat with other leg. Strive to maintain a vertical torso without side-to-side movement during the lunge.

Table 9.7 includes exercise guidelines for clients who suffer from LBP. Often, but not always, LBP may be alleviated through systematically strengthening the core muscles and posture training. Performing all exercises correctly provides the best opportunity for optimal improvement (63).

MEDICATION FOR OVERUSE INJURIES

Analgesics may be used to decrease pain and inflammation associated with tendinopathy. Although most over-the-counter analgesics are safe to use, it is important to know what type of analgesic is taken and its effect on pain, as it may mask or dampen pain that is a marker of exercise tolerance. Also, some analgesics such as NSAIDs may cause gastrointestinal (GI) bleeding with chronic use and may reduce kidney function. Although there is limited evidence that steroid injections may have some positive short-term effects, multiple studies document the adverse effects of fascial or tendon degeneration and/or rupture resulting from injections (66).

Chronic Conditions

Chronic conditions are prolonged in duration and do not resolve spontaneously and are rarely resolved completely. It is estimated that more than 75% of health care costs are due to treating chronic conditions (8). This section discusses two chronic conditions: arthritis and osteoporosis.

Arthritis

Arthritis is an inflammation of a joint. The two most common types of arthritis are rheumatoid arthritis and osteoarthritis (50).

Rheumatoid Arthritis

Rheumatoid arthritis (RA) is an autoimmune, chronic inflammatory disease affecting the synovial lining of joints and other connective tissue. RA is a slowly progressing disease that affects 1 in 12 adult women and 1 in 20 adult men in the United States with symptoms that cycle through periods of exacerbation and remission (15).

CLINICAL PRESENTATION/ASSESSMENT

Individuals with RA typically present with severe joint pain and inflammation, reduced muscle mass, decreased muscular strength and endurance, and decreased mobility and impaired physical activity. Loss of muscle strength is due to rheumatic cachexia, which creates a cytokine-driven hypermetabolism and protein degradation. RA is also associated with the increased risk of cardiovascular disease that appears to be independent of normal cardiovascular risk factors (12,84).

Assessment of RA includes a thorough client history, ROM and strength tests, and appropriate outcome measures to determine the stage of the disease and the client's functional status. These assessments should be performed by a qualified health care professional.

SAFE AND EFFECTIVE EXERCISE

Regular dynamic and isometric exercises are effective for improving muscular strength, cardiorespiratory function, and cardiovascular health in individuals with RA (72). Exercise can also reduce pain, morning joint stiffness, and fatigue. Individuals with RA can perform moderate-intensity exercises with little or no joint damage (95). Individuals with RA should be encouraged to pursue activities of daily living that require movement, as the benefits of an exercise program are lost when no longer continued (12,84). Refer to Table 9.8 for specific exercise guidelines.

Osteoarthritis

Osteoarthritis (OA) is a relatively common chronic degenerative joint disease that is more prevalent with age (45). OA first presents as deficits in articular cartilage of synovial joints (73). As OA progresses, bone remodeling and overgrowth at the joint margins also occurs. OA is thought to be the result of mechanical injury due to excessive loading or repeated low-force stressors (50). The most common anatomical locations for OA are the large weight-bearing joints, including the hips and knees, the cervical and lumbar spine, the distal interphalangeal joints of the fingers, and carpometacarpal joint of the thumb (50).

OBESITY AND OSTEOARTHRITIS

Obesity is associated with OA. It has been reported that for each kilogram of increased body mass, there is a risk of OA genesis of 14% (19). It is easy to infer how increased mass affects the large, weight-bearing joints. However, there is evidence that shows an increase of OA in the hands of those with a raised body mass index (BMI) (9). This indicates additional mechanisms are in play beyond the biomechanical. Regardless of mechanism, it is important for individuals to maintain an optimal BMI to minimize the effect of body mass on OA. Exercise training remains an important component to long-term management of obesity (34).

Table 9.8	Exercise Guidelines for Rheumatoid Arthritis and Osteoarthritis		
	Type		
	Weight-Bearing Aerobic	**Resistance**	**Flexibility/Stretching**
Type	Walking, cycling, rowing, swimming	Weight machines, isometric exercise, elastic bands	**Combination of dynamic and static stretching focused on all major joints**
Frequency	3–5 d · wk^{-1}	2–3 d · wk^{-1}	Daily
Intensity	60%–80% of maximum HRR, RPE = 11–16	Use pain tolerance to set %MVC.	
Time	Start with 5 min and build to 30 min per session.	2–3 reps × 1 set building to 10–12 reps × 3 sets	**30+ s per static stretch × 3 reps**
Special considerations for RA	With acute exacerbation, avoid high-intensity resistance exercises to minimize joint damage. Those with significant damage of large joints (assessed radiographically) should avoid moderate- to high-intensity weight-bearing exercise to avoid further damage (11,18)		
Special considerations for OA	Avoid overstretching unstable joints. Avoid high-resistance and high-impact exercise. Pain should be minimal. No strenuous exercise during acute flare-ups of OA and during periods of inflammation.		

HRR, heart rate reserve; RPE, rating of perceived exertion; %MVC, maximal voluntary contraction; reps, repetitions.

Adapted with permission from Minor M. Exercise in the treatment of osteoarthritis. *Rheum Dis Clin North Am*. 1999;25(2): 397–415.

CLINICAL PRESENTATION/ASSESSMENT

Individuals with OA often present with pain, joint stiffness, decreased strength, decreased flexibility, and decreased cardiovascular fitness. Assessments for OA include a thorough client history, ROM and strength testing, and evaluation of cardiovascular fitness. As part of the client history, pain can be evaluated using a variety of pain questionnaires including the Western Ontario and McMaster Universities Osteoarthritis Index (21).

SAFE AND EFFECTIVE EXERCISE

Evidence supports initiation or continuation of exercise for individuals with OA (23,38,73,74). Exercise improves overall function and prevents disability. Improved flexibility, muscular strength, cardiovascular fitness, and quality of life, along with decreased pain, are reported with exercise. Exercise may include land-based or aquatic-based programs. Aquatic programs provide an alternative environment that may benefit clients who do not tolerate land-based exercise because of pain or obesity (37). Individuals should exercise at times when pain from OA is minimal or when pain medication is at peak effectiveness. Individuals with OA may experience discomfort during or immediately after exercise. However, if joint pain persists or increases beyond preexercise level, duration and/or intensity should be reduced (31,93).

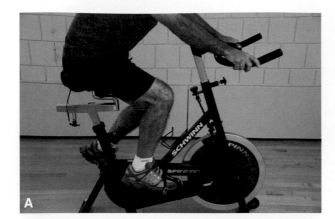

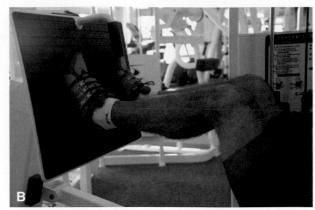

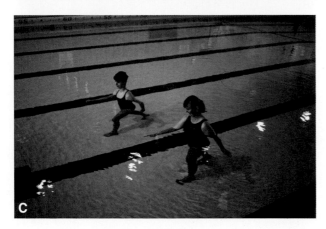

FIGURE 9.8. Types of aerobic and resistance exercises for persons with rheumatoid arthritis (RA) and osteoarthritis (OA).

Medication Effects for Rheumatoid Arthritis and Osteoarthritis

Individuals should be aware that prolonged and/or excessive use of NSAIDs can cause GI bleeding and may reduce kidney function (74). Also, RA-remitting drugs may cause secondary organ disease, including myopathy. Steroids may predispose individuals to stress fractures. Finally, oral corticosteroids may cause skeletal myopathy, truncal obesity, osteoporosis, and GI bleeding (72,73).

Exercise Guidelines for Rheumatoid Arthritis and Osteoarthritis

Examples of safe and effective aerobic and resistance exercises for RA and OA are shown in Figure 9.8. Additional details regarding exercise guidelines are supplied in Table 9.8. As indicated in the table, exercise should be avoided during periods of symptom flare-ups. However, regular, systematic exercise can be effective for preserving physical function and independence in those with RA and OA (29).

Osteoporosis

Osteoporosis, or the "silent disease," is characterized by low bone density or bone mass and deterioration of the bone microarchitecture and/or geometry that increases skeletal fragility and risk of fracture (16,39,42). It often goes undetected because early stages lack clear or overt symptoms. Diagnosis of osteoporosis is based on bone densitometry measured by dual-energy X-ray absorptiometry (DEXA or DXA) scan. Scan results are compared with those of an ethnicity- and gender-matched, 30-year-old reference. Bone density within +1.0 and −1.0 standard deviation (SD) unit (or T score) of the reference density is considered normal. A density score of -2.5 *SD* units or lower is deemed osteoporosis. *Osteopenia* is defined as bone density between normal and osteoporosis and describes those at risk for osteoporosis, with a density *SD* between -1.0 and -2.5 (22,76).

It should be noted that DEXA does not evaluate trabecular bone architecture, an indicator of overall bone strength. However, imaging technology to measure bone architecture (quantitative computed tomography or QCT; peripheral QCT or pQCT; MRI) is not used universally at this time, and thus, the definitions for bone density status rely on the more commonly used DEXA measure of bone density. Current research indicates that as much as 80% of low trauma fractures occur in those who are not diagnosed with osteoporosis but have normal or osteopenic bone density based on DEXA assessment, thus highlighting the limitations of DEXA to accurately assess bone strength (78).

Prevalence

Osteoporosis is largely preventable yet is a serious public health concern that afflicts 1 in 2 women and 1 in 5 men older than 50 years (87). Women are 3 times more likely to suffer from osteoporosis (87). In the United States, there are approximately 10 million women and men who have osteoporosis, 34 million who are at risk for developing osteoporosis, and more than 1.5 million osteoporotic fractures per year (67). Because osteoporosis often leads to fracture, it may result in loss of workdays or employment and increased hospitalizations. The economic burden of osteoporotic fractures, including loss of work, loss of independence, and cost of treatment, is substantial and has been estimated to be $20 billion in the United States and $30 billion in the European Union (16). More significantly, the loss of function in older adults due to osteoporotic fractures or related pain is a risk factor for loss of independence. The most prevalent types of osteoporotic fracture in later life are of the hip, spine, and forearm (42). Treatment and rehabilitation can translate into a long hospital visit and subsequent physical therapy before one can manage on their own. However, disuse atrophy after surgical repair compounds a potentially long, arduous recovery, and the osteoporotic fracture can easily develop into a life-threatening event for an older adult (76,88). More than 70% of osteoporotic fractures occur in those older than 70 years and present a direct threat to aging independently — a goal of most older adults. In fact, more than 25% of older adults with an osteoporotic fracture die within 5 years (5). However, even in older women with normal bone mineral density, the risk of falling and reduced quadriceps strength contributed to subsequent fracture risk (5). Therefore, activity programs for older adults should focus on bone growth and maintenance as well as lower body strength and reducing risk of falls.

Risk Factors for Osteoporosis

In addition to those who have osteoporosis, many others have low bone density or osteopenia, which predisposes one to osteoporosis. There is much still to be learned about the cause(s) of osteoporosis and osteopenia; however, research indicates a number of risk factors for developing low bone density. Table 9.9 includes both modifiable and nonmodifiable risk factors that increase the chances of developing osteoporosis. Modifiable risk factors can be influenced by lifestyle choices and indicate that we do have some control and influence over bone health.

Growth, Maturation, and Bone Density

Osteoporosis is classified as *primary* or *secondary*. Primary osteoporosis is age related, and secondary osteoporosis is due to other factors such as drug regimens for treating other diseases that can decrease bone at any time during the lifespan (61). The *female athlete triad* is an example of secondary osteoporosis and begins with disordered eating followed by amenorrhea and can result in early-onset osteoporosis (90).

Table 9.9	Risk Factors for Bone Loss, Osteoporosis, and Fracture	
Nonmodifiable Risk Factors	**Modifiable Risk Factors**	**Disorders Associated with Osteoporosis**
Female	Physical inactivity	Previous low body weight
Aging	Low calcium intake (<500–850 mg $\cdot$ d^{-1})	RA
Family history of osteoporosis or hip fracture	Vitamin D deficiency	Malabsorption syndromes (including chronic liver disease, inflammatory bowel disease)
	Smoker (current)	
White or Asian ethnicity	Excessive alcohol consumption	Primary hyperparathyroidism
	Excessive caffeine intake	
Loss of height and thoracic kyphosis	Excessive soda consumption	Long-term immobilization
Small body frame	Low strength/physical capability	
Natural or surgical menopause before age 45 yr	Low body weight (BMI <19)	
	Amenorrhea, including female athlete triad	
Previous fracture after low-energy trauma	Low testosterone in males	
	Impaired vision	
	Impaired hearing	
	Postural hypotension	
	Unstable/risky environment (low light, uneven floor, unsecured carpets)	
	Poorly fitting footwear, need for assistive devices	
	Multiple medications	

Adapted from Finigan J, Greenfield DM, Blumsohn A, et al. Risk factors for vertebral and nonvertebral fracture over 10 years: a population-based study in women. *J Bone Miner Res.* 2008;23(1):75–85; Iacono MV. Osteoporosis: a national public health priority. *J Perianesth Nurs.* 2007;22(3):175–80; Keen R. Osteoporosis: strategies for prevention and management. *Best Pract Res Clin Rheumatol.* 2007;21(1):109–22; Skinner JS, editor. *Exercise Testing and Exercise Prescription for Special Cases.* 3rd ed. Philadelphia (PA): Lippincott Williams & Wilkins; 2005. 173 p.

Peak bone density, or highest lifetime bone density, is achieved in the 20s, and loss of bone density begins around the age of 25–30 years (27). Recent longitudinal data indicate that bone loss begins earlier in men (25–39 yr) than women (40–44 yr) (4). Men and women lose bone at about the same rate until women begin to approach menopause, which occurs around the age of 52 years. Bone loss accelerates in women in late perimenopause (40–50 yr) and continues at an increased rate through early postmenopausal years (26,70,75,79,90). Although the rate of loss varies, within the early postmenopausal decade, bone loss is more evident in cortical bone and often signaled by a low-energy trauma fracture of the wrist/forearm (26,59,86,92). A low-energy trauma occurs from forces due to a fall from standing height or lower (40). On the other hand, late postmenopause (>10 yr after menopause) is marked by increased loss of trabecular bone, which comprises much of the hip and spine and contributes to the increased incidence of hip and vertebral crush fractures in older adults (26,75). Following a 5- to 10-year period of rapid postmenopausal bone loss, rate of loss returns to premenopausal values or slows down again (60). The increased rate of loss after menopause and overall lower peak bone mass in women likely contribute to the higher incidence of osteoporosis and fragility fractures in women (81). However, men are also at risk for developing osteoporosis (59). Owing to a higher lifetime peak bone density in men, increased risk of osteoporotic fracture occurs about 10 years later than in women. That is, for men, fracture risk increases after age 65 years (4).

Over the past two decades, studies of children indicate that most bone growth occurs by the end of the second decade of life, or the late teens to early 20s, with the achievement of peak bone mass and density in the 20s. The implication of this is critically important for our understanding of developing and maintaining healthy bone throughout the lifespan. Because all individuals will lose bone density and mass after the peak bone years, the goal for healthy aging of bone is to maximize the development of peak bone (achieve a high lifetime peak bone level) and minimize the rate of bone loss throughout the lifespan. In doing so, the lowest lifetime bone density, which usually occurs in later life, will still be high enough to protect from osteoporotic fracture. It appears that the age range around puberty (13–15 yr) is the time of peak bone velocity when bone growth occurs at the fastest lifetime rate. Bone growth that occurs during this critical period is inversely related with the amount of bone lost during the last four decades of life (41,56). Although genetics plays an important role in overall bone mass, nutrition and physical activity are equally important influences on the development of bone. Therefore, particular attention should be paid to these lifestyle behaviors during the critical prepubertal years (10–12 yr) when bone is most responsive to the exercise stimulus. Maximizing bone growth during puberty will confer important benefits to bone health in later life (7,56).

Inactivity and Bone Health

Cessation of bone-stimulating exercise may result in some loss of bone; however, the rate of loss and resultant bone density remains higher in young male athletes 5 years after retiring from competition, compared with their sedentary counterparts (80). The rate of loss and absolute amount of bone loss will likely vary, depending on other factors during one's lifetime (*e.g.*, bed rest, nutrition, medications, and alcohol use). Likewise, research indicates that exercise-induced bone gains in males and females, particularly during childhood and adolescence, confers benefits later in life and reduces the risk of developing osteoporosis and fragility fractures (80). In contrast, detraining studies indicate that in older adults, increased bone density due to low exercise (low exercise intensity and volume) is not long lasting but transient and may not persist after cessation of exercise (17,44,91,99). Thus, for older adults who seek to maintain bone or minimize bone loss with age, it is important to continue to exercise.

Dietary Support for Bone Health

Nutritional support for bone growth and maintenance requires adequate amounts of calcium and vitamin D. The Institute of Medicine recommendations for calcium and vitamin D intake are shown in Table 9.10 (43). However, evidence indicates that overconsumption of these nutrients may be harmful, so knowledge of these nutrient sources is important.

Medications for Bone Health

There are several pharmacological agents to increase or preserve bone or reduce bone loss. The common categories of agents to combat osteoporosis are shown in Table 9.11. Most are used in older adults, particularly postmenopausal women, and knowledge of risks associated with each drug should be considered before choosing to use a drug.

Table 9.10	Dietary Reference Intakes for Calcium and Vitamin D					
Age Group	**Calcium**			**Vitamin D**		
	Estimated Average Requirement $(mg \cdot d^{-1})$	Recommended Dietary Allowance $(mg \cdot d^{-1})$	Upper Level Intake $(mg \cdot d^{-1})$	Estimated Average Requirement $(mg \cdot d^{-1})$	Recommended Dietary Allowance $(mg \cdot d^{-1})$	Upper Level Intake $(mg \cdot d^{-1})$
0–6 mo	200	200	1,000	400	400	1,000
6–12 mo	260	260	1,500	400	400	1,500
1–3 yr	500	700	2,500	400	600	2,500
4–8 yr	800	1,000	2,500	400	600	3,000
9–13 yr	1,100	1,300	3,000	400	600	4,000
14–18 yr	1,100	1,300	3,000	400	600	4,000
19–30 yr	800	1,000	2,500	400	600	4,000
31–50 yr	800	1,000	2,500	400	600	4,000
51–70 yr males	800	1,000	2,000	400	600	4,000
51–70 yr females	1,000	1,200	2,000	400	600	4,000
>70 yr	1,000	1,200	2,000	400	800	4,000
14–18 yr pregnant/ lactating	1,100	1,300	3,000	400	600	4,000
19–50 yr pregnant/ lactating	800	1,000	2,500	400	600	4,000

Adapted from Institute of Medicine. Dietary reference intakes for calcium and vitamin D [Internet]. Washington (DC): National Academies Press; [cited 2015 Nov 11]. Available from: http://www.iom.edu/Reports/2010/Dietary-Reference-Intakes-for-Calcium-and-Vitamin-D.aspx

Exercise for Bone Health

Physical activity prevents osteoporosis by increasing bone-forming osteoblast cell activity and reducing the bone-resorbing osteoclast activity for an overall osteogenic effect of bone growth or slowing of bone loss. Bone adapts positively to sufficient and appropriate levels of stress. Strain magnitude (the quantity of load) and frequency of load (how rapidly load is imposed) on bone are imperative for bone growth and to minimize bone loss (55). Bone adaptation to stressors is site- and load-specific, meaning that only bone that is stressed appropriately will adapt favorably (17). This explains why activities such as jogging confer little benefit to appendicular bones of the upper body. Therefore, development of an appropriate and effective exercise program should consider the following: current state of bone health; site of adaptation; appropriate degree of strain via force, torque, or compression; safety of exercise for the individual; and likelihood of compliance.

Bone-growing exercise is important at all ages; therefore, it is warranted to consider the age and other needs of the client when choosing appropriate and desirable exercises. However, appropriate forms of resistance-type exercise are necessary to stimulate bone at any age (39). For example, exercises for an adolescent or young adult may include agility or plyometrics and would likely differ from those for a postmenopausal woman who is largely sedentary. Also consider other needs of the client with respect to physical function and select exercises that may satisfy more than one

Table 9.11	Pharmacological Agents for Treatment of Osteoporosis		
Agent	**Effect**	**Potential Side Effects**	**Comments**
Calcium and vitamin D	Development and maintenance of bone	Calcium — gas, constipation; vitamin D — generally none unless taking too much	Efficacy is questionable in those with already normal calcium and vitamin D levels.
Selective estrogen receptor modulators (SERM)	Prevention and treatment. Estrogen agonist in bone and fat; antagonist in breast and endometrium	Hot flashes, leg cramps, and blood clots	May not be effective for nonvertebral fractures; decreased risk for breast cancer
Hormone replacement therapy (HRT)	Prevention only; decreased risk for vertebral and non-vertebral fracture	Cancer, myocardial infarction, stroke, blood clot	Usually considered for short-term use for menopausal symptoms
Bisphosphonate	Prevention and treatment; decreased bone resorption by osteoclast inhibition	GI disturbance (can use intravenous alternative); heartburn, esophageal irritation, headache, constipation, gas, diarrhea	Generally effective at all clinical bone sites; long-term use may increase the risk of femur fracture (30,77).
Strontium ranelate	Treatment only; decreased bone resorption	GI disturbance, blood clot	Approved in Europe, not in United States
Parathyroid hormone (PTH)	Treatment only; increased bone deposition	Bone cancer in rat studies	Injection only; continuous exposure to PTH causes bone resorption
Calcitonin	Treatment only; modest reduction in the risk of vertebral fractures	Stomach upset and flushing	May relieve pain associated with bone fractures

Adapted from Deal CL. Osteoporosis: prevention, diagnosis, and management. *Am J Med*. 1997;102(1A):35S–9S; Keen R. Osteoporosis: strategies for prevention and management. *Best Pract Res Clin Rheumatol*. 2007;21(1):109–22.

objective such as exercises to improve balance and coordination and to reduce the risk of falls in older adults. Falls often result in fracture in older adults, so an exercise strategy to reduce fall risk and improve posture could indirectly benefit bone health as well as overall physical function and independence. Likewise, back strengthening exercises for older adults to reduce thoracic hyperkyphosis (dowager's hump) can reduce back pain and risk of falls (83).

Exercises that enhance bone growth and/or reduce loss of bone in children and young adults should be site-specific, be moderate-high compressive, and/or provide resistance, and be multidirectional. Although there is limited information regarding specific exercise prescription for those with or at risk for osteoporosis, it is recommended to alternate upper and lower body exercises to minimize risk of undue stress on tendons (6). Table 9.12 includes guidelines that incorporate characteristics of exercise important for improving or maintaining overall bone health. There is a wide variance in bone status among those with osteopenia and osteoporosis, and for that reason, prescribing exercise with particular attention to exercise intensity must be individualized and appropriate for each client. For middle aged to older adults, low- to moderate-impact weight-bearing exercise that is pain-free, combined with progressive resistance exercise and agility training,

Table 9.12 — Exercise Guidelines for Prevention and Treatment of Osteoporosis

Condition	Type		Balance/ Posture/ Fall Prevention
	Weight-Bearing Aerobic	**Resistance**	
Healthy skeletal status			
Frequency	3–5 d · wk^{-1}	2–3 d · wk^{-1}	Daily
Intensity	Moderate to high	Moderate to high 60%–80% estimated 1-RM, 8–12 reps, progress to 80%–90% estimated 1-RM, 5–6 reps Impact jumps from floor, height of 1–2 in Multidirectional	
Time	30–60 min · d^{-1} — total exercise time (aerobic + resistance)		
At risk for osteoporosis			
Frequency	3–5 d · wk^{-1}	2–3 d · wk^{-1}	Daily
Intensity	Moderate to high	Moderate to high 60%–80% 1-RM, 8–12 reps progress slower to 80%–90% 1-RM, 5–6 reps Impact jumps from floor, height of 1–2 in	
Time	30–60 min · d^{-1} — total exercise time (aerobic + resistance)		
Osteoporosis			
Frequency	3–5 d · wk^{-1}	2–3 d · wk^{-1}	Daily
Intensity	40%–<60% Heart rate reserve or $\dot{V}O_2$ max	Moderate Same as earlier but consider individual circumstances	
Time	30–60 min · d^{-1} — total exercise time (aerobic + resistance + balance)		

Special Considerations

Avoid explosive, high-impact exercises, dynamic abdominal exercises (*e.g.*, sit-ups) exercises that involve twisting (*e.g.*, golf swing), bending, compression, excessive flexion, or **unsupported forward flexion** of spine. Provide posture education, fall prevention education, and movement education for lifting, bending, and carrying tasks to reduce fracture risk when doing activities of daily living.

1-RM, one repetition maximum; reps, repetitions.

Adapted from Hughes JM. Exercise prescription for patients with osteoporosis. In: Swain DP, editor. *ACSM's Resource Manual for Guidelines for Exercise Testing and Prescription*. 7th ed. Philadelphia (PA): Lippincott Williams & Wilkins; 2014. p. 699–712; Nikander R, Sievanen H, Heinonen A, Daly RM, Uusi-Rasi K, Kannus P. Targeted exercise against osteoporosis: a systematic review and meta-analysis for optimising bone strength throughout life. *BMC Medicine*. 2010;8:47; Pfeifer M, Sinaki M, Geusens P, Boonen S, Preisinger E, Minne HW. Musculoskeletal rehabilitation in osteoporosis: a review. *J Bone Miner Res*. 2004;19(8):1208–14; Skinner JS, editor. *Exercise Testing and Exercise Prescription for Special Cases*. 3rd ed. Philadelphia (PA): Lippincott Williams & Wilkins; 2005.

appears to be most effective for preserving or improving bone density at the spine and hip as well as improving overall physical function (78).

Research in animals and humans indicates that whole body vibration (WBV; standing on a special, gently oscillating mechanical plate) for 10–20 minutes a day can reduce bone loss in the hip, although this is less clear for the spine (2). In addition, WBV can also increase lower limb muscle function to reduce fall risk (2). There is much still to learn about short- and long-term retention of WBV effects on bone and the dose-response relationship. Likewise, WBV is a higher risk type of exercise that must be administered under supervision and may not be appropriate for all older adults (2,55,69,71).

SUMMARY OF EXERCISE CONSIDERATIONS FOR OSTEOPOROSIS

Intervention or prevention of osteoporosis is dependent on appropriate nutritional support and regular weight-bearing physical activity. To reduce the risk of fracture in later life, strategies to enhance bone health should begin early in life and seek to do the following (48):

- Maximize bone mass.
- Maximize peak bone mass.
- Reduce age-related bone loss.
- Prevent falls.
- Avoid other risk factors for osteoporosis and fracture.
- Reduce pain.
- Reduce disability.

Working with clients who are at risk for osteoporosis should include education about risk factors for osteoporosis and nutritional support, and an individualized exercise program, including weight-bearing aerobic, resistance, and core control exercises for balance, posture, and fall prevention. Exercise should be pain-free, and the intensity should be guided by the strength and bone health status of the client. Physician clearance to exercise is warranted for a client diagnosed with osteoporosis. Furthermore, clients with osteopenia or osteoporosis who have joint replacement should be cleared by a physician to exercise, and the exercise professional should be aware of any and all physical activity limitations for these clients.

The rapidly increasing population of older adults means that osteoporosis will likely become more prevalent in the near future (76). Knowledge of the disease process, risk factors, and exercise intervention strategies is essential to develop a safe and effective physical activity program for an osteoporotic client.

Contraindicated Exercises

Exercise for which the risk of performance outweighs any perceived or derived benefit is considered to be a contraindicated exercise. Over time, the list of contraindicated exercises has grown, based largely on risk perceived to be associated with biomechanical factors inherent in the performance of the exercises. In reality, there is little scientific evidence to underscore the designation of many of these exercises as contraindicated. In fact, many of these exercises are commonly used in yoga and Pilates programs, with few apparent problems (49).

Before relegating an exercise to the "contraindicated" list, several factors should be considered with respect to your client or patient, which include the following:

- Exercise form (*e.g.*, proper exercise mechanics)
- Client fitness level (including postural habits, daily routine)
- Client tissue health (*e.g.*, previous injury, surgery)
- Client joint range of motion
- Exercise load (type, size)
- Exercise load frequency (repetitions)

Common errors in exercise form tend to occur when the magnitude of resistance exceeds the capacity of the weakest joint along the kinetic chain. In this case, often, one compensates by altering correct biomechanics to increase momentum to overcome the external load. Deviating from correct form can place undue and asymmetric stress on other joints involved in the movement, leading to tissue failure and injury (11). The imperative that correct form should rule the day cannot be overemphasized. Correct performance of an exercise promotes desired neuromotor recruitment patterns and ultimately contributes to positive adaptation of the muscles used in the movement. Improper mechanics due to poor form, excessive load, or excessive repetitions will not enhance motor recruitment patterns but will increase the risk of tissue failure and injury.

An example of a client for which otherwise acceptable exercises would be contraindicated is one who has been diagnosed with osteoporosis. For this individual, dynamic weight-bearing exercise may be risky, such as jump rope or high-intensity aerobics classes, exercises that involve quick changes of direction, or activities that involve loaded trunk flexion or twisting, such as bowling or golf. Be sure to fully understand limitations of such a client before prescribing exercise. Similarly, consider limitations of an individual who has a balance and/or vision problems when devising an exercise program. Activities that require a quick change of direction might increase the risk of falling in this case.

Ten exercises commonly identified as contraindicated (54,58,94):

1. *Yoga plough* — intended to stretch the low back but may place undue compressive forces at the cervical spine; generally considered a higher risk exercise for middle aged and older adults
2. *Neck circles with neck hyperextension* — may cause compression of the cervical nerve roots, especially in one who has degenerative disk disease, and also increases risk for compression of arteries in the neck. Neck circle done slowly through a normal range of motion is considered low risk.
3. *Bridging* — used to strengthen the neck but places excessive pressure on cervical disks and may cause disk compression and damage
4. *Straight-leg sit-up* — used to strengthen abdominal muscles but recruits abdominal muscles for only 30% of movement; places undue stress on hip flexors and contributes to stress of the low back
5. *Double-leg lift* — like the straight-leg sit-up, this exercise is used to strengthen abdominal muscles but places undue stress on the hip flexors and low back, with limited abdominal muscle recruitment.
6. *Standing toe touch* — intended as a hamstring stretch but is ineffective compared to other preferred, safer hamstring stretches. It requires one to be in unsupported forward flexion for a prolonged time and may place the low back at risk for compression of intervertebral disks.
7. *Back hyperextension* — several exercises include back hyperextension and may risk damage to the articular capsule and ligaments that surround the disk. Examples of exercises that require back hyperextension include the cobra, the donkey kick, the fire hydrant, and the "lazy" push-up (knees on ground).
8. *Hip twists* — these exercises are typically performed ballistically and cause high risk for overuse injury because the movement often exceeds the normal range of motion. Injuries or strain to capsular structures is common as well. Exercises that include this motion are windmills, leg lifts done on hands and knees with leg extended behind body, and the fire hydrant.
9. *Hurdler stretch* — intended to stretch the hamstring (of extended leg) and the quadriceps femoris (of flexed leg) but places undue stress on the medial ligaments of the unstretched (flexed) knee. The lotus position, common in yoga, includes the same type of risk.
10. *Full squat* — intended to strengthen lower body musculature and low back. Exercises with full squatting, such as the duck walk, stresses ligaments and meniscus of the knee as well as the semilunar cartilage behind the kneecap. However, with proper form, appropriate resistance, and exercise volume, an individual with healthy knees and low back can increase muscle mass, lower body, and low back strength using squat exercises.

Additional common machine-resistance exercises of concern include (11):

Lat pull-down — performing the exercise by pulling the bar down behind the neck causes excessive flexion of the cervical vertebrae and loads the shoulders at the end range of motion of external rotation. Joints are weakest at the end range of motion, so this should be avoided. Pulling the bar in front of the head to the top of the sternum, while in neutral spinal alignment, will reduce the aforementioned risks.

Upright row with barbell — intended as a deltoid exercise, elevating the humerus above 90° to the torso requires more activation of the trapezius and risks impingement of the acromion. Alternatively, using dumbbells in front of a mirror will enable achievement of the desired 90° endpoint and reduce the risk impingement.

In summary, proper form during any exercise is crucial to minimize the risk for injury. Generally, neutral spinal alignment should be maintained during all aspects of an exercise. Failure to maintain neutral spinal alignment typically indicates weakness in a specific point along the kinetic chain. Recognizing your client's joint range of motion is crucial for averting injury when using machines or weights allowing movement that may exceed the client's range of motion (10). Although the earlier exercises are commonly considered to be high-risk exercises, for trained athletes, these exercises may be appropriate given the proper training dose (repetitions, resistance) and form. Before selecting an exercise for your client, consider the value and risk of the exercise for the individual. If the value outweighs the risk, determine if your client is able and willing to perform the exercise correctly and within the constraints you deem to be appropriate. Counteracting chronic postural habits and daily movements with appropriate exercises is a good goal for most nonathlete clients. This sound reasoning should enable you to identify appropriate and effective exercises so that your clients adapt positively and with limited risk.

The Case of Mrs. Williams

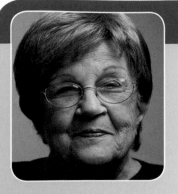

Submitted by **Travis Michael Combest, RCEP, Walter Reed National Military Medical Center at Bethesda, MD**

A 75-year-old woman was recommended for exercise programming by her primary care physician to improve mobility and function and to decrease pain of OA symptoms. Mrs. Williams's exercise program for the past year was aquatic classes 45 minutes, 2 days a week. She came to her first appointment with symptom-limited ambulation and a walker but a willingness to further her exercise program.

Narrative

A 75-year-old woman was recommended for exercise programming by her primary care physician to improve mobility and function and to decrease pain of OA symptoms. Mrs. Williams reports that her knee pain is "aching" and is 2–3/10 at rest. Notes from primary care physician indicate that Mrs. Williams has moderately severe OA in bilateral knees. She is symptom limited in walking more than 50 yards with pain of 5–6/10 and needing assistance with walking. Mrs. Williams reports for hospital visits, holding on to side rails of the walls and stopping every 50 yards. Mrs. Williams's current exercise program for the past year are aquatic classes 45 minutes, 2 days a week. She came to her first appointment at the fitness center with symptom-limited ambulation and a walker but a willingness to further her exercise program.

Physical Information

Height: 64 in
Weight: 171.7 lb
BMI: 29.5 kg · m^{-2}
Body fat percentage (measured by direct segmental bioelectrical impedance Inbody 520 by Biospace, Inc.): 51.4

Medical History from Primary Care Physician

Osteoarthritis
Type 2 diabetes
Hypertension
High cholesterol

Physical Assessments

Strength: dynamometer
Hip flexion: right, 20 lb; left, 18 lb
Leg extension: right, 15 lb; left, 10 lb
Physical activity limited by knee pain, lower body weakness

Activity Plan

Add progressive muscular and functional conditioning plan 2 days a week with aquatic aerobics.

Goals

Goal 1: Increase strength in lower extremities.
Goal 2: Increase mobility and function for quality of life.
Goal 3: Decrease pain at rest and during activity.

Exercise Program

Aerobic

Frequency: 4 days a week
Intensity: 65%–75% target heart rate (THR)
Time: 10–45 minutes
Types: Aquatic aerobics, 45 minutes, 2 days a week
Stationary recumbent bike: Level 1, speed 60–80 rpm, start with 2-minute increments work/rest ratio to 10 minutes before muscular conditioning exercises
Progression: Increase to 30 minutes continuous exercise in 3–6 months

Muscular Conditioning

Two days a week, supervised
Exercise leg band light to start two to three sets low repetitions to start
Short-term progress to medium leg band and 10–12 repetitions in 2–3 months
In 3–6 months, progress to exercise circuit machines
Incorporate upper body bands medium to start for overall conditioning two to three sets of 12–15 reps
Types: exercise leg band (cuffs) intensity light, two to three sets of five to eight repetitions exercises:
lower body exercises: leg extension, hip flexion, partial squat, hip abduction and adduction, hamstring curl, isometric hold for 20 seconds × 3 sets
Upper body exercises: medium band: lateral raise, chest fly, row, bicep curl, and triceps extension

Progression Updates

At 4 Weeks

Mrs. Williams progressed to lower body light bands: three sets of 10 repetitions, and reported able to ambulate better, pain reported with walking 5/10 and rest 2–3/10. Upper body exercises: three sets of 12–15 reps medium remained the same.

At 8 Weeks

Mrs. Williams progressed to medium lower body cuffs: three sets of 8–10 repetitions; patient reported able to walk with rest periods of approximately 100 yards and intermittently having to hold on to the handrails for support in fitness center to exercise appointments. She reported pain with walking 4–5/10 and rest 2/10. Upper body exercises: three sets of 15 reps, medium intensity remained for lateral raise, chest fly, hard intensity was increased for row, bicep curl, and tricep extension for three sets of 8–10 repetitions.

At 3 Months

Mrs. Williams progressed to circuit training machines: two to three sets of 8–10 repetitions. Lower body: hamstring curl: 10 lb, leg press: 65 lb, hip abduction: 60 lb, hip adduction: 50 lb, assisted (holding on to upper bar) reebok step up two sets of eight repetitions. Upper body: lat pull-down: 35 lb, chest press: 20 lb, incline chest press: 10 lb, lateral raise: 15 lb, bicep curl: 10 lb, tricep extension: 25 lb. She reported able to walk approximately 200 yards, one-third of way to fitness center to exercise appointment and still intermittently holding to handrails for support. The patient reported pain with activity 4/10 and rest 2/10.

At 6 Months

Mrs. Williams progressed to circuit training machines: three sets of 10 repetitions (upper three sets of 12 repetitions). Lower body: hamstring curl: 20 lb, leg press: 80 lb, hip abduction: 75 lb, hip adduction: 60 lb, assisted (holding on to upper bar) Reebok step up three sets of 10 repetitions. Upper body: lat pull-down: 45 lb, chest press: 27.5 lb, incline chest press: 20 lb, bicep curl: 15 lb, lateral raise 22.5 lb, tricep extension: 32.5 lb. Aerobic: Mrs. Williams maintained aquatic aerobics 2 days a week, 45 minutes, stationary bike increased to level 2, and she was able to perform 10 minutes without stopping, and the following 10 minutes were work/rest ratios of 2 minutes. Mrs. Williams reported able to walk approximately 600 yards to fitness center to exercise appointment and rarely need handrails for support. The patient reported pain with activity 3–4/10 and rest 1–2/10.

At 1 Year

Lower body: hamstring curl: 35 lb, leg press: 100 lb, hip abduction: 100 lb, hip adduction: 90 lb, no assistance needed Reebok step up three sets of 10 repetitions. Upper body: lat pull-down: 55 lb, chest press: 40 lb, incline chest press: 37.5 lb, bicep curl: 30 lb, lateral raise 35 lb, tricep extension: 40 lb. Aerobic: She maintained aquatic aerobics 2 days a week, 45 minutes, stationary bike increased to level 3 speed 60–80 rpm, and she was able to perform 20 minutes without stopping, and the following 10 minutes were work/rest ratios of 2 minutes. Mrs. Williams reported ability to walk approximately 600 yards to fitness center to exercise appointment and did not need handrails for support. She reports pain with activity 2–3/10 and rest 0/10. She was able to participate in community outings walking in mall with friends, walked with friends to visit museums in Washington, DC, and was able to stand entire choir practice for 1 hour.

3-Year Assessment

Physical Data

Height: 64 in
Weight: 160 lb
BMI: 27.5
Body composition: Body fat percentage: 48.1 kg · m^{-2}, Inbody 520 DSM-BIA

Fitness Data

Muscular strength: Strength: dynamometer; hip flexion: R: 35 lb, L: 35 lb; leg extension: R: 30 lb, L: 30 lb
Lower body: Three sets of 10 reps: hamstring curl: 50 lb, leg press: 135 lb, hip abduction: 115 lb, hip adduction: 110 lb, no assistance needed Reebok step up with 5 lb medicine ball, three sets of 10 repetitions, ball squat against the wall with 5-lb dumbbells.
Upper body: Three sets of 15 reps: lat pull-down: 60 lb, chest press: 50 lb, incline chest press: 40 lb, bicep curl: 35 lb, lateral raise 42.5 lb, tricep extension: 60 lb.
Aerobic: Mrs. Williams maintained aquatic aerobics 2 days a week for 45 minutes, stationary bike increased to level 3 speed 60–80 rpm and was able to perform 30 minutes without stopping.
Mrs. Williams reports ability to perform exercise 3 days a week, recumbent bike, and muscular conditioning by herself. Instructed on proper progression from American College of Sports Medicine and National Strength and Conditioning guidelines for muscular conditioning exercises and gave patient handout. Mrs. Williams reported pain in knees with walking after 2 miles 2/10, 0/10 at rest.

Conclusion

Mrs. Williams was able to progress to increase quality of life with managing OA by incorporating muscular and aerobic conditioning to routine. She was able to maintain 5 days a week for 45–60 minutes for more than 2 years, and pain was managed well. This client was motivated to increase ambulation and quality of life and was consistent with exercise programming over time. This may not be reflective of all clients but gives an example for exercise programming if a client is consistent that this will help long-term exercise prescription goals.

QUESTIONS

- What would be a good starting muscular conditioning program for a client who has OA, in terms of days per week, number of sets, and repetitions?
- How often should you increase muscular conditioning exercises for a client who has OA?

References

1. American College of Sports Medicine. *ACSM's Guidelines for Exercise Testing and Prescription*. 10th ed. Philadelphia (MD): Wolters Kluwer; 2018.
2. Baechle T, Earle R, editors. *National Strength and Conditioning Association: Essentials of Strength Training and Conditioning*. 3rd ed. Champaign (IL): Human Kinetics; 2008. 752 p.
3. Wallace JP, Ray S. Obesity. In: Durstine J, Moore G, Painter P, Roberts S, editors. *ACSM's Exercise Management for Persons with Chronic Diseases and Disabilities*. 3rd ed. Champaign (IL): Human Kinetics; 2009. 456 p.

SUMMARY

This chapter examines and provides guidelines for the exercise professional to effectively address common traumatic and overuse musculoskeletal injuries and selected chronic musculoskeletal conditions related to physical activity or inactivity. Common causes of, role of exercise on, and strategies for reducing the risk of traumatic and overuse injuries and selected chronic conditions are covered. When applicable and within the scope of practice of the exercise professional, appropriate and current exercise guidelines are discussed with particular focus on modifying the exercise prescription to address special circumstances for these conditions.

Upon completion of this chapter, the reader should understand the etiology and mechanisms of common traumatic musculoskeletal injuries (strains and sprains), overuse injuries (tendinopathy, bursitis, PF, and LBP), and chronic conditions (forms of arthritis and osteoporosis). Likewise, the reader will have knowledge of risk factors, commonly used medications, and exercise limitations and strategies to mitigate the effects of these conditions.

STUDY QUESTIONS

1. What recommendations would you make for maximizing bone health and reducing risk of osteoporosis to a client who is 55 years old? 25 years old? 12 years old?
2. Explain resistance exercise recommendations for a client diagnosed with osteoporosis of the spine who has physician clearance to exercise with appropriate limitations. What types of resistance exercises are appropriate and safe? How frequently should these exercises be performed and at what intensity?
3. A young client who is an athlete sprained her ankle (inversion) during soccer practice a day earlier, but did not want to miss a personal training session with you. She can walk, but the ankle is swollen and sore. What recommendations would you give this client regarding the injury and exercise?
4. Using the general guidelines presented, explain the progression of exercises for tendinopathies, including examples of types of exercise, frequency, and intensity.
5. Explain the difference between RA and OA, and taking into account special considerations for both, provide exercise recommendations.

REFERENCES

1. Anderson MK, Parr GP, Hall SJ. Tissue healing and wound care. In: Anderson MK, Parr GP, Hall SJ, editors. *Foundations of Athletic Training: Prevention, Assessment, and Management.* 4th ed. Philadelphia (PA): Lippincott Williams & Wilkins; 2008. p. 128–59.

2. Beck BR, Norling TL. The effect of 8 mos of twice-weekly low- or higher intensity whole body vibration on risk factors for postmenopausal hip fracture. *Am J Phys Med Rehabil.* 2010;89(12):997–1009.

3. Belyea B, Greenberger H. Physical therapy for musculoskeletal conditions. In: Pagliarulo MA, editor. *Introduction to Physical Therapy.* 4th ed. St. Louis (MO): Mosby; 2011. p. 173–212.

4. Berger C, Langsetmo L, Joseph L, et al. Change in bone mineral density as a function of age in women and men and association with the use of antiresorptive agents. *CMAJ.* 2008;178(13):1660–8.

5. Bliuc D, Nguyen ND, Nguyen TV, Eisman JA, Center JR. Compound risk of high mortality following osteoporotic fracture and refracture in elderly women and men. *J Bone Miner Res.* 2013;28(11):2317–24.

6. Booher J, Thibodeau G. Athletic injuries and related skin conditions. In: Booher J, Thibodeau G, editors. *Athletic Injury Assessment.* 4th ed. Boston (MA): McGraw-Hill; 2000. p. 77–106.

7. Bradney M, Pearce G, Naughton G, et al. Moderate exercise during growth in prepubertal boys: changes in bone mass, size, volumetric density, and bone strength: a controlled prospective study. *J Bone Miner Res.* 1998;13(12):1814–21.

8. Centers for Disease Control and Prevention. Chronic diseases: The power to prevent, the call to control: at a glance 2009 [Internet]. Atlanta (GA): Centers for Disease Control and Prevention; [cited 2009]. Available from: https://www.cdc.gov/chronicdisease/pdf/2009-Power-of-Prevention.pdf. Accessed January 2017.

9. Cicuttini F, Baker J, Spector TD. The association of obesity with osteoarthritis of the hand and knee in women: a twin study. *J Rheumatol.* 1996;23(7):1221–6.

10. Colado JC, Garcia-Masso X. Technique and safety aspects of resistance exercises: a systematic review of the literature. *Phys Sports Med.* 2009;37(2):104–11.

11. Contraindicated exercises. [cited 2015 Aug 11]. Available from: https://www.ncsf.org/enew/articles/articles-contraindicated exercises.aspx#

12. Cooney JK, Law RJ, Matschke V, et al. Benefits of exercise in rheumatoid arthritis. *J Aging Res.* 2011;2011:681640.

13. Cosca D, Navazio F. Common problems in endurance athletes. *Am Fam Physician.* 2007;76(2):237–44.

14. Covey CJ, Mulder MD. Plantar fasciitis: how best to treat? *J Fam Practice.* 2013;62(9):466–71.

15. Crowson C, Matteson E, Myasoedova E, et al. The lifetime risk of adult-onset rheumatoid arthritis and other inflammatory autoimmune rheumatic diseases. *Arthritis Rheum.* 2011;63(3):633–9.

16. Cummings SR, Melton LJ. Epidemiology and outcomes of osteoporotic fractures. *Lancet.* 2002;359(9319):1761–7.

17. Dalsky GP, Stocke KS, Ehsani AA, Slatopolsky E, Lee WC, Birge SJ Jr. Weight-bearing exercise training and lumbar bone mineral content in postmenopausal women. *Ann Intern Med.* 1988;108(6):824–8.

18. de Jong Z, Vliet Vlieland T. Safety of exercise in patients with rheumatoid arthritis. *Curr Opin Rheumatol.* 2005;17:177–82.

19. Denning WM, Winward JG, Pardo MB, Hopkins JT, Seeley MK. Body weight independently affects articular cartilage catabolism. *J Sport Sci Med.* 2013;14:290–6.

20. DiGiovanni BF, Nawoczenski DA, Lintal ME, et al. Tissue-specific plantar fascia-stretching exercise enhances outcomes in patients with chronic heel pain. A prospective, randomized study. *J Bone Joint Surg Am.* 2003;85-A(7):1270–7.

21. Ehrich EW, Davies GM, Watson DJ, Bolognese JA, Seidenberg BC, Bellamy N. Minimal perceptible clinical improvement with the Western Ontario and McMaster Universities osteoarthritis index questionnaire and global assessments in patients with osteoarthritis. *J Rheumatology.* 2000;27(11):2635–41.

22. Epstein S. Update of current therapeutic options for the treatment of postmenopausal osteoporosis. *Clin Ther.* 2006;28(2):151–73.

23. Ettinger WH Jr, Burns R, Messier SP, et al. A randomized trial comparing aerobic exercise and resistance exercise with a health education program in older adults with knee osteoarthritis. The Fitness Arthritis and Seniors Trial (FAST). *JAMA.* 1997;277(1):25–31.

24. Fairbank J, Pynsent P. The Oswestry Disability Index. *Spine.* 2000;25(22):2940–53.

25. Faries M, Greenwood M. Core training: stabilizing the confusion. *Strength Cond J.* 2007;29(2):10–25.

26. Finkelstein JS, Brockwell SE, Mehta V, et al. Bone mineral density changes during the menopause transition in a multiethnic cohort of women. *J Clin Endocrinol Metab.* 2008;93(3):861–8.

27. Firooznia H, Golimbu C, Rafii M, Schwartz MS, Alterman ER. Quantitative computed tomography assessment of spinal trabecular bone. I. Age-related regression in normal men and women. *J Comput Tomogr.* 1984;8(2):91–7.

28. Flokowski P, Brunt D, Bishop M, Woo R, Horodyski M. Intrinsic pedal musculature support of the medial longitudinal arch: an electromyography study. *J Foot Ankle Surg.* 2003;42(6):327–33.

29. Goksel Karatepe A, Gunaydin R, Turkmen G, Kaya T. Effects of home-based exercise program on the functional status and the quality of life in patients with rheumatoid arthritis: 1-year follow-up study. *Rheumatol Int.* 2011;31(2):171–6.

30. Gudena R, Werle J, Johnston K. Bilateral femoral insufficiency fractures likely related to long-term alendronate therapy. *J Osteoporos.* 2011;2011:810697.

31. Hall C, Thein-Brody L. Functional approach to therapeutic exercise for physiologic impairments. In: Hall C, Thein-Brody L, editors. *Therapeutic Exercise.* Philadelphia (PA): Lippincott Williams & Wilkins; 1999. p. 43–69.

32. Hart L. Exercise and soft tissue injury. *Baillieres Clin Rheumatol.* 1994;8(1):137–48.

33. Headlee D, Leonard J, Hart J, Ingersoll C, Hertel J. Fatigue of the plantar intrinsic foot muscles increases navicular drop. *J Electromyogr Kinesiol.* 2007;18(3):420–5.

34. Headley S, Wood RE. Exercise prescription for patients with comorbidities and other chronic diseases. In: Swain DP, editor. *ACSM's Resource Manual for Guidelines for Exercise*

Testing and Prescription. 7th ed. Philadelphia (PA): Lippincott Williams & Wilkins; 2014. p. 682–98.

35. Herring S, Nilson KL. Introduction to overuse injuries. *Clin Sports Med.* 1987;6:225–39.

36. Herzog R. Radiologic imaging in rehabilitation. In: Kibler W, Herring S, Press J, editors. *Functional Rehabilitation of Sports and Musculoskeletal Injuries.* Gaithersburg (MD): Aspen Publishers; 1998. p. 20–70.

37. Hinman R, Heywood S, Day A. Aquatic physical therapy for hip and knee osteoarthritis: results of a single-blind randomized controlled trial. *Phys Ther.* 2007;87:32–43.

38. Hopman-Rock M, Westhoff M. The effects of a health educational and exercise program for older adults with osteoarthritis for the hip or knee. *J Rheumatol.* 2000;27(8):1947–54.

39. Howe TE, Shea B, Dawson LJ, et al. Exercise for preventing and treating osteoporosis in postmenopausal women. *Cochrane Database Syst Rev.* 2011;(7):CD000333.

40. Hughes JM. Exercise prescription for patients with osteoporosis. In: Swain DP, editor. *ACSM's Resource Manual for Guidelines for Exercise Testing and Prescription.* 7th ed. Philadelphia (PA): Lippincott Williams & Wilkins; 2014. p. 699–712.

41. Hui SL, Slemenda CW, Johnston CC Jr. The contribution of bone loss to postmenopausal osteoporosis. *Osteoporos Int.* 1990;1(1):30–4.

42. Iacono MV. Osteoporosis: a national public health priority. *J Perianesth Nurs.* 2007;22(3):175–80.

43. Institute of Medicine. Dietary reference intakes for calcium and vitamin D [Internet]. Washington (DC): National Academies Press; [cited 2015 Nov 11]. Available from: http://www.iom.edu/Reports/2010/Dietary-Reference-Intakes-for-Calcium-and-Vitamin-D.aspx

44. Iwamoto J, Takeda T, Ichimura S. Effect of exercise training and detraining on bone mineral density in postmenopausal women with osteoporosis. *J Orthop Sci.* 2001;6(2):128–32.

45. Jan M-H, Lin J-J, Liau J-J, Lin Y-F, Lin D-H. Investigation of clinical effects of high and low-resistance training for patients with knee osteoarthritis: a randomized controlled trial. *Phys Ther.* 2008;88(4):427–36.

46. Janda V. *Muscle Function Testing.* London (UK): Butterworths; 1983. 260 p.

47. Jung D-Y, Kim M-H, Koh E-K, Kwon O-Y. A comparison in the muscle activity of the abductor hallucis and the medial longitudinal arch angle during toe curl and short foot exercises. *Phys Ther Sport.* 2011;12(1):30–5.

48. Keen R. Osteoporosis: strategies for prevention and management. *Best Pract Res Clin Rheumatol.* 2007;21(1):109–22.

49. Kemper K, Ferguson M. Contraindicated exercises revisited. San Diego (CA): IDEA; [cited 2007 May 1]. Available from: http://www.ideafit.com/fitness-library/search?query=contraindicated-exercises-revisited

50. Kisner C, Colby L. *Therapeutic Exercise Foundations and Techniques.* 5th ed. Philadelphia (PA): F.A. Davis; 2007. 309 p.

51. Kolber M, Beekhuizen K. Lumbar stabilization: an evidence-based approach for the athlete with low back pain. *Strength Cond J.* 2007;29(2):26–37.

52. Koplan JP, Powell KE, Sikes RK, Shirley RW, Campbell CC. An epidemiologic study of the benefits and risks of running. *JAMA.* 1982;248:3118–21.

53. Kubo K, Ikebukuor T, Yata H, Tsundoa N, Kanehisa H. Time course of changes in muscle and tendon properties during strength training and detraining. *J Strength Cond Res.* 2010;24(2):322–31.

54. Liemohn W, Haydu T, Phillips D. Questionable exercises. *PCPFS Res Digest.* 1999;3(8):1–8.

55. Liu PY, Brummel-Smith K, Ilich JZ. Aerobic exercise and whole-body vibration in offsetting bone loss in older adults. *J Aging Res.* 2011;2011:379674.

56. Lloyd T, Petit MA, Lin HM, Beck TJ. Lifestyle factors and the development of bone mass and bone strength in young women. *J Pediatr.* 2004;144(6):776–82.

57. Lorenz D, Reiman M. The role and implementation of eccentric training in athletic rehabilitation: tendinopathy, hamstring strains, and ACL reconstruction. *Int J Sports Phys Ther.* 2011;6(1):27–44.

58. Lubell, A. Potentially dangerous exercises: are they harmful to all? *Phys Sports Med.* 1989;17(1):187–92.

59. Maggio D, Pacifici R, Cherubini A, et al. Age-related cortical bone loss at the metacarpal. *Calcif Tissue Int.* 1997;60(1):94–7.

60. Mazess RB. Bone mineral content in early-postmenopausal and postmenopausal osteoporotic women. *Radiology.* 1987; 165(1):289–91.

61. Mazziotti G, Canalis E, Giustina A. Drug-induced osteoporosis: mechanisms and clinical implications. *Am J Med.* 2010;123(10):877–84.

62. McGill S. *Low Back Disorders.* Champaign (IL): Human Kinetics; 2002. 210 p.

63. McGill S. Opinions on the links between back pain and motor control: the disconnect between clinical practice and research. In: Hodges PW, Cholewicki J, vanDieen JH, editors. *Spinal Control: The Rehabilitation of Back Pain: State of the Art and Science.* New York (NY): Churchill Livingstone; 2013. p. 75–87.

64. McGill S. *Ultimate Back Fitness and Performance.* 3rd ed. Waterloo (Canada): Backfitpro; 2006. 221 p.

65. McKenzie RA, May S. *The Lumbar Spine: Mechanical Diagnosis and Therapy.* 2nd ed. Waikanae (New Zealand): Spinal Publications; 2003. 700 p.

66. McPoil T, Martin R, Cornwall M, Wukichj D, Irrgang J, Godges J. Heel pain: plantar fasciitis. *J Orthop Sports Phys Ther.* 2008;38(4):A1–18.

67. Melton L. Adverse outcomes of osteoporotic fractures in the general population. *J Bone Miner Res.* 2003;18(6):1139–41.

68. Melzack R. The McGill pain questionnaire: major properties and scoring methods. *Pain.* 1975;1(3):277–99.

69. Merriman H, Jackson K. The effects of whole-body vibration training in aging adults: a systematic review. *J Geriatr Phys Ther.* 2009;32(3):134–45.

70. Meunier P, Courpron P, Edouard C, Bernard J, Bringuier J, Vignon G. Physiological senile involution and pathological rarefaction of bone. Quantitative and comparative histological data. *Clin Endocrinol Metab.* 1973;2(2):239–56.

71. Mikhael M, Orr R, Fiatarone Singh MA. The effect of whole body vibration exposure on muscle or bone morphology and function in older adults: a systematic review of the literature. *Maturitas.* 2010;66(2):150–7.

72. Millar AL. Exercise prescription for patients with arthritis. In: Swain DP, editor. *ACSM's Resource Manual for Guidelines for Exercise Testing and Prescription.* 7th ed.

Philadelphia (PA): Lippincott Williams & Wilkins; 2014. p. 713–28.

73. Minor M. Exercise in the treatment of osteoarthritis. *Rheum Dis Clin N Am.* 1999;25(2):397–415.

74. Minor M, Kay D. Arthritis. In: Durstine J, Moore G, editors. *ACSM's Exercise Management for Persons with Chronic Diseases and Disabilities.* 2nd ed. Champaign (IL): Human Kinetics; 2003. p. 259–65.

75. Mosekilde L. Sex differences in age-related loss of vertebral trabecular bone mass and structure — biomechanical consequences. *Bone.* 1989;10(6):425–32.

76. Mosely K, Jan de Beur S. Osteoporosis in men and women. In: Legato M, editor. *Principles of Gender-Specific Medicine.* 2nd ed. Cambridge (MA): Elsevier; 2010. p. 716–36.

77. Neviaser AS, Lane JM, Lenart BA, Edobor-Osula F, Lorich DG. Low-energy femoral shaft fractures associated with alendronate use. *J Orthop Trauma.* 2008;22(5):346–50.

78. Nikander R, Sievanen H, Heinonen A, Daly RM, Uusi-Rasi K, Kannus P. Targeted exercise against osteoporosis: a systematic review and meta-analysis for optimising bone strength throughout life. *BMC Medicine.* 2010;8:47.

79. Nilas L, Christiansen C. Rates of bone loss in normal women: evidence of accelerated trabecular bone loss after the menopause. *Eur J Clin Invest.* 1988;18(5):529–34.

80. Nordström A, Karlsson C, Nyquist F, Olsson T, Nordström P, Karlsson M. Bone loss and fracture risk after reduced physical activity. *J Bone Miner Res.* 2005;20(2):202–7.

81. O'Flaherty EJ. Modeling normal aging bone loss, with consideration of bone loss in osteoporosis. *Toxicol Sci.* 2000; 55(1):171–88.

82. Pfefer M, Cooper S, Uhl N. Chiropractic management of tendinopathy: a literature synthesis. *J Manipulative Physiol Ther.* 2009;32(1):41–52.

83. Pfeifer M, Sinaki M, Geusens P, Boonen S, Preisinger E, Minne HW. Musculoskeletal rehabilitation in osteoporosis: a review. *J Bone Miner Res.* 2004;19(8):1208–14.

84. Plasqui G. The role of physical activity in rheumatoid arthritis. *Physiol Behav.* 2007;94(2):270–5.

85. Potach D, Ellenbecker T. Clients with orthopedic, injury, and rehabilitation concerns. In: Earle R, Baechle T, editors. *NSCA's Essentials of Personal Training.* Champaign (IL): Human Kinetics; 2004. p. 533–56.

86. Rannevik G, Jeppsson S, Johnell O, Bjerre B, Laurell-Borulf Y, Svanberg L. A longitudinal study of the perimenopausal transition: altered profiles of steroid and pituitary hormones, SHBG and bone mineral density. *Maturitas.* 1995;21(2):103–13.

87. Sambrook P, Cooper C. Osteoporosis. *Lancet.* 2006;367(9527): 2010–8.

88. Sexson SB, Lehner JT. Factors affecting hip fracture mortality. *J Orthop Trauma.* 1987;1(4):298–305.

89. Simmonds M, Dreisinger T. *Lower Back Pain Syndrome.* 2nd ed. Champaign (IL): Human Kinetics; 2003. 218 p.

90. Smith R, Cullen D. Osteoporosis. In: LeMura L, von Duvillard S, editors. *Clinical Exercise Physiology.* Philadelphia (PA): Lippincott Williams & Wilkins; 2004. p. 485–502.

91. Snow CM, Shaw JM, Winters KM, Witzke KA. Long-term exercise using weighted vests prevents hip bone loss in postmenopausal women. *J Gerontol A Biol Sci Med Sci.* 2000;55(9): M489–91.

92. Sornay-Rendu E, Munoz F, Duboeuf F, Delmas PD. Rate of forearm bone loss is associated with an increased risk of fracture independently of bone mass in postmenopausal women: the OFELY study. *J Bone Miner Res.* 2005;20(11):1929–35.

93. Thompson W, Gordon N, Pescatello L, editors. *Exercise Prescriptions for other Clinical Populations.* 8th ed. Philadelphia (PA): Lippincott Williams & Wilkins; 2009.

94. Timmermans, HM, Martin M. Top ten potentially dangerous exercises. *JOPERD* 1987;58(6):29–33.

95. van den Ende CH, Breedveld FC, le Cessie S, Dijkmans BA, de Mug AW, Hazes JM. Effect of intensive exercise on patients with active rheumatoid arthritis: a randomised clinical trial. *Ann Rheum Dis.* 2000;59:615–21.

96. Wasielewski NJ, Kotsko KM. Does eccentric exercise reduce pain and improve strength in physically active adults with symptomatic lower extremity tendinosis? *A systematic review. J Athletic Training.* 2007;42(3):409–21.

97. Williams D III. *Foot and Ankle.* London (UK): Churchill Livingstone; 2003. 451 p.

98. Wilson J, Best T. Common overuse tendon problems: a review and recommendations for treatment. *Am Fam Physician.* 2005;72(5):811–8.

99. Winters KM, Snow CM. Detraining reverses positive effects of exercise on the musculoskeletal system in premenopausal women. *J Bone Miner Res.* 2000;15(12):2495–503.

100. Zulia P, Prentice W. *Rehabilitation of the Elbow.* New York (NY): McGraw-Hill; 2001. 466 p.

10

Exercise Programming Across the Lifespan: Children and Adolescents, Pregnant Women, and Older Adults

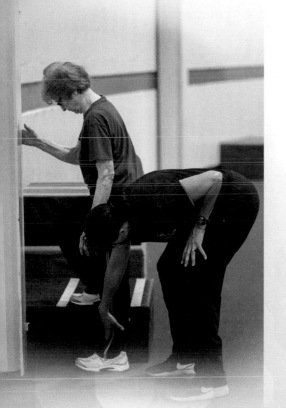

OBJECTIVES

- To understand the physical and selected physiological changes during the aging process (childhood to older adult).

- To understand the adaptations to training for children, adolescents, older adults, and pregnant women.

- To understand the differences in exercise prescriptions between children, adolescents, older adults, and pregnant women.

- To apply the American College of Sports Medicine (ACSM), American Heart Association (AHA), and Centers for Disease Control and Prevention (CDC) guidelines to exercise prescriptions for children, adolescents, older adults, and pregnant women.

INTRODUCTION

Individuals at any phase of the lifespan can respond positively to exercise training assuming the stimulus is appropriate and there is adequate time for recovery between stressors. However, placing an inappropriately low or high load on a developing, frail, or compromised system is ineffective or even contraindicated. Therefore, the goal of this chapter is to describe the changes with aging and pregnancy on selected physiological systems as well as the effect of training on those systems. This chapter summarizes the practical applications of exercising programming across the lifespan.

This chapter focuses on three separate populations: children and adolescents, pregnant women, and older adults. Each population will be addressed in terms of physical and physiological changes, the impact of chronic exercise, and relevant exercise programming (*e.g.*, including specific exercise considerations and meeting activity recommendations). In accordance with the American College of Sports Medicine's (ACSM) *Guidelines for Exercise Testing and Prescription* (4), "children" are those who are younger than 13 years, "adolescents" are 13 through 17 years, and "older adults" are those 65 years and older and 50 to 64 years with significant physical or physiological limitations that affect physical movement or capacity.

An understanding of physical and physiological changes across the lifespan is important when prescribing exercise for children, adolescents, pregnant women, and older adults. However, it is not the purpose of this chapter to provide a comprehensive discussion of growth, development, and aging. For a complete description of these topics, see Malina et al. (28) for youth, Skinner (43) and Chodzko et al. (9) for aging, and Mottola (37,38) for pregnancy. Instead, this chapter focuses on those areas that are pertinent to the safe and effective prescription of exercise by the certified exercise physiologist (EP-C) for children, adolescents, older adults, and pregnant women. Those pertinent areas include musculoskeletal system status and function, alterations in body composition, the function of the cardiorespiratory system during rest and exercise, endocrine system alterations, thermoregulation, and motor performance.

Children and Adolescents

Children and adolescents quite simply are not miniature adults. In fact, most physiological systems are very different from adults, and this directly impacts exercise prescription in this population. In addition, many exercise measurement methods originally designed for adults are not scalable to children solely on the basis of body size. It is important to note that behavioral and psychological issues should be considered when prescribing exercise for children and adolescents in order to ensure maximal participation.

Physical and Physiological Changes

Body Size and Composition

The obvious physical change observed during childhood and adolescence is the increase in body size. Besides weight and height increasing with age, normal growth occurs across the lifespan with rapid growth in infancy, steady increases in early childhood, an accelerated period at puberty (about 12 yr for girls and 14 yr for boys), and slow gains until adult height and weight are attained (31). In general, girls stop growing in stature by 15 years of age, and boys reach their adult height by about 17 years of age (31). The longer period of growth in boys results in a gender difference, which makes adult males about 10–12 cm, or 4–5 in, taller than average adult females (31). The increase in height during childhood is achieved by long bone growth, where a layer of cartilage called the growth plate undergoes proliferation and subsequent ossification, resulting in longitudinal progression of the bone. This process eventually ceases once adult height is achieved (27).

There are also noticeable and important changes in the tissues that constitute body weight, which are bone mass, fat mass, and fat-free mass (27). Lower and upper extremity bone mass increases in childhood with accelerated growth in adolescence, whereas head and trunk bone mass remain fairly constant during these same periods (27). Although total body bone mass increases similar to height increase with age, the increase continues until 20 years of age in males (27). Fat-free mass, primarily skeletal muscle, increases in a manner similar to height in boys and girls, resulting in adult females having about 30% less skeletal muscle mass than males. Fat mass increases for boys and girls, whereas percentage body fat increases in girls but decreases in boys because of the previously described increases in fat-free mass for boys (26).

Cardiorespiratory Function

As children grow, their cardiorespiratory system continues to develop. At birth, children have a high heart rate and respiration rates, which decline with age as the nervous system innervations of these organs mature. The heart rate of young children seated and at rest ranges between 100 and 110 beats $\cdot$ minute^{-1}, and maximal heart rate is higher than adults. Respiratory frequency is also elevated in children relative to adults but also decreases throughout childhood and adolescence until adult values are achieved (29). Lung function measures increase with age, mainly as a function of height (29). Due to increased metabolism, children recover faster from a bout of exercise compared with adults; thus, heart rate, oxygen consumption, and minute ventilation return to resting values more quickly than adults (23).

Although heart rate is higher in children, stroke volume is lower, resulting in cardiac output values lower than adults (23). Systolic blood pressure, and to a lesser extent diastolic blood pressure, is lower in children than in adults at rest and during exercise. As children age, resting blood pressure, especially systolic, increases mainly due to changes in compliance of vessel walls (29). Hemoglobin concentration and red blood cell count increase during childhood, with an accelerated increase at puberty, with boys' values exceeding girls'. However, children have greater blood flow and oxygen extraction at the periphery during exercise (23). Despite this, children and adolescents have a greater oxygen cost during exercise than adults even after accounting for size differences. The relative inefficiency may be due to immature motor patterns, nervous system, and hormone response, which improve with age. Peak volume of oxygen consumed per unit time ($\dot{V}O_2$) measured in children is lower than in adults but increases with age once size, adiposity, and gender are considered (23). A gender difference exists in $\dot{V}O_2$ measures with girls demonstrating lower peak $\dot{V}O_2$ measures, most likely due to body composition and blood hemoglobin, and more sedentary behaviors especially around puberty (23).

Muscular Strength, Flexibility, and Motor Performance

In boys and girls, muscular strength increases with age and is related to the increases in body weight, height, fat-free mass, and muscle mass (30). This increase in size is accelerated in boys during puberty but plateaus in girls in proportion to the fat-free mass and muscle mass (26). Motor performance measures tend to follow the same pattern of improving with physical maturation (32). The smaller increases in girls, especially for weight-dependent performance measures such as vertical jump and long jump, may be due to the increase in fat mass at puberty. The decrease in physical activity among girls at puberty also contributes to this trend. However, girls tend to outperform boys in flexibility measures and some measures of balance (32).

Perceived Exertion

Children and adolescents are able to distinguish between different levels of effort just as can adults. However, children tend to rate exertion lower than adolescents and adults; adolescents also rate exertion lower than adults (23). Children may not be as able to reproduce an exercise intensity that corresponds to a particular exertion rating as are adults, although some studies have shown that they can do so during cycling exercise using the child-friendly OMNI scale (23). This scale is a 0–10 rating scale with pictures corresponding to different levels of effort for walking/jogging and for cycling. A scale also exists for the perceived exertion of resistance exercise (17). A 6–20 scale or a 0–10 scale, however, without illustrations, has been less useful for children.

Thermoregulation

During exercise in hot environments, the evaporation of sweat is the main avenue for heat dissipation in humans. However, in children, the ability to produce sweat is less than that of adults (23). Although children have more sweat glands, the output of each gland is lower than adults and the temperature when sweating initiates is higher than in adults (23). The result is that children cannot sustain exercise for as long as adults when temperatures exceed 40°C, or approximately 100°F. Inability to thermoregulate is exacerbated when the child is not well hydrated, thus further limiting the ability of a child to produce sweat (23). Children or adolescents who are at special risk are those for whom proper hydration is not well maintained because of cognitive or physiological conditions. Staying well hydrated, particularly in warm conditions, should always be emphasized and encouraged by the EP-C.

Obese children tend to acclimatize to heat stress more slowly and have a lower threshold for core temperature regulation. Although lean and obese children do not show a difference in heat tolerance, obese children exercising in the heat have increased core temperatures and higher heart rates at submaximal workloads (13). Mechanisms for lower heat tolerance in obese children have not fully been examined, but adiposity has been shown to decrease abdominal heat transfer in adults and therefore may contribute to increased core temperature in children as well.

The Impact of Chronic Exercise

Exercise has been shown to be beneficial for most people, including children and adolescents (41). Specifically, physically active youth will reap benefits such as improved cardiorespiratory and muscular fitness, metabolic health, cardiometabolic profiles, body composition, and, for some, mental health (14,41). Children performing exercise and training for certain sports can improve motor performance and efficiency and increase muscular strength and endurance, and those who include more intense aerobic activity can improve cardiorespiratory fitness and aerobic performance (15,41). Chronic exercise and physical activity combined with reduced sedentary time and healthy eating can prevent and treat obesity in children (6,11). As with adults, there is a dose-response effect in the benefits of exercise. Increases in the quantity and quality of exercise will result in more health-related improvements (15,41).

There is no evidence that exercise, including resistance training, weightlifting, and plyometric training, has any adverse effects on children and adolescents when exercises are performed properly and are supervised by qualified adults (15,16,25,41). In fact, resistance training and sports conditioning have been shown to reduce the rate of sports-related injuries (15). There is always the possibility, as with any activity, an injury of the epiphyseal or growth plate may occur, which could negatively impact growth. A few children with undetected medical conditions may suffer adverse reactions, even sudden cardiac death, to physical activity; however, the preponderance of evidence suggests exercise is safe and the benefits outweigh the risks. Precautions should be taken, especially for children who have cardiometabolic risk factors, who cannot adequately follow directions, or who are exercising in hot environments, to reduce the risk of injury or sudden death.

Exercise Programming and Specific Exercise Considerations

The recommended amount of activity for children and adolescents to reap health benefits is described in detail by the Physical Activity Guidelines Advisory Committee (41). The Advisory Committee reports that children and adolescents should perform at least 60 minutes of moderate or vigorous activity daily, with vigorous activity included at least 3 days a week. In addition, sedentary activities such as watching television, using a computer, or playing video games should be limited to less than 2 hours $\cdot$ day^{-1} (13). Examples of moderate aerobic activity are brisk walking, hiking, casual biking, or activities that result in an effort of 5–6 on a rating of perceived exertion (RPE) scale of 0–10. Vigorous aerobic activities are those that are a 7–8 RPE such as running, skipping, and jumping; chasing games such as tag and jump rope; or playing sports such as soccer or field hockey. Active video games may provide another option for obtaining the recommended amount of exercise. A recent review shows that most active video games provide light or moderate activity; however, there is not yet enough evidence to draw conclusions concerning the long-term role of these games for increasing exercise in youth (8). For youth who do not meet the guidelines for activity, the intensity and duration of activities should be progressed gradually until the minimum levels are achieved (41,51).

Muscle and bone strengthening activities should be included at least 3 days $\cdot$ week^{-1} (41). Muscle strengthening exercises require moving against resistance and can include resistance from body weight (push-ups, pull-ups, squats), free weights (dumbbells and barbells), or weight machines. Other examples of resistance training are playing on jungle gyms, using climbing walls, tree climbing, and playing tug of war. Bone strengthening exercises are those that result in a physical impact on the skeletal system, such as jumping, running, hopping, jumping rope, or gymnastics. Guidelines and recommendations exist for resistance training and plyometric training for youth (15,25,41). In general, a muscle strengthening program should target large muscles of the whole body and should include a 5- to 10-minute warm-up and end with a cool-down. These exercises can be body weight exercises or machine-based exercises, depending on the child's ability to safely perform the exercises with proper form. For each exercise, 6–15 repetitions to fatigue can be performed in one to three sets on nonconsecutive days. One to three sets of power exercises can be performed for 3–6 repetitions. The EP-C should monitor proper form, start with light weights, and progress the intensity gradually by 5%–10%. One repetition maximum (1-RM) testing can also be performed under direct supervision by an EP-C, ensuring to follow all recommended procedures (18). For all exercises, proper form with light weight should be emphasized first, followed by progression to heavier weights as tolerated by the child or adolescent. If a child consistently fails to perform resistance exercises safely, the child may not be emotionally of physically mature enough to safely engage in resistance training, and consideration should be given to delay the onset of resistance training for that child.

Children

Parents and the EP-C should encourage physical activities that are age-appropriate and enjoyable for children. Families should be encouraged to engage in active and fun activities together to establish positive lifelong physical activity habits. To this end, the EP-C should realize that activity for children must be fun and intermittent in order for a child to continue participation. Physical activity programs for children should emphasize games, fun activities, and unstructured play. Rather than using an adult prescription paradigm, children should be allowed to self-regulate the intensity and the duration of their activity (51). With this in mind, games and activities should have intermittent rest opportunities as part of the game. Games that eliminate children from participation based on poor performance should be avoided. A high-intensity game can be alternated with a low-intensity game, or safe zones can be included for children to have recovery time and still be included in the game. This is especially important for obese children whose cost of locomotion is higher than a nonobese child. It is also important to focus on limiting sedentary behavior among children.

Adolescents

As children become adolescents, the activity paradigm can become more structured but should still emphasize enjoyment (51). More complex games and activities requiring more maturity can be included. Rather than play-based strengthening activities used for very young children, older children and adolescents prefer a more structured resistance training program. The use of child-sized resistance equipment and dumbbells can be incorporated on the basis of how well children follow directions. Children as young as 7 or 8 years can be successful in a structured resistance training program (15). Medicine balls and resistance bands can be incorporated as long as the child can respect the rules given by the teacher. This will vary depending on the child's ability to follow directions; most adolescents are mature enough to participate in a resistance training program that includes free weights, medicine balls, resistance bands, and weightlifting. Because adolescents of the same chronological age can have different biological ages, it is important to consider the biological age when determining appropriate exercises for this population.

Many children, their parents, or pediatricians are increasingly concerned about weight status during childhood and adolescence. The Summary Report from the American Academy of Pediatrics Expert Committee on the Prevention, Assessment and Treatment of Child and Adolescent Overweight and Obesity is a good resource for the EP-C and other professionals who work with youth (6). The Expert Committee recommends that all children be encouraged to engage in specific healthy eating behaviors, reduce screen time, and increase physical activity. The recommendations stress the importance of children being taught to self-regulate these behaviors with the help of their parents. For those who are overweight or obese, several strategies are presented depending on the age of the child and their weight status. Generally, youth who are older and more obese are candidates to engage in more aggressive weight loss strategies such as caloric restriction and higher levels of activity. Younger children, even those who are obese, should not restrict calories in an effort to lose weight but should be encouraged to improve healthy behaviors to improve weight status (6). In all cases, the parents, the family, and the pediatricians are all active participants in promoting behaviors that produce a healthy weight.

 Pregnant Women

Physical and Physiological Changes

Many changes occur to a woman's body during pregnancy, the most visible of which is an increase in body weight. Overall, appropriate gestational weight gain depends on maternal body mass index (BMI) prior to pregnancy: underweight 28–40 lb, normal weight 25–35 lb, overweight 15–25 lb, and all obese 11–20 lb (47). The change in the distribution of gestational weight gained is mainly due to the growing fetus within the uterus and thus causes the maternal abdomen to protrude and shifts the center of gravity more anterior and superior than in the nonpregnant state. As a result of this anterior and superior shift of maternal center balance, half of pregnant women suffer with lower back and pelvic pain (1,2). Significant hormonal changes also occur, including increases in estrogen and aldosterone, which contribute to water retention and increased blood volume. Due to possible laxity of joints, caution should be used during flexibility exercises so as not to overstretch the joints. Fatigue and nausea can also occur, especially during the first trimester, most likely due to the hormonal changes accompanying pregnancy. Often, after the first trimester the feelings of fatigue and nausea are attenuated (49). Especially during times of nauseousness, interest in physical activity may be diminished. It is important to note, the energy cost of pregnancy requires additional food, depending on gestational age: $114 \, \text{kcal} \cdot \text{day}^{-1}$ from 0 to 10 weeks, $379 \, \text{kcal} \cdot \text{day}^{-1}$ from 10 to 20 weeks, $421 \, \text{kcal} \cdot \text{day}^{-1}$ from 20 to 30 weeks, and $322 \, \text{kcal} \cdot \text{day}^{-1}$ from 30 to 40 weeks gestation (24).

The maternal cardiovascular system changes during pregnancy to accommodate the demands of the fetoplacental unit. In order to meet the needs to the increased tissue and metabolism, pregnancy causes an increased blood volume. At rest, cardiac output, stroke volume, and heart rate increase, while vascular resistance decreases. Additionally, resting oxygen uptake increases to allow for fetal and placental growth (36). Slight hypertrophy of the maternal heart may occur as a result of the elevated heart rate and stroke volume (49). Despite these cardiovascular changes, lying supine after 16 weeks of pregnancy may compress the inferior vena cava, causing a reduced venous return or less blood back to the heart, due to the expanded fetoplacental unit (36). This is an important consideration for the EP-C working with pregnant women, as supine exercise during the third trimester may lead to hypotension and dizziness. The EP-C must also be aware that the decreased peripheral vascular resistance makes women more prone to hypotension with changes in body position (36,49).

Exercising during pregnancy causes similar and somewhat different physiological responses. For example, heart rate is higher at low intensities, but maximal heart rate is lower compared to the nonpregnant state (36,46). Therefore, the heart rate reserve, or the range of heart rate response, is smaller during pregnancy (36). Oxygen consumption during submaximal exercise is higher when pregnant, more than would be expected from the increase in body weight. This is largely due to the increased oxygen cost of the maternofetoplacental unit and the increased oxygen cost of respiration (52). In general, the caloric requirements of pregnancy increase with amount of time participating in physical activity (24).

The Impact of Chronic Exercise

Exercise is beneficial for those who exercised prior to pregnancy and for those who start after becoming pregnant (33). Chronic exercise confers the same benefits to pregnant woman as it does for the general population, although there are benefits specific to pregnancy. Similar to the nongravid state, exercise improves circulation and helps decrease pregnancy-related edema that often occurs in the extremities (49). Similarly, participation in aerobic exercise throughout pregnancy improves overall maternal cardiovascular function (45). Exercise also improves mood and helps alleviate some discomforts associated with pregnancy (33). Exercise training can reduce the risk of developing preeclampsia (high blood pressure and protein in the urine) and gestational diabetes (49). Chronic exercisers are more likely to delivery normal size (weight) babies and less likely to have delivery complications (49). Similar to aerobic exercise, resistance training has a similar physiologic response; therefore, participation in resistance training leads to no adverse pregnancy outcomes or injuries (44) and no difference in type of delivery (5). Lastly, participation in combination exercise, including aerobic and resistance components, have decreased incidence of gestation conditions (*i.e.*, hypertension, diabetes), less complications with delivery, and similar birth weights relative to nonexercisers (34).

The general consensus based on the expanding research is that exercise training is safe and does not increase maternal or fetal risk of adverse outcomes (3). Any woman with a low-risk pregnancy, approved by obstetric provider, can start exercising or continue exercising (3). Furthermore, research suggests improved cardiovascular and nervous system maturation before and after birth in the offspring of women who did aerobic exercise throughout pregnancy compared with offspring of women who were not active (33,35). Other studies found increased resistance training was associated with increased cardiac autonomic maturation as well as decreased likelihood of fetal complication during pregnancy (7). Research regarding combination (aerobic and resistance) regimens during pregnancy found no significant differences in birth weight of offspring (21,42) and increased cardiac autonomic maturation (35) between combination exercise and control groups. In fact, all types of exercise should be encouraged during pregnancy due to the benefits for improved maternal health, delivery outcomes, and possible benefits for the child.

Exercise Programming and Specific Exercise Considerations

The American Congress of Obstetricians and Gynecologists (ACOG) (3) recommends that pregnant women accumulate 30 minutes of moderate-intensity exercise on all or most days of the week. This recommendation applies to all healthy pregnant women who have no absolute or relative contraindications (Table 10.1) for exercise (3). The PARmed-X for Pregnancy health screening tool, developed by the Canadian Society for Exercise Physiology (available from www.csep.ca), should be used to screen all pregnant women seeking to start or continue exercising during pregnancy. All EP personnel should make sure they keep a clearance letter (*i.e.*, PARmed-X) prior to a woman's participating in exercise and be familiar with the contraindications to exercise during pregnancy (Table 10.1). If a pregnant client develops a medical condition, then the exercise program should be discontinued until she receives approval from her health care provider.

Although any activity is encouraged, a moderate intensity, or 40%–60% of heart rate reserve, is recommended to achieve health benefits (4). Because pregnancy alters heart rate response to exercise, exercise intensity can be monitored by using RPE or a combination of tools (46). On a 6–20 scale, moderate intensity is the equivalent of 12–14 RPE, or of maintaining the ability to converse while exercising. Exercise target heart rate zones for pregnancy have also been determined based on age, BMI, and fitness level (12,38).

Activities should include aerobic and resistance exercise and include 10–15 minutes of warm-up and cool-down with low-intensity activity and stretching (4). During all exercises, the EP-C must coach the pregnant client to breathe appropriately to avoid the Valsalva maneuver and hypotension/dizziness. Pregnant women can safely participate in aerobic, resistance, and combination types exercises, but ACOG recommends avoiding activities that may cause trauma to the abdomen (*i.e.*, ice hockey, soccer, and basketball) or have a high risk of falling (horseback riding, downhill skiing, gymnastics, or vigorous racquet sports) (3,4). Furthermore, scuba diving or exercise at altitudes higher than 6,000 ft should be avoided to ensure appropriate fetal oxygen supply, unless a woman already lives at high altitude (3). Exercising in a cool comfortable environment is important to prevent fetal harm due to hyperthermia (3). Moreover, women should ensure that they are properly hydrated by ingesting a pint (16 oz or 500 mL) of water prior to exercise and a cup every 20 minutes during exercise with the goal of replacing any fluid lost during exercise (45,48). This will help ensure maximal thermoregulatory ability.

Women who develop a contraindication for exercise should stop exercise immediately and consult their obstetric provider to determine if exercise should be continued during the pregnancy. All women, whether novice or experienced, who exercise while pregnant should be aware of the warning signs when exercise should be terminated and a physician consulted (3): vaginal bleeding, shortness of breath prior to exertion, dizziness, headache, chest pain, muscle weakness, calf pain

Table 10.1	Contraindications for Exercise during Pregnancy
Relative Contraindications	**Absolute Contraindications**
Severe anemia	Hemodynamically significant heart disease
Unevaluated maternal cardiac arrhythmia	Restrictive lung disease
Chronic bronchitis	Incompetent cervix/cerclage
Poorly controlled Type 1 diabetes mellitus	Multiple gestation at risk for premature labor
Extreme morbid obesity	Persistent second- or third-trimester bleeding
Extreme underweight (BMI <12)	Placenta previa after 26 wk of gestation
History of extremely sedentary lifestyle	Premature labor during the current pregnancy
Intrauterine growth restriction in current pregnancy	Ruptured membranes
Poorly controlled hypertension	
Orthopedic limitations	
Poorly controlled seizure disorder	
Poorly controlled hyperthyroidism	
Heavy smoker	

Reprinted with permission from American College of Obstetricians and Gynecologists. ACOG Committee Opinion No. 650: Physical activity and exercise during pregnancy and the postpartum period. *Obstet Gynecol.* 2015;650:2.

or swelling, preterm labor, decreased fetal movement, or a leaking of amniotic fluid. Beside the additional caloric need of pregnancy (second and third trimesters), exercise results in an additional caloric cost. Caloric intake should therefore be adjusted so that appropriate gestational weight gain is achieved (24,46).

Finally, those women who begin exercising while pregnant should gradually increase the intensity and duration of exercise or activity until they meet the recommendations. All pregnant women should avoid extended periods of motionless standing and any activity that is conducted in a supine position, especially after the first trimester when venous return can become compromised (3). Resistance training, provided that all of the earlier recommendations are met, is also acceptable, although exercises should be modified to avoid the supine position and the Valsalva maneuver. If resistance training is conducted, exercises should be dynamic in nature and focus on the large muscles of the whole body. A resistance that produces a moderate level of muscular fatigue within 12 to 15 repetitions is recommended, as is maintaining an RPE between 12 to 14, within target heart range, and being able to converse while exercising (4,46).

Maternal physiology is able to adapt to pregnancy as well as exercise during pregnancy. Moderate-intensity exercise is safe and recommended during pregnancy. To date, exercise during pregnancy has been shown to be beneficial for maternal health, pregnancy outcome, as well as that of the developing fetus. Maternal physiology demonstrates the unique capability to adapt to various anatomical, physiological, and hormonal changes as a result of pregnancy, and understanding this normal process is important in healthy women but may help in understanding disease processes specific to pregnancy. EP professionals should be familiar with the clearance process for pregnancy and exercise, current ACOG recommendations for maternal exercise, as well as contraindications for exercise.

Based on current research and exercise principles, the following prescription is appropriate for exercise during pregnancy after medical screening by a health care provider (34): Frequency: 3–4 days $\cdot$ week^{-1}; Intensity: moderate intensity within 12–14 RPE (6–20 scale), target heart rate zone (12,38), and "talk test" (able to converse with some slight effort during workout); Time: 30–60 minutes per session (previously sedentary women start with 15 minutes, 3 sessions per week and progress to at least 30 min three times per week); Type: include aerobic and strength exercises, that is, walking and resistance bands, or other enjoyable activity. Every exercise session must include 10- to 15-minute warm-up and cool-down with low-intensity activity and stretching. Pregnant women should always exercise in a comfortable, cool environment and stay well hydrated. While exercising, pregnant women should wear loose-fitting clothing with a supportive bra.

 Older Adults

Older adults and those who are younger but severely deconditioned present fitness professionals with unique challenges. The process of aging affects every system to some extent and these changes are inevitable. Of course, a healthy lifestyle in most people alters the rate of these changes resulting in increased longevity and better physical functioning. However, the older adult populations tend to have more disease conditions and also tend to be further progressed in those conditions. Several disease states are discussed in Chapters 8 and 9 in this book. The discussion here focuses on the relatively healthy older adult who is free from the advanced stages of disease but may be sedentary and generally deconditioned.

Physical and Physiological Changes

Body Composition and Musculoskeletal Function

During adulthood, individuals tend to gain body weight and fat mass and tend to lose fat-free mass, height, and bone (9,43). However, the increases in percentage fat and body weight in older adults may be largely lifestyle related rather than a natural consequence of aging (43). Mirroring the loss of fat-free mass is a loss of muscular strength and the associated decreases in physical function (9,10). The loss of strength, muscle mass, and bone density are larger in women than in men (9,10). In the very old adult, there is also a loss of body weight and body cell mass (20), and this loss of weight is associated with a higher mortality rate (40). As the total body water content decreases with age, so does the elasticity and pliability of tissues such as cartilage and connective tissues that are found within joints among other places. Range of motion becomes reduced, the effects of which are compounded by the low levels of activity in many older adults (9,43,50). Neuromotor function also deteriorates with age because of a reduction in the number of neurons resulting in reduced coordination, slower walking speed, shorter stride length, slower reaction time, poorer balance, and lower agility (9,43,50).

Cardiorespiratory Function and Thermoregulation

The cardiorespiratory system is affected by aging and by a sedentary lifestyle. Vessels become stiffer, and elasticity is lost in cardiac tissue, including the heart valves. This results in higher blood pressure and higher resistance to flow, which creates more work for the heart (9,43). During submaximal exercise, aging tends to result in higher ventilation, blood pressure, lower cardiac output and stroke volume, and little change in heart rate and oxygen uptake (9,43). At maximal levels of exercise, oxygen uptake, ventilation, cardiac output, heart rate, stroke volume, oxygen extraction, and lactic acid concentrations are lower, whereas total peripheral resistance and blood pressure is higher than in a younger person (9,43). Because collagen fibers in the lungs also lose elasticity and

EXERCISE IS MEDICINE CONNECTION

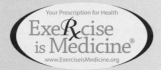

Figueroa A, Park SY, Seo DY, Sanchez-Gonzalez MA, Baek YH. Combined resistance and endurance exercise training improves arterial stiffness, blood pressure, and muscle strength in post-menopausal women. *Menopause*. 2011;18(9):980–4.

Figueroa and colleagues (2011) conducted a study in which postmenopausal women engaged in resistance and endurance exercise over 12 weeks. Arterial stiffness (at the ankle), blood pressure, and muscle strength were evaluated. This randomized controlled trial compared the control group with the treatment group who completed a circuit resistance training program followed by endurance (aerobic) training at 60% of age-predicted maximal heart rate (HR_{max}) 3 days · week^{-1}. Participants included 24 postmenopausal women who were between 47 and 68 years of age. Results indicated that postmenopausal women in the treatment group had significantly better ankle blood flow, lower mean systolic and diastolic blood pressure, and greater dynamic leg strength and isometric handgrip strength than those in the control group. The authors of this study reported that combined resistance and aerobic training had favorable outcomes on risk factors associated with hypertension and frailty in postmenopausal women.

bronchioles lose their tone, less air can be moved per minute in an older adult (9,50). The result of these processes, and what is important for the EP-C to recognize, is that older individuals have a lower overall exercise capacity and that any given absolute submaximal exercise intensity represents a higher percentage of their maximum.

Thermoregulatory ability also declines with aging (9). The number and activity of sweat glands decreases with age and the capillary density also decreases. This results in a lower ability of the body to benefit from evaporative or radiant cooling. Older adults, as well as younger groups, also cannot withstand the cold because of a reduced ability to divert blood flow toward deeper tissues (9). In the very old, this is exacerbated by the loss of subcutaneous body fat (50).

The Impact of Chronic Exercise

It is not the purpose of this discussion to provide a comprehensive literature review on the benefits of chronic exercise because this has been well documented elsewhere (9,19,22,39,41). However, there is strong evidence that an adequate amount and type of exercise lowers the risks of several cancers, cardiovascular disease, some metabolic diseases, and premature death in older adults (9,19,22,39,41). Exercise results in a more favorable cardiovascular risk profile, increases physical function, prevents falls, improves some mental health outcomes, improves fitness, and helps with achieving a healthy weight (9,19,22,39,41). In fact, many of the age-related declines in fat-free mass, strength, and motor performance are at least partially reversible with the onset of a regular exercise program (9,39,43). There is evidence that these benefits can be reaped even in sedentary older adults who initiate an exercise program late in life (9,19,39,41).

Nelson et al. (39) outlines in detail the benefits of regular exercise in older adults. Specifically, in addition to the benefits that are reaped for all adults, regular exercise in older adults reduces the risk of falls, injuries from falls, and functional limitations and improves the management of many conditions, including dementia, anxiety, and back pain. There is some evidence that exercise improves sleep in older adults and can prevent or delay the negative cognitive changes that often occur with aging (39).

Exercise Programming and Specific Exercise Considerations

As is the case for all adults, the EP-C should perform proper baseline assessments, health screenings, and risk factor stratification for an older adult to determine whether contraindications for exercise exist as well as to determine the type, intensity, and quantity of exercise that can be safely performed. Individualized approaches to promoting exercise can be designed on the basis of this risk. This process is discussed in Chapter 3 and is described in *ACSM's Guidelines for Exercise Testing and Prescription* (4). *ACSM's Resource Manual for Guidelines for Exercise Testing and Prescription* presents an evaluation tool to help an exercise professional determine the appropriateness of exercise prescription in older adults (10). The general guidelines in the following text are recommended for older adults who are healthy but may be deconditioned.

For all components of fitness, the EP-C should ensure that the choice of exercise is appropriate for the older adult given any prior injuries, orthopedic concerns, vision concerns, or deficits in balance and agility (4). Exercise in water or using a weight support machine such as a cycle might be more appropriate than walking and running for those with poor balance. A treadmill with a handrail will offer more stability than other modes of exercise for someone who is visually impaired or who has balance issues. Exercises that provide support such as weight machines are more appropriate for the very deconditioned than exercises that require more balance and skill such as free weights. Exercises should be individualized and tailored for each older adult to allow for successful completion before progressing to more challenging exercises.

Aerobic Activity

Older adults should strive for the same amount of aerobic activity that is recommended for all adults: Accumulate at least 30 minutes and up to 60 minutes of moderate-intensity activity on 5 or more days a week in bouts of at least 10 minutes, or at least 20 minutes of vigorous activity for 3 days a week, or a combination of vigorous and moderate activity for 3–5 days a week (20) — see also Chapter 3. Those who are very deconditioned should start with lighter intensity activities and progress to higher intensity activities until the mentioned guidelines are met. Greater levels of activity should be encouraged in those who are able to do so safely, as exceeding these minimal recommendations will result in further health benefits and will improve an older adult's ability to manage existing conditions and further reduce disease risk (39). However, any person who is at high risk should be medically cleared before engaging in vigorous activity (4).

Because of the heterogeneity of aerobic capacities in the older adult population, a different definition of moderate versus vigorous intensity is required (39). Because the subjective rating of an activity may be vastly different for an unconditioned person compared with a well-conditioned person, an exercise that is easy for one person may be very difficult for another. For adults, intensity is defined in absolute terms, but for older adults, a subjective rating system is used to determine the intensity of exercise, which accounts for differences in the level of conditioning. Moderate intensity is a 5 or 6 on a 0–10 scale (where 0 is sitting and 10 is a maximal effort) and is that which produces a noticeable change in breathing and heart rate. A vigorous effort would be a 7 or 8 on the same scale and would produce large increases in heart rate and breathing. It should also be noted that any activity is beneficial, so the EP-C should also emphasize reducing sedentary behaviors as well as a gradual approach to adopting exercise. Very deconditioned adults may initially aim for light-intensity activity (<5 subjective rating of effort) and perform exercise in shorter bouts until more continuous exercise can be sustained (39).

Muscle-Strengthening Activity

All adults are recommended to perform muscle-strengthening activities on at least 2 nonconsecutive days a week, targeting the major muscle groups in 8–10 exercises (9,19,39) (see also

Chapter 4). Older adults should choose a weight or resistance that can be performed 8–12 times, which produces a level of effort that is moderate to high. A perception rating of 5–6 is moderate and a 7–8 is considered high on a 10-point scale (where 0 is no movement and 10 is a maximal muscular effort) (39). As with all individuals, a lighter initial weight with a focus on proper form followed by progressively increasing loads based on each person's ability is recommended. Achieving more than the minimum recommendations for muscle strengthening activity will confer proportionally greater health benefits and should be encouraged, if possible, on the basis of how well exercise is tolerated (39).

Flexibility Activity and Neuromotor Exercises

Exercises that target joint mobility are recommended for all adults. Stretching exercises that are held for 10–30 seconds to a point of tightness or mild discomfort for the major muscle groups (after a warm-up) and performed 2–3 days a week are recommended (9,19,39) (see also Chapter 5). For older adults, stretches may produce greater benefits when they are held for 30–60 seconds. The total time for flexibility training should reach about 10 minutes per session and should occur on at least 2 days a week. Neuromotor exercises that help improve balance, coordination, agility, gait, and proprioception are recommended for older adults to reduce the number and severity of falls, aid in functional tasks, and improve the quality of life (19,39). Tai chi, qigong, and yoga have been studied and have been shown to reduce falls, but there is not enough evidence to recommend a frequency, duration, or intensity for these activities (4,19).

Thermoregulation

As with children and other vulnerable populations, the EP-C should protect against a heat injury in the older adult by conducting exercise in a thermoneutral environment and encouraging clients to avoid exercise in the hottest times of day. It is also important to ensure adequate hydration so that evaporative cooling is maximized. For exercise in the cold, older adults should dress in layers for increased warmth and for the ability to add or remove layers as needed.

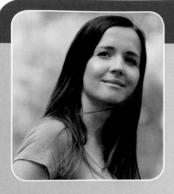

The Case of Katie

Submitted by **Kim DeLaFuente, MA, ACSM-PD, Spectrum Health Healthier Communities Department, Grand Rapids, MI**

Katie is a 26-year-old pregnant mother of one with a history of gestational diabetes. She is interested in exercising safely during her pregnancy while maintaining her endurance and strength levels.

Narrative

Katie is a 26-year-old woman who is 15 weeks pregnant with her second child. She is a part-time nurse who works 24 hours a week on an intensive care unit (ICU) floor. Her work is stressful and demands a lot of time on her feet with limited rest periods. In addition, she has a young child at home that requires much of her attention.

Health Appraisal

Age: 26 years old
Family history: none
Cigarette smoking: none
Sedentary lifestyle: regularly participated in an exercise program until becoming pregnant. She suffered from morning sickness during the first trimester of her pregnancy and did little physical activity during this time.
Obesity: none; BMI was 26.7 (overweight) before becoming pregnant
Hypertension: none
Dyslipidemia: none
Diabetes: history of gestational diabetes with first pregnancy and family history of diabetes
Risk classification: low risk, after consultation with physician to determine blood glucose level

Physical Data

Height: 5′4″
Weight: 155 lb (before pregnancy); 162 lb (current weight)
% Body fat: NA
BMI: 26.6 kg · m^{-2} before pregnancy (overweight)
Blood pressure: 120/74 mm Hg
Resting heart rate: 86 bpm
Fasting blood sugar: 96
No exercise test was done.

To date, Katie's pregnancy is uncomplicated. During her first pregnancy, Katie gained 50 lb, and she was not physically active outside of work and activities of daily living. She has a family history of type II diabetes and a diagnosis of gestational diabetes in her first pregnancy. She became motivated to exercise regularly and has maintained an exercise program that consists of jogging for 30 minutes, 4 days a week, at an RPE of 15 and resistance training 2 days a week. Nausea and vomiting during the first trimester has reduced her exercise to walking a few times a week. Now that she is feeling better, Katie is interested in increasing her exercise again. Because she did not exercise during her first pregnancy, she is unsure how much or what type of exercise she should be doing.

Goals

Her goals include healthy weight gain, maintaining endurance and strength levels and safe exercise.

Goal 1: In addition to walking (2 days · week^{-1}), start a prenatal water aerobics class, 2 days · week^{-1} (RPE 12).

Goal 2: Restart a muscular strength program, 2 days · week^{-1}, using resistance bands and a stability ball.

Goal 3: Learn and apply exercise guidelines related to pregnancy. What other considerations need to be made with physical activity during pregnancy?

QUESTIONS

- Identify exercise precautions that should be taken during pregnancy.
- Identify four symptoms that would require exercise be terminated if a woman is pregnant.
- Identify four appropriate modes of exercise during pregnancy.

References

1. American College of Sports Medicine. *ACSM's Guidelines for Exercise Testing and Prescription.* 10th ed. Philadelphia (PA): Wolters Kluwer; 2017.
2. American Congress of Obstetrics and Gynecology. *Exercise during Pregnancy* [Internet]. 2011 [cited 2016 Jan 15]. Available from: http://www.acog.org/Patients/FAQs/Exercise-During-Pregnancy
3. Colberg SR, Albright AL, Blissmer BJ, et al. Exercise and type II diabetes: American College of Sports Medicine and the American Diabetes Association: joint position statement. *Med Sci Sports Exerc.* 2010;42(12):2282–303.

SUMMARY

Exercise is beneficial for all individuals regardless of age or activity status; however, the EP-C must be aware of the unique concerns of older individuals, the young, and pregnant women. Benefits can be achieved for each of these populations once exercise type, quantity, and intensity have been adjusted on the basis of unique individual needs.

STUDY QUESTIONS

1. Which modes of exercise should be avoided by children for safety reasons?
2. Describe how exercise should be modified for pregnant women.
3. Under what conditions should a pregnant woman stop exercising?
4. What are different ways exercise intensity should be gauged for older adults and why?
5. What are some exercise precautions that should be taken when children, pregnant women, or older adults are exercising in the heat?

REFERENCES

1. Aldabe D, Milosavljevic S, Bussey MD. Is pregnancy related pelvic girdle pain associated with altered kinematic, kinetic and motor control of the pelvis? A systematic review. *Eur Spine J.* 2012;21(9):1777–87.

2. Aldabe D, Ribeiro DC, Milosavljevic S, Dawn Bussey M. Pregnancy-related pelvic girdle pain and its relationship with relaxin levels during pregnancy: a systematic review. *Eur Spine J.* 2012;21(9):1769–76.

3. American College of Obstetricians and Gynecologists. ACOG Committee Opinion Number 267, January 2002: exercise during pregnancy and the postpartum period. *Obstet Gynecol.* 2002;99(1):171–3.

4. American College of Sports Medicine. *ACSM's Guidelines for Exercise Testing and Prescription.* 10th ed. Philadelphia (PA): Wolters Kluwer; 2018.

5. Barakat R, Ruiz JR, Stirling JR, Zakynthinaki M, Lucia A. Type of delivery is not affected by light resistance and toning exercise training during pregnancy: a randomized controlled trial. *Am J Obstet Gynecol.* 2009;201(6):590.e1–6.

6. Barlow SE. Expert committee recommendations regarding the prevention, assessment, and treatment of child and adolescent overweight and obesity: summary report. *Pediatrics.* 2007;120(Suppl 4):S164–92.

7. Beilock SL, Feltz DL, Pivarnik JM. Training patterns of athletes during pregnancy and postpartum. *Res Q Exerc Sport.* 2001;72(1):39–46.

8. Biddiss E, Irwin J. Active video games to promote physical activity in children and youth: a systematic review. *Arch Pediatr Adoles Med.* 2010;164(7):664–72.

9. Chodzko WJ, Proctor DN, Fiatorone Singh MA, et al. American College of Sports Medicine position stand. Exercise and physical activity for older adults. *Med Sci Sports Exerc.* 2009;41(7):1510–30.

10. Coe DP, Fiatarone-Singh MA. Exercise prescription for special populations: women, pregnancy, children and older adults. In: Swain DP, editor. *ACSM's Resource Manual for Guidelines for Exercise Testing and Prescription.* 7th ed. Baltimore (MD): Lippincott Williams & Wilkins; 2014. p. 565–97.

11. Daniels SR, Hassink SG. The role of the pediatrician in primary prevention of obesity. *Pediatrics.* 2015;136(1):e275–92.

12. Davenport MH, Charlesworth S, Vanderspank D, Sopper MM, Mottola MF. Development and validation of exercise target heart rate zones for overweight and obese pregnant women. *Appl Physiol Nutr Metab.* 2008;33(5):984–9.

13. Dougherty KA, Chow M, Kenney WL. Critical environmental limits for exercising heat-acclimated lean and obese boys. *Eur J Appl Physiol.* 2010;108(4):779–89.

14. Expert Panel on Integrated Guidelines for Cardiovascular Health and Risk Reduction in Children and Adolescents, National Heart, Lung, and Blood Institute. Expert panel on integrated guidelines for cardiovascular health and risk reduction in children and adolescents: summary report. *Pediatrics.* 2011;128(Suppl 5):S213–56.

15. Faigenbaum AD, Kraemer WJ, Blimkie CJR, et al. Youth resistance training: updated position statement paper from the National Strength and Conditioning Association. *J Strength Cond Res.* 2009;23(5):S60–79.

16. Faigenbaum AD, McFarland J. Relative safety of weightlifting movements for youth. *Strength Cond J.* 2008;30(6):23–5.

17. Faigenbaum AD, Milliken LA, Cloutier G, Westcott WL. Perceived exertion during resistance exercise in children. *Percept Mot Skills.* 2004;98(2):627–37.

18. Faigenbaum AD, Milliken LA, Westcott W. Maximal strength testing in children. *J Strength Cond Res.* 2003;17(1):162–6.

19. Garber CE, Blissmer B, Deschenes MR, et al. American College of Sports Medicine position stand. Quantity and quality of exercise for developing and maintaining cardiorespiratory, musculoskeletal, and neuromotor fitness in apparently healthy adults: guidance for prescribing exercise. *Med Sci Sports Exerc.* 2011;43(7):1334–59.

20. Going S, Williams DP, Lohman TG. Aging and body composition: biological changes and methodological issues. *Exerc Sport Sci Rev.* 1995;23:411–58.

21. Hall DC, Kaufmann DA. Effects of aerobic and strength conditioning on pregnancy outcomes. *Am J Obstet Gynecol.* 1987;157(5):1199–203.

22. Haskell WL, Lee IM, Pate RR, et al. Physical activity and public health: updated recommendation for adults from the American College of Sports Medicine and the American Heart Association. *Med Sci Sports Exerc.* 2007; 39(8):1423–34.

23. Hebestreit HU, Bar-Or O. Differences between children and adults for exercise testing and prescription. In: Skinner JS, editor. *Exercise Testing and Exercise Prescription for Special Cases.* 3rd ed. Baltimore (MD): Lippincott Williams & Wilkins; 2005. p. 68–84.

24. Institute of Medicine, Committee on the Nutritional Status During Pregnancy and Lactation. *Nutrition During Pregnancy: Part I Weight Gain: Part II Nutrient Supplements.* Washington (DC): National Academies Press; 1990. 480 p.

25. Johnson BA, Salzberg CL, Stevenson DA. A systematic review: plyometric training programs for young children. *J Strength Cond Res.* 2011;25(9):2623.

26. Malina RM, Bouchard C, Bar-Or O. Body composition. In: *Growth, Maturation, and Physical Activity.* 2nd ed. Champaign (IL): Human Kinetics; 2004. p. 101–19.

27. Malina RM, Bouchard C, Bar-Or O. Bone tissue in skeletal growth and body composition. In: *Growth, Maturation, and Physical Activity.* 2nd ed. Champaign (IL): Human Kinetics; 2004. p. 121–35.

28. Malina RM, Bouchard C, Bar-Or O. *Growth, Maturation, and Physical Activity.* 2nd ed. Champaign (IL): Human Kinetics; 2004. 728 p.

29. Malina RM, Bouchard C, Bar-Or O. Heart, blood and lungs. In: *Growth, Maturation, and Physical Activity.* 2nd ed. Champaign (IL): Human Kinetics; 2004. p. 181–93.

30. Malina RM, Bouchard C, Bar-Or O. Skeletal muscle tissue. In: *Growth, Maturation, and Physical Activity.* 2nd ed. Champaign (IL): Human Kinetics; 2004. p. 137–57.

31. Malina RM, Bouchard C, Bar-Or O. Somatic growth. In: *Growth, Maturation, and Physical Activity.* 2nd ed. Champaign (IL): Human Kinetics; 2004. p. 41–81.

32. Malina RM, Bouchard C, Bar-Or O. Strength and motor performance. In: *Growth, Maturation, and Physical Activity.* 2nd ed. Champaign (IL): Human Kinetics; 2004. p. 215–33.

33. May LE. *Physiology of Prenatal Exercise and Fetal Development.* New York (NY): Springer; 2012. viii, 44 p.

34. May LE, Allen JJB, Gustafson KM. Fetal and maternal cardiac responses to physical activity and exercise during pregnancy. *Early Hum Dev.* 2016;94:49–52.

35. May LE, Strickland D, Newton E, Gross-McMillan A, Steed D, Biko D. *FASEB J.* 2015; 29(1 Suppl):1055.28.

36. Melzer K, Schutz Y, Boulvain M, Kayser B. Physical activity and pregnancy: cardiovascular adaptations, recommendations and pregnancy outcomes. *Sports Med.* 2010;40(6):493–507.

37. Mottola MF. Exercise prescription for overweight and obese women: pregnancy and postpartum. *Obstet Gynecol Clin North Am.* 2009;36(2):301–16, viii.

38. Mottola MF, Davenport MH, Brun CR, Inglis SD, Charlesworth S, Sopper MM. VO2peak prediction and exercise prescription for pregnant women. *Med Sci Sports Exerc.* 2006;38(8):1389–95.

39. Nelson ME, Rejeski WJ, Blair SN, et al. Physical activity and public health in older adults: recommendation from the ACSM and the AHA. *Circulation.* 2007;116(9):1094–104.

40. Newman AB, Yanez D, Harris T, et al. Weight change in old age and its association with mortality. *J Am Geriatr Soc.* 2001;49(10):1309–18.

41. Physical Activity Guidelines Advisory Committee. *Physical Activity Guidelines Advisory Committee Report, 2008.* Washington (DC): U.S. Department of Health and Human Services; 2008.

42. Price BB, Amini SB, Kappeler K. Exercise in pregnancy: effect on fitness and obstetric outcomes—a randomized trial. *Med Sci Sports Exerc.* 2012;44(12):2263–9.

43. Skinner JS. Aging for exercise testing and exercise prescription. In: Skinner JS, editor. *Exercise Testing and Exercise Prescription for Special Cases.* 3rd ed. Baltimore (MD): Lippincott Williams & Wilkins; 2005. p. 85–99.

44. SMA statement the benefits and risks of exercise during pregnancy. Sport Medicine Australia. *J Sci Med Sport.* 2002; 5(1):11–9.

45. Stevenson L. Exercise in pregnancy. Part 1: update on pathophysiology. *Can Fam Physician.* 1997;43:97–104.

46. Stevenson L. Exercise in pregnancy. Part 2: recommendations for individuals. *Can Fam Physician.* 1997;43:107–11.

47. Truong YN, Yee LM, Caughey AB, Cheng YW. Weight gain in pregnancy: does the Institute of Medicine have it right? *Am J Obstet Gynecol.* 2015;212(3):362.e1–8.

48. Wang TW, Apgar BS. Exercise during pregnancy. *Am Fam Physician.* 1998;57(8):1846–52.

49. Williamson P. Exercise during pregnancy. In: *Exercise for Special Populations.* Baltimore (MD): Lippincott Williams & Wilkins; 2011. p. 46–81.

50. Williamson P. Exercise for senior adults. In: *Exercise for Special Populations.* Baltimore (MD): Lippincott Williams & Wilkins; 2011. p. 121–78.

51. Williamson P. Exercise for youth. In: *Exercise for Special Populations.* Baltimore (MD): Lippincott Williams & Wilkins; 2011. p. 82–120.

52. Wolfe LA. Pregnancy. In: Skinner JS, editor. *Exercise Testing and Exercise Prescription for Special Cases.* 3rd ed. Baltimore (MD): Lippincott Williams & Wilkins; 2005. p. 377–91.

Additional Resources

1. Swain DP, editor. *ACSM's Resource Manual for Guidelines for Exercise Testing and Prescription.* 7th ed. Baltimore (MD): Lippincott Williams & Wilkins; 2014.

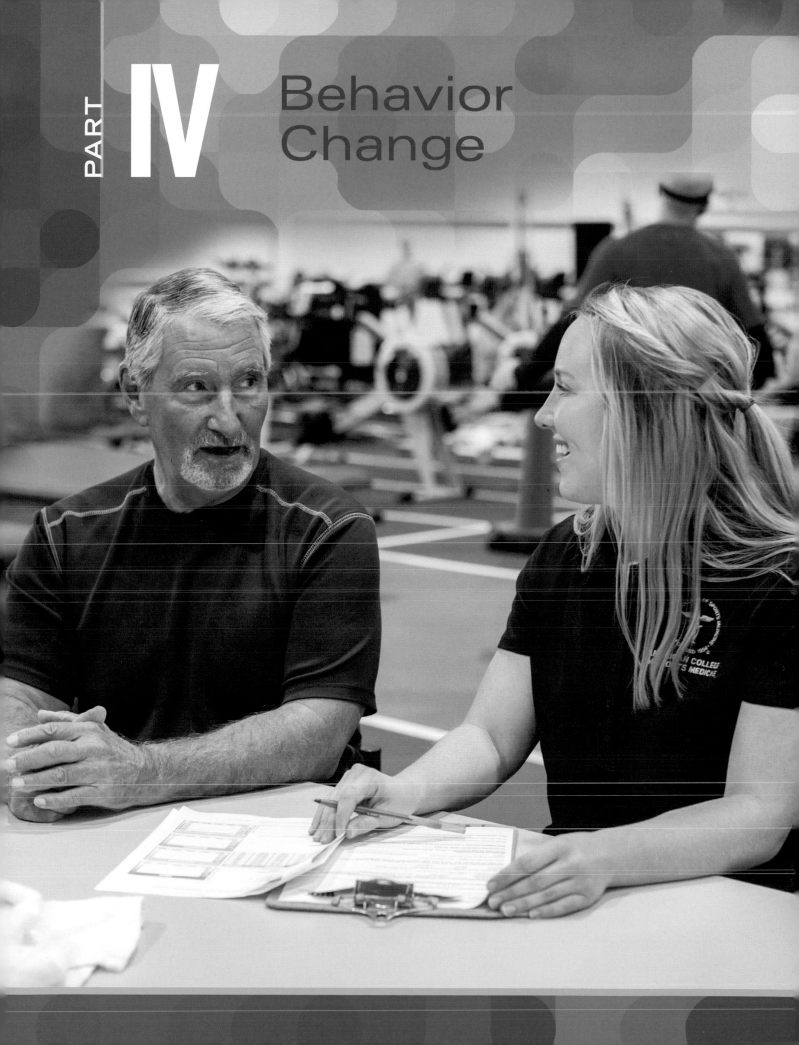

PART IV

Behavior Change

11

Theories of Behavior Change

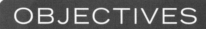

OBJECTIVES

- To identify and describe the theories and models used to explain physical activity behaviors.

- To understand key terminology as it relates to behavior change.

- To summarize the empirical support for the theories and models.

- To understand the practical application of the concepts presented in the chapter.

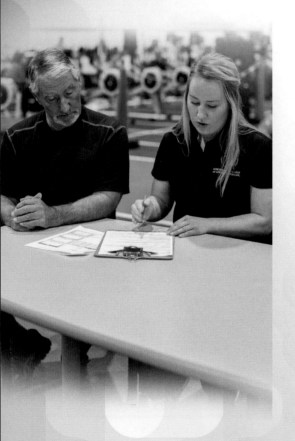

INTRODUCTION

This chapter summarizes theories and models important for physical activity behavior change, including the transtheoretical model (TTM), social cognitive theory (SCT), social ecological model, health belief model, theory of planned behavior (TPB), self-determination theory (SDT), and hedonic theory. The evidence supporting each of the theories will also be briefly outlined. In addition, the practical application of the theories will be briefly described. Chapter 12 will expand on this chapter by summarizing how concepts from these theories and models are applied to interventions designed to motivate individuals to adopt physical activity. Before the specific models and theories are reviewed, the difference between and importance of models and theories will be explored.

 ## What Is the Difference between a Theory and a Model?

A theory refers to a systematic view of a behavior by specifying relationships between variables and predicting specific behaviors and situations (29). Theories typically share three essential elements, namely (a) variables that influence the particular behavior, (b) the relationship between the variables, and (c) understanding the conditions in which the relationships occur or do not occur (57). Specifically related to physical activity, a theory would explain the variables that influence physical activity, how these variables interact with one another to influence physical activity, and the conditions under which physical activity occurs. Theories can also help in designing interventions for physical activity promotion. A model, on the other hand, is defined as a hypothetical depiction of a behavior or situation (30). Models do not attempt to understand the variables underlying a particular behavior but rather to represent what is happening with a particular behavior. It is important to note that these definitions are general guidelines, and researchers will occasionally use the terms *theory* and *model* interchangeably.

 ## Importance of Theories and Models

There are a number of reasons why it is important to utilize theories and models for physical activity. First, theories and models provide a framework for better understanding physical activity adoption. For example, practitioners may identify that their clients have low self-efficacy toward physical activity, which refers to one's confidence in his or her ability to engage in physical activity. Self-efficacy is derived from a specific and prominent theory, which will be discussed later in this chapter. The practitioner may be more successful at increasing the client's physical activity after discussing with him or her different strategies to increase self-efficacy. Second, theories and models can help practitioners understand why a client has stopped his or her physical activity participation. For example, the barrier of time is a frequently reported variable for stopping physical activity and thus could be addressed with the client. Third, theories and models allow the practitioner to identify which types of clients respond to which types of physical activity promotion strategies. For example, it may be especially important for adults with children to have spousal support for engaging in physical activity; yet, this may not be necessary for people without children living at home. In summary, models and theories provide the foundation for better understanding physical activity adoption and maintenance and can provide helpful tools for practitioners attempting to increase physical activity among their clients.

Transtheoretical Model

When discussing theories or models, it is important to understand that both cognitive and behavioral processes are relevant to behavior and behavior change. Cognitive processes are used to change the way we think about activity, whereas behavioral processes are used to change or initiate the actual behavior itself.

The TTM has been used to explain a variety of health behaviors (16,63,68,93), understand physical activity behavior, and to create physical activity interventions (48). Research indicates that physical activity interventions based on the TTM are efficacious for increasing physical activity among sedentary adults (19,50,51,56,61,65) and other groups (8,13,44). The TTM proposes that individuals move through a series of "stages of change" during physical activity adoption (18,62): (a) precontemplation, (b) contemplation, (c) preparation, (d) adoption, and (e) maintenance (48). These specific stages are outlined in Table 11.1.

Table 11.1	The Transtheoretical Model: Stages of Change	
Stage of Change	**Progression Through the Five Stages**	**Application to Physical Activity**
Precontemplation	Individuals in this stage are not intending to take action within the next 6 mo. There may be a variety of reasons why an individual would be in the precontemplation stage — uninformed about the health effects of a sedentary lifestyle, uninformed about the consequences, not motivated to make changes, or have made several failed attempts at physical activity adoption and is now discouraged or debilitated.	Stage 1: Inactive and not thinking about becoming more active These individuals do not currently engage in physical activity and do not plan on doing so in the near future.
Contemplation	Individuals in this stage are intending to alter their behavior within the next 6 mo. They may be becoming more aware of the pros of engaging in physical activity; however, the costs associated with physical activity may still outweigh the benefits.	Stage 2: Inactive and thinking about becoming more active These individuals are thinking about adopting physical activity and are planning to become more physically active within a reasonable time frame.
Preparation	Individuals in this stage are intending to increase their physical activity in the immediate future. These individuals may have a specific plan to change behavior and may be seeking out resources for assistance.	Stage 3: Doing some physical activity These individuals are currently doing physical activity but are not meeting the standards and guidelines identified by the American College of Sports Medicine.
Action	Individuals in this stage have made specific, measureable changes in their physical activity in the past 6 mo.	Stage 4: Doing enough physical activity These individuals are currently engaging in physical activity 5 d · wk^{-1} for at least 30 min each session. These individuals have participated in regular physical activity for <6 mo.
Maintenance	Individuals in this stage are maintaining their physical activity and are working to prevent relapse to old habits.	Stage 5: Making physical activity a habit These individuals have been participating in regular physical activity at the recommended levels for at least 6 mo.

Specific behavioral and cognitive processes occur and are utilized as individuals move through these stages of change. The various processes are thought to receive differential emphasis during particular stages of change (17,18,62,64). Cognitive processes of change include increasing knowledge, being aware of risks, caring about consequences to others, comprehending benefits, and increasing healthy opportunities. Behavioral processes of change include substituting alternatives, enlisting social support, rewarding yourself, committing yourself, and reminding yourself (45). These processes represent principles of change in behavior and are considered critical for movement through the various stages of the TTM.

Sufficient evidence exists to support the use of the TTM in facilitating physical activity behavior change regardless of the type of physical activity intervention (49,91). Both print- and telephone-based exercise interventions have been guided by the TTM, and each type of intervention has led to increasing levels of moderate-intensity physical activity for at least 6 months, especially relative to controls. Similarly, more technology rich physical activity interventions based on the TTM have also shown promise (13,83). This evidence supports the view that receiving a physical activity intervention guided by the TTM typically leads to increases in behavioral strategies, cognitive processes, self-efficacy, and positive changes in decisional balance (*i.e.*, relatively more pros than cons for becoming physically active when moving through the stages).

Social Cognitive Theory

SCT (5–7), first known as social learning theory, is one of the most popular theoretical frameworks for understanding physical activity adoption (52,81). SCT emphasizes reciprocal determinism, which is the interaction between individuals and their environments (Fig. 11.1). SCT identifies three main factors that influence behavior and behavioral choices: (a) the environment (*e.g.*, neighborhood and proximity to gym), (b) individual personality characteristics and/or experience (including cognitions), and (c) behavioral factors. According to SCT, behavior is the product of the interplay between these three factors. In other words, the environment can influence individuals and groups, but individuals and groups can also influence their environments, and in turn, govern their own behaviors.

A key concept related to SCT is self-efficacy (4–6). Self-efficacy refers to one's belief in his or her ability to successfully engage in and perform a specific behavior. The more confident one feels in his or her capabilities and skills to succeed (*i.e.*, higher self-efficacy), the more likely he or she will engage in that behavior (6). Capabilities and skills refer to the organization and execution of the necessary course of action required to produce the desired results. Intervention studies indicate that self-efficacy is likely an important component of physical activity behavior change for apparently healthy adults (45), children and older adults (19,47,82,86), and those with controlled disease (28,32,52,53,76).

Self-efficacy is a position of situation-specific confidence that is a product of, and therefore can be influenced by, four sources of information: (a) mastery experience, (b) vicarious experience, (c) verbal persuasion, and (d) physiological or affective states (6). First, mastery experience is the successful performance of the target behavior (in this case, physical activity), which should enhance perceptions of confidence, whereas failure to perform the behavior typically decreases confidence.

FIGURE 11.1. Reciprocal determinism: based on Bandura's social cognitive theory. (Reproduced with permission from Bandura A. *Social Foundations of Thought and Action: A Social Cognitive Theory.* Englewood Cliffs [NJ]: Prentice-Hall Inc.; 1986. 544 p.)

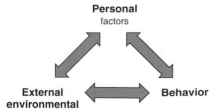

| **HOW TO** | **Determine an Individual's Stage or Change for Physical Activity** |

According to the TTM, interventions should be tailored to the individual depending on his or her stage of change. Specific to physical activity, it may be helpful to ask the following questions to determine an individual's stage of change:

1. Are you currently accumulating at least 150 min of moderate-intensity physical activity each week? (If yes, present stage is action or maintenance, and go to question 2; if no, go to question 3.)

2. Have you been regularly physically active over the past 6 months? (If yes, present stage is maintenance, and stop questions; if no, in action stage and stop questions.)

3. Are you doing any physical activity? (If yes, present stage is preparation and stop questions; if no, go to question 4.)

4. Have you made any actions and/or concrete plans in increasing your physical activity (*i.e.*, gym membership, purchasing exercise equipment, and hiring a trainer)? (If yes, present stage is preparation and stop questions; if no, go to question 5.)

5. Do you plan on becoming more physically active over the next 6 months? (If yes, present stage is contemplation; if no, present stage is precontemplation.)

For example, an individual who is able to successfully maintain a regular physical activity program for 6 weeks would demonstrate higher levels of perceived self-efficacy. Second, vicarious experience refers to seeing a similar individual successfully perform a behavior and comparing one's own performance with the performance of the other individual. Third, verbal persuasion occurs when others express faith in the individual's capabilities. Finally, the presence of an optimal emotional and affective state positively influences self-efficacy. Researchers have determined that mastery experience, verbal self-persuasion, and reduction in negative affective states as the most important predictors of high self-efficacy for physical activity among older adults (84).

Answers to these questions can facilitate the development of a more optimal plan of action specific to each client and tailored to the client's current stage or readiness. For those clients in the maintenance stage, the plan might just involve introducing new exercises or goals. For those in the contemplation or preparation stages, the plan will need to be more detailed and include guidance on how to handle setbacks.

Substantial evidence supports the SCT as an effective means of influencing human behavior and consequently, a viable resource for intervention design (80). Results compiled from multiple studies indicate that the most successful behavioral interventions for enhancing self-efficacy were found when vicarious experiences and feedback techniques (*e.g.*, providing feedback by comparing participants' performance with the performance of others, providing feedback on the participants' past performances) were used in an intervention (3). In addition, monitoring an individual's behavior and performance based on task mastery and skill development may also have a positive influence on self-efficacy. Setting a specific detailed plan and encouraging individuals to set a specific intention of how to adopt physical activity are common among successful intervention programs (89).

Interestingly, there is emerging literature indicating that focusing on relapse prevention techniques and identifying physical activity barriers may actually have a negative impact on physical activity and therefore are not recommended to enhance physical activity self-efficacy. Instead, the focus of interventions should be on what the individual can do to achieve the desired behavior change rather than emphasizing what they cannot do. This is believed to be the most effective means of improving self-efficacy toward physical activity (3,59,89).

EXERCISE IS MEDICINE CONNECTION

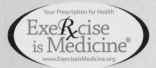

Wilcox S, Dowda M, Leviton LC, et al. Active for life: final results from the translation of two physical activity programs. *Am J Prev Med.* 2008;35:340–51.

Research now demonstrates that theory-based physical activity interventions are efficacious when translated into real-world settings. The interventions were "Active Choices" and "Active Living Everyday." Both interventions were based on SCT and the TTM. Active Choices lasted 6 months and included a face-to-face contact and up to eight telephone contacts. Participants were given a physical activity log, a pedometer, and a resource guide at the face-to-face visit. Participants set physical activity goals and were given strategies on the basis of SCT and TTM (*e.g.*, overcoming barriers and self-monitoring). Active Living Everyday was a 12-week program, whereby the physical activity program was delivered in small groups. There were nine organizations that disseminated the programs. Examples included Blue Shield of California, the Council on Aging of Southwestern Ohio, and the Berkeley Public Health Department. Participants included individuals who were at least 50 years of age and who were sedentary or underactive. Results indicated that the number of individuals meeting or exceeding the American College of Sports Medicine (ACSM)/Centers for Disease Control and Prevention (CDC) physical activity guidelines increased from pre- to posttest. The researchers reported that the interventions were adapted to meet the needs of the organization while maintaining high treatment fidelity. This study indicated that theory-based efficacious physical activity interventions can be successfully disseminated into real-world settings. Although these protocols do work for the period of time enlisted, there are still questions that arise in terms of whether there is continuation of necessary activity needs when the program ends? If there are a great number who do continue postprogram exercise, what are the underlining reasons for doing so and how can we all make that number grow and spread?

Although there are numerous correlates of physical activity, such as attitudes, perceived barriers, enjoyment, and expected benefits, the prevailing evidence supports self-efficacy as an important component of physical activity behavior change (81). However, despite this strong evidence, results of various self-efficacy–based interventions have been inconsistent. In general, there are consistent increases in physical activity (89) but inconsistent improvements in self-efficacy (34,35,45).

On the basis of SCT, there is still sufficient evidence to support the certified exercise physiologist (EP-C) focusing on increasing physical activity self-efficacy. Some techniques that could be used in building physical activity self-efficacy include the following:

- Verbal persuasion to reinforce task mastery.
- Provide exposure to positive vicarious experiences.
- Explain and reinforce the positive physiological states achieved from exercise.
- Encourage various forms of physical activity, noting what is most enjoyed.
- Encourage client recall of previous successful behavior change.
- Maintain a physical activity log to help track successes and progressions.
- Encourage reasonable, specific physical activity goals that can be achieved in a short time.
- Encourage perseverance and praise efforts to achieve goals, not just the attainment of goals.

Social Ecological Model

The social ecological model is a comprehensive approach integrating multiple variables and layers that influence behavior. These layers include intrapersonal and interpersonal factors, community and organizational factors, institutional factors, environmental factors, and public policies (Fig. 11.2). Within this model, each layer has a resulting impact on the next layer. For example, an individual's social environment of family, friends, and workplace are embedded within the physical environment of geography and community facilities. This is then embedded within and influenced by the policy environment of government or other official bodies. All levels of the social ecological model influence the behavior of the individual (12).

There are many versions of the social ecological model for physical activity, including systems theory, ecological model of health behavior, and social ecology model for health promotion. Each of these applications uses slightly different classifications of environmental influences. Systems theory uses the "microsystem" (*e.g.*, personal interactions between family members, work groups), "mesosystem" (physical settings for family, school, and work), and "exosystem" (the larger social influences including economics, policies, culture, and politics) (12). The social ecological model is specific to an individual's health behaviors and includes factors such as intrapersonal, interpersonal processes, institutional influences, community factors, and public policies (54). The social ecology model is specific to the promotion of health behaviors and focuses on assumptions related to influencing the physical and social environments; multidimensional environments; interactions between individuals, families, communities, and how individuals influence their surroundings (77,78).

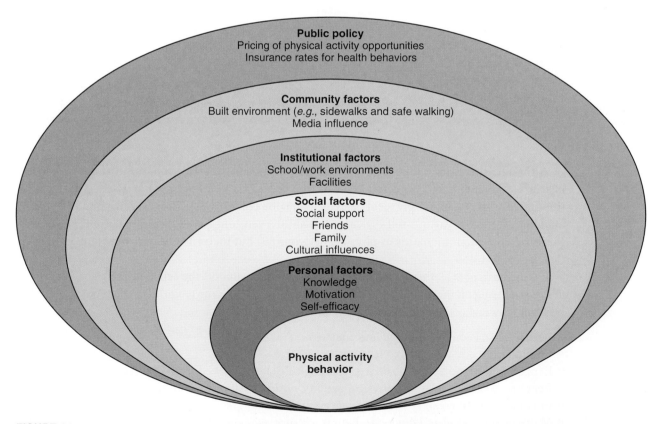

FIGURE 11.2. Social ecological model of physical activity behavior: based on Bronfenbrenner's social ecological model. (Reproduced with permission from Bronfenbrenner U. *The Ecology of Human Development: Experiments by Nature and Design.* Cambridge [MA]: Harvard University Press; 1979. 352 p.)

Many of the traditional ecological models were meant to apply broadly across a variety of behaviors; yet, more recent models have been developed to apply specifically to health behaviors (54,77,78). Researchers and practitioners have begun to acknowledge the significant role that the environment plays on health behaviors. Many health behaviors, including physical activity, are too complex to be adequately evaluated and understood by simply addressing the individual. Research suggests that coordinating and planning efforts among the agencies responsible for transportation, urban planning, school zoning, access to facilities and programs, and supporting social environments that encourage activity (*e.g.*, walking and biking trails, sidewalks, and reduction of crime) may help to optimize physical activity behavior (15,25,37,73,74).

Uncovering the motivational factors that underlie the successful adoption and maintenance of physical activity programs requires a multidimensional approach that considers not only behavioral change and intrapersonal factors but also social and environmental factors. The socioeconomic approach incorporates these considerations; however, the application of socioeconomic models can be difficult, as they need to be tailored and refined to meet the needs of specific behaviors and populations. A number of multidimensional models, specific to the physical activity domain, have been proposed and empirically supported (11,24,72). Research specific to adolescent girls described a framework that was created to promote physical activity behavior (24). This framework guided the intervention known as trial of activity for adolescent girls (TAAG) and adopted principles from behavioral modification, social cognitive, and organizational change theories to influence physical activity behavior in adolescent girls' intrapersonal, school, and community environments. The TAAG approach has been used to promote positive physical activity behaviors in middle school girls, and when incorporated in a school and community-based environment, girls in the intervention schools demonstrated a trend of increased physical activity in comparison with those in the schools that did not receive the program (24,85).

The social ecological model provides a useful framework for better understanding the multiple factors and barriers that influence physical activity behavior. Empirical evidence suggests that the social, physical, and policy environments influence physical activity participation. Behavior can be difficult to change, especially in an environment that does not support change. To increase physical activity, efforts may need to focus on both the behavior choices of each individual and factors that influence those choices. The social ecological model helps identify opportunities to promote participation in physical activity by recognizing the multiple variables that may influence an individual's choices.

As advocates of regular physical activity, EP-C may find that they are more successful at influencing an individual's physical activity when multiple levels of influence are addressed at the same time. According to this model, in order for physical activity interventions to be effective, the EP-C must go beyond simple exercise prescriptions. Other factors that influence physical activity behavior choices must also be addressed. For example, the EP-C may help the client choose new exercise equipment for the home, employ family members to join the physical activity program, decrease overall sedentary behavior, and assist in identifying possible environmental barriers to exercise. This holistic approach in providing physical activity guidance may help the EP-C develop more appropriate, sensitive, and effective motivational and intervention strategies.

Additional strategies the EP-C can use to create an environment that promotes physical activity include the following:

- Assist clients in identifying the wide variety of physical activity options that exist within proximity to their home. This may include parks, gyms, community centers, clubs, hiking trails, and the like.
- Discuss with your client the existing potential environmental barriers that deter him or her from regular physical activity.
- Encourage your client to join a walking or jogging club or training group.

Health Belief Model

The health belief model is a conceptual framework that outlines an individual's health behavior based on his or her health beliefs (70). The model suggests that as individuals take greater investment in their personal health, they are more likely to make relevant and meaningful behavior changes. The model identifies four main components that may influence an individual's health behavior choices as follows:

1. Perception of susceptibility or risk of the identified health threat
2. Perception of the severity of the identified health threat, including clinical and/or medical and social consequences
    a. Combined, these two factors create a "perceived threat" to each individual that will largely determine their level of interest in initiating change
3. Perception of the benefits from taking action to reduce the identified health threat
4. Perception of barriers and/or costs of taking action to reduce the identified health threat
    a. Combined, these two factors create a potential action plan for any given individual, assuming the perceived threat is great enough to create the need for action

According to the health belief model, an individual examines the negative aspects of a particular health action and/or behavior and weighs those "costs" with the benefits of the health action. If benefits outweigh the costs, then the individual is more likely to participate in the health action. For example, an individual may weigh the barriers of physical activity (*e.g.*, time-consuming, inconvenience, cost, and unpleasant) against the perceived benefits of physical activity (*e.g.*, reduction in risk of disease, weight management, and social connection). If the individual decides that the reduction in disease risk and weight loss (benefits) outweighs the cost of the inconvenience of physical activity, then that individual would experience higher levels of motivation to begin and/or maintain a regular exercise program. This can also be considered an equation in which (a) (susceptibility + seriousness) = perceived threat, (b) (benefits + barriers) = outcome expectation, and (c) (threat + expectations) = likelihood of action.

A comprehensive review of literature notes that the most powerful determinants of health behaviors were the perception of barriers and the costs of taking action (39). Perceived severity was the least powerful predictor of health behaviors; yet, the health belief model has been shown to have support when examining health behaviors and compliance with medical recommendation, particularly in older persons (10,36). However, the support for the health belief model applied to physical activity has been mixed (55,58).

Research examining the health belief model in women with Type 2 diabetes mellitus found that women who exercised regularly reported fewer barriers to exercise and perceived greater benefits from adhering to a regular exercise regimen than women who reported lower levels of physical activity (41). In addition, women indicated that the belief in the perceived benefits of exercise (health belief) was most strongly linked to desired behaviors (regular physical activity).

Although empirical evidence is inconclusive regarding the importance of the health belief model for physical activity adoption, practitioners can benefit from principles based on the model. On the basis of the health belief model's hypothesis of predicting health-related behaviors, the EP-C can do the following to assist his or her clients in adopting and maintaining a regular fitness regime:

1. Assist clients in identifying their personal susceptibility and potential severity of disease if regular physical activity does not become a lifestyle behavior.
2. Educate clients regarding the risk of a sedentary lifestyle on the basis of empirically supported research.
3. Assist clients in identifying the potential benefits of a regular physical activity program on the basis of their personal goals and motivation.
4. Prepare clients for the potential barriers of maintaining a regular physical activity program (*e.g.*, time, cost, sickness, family-related obligations, and work) and develop a plan for maintaining physical activity even when potential barriers appear to outweigh the benefits.

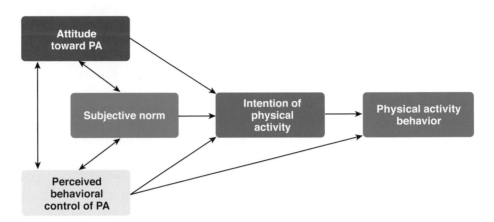

FIGURE 11.3. Theory of planned behavior: based on Ajzen's theory of planned behavior. (Adapted from Ajzen I. The theory of planned behavior. *Organ Behav Hum Decis Process.* 1991;50[2]:179–211 and Marcus BH, Forsyth LH. *Motivating People to Be Physically Active.* 2nd ed. Champaign [IL]: Human Kinetics; 2009. 216 p.)

 ## Theory of Planned Behavior

The TPB is an intention-based model used to explain physical activity behavior (1,33). The TPB is an extension of the theory of reasoned action (26) and identifies intention as the primary influence in determining behavior (see Fig. 11.3). Intention directly reflects the individual's level of motivation (*i.e.*, willingness and amount of effort exerted) to perform the desired behavior. According to the TPB, one's attitude, subjective norms, and perceived behavioral control influence intention, which then influences actual behavior. Specifically related to physical activity, attitude is defined as a positive or negative evaluation of physical activity. Subjective norm is the individual's perception of social pressure to participate, or not, in physical activity. Perceived behavioral control is the individual's perception of the ease or difficulty for engaging in physical activity. This can be perceived as similar to self-efficacy because it involves an individual's perception that he or she has the ability to execute the desired behavior.

The research literature is mixed in terms of support for intention predicting physical activity behavior (2,20,43). Although intention appears to be the most influential factor in predicting behavior, perceived behavioral control significantly adds to the prediction of actual behavior (31). Importantly, TPB predicts that perceived behavioral control may also directly impact behavior itself (20). Therefore, each can stand on its own to predict behavior; however, combined, they have a much stronger effect.

In using the TPB in practice, the EP-C may assist the client in identifying and developing their intentions. These intentions will then be influenced by the individual's attitude, perceived level of behavioral control, and subjective norm. An EP-C can encourage physical activity behavior by assisting in the development of self-efficacy, helping the client create an environment of support by recruiting coworkers and friends to provide encouragement and reminders for physical activity (subjective norm), and making physical activity easily accessible (perceived behavioral control). With these changes, the client's intention for physical activity behavior will be increased, causing an improvement in actual physical activity behavior.

Self-Determination Theory

SDT is built around the premise that individuals have three basic psychological needs that must be met in order to be motivated to engage in a behavior: (a) competence, (b) relatedness, and (c) autonomy (71). Competence is the sense of being capable of completing an activity or mastering a task and the perception of being effective in that task. Relatedness is the need to be connected and involved with the social world. Autonomy is characterized by maintaining a perceived internal locus of control and a sense that behaviors are freely chosen. When a behavior is self-determined, an individual perceives that the locus of control is internal to self. However, when an individual feels that a behavior is controlled, then they perceive the locus of control to be external to self. The more the individual feels he or she is engaging in self-directed behavior with a perceived internal locus of control, the more likely that individual will continue the desired behavior. For example, when individuals have an opportunity to freely choose which physical activities they engage in (perceived internal locus of control) versus being told specifically which mode of physical activity to engage in (perceived external locus of control), according to SDT, those individuals will be more likely to adhere with the desired physical activity behavior.

SDT proposes that the extent to which the needs (*i.e.*, competence, relatedness, and autonomy) are met describes how motivated an individual is to complete a task. In other words, when individuals in a social context feel competent, related, and autonomous, they will be motivated to participate in an activity and the motivation will be based on self-determination rather than an external factor.

Motivation is described as a continuum and ranges from amotivation, or a complete lack of motivation, to intrinsic motivation, or motivation based on enjoyment and excitement. According to SDT, motivations more proximal to intrinsic motivation are more likely to produce a motivational state that is conducive to desired behavior and adherence than motives more proximal to amotivation. An individual who is intrinsically motivated to participate in physical activity would be motivated by the genuine love of physical activity. An extrinsically motivated individual would engage in physical activity for reasons such as weight control and stress reduction. An amotivated person would not engage in physical activity because he or she has no motivation at all.

Also within the motivation continuum exists a threshold of autonomy, as not all extrinsic motives are the same and there may be a nonlinear prediction along the continuum. In addition, it is important to note that truly intrinsic motivation toward physical activity, or many other behaviors, may be somewhat rare and should not be considered necessary for successful change and continuation of exercise behavior. In fact, a person can exercise to avoid disease or exercise because being healthy is important; these may seem similar on the surface, but they are very different from a theoretical perspective. That is, exercising to avoid disease presumes some amount of pressure and coercion, whereas exercising to be healthy presumes free choice and autonomy.

SDT is a holistic, inclusive approach that can help gain a stronger understanding of exercise behavior and a better understanding of the intrapersonal (*e.g.*, psychological needs) and interpersonal (*e.g.*, influence of exercise environment) factors that influence physical activity. This theory considers the social context in which the individual operates. According to SDT, individuals who are in an autonomy supportive climate (a climate in which the client plays an active role in choosing how and/or what he or she learns) are more likely to feel like their needs of autonomy, relatedness, and competence are being met (71), which promotes greater intrinsic motivation. In addition, events that are interpreted by the individual to be informational, rather than controlling, will result in the endorsement of intrinsic motivating behaviors. According to this theory, sociocontextual variables can be manipulated to create an environment conducive to exercise. Therefore, this theory can provide insight into why individuals intend to adopt and maintain physical activity, as preliminary research supports SDT as a predictor of individual motivation to engage in physical activity (22,90).

SDT offers promise in explaining the behaviors that influence an individual's motivation. On the basis of the foundational principles of SDT, the EP-C may see improved levels of motivation for physical activity if the three innate psychological needs of autonomy, competence, and relatedness are met. Autonomy can be encouraged by allowing the client to have input on the physical activity plan, including choice of activity mode and intensity. Competence can be encouraged by making sure the client is entering a physical activity environment in which he or she will feel challenged but can be successful. For example, if working with a client who is just returning to running, encourage him or her to join a beginner group that would likely lead to success. Finally, the EP-C should encourage clients to exercise with others to meet the relatedness need component of SDT.

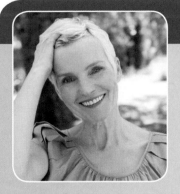

The Case of Anna

Submitted by **Steve McClaran, PhD, ACSM EP-C, Associate Professor, Colorado State University-Pueblo, Pueblo, CO**

Anna was an almost 60-year-old woman who could barely walk four blocks before beginning an exercise program. Anna had a history of attempting an exercise program in the past but had low adherence to these programs.

Narrative

When I first met Anna, we decided to go for a walk — she barely made it four blocks. Five years later after exercising regularly, she had lost more than 150 lb and walked a half marathon in 4 hours! She was almost 60 years when we started our project, and we concentrated on the process of behavior change. What were the best practices to stay motivated for exercise? We started with three questions:

1. Where are you now? To help with this question, we did a fitness assessment. As a note, we redid the fitness assessment after the first 3 months, again after 6 months, after a year, and then yearly for the next 5 years.
2. Where do you want to go? To help with this, we felt that first we wanted to personalize the goal. Anna had tried many times to be successful and had failed a lot! We started off slowly and used short-term goals every month. Of course, we had long-term goals, but we concentrated on the short-term goals to keep building her confidence in the long-term success. We continuously asked what the potential positive outcome was and then molded the goal to optimize the long-term outcome. Lastly, and maybe most importantly, we concentrated on focusing goals on specific and measurable behaviors rather than specific fitness outcomes. There was a strong sense that in Anna's past attempts, she concentrated on the outcomes as opposed to the behaviors that would lead to these positive outcomes. I feel that the behavior goals are the important and sustainable pieces of long-term behavior change.
3. How are you going to get there? We found that attention to behavior change skills was extremely helpful.

I know this has been discussed a lot, but we concentrated on discussion of benefits of physical activity, barriers or obstacles to long-term success, goal setting, social support, and monitoring her activities. It started with a commitment: We devised together a behavior change contract, and our responsibilities to the cause were delineated and signed. As far as benefits, not only is it the knowledge of what the benefits are but there was also a discussion of what she was feeling toward our original list of benefits every time during our weekly exercise walks. We felt that realizing the benefits during the behavior change process was critical for continued motivation. Social support strategies include practical support (logistics will be discussed later in the barriers section), technical support (I found a lot of shared experiences on the Internet and would find something each month to discuss during our weekly walks), group support (she joined a gym and did aerobics classes at the senior center), and emotional motivational support (she shared the experience with her sister, daughter, son, and her colleagues at work).

Barriers or obstacles were our next order of business to solve. We started with a list of five obstacles and then came up with creative and workable solutions to each of the issues. We looked on each of the obstacles as a challenge, and we revisited the five every 3 months to determine our progress. We also felt that logistics were the practical steps she needed to be successful with behavior change. As obvious and simple as logistics are, any failure to pay attention to logistical details is often a cause of relapse. If plan A didn't work for some reason, having plans B and C ready helped our chances of success. Planning for weather changes was essential for exercise; walking in cold weather means you need either different gear or an inside track. We found that scheduling exercise before work was logistically more effective than planning to do it later, when complications may interfere.

Logistical problems were never completely solved, so you want to help your client adopt the mindset of finding a solution to any problem that arises. We felt that environment control was an important consideration. First, we discussed removing herself from the presence of temptation. Anna owned her own business with four other women. Prior to her starting her journey toward the half-marathon, there was always some form of fattening pastries at the office, so she asked her partners if it was all right to bring in fruit and vegetable platters to replace the pastries, and they all agreed. Maybe more importantly was putting her in the presence of the desired behavior: She joined a gym and signed up for aerobics classes at the senior center. Concentrating on emotional control reduced both the risk of returning to the old behavior and increased the opportunity to engage in the new behavior. Anna also sets up a stationary bike and a Bowflex in the basement, which helped with those times that weather was an issue. As a further note, Anna found music when exercising in her basement! She would often share with me those songs that were the most inspirational. By the end of the third year, she had a library of more than 500 songs she could use and rock out to in her basement.

Reward systems worked for us. It seems that some people simply make a decision to do something, and do it, with no other need for rewards. Most of us need a system of reward that includes external incentives followed by internal ones. Some of us use disincentives, or punishments. A further variation is a balance system of earning rewards, such as working out to use the number of calories in the dessert we plan to have after dinner. Anna liked to put stickers on her calendar when she completed a desired behavior and then she gave herself a reward when she earned a certain number of stickers. Eventually, her continued success brought its own reward, and we felt that external rewards became more unnecessary. Another idea she came up with was to give her clothes away to charity as she lost weight and waist size. Anna felt that giving the clothes away would close that part of her life and make it more difficult to go back to the fit of those clothes.

Maybe one of the biggest reasons for Anna's success was the continued monitoring and reporting she did. Once she had completed her exercise for the week, she e-mailed me every Sunday evening. She is a pretty competitive person that in the first year and a half, she would sometimes exercise later in the week just so she wouldn't have to send in a low-volume exercise report. This I believe worked to help the new behavior become a habit. One interesting part about our monitoring and reporting plan was the first and second yearly summaries. After the first year, I used a computer graphing package to make a picture of how much she exercised every week — I made an average weekly amount of exercise line that went through each of the 52 bars that represented the amount of exercise for that week. As all of the weekly volume bars were on one page, both of us could see when the good and less good periods were. We then made some goals that would improve the amount of exercise time for those periods for the next year. This helped a lot with motivation. Eventually, we went with pedometers, which we believed significantly help by reminding and challenging her to achieve success. I crossed that finish line at the end of the half-marathon with Anna and her daughter.

It is difficult to describe how great it was to see how happy she was at accomplishing those many goals along her journey. Her daughter had cameras and video evidence, and many family members were there to help her celebrate. I have since moved half way across the country, but we still keep in touch. She sends me postcards from Africa, South America, and Europe as she and her sister do many hiking adventures that were essentially unavailable to her before she went on her successful exercise journey.

QUESTIONS

- How important are benefits?
- What is the process of successful behavior change?
- What were the most important aspects of the process you emphasized?

Hedonic Theory

A theoretical perspective that has received some attention but less than others discussed thus far is hedonic theory (40,92). Hedonic theory has been applied to better understanding several health behaviors; however, the application of hedonic theory to physical activity is a relatively new research area. Hedonic theory is an evolution of learning theory (79) and refers to individuals becoming accustomed to a positive or negative stimulus. This theory is based on the concept of "hedonic psychology," which states that the perceived utility of a behavior or experience is defined by an individual's affective response to the behavior (40). Within the context of physical activity, this means that feeling good in response to physical activity is more likely to lead to adherence. Individuals seeking to enhance or prolong pleasure and avoid or minimize pain are engaging in what is known as "the hedonic principle." Therefore, an individual's decision to engage in physical activity is due to the affective consequences or affective anticipation (*i.e.*, expectations) of the physical activity experience.

Research suggests that feelings can play an important role in accounting for exercise behavior (66). For example, researchers have found that sedentary participants who reported positive affective responses to a single session of moderate-intensity exercise at baseline reported more minutes of physical activity 6 months and a full year later (88). Additionally, research demonstrates that exercising at or just below the ventilatory threshold produces positive affect and pleasure, whereas intensities above the ventilatory threshold produces less pleasure (23). Other research demonstrates that allowing exercisers to self-select and maintain that intensity report more stable and positive affect in comparison to exercise imposed at a slightly higher intensity. However, participants who were told what intensity to use reported a decrease in positive affect (46). Additionally, research has noted that increases in positive affect during treadmill exercise predicted exercise behavior 3 months later (42). Taken together, these studies suggest that individuals may be more likely to adhere to self-paced exercise than higher intensity prescription-based exercise, especially sedentary adults (87).

Affective expectations have also been found to be predictive of physical activity behavior. For example, research indicates that participants exposed to a positive affective expectation manipulation prior to 10 minutes of exercise had a better postexercise mood and higher exercise intentions compared to a no-expectation condition (38). This study suggests that postexercise feelings, intentions, and, consequently, physical activity behaviors can be altered by exposure to an affective expectation manipulation. These results support previous research indicating that expecting exercise to improve affect predicts higher levels of exercise (21,27).

In summary, research suggests that exercise may be reinforcing for individuals who experience or expect positive affect as a result of exercise. Consequently, individuals who experience positive affect after exercise may be more likely to adhere to exercise programs. Although some individuals experience improvements in affect during exercise, others may experience no change or even an increase in negative affect (60). This may depend on contextual factors (*e.g.*, the setting in which the exercise takes place), stimulus factors (*e.g.*, exercise intensity), and individual differences (*e.g.*, the individual's current exercise level; 67). Additional research is needed that examines the application of hedonic theory to exercise behavior, but existing research provides encouragement that this concept can be used to improve the efficacy of physical activity interventions.

Based on the research thus far, the EP-C can engage in the following strategies based on hedonic theory to help his or her clients adopt and maintain physical activity:

1. Work with clients to determine their personal preferences regarding intensity level.
2. Brainstorm with the client to create a list of new types of exercise and encourage the client to try these new exercises.
3. Discuss with the clients various strategies that would make exercise more enjoyable. For example, listening to music while walking or buying more comfortable workout clothing.

4. Determine the time of day that elicits the most positive affect for the client following exercise.
5. Prior to an exercise session, work with the client to generate a list of positive associations with exercise and actively reframe negative associations with exercise.
6. As the EP-C, work with the client to identify positive outcomes that occur immediately after exercise and throughout the day (*e.g.*, more energy, better sleep).

SUMMARY

In recent years, an expansion has occurred in the number and type of factors examined as correlates and determinates of physical activity behaviors, moving past individual factors and adopting multidimensional models and theories of behavior change (9). The TTM, SCT, social ecological model, health belief model, TPB, and SDT have been used to better understand physical activity behavior. The TTM has been researched most frequently followed by SCT and the TBP (69). Self-determination and hedonic theories are newer but have received greater interest recently (14,75). Even though there is less support for the social ecological model, health belief model, and the TBP, EP-Cs can use tools from these models to motivate individuals to adopt physical activity. For any EP-C, there is a need to fully understand the psychological processes that influence the adoption and maintenance of physical activity across all populations. Otherwise, simply prescribing an exercise prescription without considering the behavioral aspects of why someone may or may not fully engage in physical activity will likely lead to low retention rates.

The purpose of this chapter was to outline the basic tenets of various theories and models that have been applied to physical activity behavior. Chapter 12 will explore in more detail how these theories have been specifically applied to interventions and how the EP-Cs can provide these theory-based interventions to physical activity behavior change among their clients.

STUDY QUESTIONS

1. What is the difference between a theory and a model?
2. What are the five stages of change, as identified by the TTM? How would an EP-C use the five stages of change to assess his or her client's readiness to participate in physical activity?
3. What are the four sources of self-efficacy? What techniques would an EP-C use to improve self-efficacy?
4. Briefly describe other models of change (SCT, health belief model, SDT) and how the EP-C could use them to increase physical activity participation.
5. How does the hedonic theory explain promotion and adherence to physical activity?

REFERENCES

1. Ajzen I. The theory of planned behavior. *Organ Behav Hum Decis Process*. 1991;50(2):179–211.
2. Armitage C. Can the theory of planned behavior predict the maintenance of physical activity? *Health Psychol*. 2005;24(3):235–45.
3. Ashford S, Edmunds J, French DP. What is the best way to change self-efficacy to promote lifestyle and recreational physical activity? A systematic review with meta-analysis. *Br J Health Psychol*. 2010;15(2):265–88.
4. Bandura A. Self-efficacy mechanism in psychobiologic functioning. In: Schwarzer R, editor. *Self-efficacy: Thought Control of Action*. Washington (DC): Hemisphere Publishing; 1992. p. 355–94.
5. Bandura A. *Self-Efficacy: The Exercise of Control*. New York (NY): W.H. Freeman and Company; 1997. 604 p.
6. Bandura A. Self-efficacy: toward a unifying theory of behavioral change. *Psychol Rev*. 1977;84(2):191–215.
7. Bandura A. *Social Foundations of Thought and Action: A Social Cognitive Theory*. Englewood Cliffs (NJ): Prentice-Hall; 1986. 544 p.
8. Bassilios B, Judd F, Pattison P, Nicholas A, Moeller-Saxone K. Predictors of exercise in individuals with schizophrenia: a test of the transtheoretical model of behavior change. *Clin Schizophr Relat Psychoses*. 2015;8(4):173A–82.
9. Bauman AE, Reis R, Sallis JF, Wells JC, Loos R, Martin BW. Correlates of physical activity: why are some people physically active and others not? *The Lancet*. 2012;380(9838):258–71.
10. Becker MH, Maiman LA, Kirscht JP, Don PH, Drachman RH. The health belief model and prediction of dietary compliance: a field experiment. *J Health Soc Behav*. 1977;18(4):348–66.
11. Booth SL, Sallis JF, Ritenbaugh C, et al. Environmental and societal factors affect food choice and physical activity: rationale, influences, and leverage points. *Nut Rev*. 2001;59(3):S21–36.
12. Bronfenbrenner U. *The Ecology of Human Development: Experiments by Nature and Design*. Cambridge (MA): Harvard University Press; 1979. 352 p.
13. Carlson J, Sallis J, Ernesto R, Ramirez K, Norman GJ. Physical activity and dietary behavior change in Internet-based weight loss interventions: comparing two multiple-behavior change indices. *Prev Med*. 2012;54(1):50–4.
14. Chatzisarantis NL, Hagger MS. Effects of an intervention based on self-determination theory on self-reported leisure-time physical activity participation. *Psychol Health*. 2009;24(1):29–48.
15. Davison K, Lawson C. Do attributes in the physical environment influence children's physical activity? A review of the literature. *Int J Behav Nut Phys Act*. 2006;3(1):19.
16. de Menezes MC, Mingoti SA, Cardoso CS, de Deus Mendonça R, Lopes ACS. Intervention based on transtheoretical model promotes anthropometric and nutritional improvements — a randomized controlled trial. *Eat Behav*. 2015;17:37–44.
17. DiClemente CC, Prochaska JO. Self-change and therapy change of smoking behavior: a comparison of processes of change in cessation and maintenance. *Addict Behav*. 1982;7(2):133–42.
18. DiClemente CC, Prochaska JO, Fairhurst SK, Velicer WF, Velasquez MM, Rossi JS. The process of smoking cessation: an analysis of precontemplation, contemplation, and preparation stages of change. *J Consult Clin Psychol*. 1991;59(2):295–304.
19. Dishman RK, Motl RW, Saunders R, et al. Self-efficacy partially mediates the effect of a school-based physical-activity intervention among adolescent girls. *Prev Med*. 2004;38:628–36.
20. Duncan MJ, Rivis A, Jordan C. Understanding intention to be physically active and physical activity behaviour in adolescents from a low socio-economic status background: an application of the theory of planned behaviour. *J Adolesc*. 2011;35(3):761–4.
21. Dunton GF, Vaughan E. Anticipated affective consequences of physical activity adoption and maintenance. *Health Psychol*. 2008;27(6):703–10.
22. Edmunds J, Ntoumanis N, Duda JL. Testing a self-determination theory-based teaching style intervention in the exercise domain. *Eur J Soc Psychol*. 2008;38(2):375–88.
23. Ekkekakis P, Hall EE, Petruzzello SJ. Practical markers of the transition from aerobic to anaerobic metabolism during exercise: rationale and a case for affect-based exercise prescription. *Prev Med*. 2004;38(2):149–59.
24. Elder JP, Lytle L, Sallis JF, et al. A description of the social-ecological framework used in the trial of activity for adolescent girls (TAAG). *Health Educ Res*. 2007;22(2):155–65.
25. Ewing R, Schmid T, Killingsworth R, Zlot A, Raudenbush S. Relationship between urban sprawl and physical activity, obesity, and morbidity. *Am J Health Promot*. 2003;18(1):47–57.
26. Fishbein M, Ajzen I. *Belief, Attitude, Intention, and Behavior: An Introduction to Theory and Research*. Reading (MA): Addison-Wesley; 1975. 480 p.
27. Gellert P, Ziegelmann JP, Schwarzer R. Affective and health-related outcome expectancies for physical activity in older adults. *Psychol Health*. 2012;27(7):816–28.
28. Ginis KA, Latimer AE, Arbour-Nicitopoulos KP, Bassett RL, Wolfe DL, Hanna SE. Determinants of physical activity among people with spinal cord injury: a test of social cognitive theory. *Ann Behav Med*. 2011;42(1):127–33.
29. Glanz K, Lewis FM, Rimer BK. Theory, research, and practice in health behavior and health education. In: Glanz K, Rimer BK, Lewis FM, editors. *Health Behavior and Health Education: Theory, Research, and Practice*. 3rd ed. San Francisco (CA): Jossey-Bass; 2002. 592 p.
30. Glanz K, Rimer BK. *Theory at a Glance: A Guide for Health Promotion Practice (NIH Pub. No. 95-3896)*. Washington (DC): National Cancer Institute; 1995. 94 p.
31. Godin G, Kok G. The theory of planned behavior: a review of its applications to health-related behaviors. *Am J Health Promot*. 1996;11(2):87–98.
32. Haas BK. Fatigue, self-efficacy, physical activity, and quality of life in women with breast cancer. *Cancer Nurs*. 2011;34(4):322–34. doi:10.1097/NCC.0b013e3181f9a300.
33. Hagger MS, Chatzisarantis NLD, Biddle SJH. A meta-analytic review of the theories of reasoned action and planned behavior in physical activity: predictive validity and the contribution of additional variables. *J Sport Exerc Psychol*. 2002;24(1):3–32.

34. Hallam J, Petosa R. A worksite intervention to enhance social cognitive theory constructs to promote exercise adherence. *Am J Health Promot.* 1998;13(1):4–7.

35. Hallam JS, Petosa R. The long-term impact of a four-session work-site intervention on selected social cognitive theory variables linked to adult exercise adherence. *Health Educ Behav.* 2004;31(1):88–100.

36. Harrison JA, Mullen PD, Green LW. A meta-analysis of studies of the health belief model with adults. *Health Educ Res.* 1992;7(1):107–16.

37. Heath GW, Brownson RC, Kruger J, et al. The effectiveness of urban design and land use and transport policies and practices to increase physical activity: a systematic review. *J Phys Act Health.* 2006;3(Suppl 1):S55–76.

38. Helfer SG, Elhai JD, Geers AL. Affect and exercise: positive affective expectations can increase post-exercise mood and exercise intentions. *Ann Behav Med.* 2015;49(2):269–79.

39. Janz NK, Becker MH. The health belief model: a decade later. *Health Educ Behav.* 1984;11(1):1–47.

40. Kahneman D, Diener E, Schwarz N, editors. *Well-Being: Foundations of Hedonic Psychology.* New York (NY): Russell Sage Foundation; 1999. 605 p.

41. Koch J. The role of exercise in the African-American woman with type 2 diabetes mellitus: application of the health belief model. *J Am Acad Nurse Pract.* 2002;14(3):126–30.

42. Kwan BM, Bryan AD. Affective response to exercise as a component of exercise motivation: attitudes, norms, self-efficacy, and temporal stability of intentions. *Psychol Sport Exer.* 2010; 11(1):71–9.

43. Kwan MYW, Bray SR, Ginis KA. Predicting physical activity of first-year university students: an application of the theory of planned behavior. *J Am Coll Health.* 2009;58(1):45–52.

44. Lewis BA, Gjerdingen DK, Avery MD, et al. A randomized trail examining a physical activity intervention for the prevention of postpartum depression: the healthy mom trial. *Ment Health Phys Act.* 2014;7(1):42–9.

45. Lewis BA, Marcus BH, Pate RR, Dunn AL. Psychosocial mediators of physical activity behavior among adults and children. *Am J Prev Med.* 2002;23(2 Suppl 1):26–35.

46. Lind E, Ekkekakis P, Vazou, S. The affective impact of exercise intensity that slightly exceeds the preferred level 'pain' for no additional 'gain.' *J Health Psychol.* 2008;13(4): 464–8.

47. Manley D, Cowan P, Graff C, et al. Self-efficacy, physical activity, and aerobic fitness in middle school children: examination of a pedometer intervention program. *J Pediatr Nurs.* 2014;29(3):228–37.

48. Marcus BH, Forsyth LH. *Motivating People to Be Physically Active.* 2nd ed. Champaign (IL): Human Kinetics; 2009. 216 p.

49. Marcus BH, Napolitano MA, King AC, et al. Telephone versus print delivery of an individualized motivationally tailored physical activity intervention: project STRIDE. *Health Psychol.* 2007;26(4):401–9.

50. Marcus BH, Rossi JS, Selby VC, Niaura RS, Abrams DB. The stages and processes of exercise adoption and maintenance in a worksite sample. *Health Psychol.* 1992;11(6):386–95.

51. Marshall S, Biddle S. The transtheoretical model of behavior change: a meta-analysis of applications to physical activity and exercise. *Ann Behav Med.* 2001;23(4):229–46.

52. McAuley E, Blissmer B. Self-efficacy determinants and consequences of physical activity. *Exerc Sport Sci Rev.* 2000; 28(2):85–8.

53. McAuley E, White SM, Rogers LQ, Motl RW, Courneya KS. Physical activity and fatigue in breast cancer and multiple sclerosis: psychosocial mechanisms. *Psychosom Med.* 2010;72(1):88–96.

54. McLeroy KR, Bibeau D, Steckler A, Glanz K. An ecological perspective on health promotion programs. *Health Educ Behav.* 1988;15(4):351–77.

55. Mirotznik J, Feldman L, Stein R. The health belief model and adherence with a community center-based, supervised coronary heart disease exercise program. *J Community Health.* 1995;20(3):233–47.

56. Nigg CR, Courneya KS. Transtheoretical model: examining adolescent exercise behavior. *J Adolesc Health.* 1998;22(3):214–24.

57. Nutbeam D, Harris E. *Theory in a Nutshell: A Guide to Health Promotion Theory.* Sydney (Australia): The McGraw-Hill Companies Inc.; 1999. 96 p.

58. O'Connell JK, Price JH, Roberts SM, Jurs SG, McKinley R. Utilizing the health belief model to predict dieting and exercising behavior of obese and nonobese adolescents. *Health Educ Behav.* 1985;12(4):343–51.

59. Olander EK, Fletcher H, Williams S, Atkinson L, Turner A, French DP. What are the most effective techniques in changing obese individuals' physical activity self-efficacy and behaviour: a systematic review and meta-analysis. *Int J Behav Nutr Phys Act.* 2013;10(29):1–15.

60. Parfitt G, Rose EA, Burgess WM. The psychological and physiological responses of sedentary individuals to prescribed and preferred intensity exercise. *Brit J Health Psych.* 2006;11(1):39–53.

61. Plotnikoff RC, Lubans DR, Costigan SA, et al. A test of the theory of planned behavior to explain physical activity in a large population sample of adolescents from Alberta, Canada. *J Adolesc Health.* 2011;49(5):547–9.

62. Prochaska JO, DiClemente CC. Stages and processes of self-change of smoking: toward an integrative model of change. *J Consult Clin Psychol.* 1983;51(3):390–5.

63. Prochaska JO, DiClemente CC, Norcross JC. In search of how people change: applications to addictive behaviors. *Am Psychol.* 1992;47(9):1102–14.

64. Prochaska JO, Velicer WF, DiClemente CC, Fava J. Measuring processes of change: applications to the cessation of smoking. *J Consult Clin Psychol.* 1988;56(4):520–8.

65. Prochaska JO, Velicer WF, Rossi JS, et al. Stages of change and decisional balance for 12 problem behaviors. *Health Psychol.* 1994;13(1):39–46.

66. Reed J, Buck S. The effect of regular aerobic exercise on positive-activated affect: a meta-analysis. *Psych Sport Exer.* 2009; 10:581–94.

67. Reed J, Ones DS. The effect of acute aerobic exercise on positive activated affect: a meta-analysis. *Psychol Sport Exerc.* 2006;7(5):477–514.

68. Reisenhofer S, Taft A. Women's journey to safety — the transtheoretical model in clinical practice when working with women experiencing intimate partner violence: a scientific review and clinical guidance. *Patient Educ Couns.* 2013;93(3): 536–48.

69. Rhodes RE, Pfaeffli LA. Mediators of physical activity behavior change among adult non-clinical populations: a review update. *Int J Behav Nut Phys Act*. 2010;7:37.

70. Rosenstock I. Historical origins of the health belief model. *Health Educ Monogr*. 1974;2:328–35.

71. Ryan RM, Deci EL. Self-determination theory and the facilitation of intrinsic motivation, social development, and well-being. *Am Psychol*. 2000;55(1):68–78.

72. Saelens B, Sallis J, Frank L. Environmental correlates of walking and cycling: findings from the transportation, urban design, and planning literatures. *Ann Behav Med*. 2003;25(2):80–91.

73. Sallis JF, Bauman A, Pratt M. Environmental and policy interventions to promote physical activity. *Am J Prev Med*. 1998;15(4):379–97.

74. Sallis JF, Floyd MF, Rodríguez DA, Saelens BE. Role of built environments in physical activity, obesity, and cardiovascular disease. *Circulation*. 2012;125(5):729–37.

75. Silva MN, Vieira PN, Coutinho SR, et al. Using self-determination theory to promote physical activity and weight control: a randomized controlled trial in women. *J Behav Med*. 2009;33:110–22.

76. Snook EM, Motl RW. Physical activity behaviors in individuals with multiple sclerosis: roles of overall and specific symptoms, and self-efficacy. *J Pain Symptom Manage*. 2008;36(1):46–53.

77. Stokols D. Establishing and maintaining healthy environments: toward a social ecology of health promotion. *Am Psychol*. 1992;47(1):6–22.

78. Stokols D, Grzywacz JG, McMahan S, Phillips K. Increasing the health promotive capacity of human environments. *Am J Health Promot*. 2003;18(1):4–13.

79. Thorndike EL. The law of effect. *Am J Psychol*. 1927;39:212–22.

80. Tougas ME, Hayden JA, McGrath PJ, Huguet A, Rozario S. A systematic review exploring the social cognitive theory of self-regulation as a framework for chronic health condition interventions. *PLoS One*. 2015;10(8):e0134977.

81. Trost SG, Owen N, Bauman AE, Sallis JF, Brown W. Correlates of adults' participation in physical activity: review and update. *Med Sci Sports Exerc*. 2002;34(12):1996–2001.

82. Valois RF, Umstattd MR, Zullig KJ, Paxton RJ. Physical activity behaviors and emotional self-efficacy: is there a relationship for adolescents? *J Sch Health*. 2008;78(6):321–7.

83. Van den Berg MH, Schoones JW, Vlieland TP. Internet-based physical activity interventions: a systematic review of the literature. *J Med Internet Res*. 2007;9(3):e26.

84. Warner LM, Schüz B, Wolff JK, Parschau L, Wurm S, Schwarzer R. Sources of self-efficacy for physical activity. *Health Psych*. 2014;33(11):1298–308.

85. Webber LS, Catellier DJ, Lytle LA, et al. Promoting physical activity in middle school girls: trial of activity for adolescent girls. *Am J Prev Med*. 2008;34(3):173–84.

86. White SM, Wójcicki TR, McAuley E. Social cognitive influences on physical activity behavior in middle-aged and older adults. *J Gerontol B Psychol Sci Soc Sci*. 2011;67(1):18–26.

87. Williams DM. Exercise, affect, and adherence: an integrated model and a case for self-paced exercise. *J Sport Exer Psychol*. 2008;30(5):471–96.

88. Williams DM, Dunsiger S, Ciccolo JT, Lewis BA, Albrecht AE, Marcus BH. Acute affective response to a moderate-intensity exercise stimulus predicts physical activity participation 6 and 12 months later. *Psychol Sport Exer*. 2008;9(3):231–45.

89. Williams SL, French DP. What are the most effective intervention techniques for changing physical activity self-efficacy and physical activity behaviour — and are they the same? *Health Educ Res*. 2011;26(2):308–22.

90. Wilson PM, Rodgers WM. The relationship between perceived autonomy support, exercise regulations and behavioral intentions in women. *Psychol Sport Exerc*. 2004;5(3):229–42.

91. Yang HJ, Chen KM, Chen MD, et al. Applying the transtheoretical model to promote functional fitness of community older adults participating in elastic band exercises. *J Adv Nurs*. 2015;71(10):2338–49.

92. Young PT. The role of hedonic processes in the organization of behavior. *Psych Review*. 1952;59(4):249.

93. Yusufov M, Rossi JS, Redding CA, et al. Transtheoretical model constructs' longitudinal prediction of sun protection over 24 months. *Int J Behav Med*. 2016;23(1):71–3.

12 Facilitating Health Behavior Change

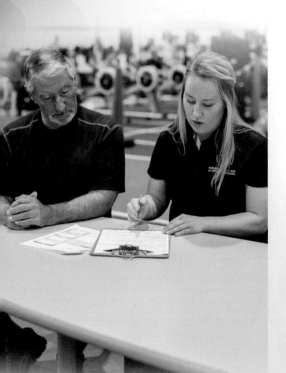

- To describe common strategies useful in facilitating positive health behavior change, especially as it concerns exercise and physical activity.

- To evaluate common threats to successful behavior change and maintenance and how these threats can be overcome.

- To encourage review and evaluation of current and future research on facilitators and barriers to health behavior change for the evidence-based practitioner.

INTRODUCTION

Theory-based behavioral interventions are an effective means for increasing physical activity among sedentary adults (16,23). These interventions can provide the health fitness professional with a framework for helping clients adopt a new exercise program or adhere to an existing exercise program. More specifically, theory-based interventions that are tailored to each individual's specific interests, preferences, and readiness for change can teach behavioral skills that help individuals incorporate exercise into their daily routines. The purpose of this chapter is to expand on Chapter 11, which discussed various theories related to exercise promotion, by applying theory to practice. This chapter summarizes several intervention strategies, including using self-regulation strategies (*e.g.*, self-monitoring, goal setting, self-control); overcoming barriers to exercise; increasing social support; identifying outcome expectancies; and engaging in motivational interviewing, relapse prevention, and effective communication.

Understanding Client Behavior

An idea asserted in recent years is that exercise is medicine. Indeed, exercise can be a powerful tool for promoting health, but benefits from this medication are only experienced when the medication is taken regularly. Thus, we must examine ways to facilitate exercise adoption and maintenance to more fully realize the medicinal power of exercise. These efforts are especially important in light of the difficulties many people face in changing their exercise and physical activity behavior. Research indicates that the vast majority of Americans are not meeting minimal physical activity guidelines (32). This large majority is not only those who do not desire to live an active lifestyle but also those who have intention to be active but do not have the skills and abilities to successfully self-regulate the behavior (1).

Self-regulation is the process of monitoring and changing one's behavior when normalcy is interrupted. Normal for many people is an inactive lifestyle, often paired with a poor diet, stress, and poor sleep. This lifestyle is habitual, automatic, and comfortable. Normal is having a sedentary job and a day-to-day routine that tends to all other priorities (*e.g.*, work, family, hobbies), instead of giving time and attention to being physically active. When this normalcy is interrupted, such as with a medical diagnosis and exercise prescription, many individuals initiate a process of trying to monitor and change their behavior to align with their new healthy lifestyle goals. However, many do not have the self-regulatory abilities to successfully carry out the behavior change thus are at risk for falling back to where they are more comfortable—normalcy.

An Evidence-Based Practice

Health fitness professionals must have the knowledge and understanding to help facilitate behavior change in their clients during these difficult times. Thus, in this chapter, key factors associated with facilitating and guiding healthy behavior change are presented. This chapter will also explore strategies to overcome the threats that can undermine successful behavioral efforts. Although, examples are provided, many of which are related to physical activity, the professional should consider his or her own examples across multiple health behaviors and based on specific situations and populations of interest. In addition, as an evidence-based practitioner, the professional should stay attune to the research evidence, as well as further explore the research presented in this chapter. In doing so, health fitness professionals can better meet specific practice needs.

Facilitating Behavior Change

Self-Monitoring

Behavior change begins with self-monitoring, which brings about awareness of positive and negative behaviors and cognitions through "paying attention on purpose." It is beneficial for clients to use self-monitoring to maintain their awareness, thus creating opportunity for change. Without self-monitoring, clients might not be aware of behaviors or cognitions that are hindering their behavioral efforts or able to alter behaviors and cognitions to keep them on track to their goals. With self-monitoring, clients can increase their opportunity to facilitate behavior change. For example, regular self-monitoring of weight by way of weighing oneself on a schedule is associated with weight loss and the prevention of weight gain (56,57). As such, self-monitoring of physical activity can be a fruitful facilitator of behavior change. However, there are some key features to self-monitoring, especially concerning physical activity and exercise that will optimize its effectiveness (28).

Self-Monitoring Recommendations

1. Provide prompt self-monitoring of behavior as an explicitly stated, important component of the client's efforts.
2. Provide prompt intention formation so that clients are explicitly encouraged to form intentions, make plans, and commit to doing the behavior.
3. Provide immediate feedback on performance, which involves providing clients with data about and commenting on their recorded behavior.
4. Provide self-monitoring tasks that do not require excessive amounts of thought and energy to lessen the self-regulatory and self-control demands and increase the odds of successful usage.
5. Provide prompt goal setting and review that includes behavioral goals, such as the target number of steps to engage in each day (*e.g.*, ≥7,500).
6. Encourage use of consistent self-monitoring, which is better than intermittent self-monitoring (33).

It is advised to recognize the perceived advantages, barriers, facilitators, and consequences of self-monitoring. Consider physical activity monitoring as an example. *Perceived advantages* of monitoring physical activity might be the reassurance that activity goals are being met, or feeling that such monitoring can help them assess the effects of behavior. *Perceived barriers* of monitoring physical activity might be lack of specific instructions, or the threat of monitoring reminding the client of his or her poor fitness or health. *Facilitators* enhance the use of self-monitoring, such as providing instructions on self-monitoring or encouraging the client through positive messages and feedback to the client. *Consequences* of self-monitoring can be either positive (*e.g.*, improved behavior or clinical outcomes) or negative (*e.g.*, dislike of the monitoring process). Awareness of these key factors can help clients' use of self-monitoring be more effective in facilitating behavior change.

Physical Activity Monitors

As new activity monitoring technology continues to emerge, pedometers have ample support to facilitate behavior change, especially when a step goal is provided (17). Pedometers can be a simple, convenient, and cost-efficient method of physical activity monitoring for adult clients, alongside the easy-to-follow guidelines for meeting physical activity recommendations for physical activity (≥7,500 steps per day), exercise (3,000 of total daily steps at 100 steps per minute), and limiting sitting time (>5,000 steps per day) (50,51). Guidelines have also been established for older adults (48) and children/adolescents (49). In addition, 3 days of self-monitoring with pedometer can provide sufficient estimate of the number of steps one gets per day, thus useful in physical activity assessment of clients (47).

Other physical activity monitors are also showing promise, although the research cannot keep up with the growing market. With this growth, the exercise professional can be excited but wary that all of these new monitors are valid measures of physical activity. That is, not every monitor is valid or accurately assesses activity amounts. Of the more popular consumer-grade monitors, the Fitbit accelerometer is showing promise as a valid measure of steps and energy expenditure (5,19). Like the Fitbit and other similar wearable monitors, smart phones use accelerometer technology to measure movement and research evidence is providing support that phone-based monitoring tools can provide valid and reliable physical activity information (15,30). Worthwhile goals of the health fitness professional are to have good familiarity with the various products and technology used in monitoring and to stay current on the research that evaluates the scientific validity of these tools. Similarly, the exercise professional should be comfortable discussing complimentary self-monitoring values, such as heart rate ranges or ratings of perceived exertion (RPE), during exercise. In addition, clients are becoming armed with more, evolving health information related to monitoring their behavior, progress, and/or outcomes; thus, the exercise professional should also ensure that clients are adequately and correctly informed to self-monitor.

Goal Setting and Shaping

Behavior cannot be understood without being aware of the standard or goal that the client holds. For example, is the goal to improve health parameters look like a fitness model, achieve a weight held back in college, or fit into a particular piece of clothing? Perhaps the client's goal is to actually be inactive and continue to eat a preferred yet unhealthy diet. Thus, it is important to understand the goals that clients have to properly understand their thoughts and behavioral choices. At the same time, the health fitness professional is tasked with helping clients achieve new, healthy goals. Thus, there are some key features of goals that can enhance the effectiveness of facilitating behavior change and maintenance.

Goal setting has long been established as an effective strategy for exercise adherence (42). Therefore, goal setting is an important component of the overall exercise prescription plan. Goals refer to inherently valued, futuristic outcomes that are derived from a level of dissatisfaction with the present condition or circumstance. Goals should direct effort and attention toward activities that are goal-relevant and away from those that are irrelevant (22). Goals also increase persistence, knowledge, and skill attainment. The strategies and tools used to set health behavior–related goals vary; however, the majority of goals should address the following key components to ensure that goals are SMART:

- *Specific:* carefully identify the what, where, and how aspect of the goal
- *Measureable:* ensure that change and progress are clearly noted
- *Attainable:* set up goals that are challenging but within reach with good effort
- *Relevant:* focus energy toward goals that help achieve outcomes that are highly valued
- *Time-bound:* explicitly state dates for goal completion

Explicit goals that state the desired outcome exactly reduce the ambiguity of the task, which makes the achievement of the goal more likely. In contrast, setting goals that are too vague, complex, or difficult can limit success and therefore negatively impact one's confidence to exercise (43). Setting specific short-term goals in the context of a long-term goal is a more successful approach to enhancing performance than setting a long-term goal in isolation (20). Effective goal setting also requires clients to monitor progress and assess capabilities, adjust the strategy and goal as needed, and set a new goal as needed. It is important for the health fitness professional to provide regular feedback and encouragement regarding the individual's progress toward his or her goals and work with the individual to create new goals when the previous goals are attained (22).

Social Support

Behavior change efforts are challenging, but the support of others can enhance the opportunity for success. This support from significant others, such as family and friends, is referred to as social support and is described as the perceived and actual caring and assistance received by the individual engaging in behavior change efforts. Four primary types of social support have been identified (52):

- Instrumental: providing tangible, practical assistance for goal achievement (*e.g.*, driving a spouse to a cardiac rehabilitation appointment; providing child care for a mother)
- Emotional: expressing encouragement, empathy, and concern (*e.g.*, praising an exerciser for his or her efforts; demonstrating compassion for sore muscles)
- Informational: giving instructions, advice, and feedback (*e.g.*, providing exercise tips; giving valuable health-related information)
- Companionship: providing a sense of belonging and connectedness (*e.g.*, making oneself available as an exercise partner or group)

These types of support can be provided by a variety of sources, including family, significant others, and health fitness professionals, with each source of social support having the potential to provide benefit. One other important consideration within social support is whether the support is actually received or is instead perceived. Although support that is real and tangible is valuable in the promotion of healthy behaviors and behavior change, research demonstrates that perceptions of support or nonsupport are also critical elements in health behavior (11). That is, perceptions of support can be more important than actual or received support. This reality necessitates careful consideration of what the individual working toward change perceives about the support provided by their available resources.

A critical aspect of social support is that the relative importance, of type of support, source of support, and whether the support is actual or perceived, may be influenced in part by the specifics of the individual circumstance. The combination of support most influential and beneficial for one person may not be the same for others. As such, the characteristics of social support perhaps most beneficial for a busy single mother employed full-time might be tangible and instrumental support provided by her friend. In contrast, perceived emotional support from a spouse might be of greatest value to a newly enrolled cardiac rehabilitation patient. Social support is varied in how it manifests, which produces a circumstance where needs and resources of the individual working toward healthful behaviors must be fully considered. Informal communications with individual clients and patients can provide the information needed to deliver the social support and positively impact health behavior.

Self-Control

Self-control, defined as the ability to override one response to make another response possible, is a key ability in those seeking to adopt and maintain health behavior. As previously mentioned, clients just starting out might be habituated to being inactive. Despite the intention to be more active, the desires toward enjoying a sedentary lifestyle remain salient and may be difficult to overcome. The client must exhibit self-control over those desires and behaviors in order to stay in line with a new goal of creating a healthy lifestyle.

Self-control, however, is based on a limited resource or energy, called *willpower*, and when someone has to perform several acts of self-control, their willpower is depleted (2). This depletion of willpower, or self-control strength, is also called "ego-depletion" because the "ego" refers to the classic psychological term for the rational, decision-making component of personality. Just as athletes might conserve their strength following repeated muscular exertions, people will seek to maintain their willpower and self-regulatory resources as it has been used up. Thus, the act of self-control can make subsequent acts of self-control more difficult (*e.g.*, facing challenges or demands), thus increasing the probability that one will choose the option that he or she wants to self-control — most likely the behavior that is not in line with new, healthy goal(s).

Suppose, for example, that a client has had a stressful day at work, not unlike every other day. In the past, this client has always passed the gym and opted for a favorite fast-food meal for dinner. The client now has new goals to stop by the gym on the way home to exercise and then prepare a healthy meal at home. However, the stresses of the workday and repeated acts of self-control have left the client ego-depleted by the end of the workday. So, even though the client wants to self-control the strong desire to stop at fast food and pass the exit for the gym, the client does not have the willpower to do so. Instead of staying in line with the new goals, the client then falls back into old, unhealthy habits.

In this example, the client would have benefited from some self-control, and research indicates that replenishment of depleted willpower can be accomplished in a multitude of ways, including glucose consumption (9), prayer (8), positive feelings states (44), and mindfulness meditation (7). Importantly, the client could be taught these methods in order to have the willpower needed to make the healthier decision on the next trip home from work. The client could eat a healthy snack 30 minutes before leaving the office or could positively reframe the stressful workday into positive thoughts, thus enhancing mood. The client could also spend a few minutes after the workday to decompress, pray, and meditate to provide the needed willpower and outlook to take the exit to the gym and make it home for a healthy meal. Tactics such as these can be useful to implement, when needed, to provide acute benefits as needed, and potentially act as training of the client's "mental muscles" to handle future adversity and acts of self-control.

Emotional Regulation

Emotions play a key role in one's level of motivation, effort, and behavioral choice (4). First, positive emotions can be generally related to continued motivation to keep going, whereas negative emotions might promote motivation to change, try harder, or give up. Interestingly, specific emotions, especially around awareness to not meeting up to a self-held standard, can lead to quite different levels of effort. For example, frustration and anger appear to be effort-enhancing type emotions, whereas feelings of sadness, depression, or despondency might be related to less effort (3). Thus, the health fitness professional must be attentive to how clients feel, especially when they did not reach a highly valued goal. The professional can then more adequately aid to place the client in an emotional state that is more productive for behavior change, thus helping the clients maintain their behavioral efforts.

Of course, clients have to regulate their emotions on their own, day-to-day, and should be equipped to do so. Emotional regulation is a form of self-control, as certain emotions are overridden in order to allow another more compatible emotional response possible (45). As clients experience stressful and busy days, while diligently trying to stay in line with their health goals, emotional distress can undermine their efforts. The implications are important, because when a client is upset and under emotional distress, the immediate impulse will most likely be engage in a behavior to feel better, even if it is in contradiction with health goals (46).

In addition, exercise and healthy eating behaviors can also lead to negative feelings. For example, the client might question whether or not the healthy food option tastes good. How does the client respond to not being able to stop at a fast-food restaurant on the way home from work, especially when craving it? Similarly, how does exercise make the client feel: positive or negative; encouraged or discouraged? Exercise provides an array of physiological feedback to be interpreted by the brain, and individuals tend to interpret this differently. A new exerciser or postrehabilitation client might interpret such feelings of rapid heart rate, hyperventilation, sweat, and muscle fatigue in a negative way, thus resulting in a "terrible workout." In contrast, an avid exerciser may feel all of the same stimuli but think, "Wow, that was a great workout!"

To help, the health fitness professional could maximize the self-efficacy or confidence in clients' abilities during and following such exercise sessions. For example, research supports that efficacy-building feedback after exercise can reduce anxiety and improve emotional experiences, whereas low-efficacy feedback might not (25,27). What are the implications? The positive feelings experienced from a single bout of exercise can predict physical activity levels a year later (35,55). Importantly, research indicates each unit of increase in positive feelings translates to significantly more physical activity over time. The health fitness professional's goal, then, should be to maximize positive feelings states with exercise and understand the complexity of such responses. Also, it is important that clients understand that health behavior change can be an emotional journey, and proper understanding and handling of these emotions can facilitate goal-directed behaviors.

Communication

Communication skills, as they relate to behavior change, are extremely important for a number of reasons. First, the health fitness professional is faced with a challenging task of extracting a client's thoughts and experiences and then being able to take the client's words and applying them back to psychological and behavioral concepts that can aid in developing interventions to facilitate behavior change. For example, Chapter 11 introduced self-efficacy and ways to improve it. However, a client is unlikely to state, "I do not feel very *efficacious* in doing those exercises on my own, thus I need more mastery experience to enhance my feelings of efficacy." Rather, the client might say something like, "I am not too sure I can exercise this week with how busy I am" or "I do not feel very confident when I am at the gym." The health fitness professional must then discern that the client is actually talking about self-efficacy, and knowing this information, the professional can then develop interventions and communicate with the client to enhance perceptions of self-efficacy using one of several different strategies.

This important dynamic of communication between health fitness professional and client or patient is vital in the behavior change process. *Communication* as it is most often considered involves two parties: sender and receiver. The sender conveys the message and the receiver interprets and responds. Messages are sent verbally through oral communication, primarily by speaking aloud. Messages can also be sent nonverbally by way of body language, visual engagement, and hand gestures. Although the natural tendency is to presume that verbal communication is far and away the most important channel for communication, nonverbal factors are key in the overall interpretation of interpersonal communication. Listening is also of great importance within communication, which can be as important as speaking in the communication process. Active listening is a specific type of listening that demonstrates complete comprehension of the message by listening with undivided attention and repeating back to the speaker a summary of the message that was heard, which enhances accuracy of interpretation. Effective listening provides important assurances that the message is receiving appropriate attention and consideration, which helps to build rapport between the professional and the client or patient. Facilitation of quality communication is, therefore, key to promoting change. The health fitness professional strives to convey messages in a manner that encourage, inspire, and motivate. Additionally, no single communication style should be used exclusively. Fitness professionals should adapt and tailor their communication style to the needs to the client.

Using Motivational Interviewing

One effective approach to motivating change involves utilization of motivational interviewing (MI), which is person-centered, and intends to facilitate autonomy and strengthen motivation for change (29). A basic premise of MI is that behavior change is more successful when the client takes the lead in discovering and fully considering all the factors that impact action and inaction toward a specific behavior. Such an approach is more participatory and autonomy-supportive than most traditional counseling orientations that focus on the expert or professional directing and instructing the client toward change. The strategies associated with MI have been shown to be effective for promoting a variety of healthy behaviors, including exercise (26,38).

A key feature within MI is helping clients overcome their feelings of ambivalence for change. That is, many inactive individuals have contemplated increasing their activity but are unsure if they really want to make a commitment to change. The purpose of an MI intervention is to help clients explore and work through their ambivalence about change (37). Four general principles underlie MI, and each is important in the facilitation of behavior change:

- Express empathy: reflect an attitude of acceptance, utilize skillful listening, demonstrate understanding
- Develop discrepancies: clarify the difference between current and preferred behavior, encourage exploration of likely outcomes in life with and without change
- Roll with resistance: avoid arguing, offer new perspectives, demonstrate patience and flexibility
- Support self-efficacy: instill confidence in ability to change, limit and redirect negativity, affirm appropriate goals

As individuals discuss their ambivalence about behavior change, they typically produce two types of talk regarding their behavior: sustain talk and change talk. Sustain talk refers to talking about the costs of changing and the benefits of not changing. Sustain talk is used as a way for the client to not feel obligated to adopt any change. Change talk refers to talk about the benefits of changing a client's behavior and the costs of not changing. The goal of an MI intervention is to generate change talk, as this indicates client movement toward readiness to adopt change. This is accomplished by asking open-ended questions, summarizing, and skillfully using reflective listening to express empathy, with the goal of guiding the conversation toward more change talk. Change talk is facilitated by communication that focuses on observations made by the health fitness professional and is hindered when the focus shifts toward judgment, interpretation, and evaluation, which inhibits open and relaxed communication. Utilization of good MI technique provides a pathway for change that is directed by the individual, which enhances the likelihood of success.

 ## Threats to Exercise Behavior

Barriers to Physical Activity

Beyond the common barriers of time, cost, and motivation, clients have an array of barriers to exercise. Actual barriers are those that are objectively manifested, such as a client not having a ride to the gym. Perceived barriers are those that are subjectively manifested from the client's perspective. For example, researchers have found that actual time commitments did not predict lack of time for physical activity in women, suggesting that clients might perceive that they do not have time to be active, but in actuality, they do (14). However, perceived barriers are powerful and hinder behavior change as much as actual barriers. In other words, the barrier does not have to be real or objectively manifested to be a hindrance to the client. Rather, if the client *perceives* it to be a barrier, then that perceived barrier can negatively affect behavior change.

Environmental Barriers

The environment is another potential barrier to exercise, such as bad weather, lack of exercise facilities, cost, and safety issues. In addition, living in rural, suburban, and urban areas brings about specific barriers. For example, a more prominent barrier for an older adult in a rural area might be lack of sidewalks, inadequate lighting, lack of access to facilities, or unattended dogs, whereas concerns related to safety might be a prominent barrier in an urban area (54). When addressing environmental challenges, exercise should be tailored to accommodate these and other environmental constraints specific to the client. It is important for the health fitness professional to help the client find alternatives when impacted by these factors. Where there is a lack of exercise facilities, walking might be the best option. In locations where the weather is a challenge, finding indoor alternatives is essential. Also, terrain can be an issue if someone lives in a particularly hilly area, and therefore, exercise plans might need to be adjusted accordingly.

Body-Related Barriers

Clients commonly will have body-related barriers to exercise, such as social physique anxiety, which is a form of anxiety linked to discomfort with having one's body on display for others to see (12). For many individuals, the physique anxiety experiences incurred within physical activity is an important barrier that creates the need for strategies aimed at reducing such experiences (39). To better understand anxiety, the health fitness professional should be aware of the more general concept of self-presentation, which refers to a process of monitoring and controlling how one is perceived by other people. Self-presentation can impact (a) motivation to engage in exercise, (b) choices of activity and activity contexts, (c) quality of performance, and (d) emotional reactions to participating in physical activity or exercise (21). Importantly, clients can experience improvements in perceived body image with their exercise behavior (13), thus potentially reducing the effect of body image–related barriers.

The physical body–related barriers associated with exercise common in clinical populations (*e.g.*, difficulty breathing, low back or knee pain, arthritis, and/or other orthopedic complications) could provide a substantial barrier to exercising. First, they can make exercise or specific exercises difficult or even contraindicated. Second, such barriers can negatively affect the client's motivation to be active, especially in light of the discomfort they expect to experience. Modifying the exercise prescription to adjust for these times could help clients maintain motivation and positive perceptions of exercise.

Exercise Environments

Certain exercise environments have been shown to negatively impact both physique anxiety and self-presentational views. Environmental variables observed to create challenges include the use of mirrors, aggressive colors within the gym setting (*e.g.*, red, black), intimidating group exercise environment, and revealing instructor clothing. Such environments not only impact one's view of self but might also undermine confidence to control the perceptions by others (*e.g.*, self-presentation efficacy), thus discouraging participation. Also, navigating social norms of a fitness facility can be an intimidating barrier to exercising, especially if the client is disrupted by the lack of knowledge, comfort, and confidence to navigate these norms. For example, clinical environments have been found to intensify self-presentational concerns in women due to inadequate views of their physical appearance, the presence of men or younger women in the clinic, perceived inability to perform exercise as well as expected, and mirrors/windows in the clinic (6). In addition, the anxiety did not appear to diminish over time in the clients, thus promoting the use of avoidance coping strategies (*e.g.*, hiding behind equipment) to deal with their anxious and apprehensive feelings. Thus, the health fitness professional should ensure that the client is not placed in a situation or environment that could exacerbate any perceived feelings of physique anxiety or self-presentational concerns while being encouraged to participate in a nonintimidating or anxiety-producing environment.

Perceived Access to and Options for Physical Activity

Suppose a client has been walking around the neighborhood three times a week for the last 2 weeks. Today is a day to walk, but it is raining. What does the client do? Unfortunately, like many clients, a common response might be to do nothing. One major reason might be the perceived lack of other options to be physically active in this type of scenario. To facilitate behavior change, clients need to perceive additional options to be active. In this example, other options would have helped the client meet daily physical activity goal. With options, the client could have walked at the mall, used a gym membership, or enjoyed a favorite exercise video. Thus, the perception of options for physical activity could increase the odds that clients will be active. Research supports this suggestion, as having four places for physical activity was related to 1,000% increase in the odds of adult women *meeting* physical activity guidelines of 150 minutes per week, compared to those with no perceived options (31).

Options for physical activity can also facilitate autonomy, or the belief that the client is the origin of his or her own actions, and has the power to choose. Autonomy is a key innate need that all humans possess and is crucial in helping facilitate more self-determined forms of motivation (see Chapter 11). In seeking ways to encourage, support, and enhance autonomy, the health fitness professional can provide more physical activity options for the client to choose from. This could be as simple as letting a client choose from a list of exercises during a training session, instead of dictating what exercises must be completed.

Options also allow clients to tap into another important source of intrinsic motivation — to experience stimulation, fun, and pleasure. For example, the health fitness professional could provide the client with a large list of moderate-intensity physical activities. The client could then highlight the physical activities that are enjoyable, alongside others he or she would like to try. A choice can be then be made from options that are self-determined, rather than those forced on the client by the professional or someone else, while providing an ample list of activities to choose from when difficult times arise.

The health fitness professional should also be aware of clients' perceptions of access to physical activity, which can vary across urban, suburban, and rural environments. The practitioner can help the client assess perceptions give consideration to how supportive a rural environment is perceived to be for physical activity (53). Similarly, there are ways to assess the perceived nutritional environment (10), which could greatly vary between urban or suburban areas where clients might have more access, compared to a rural setting with limited access to a single convenience store and fast food outlet (41). An interesting factor is the home environment, which could be the culprit of unhealthy eating habits. A client could be asked, "How easy is it for you to eat unhealthy in your home?" If it is really easy to eat unhealthy in the client's house, then it will pose as a powerful barrier to eat healthy, while increasing the need of self-control to override the urges to eat the easily accessible, unhealthy foods.

Outcome Expectations

A key feature in behavior change is the outcome expectation associated with performing the behavior. This concept is linked to social cognitive theory described in Chapter 11 and has significant relevance to exercise behavior. Importantly, increased physical activity is more likely to occur when a highly desirable outcome is expected in response to participation. For example, individuals who would like to have an improved mood after exercising are more inclined to initiate physical activity if they hold a firm expectation that exercise can produce this outcome. In contrast, overweight individuals who do not believe that exercise can help to improve their weight status are not likely to start a training program. An important consideration is that expectations of outcomes are the stimulus for initiating the activity, although actual outcomes are key to long-term maintenance of the behavior. A task of the health fitness professional is to ensure that clients are fully aware of the benefits that can be reasonably expected in response to exercise participation. Given the numerous benefits of exercise, there is a great likelihood that one or more of those outcomes would be highly valued and could therefore help initiate the adoption of regular exercise. Importantly, research involving a wide range of individuals indicates that outcome expectations are linked to exercise behavior (36,40).

Addressing Relapse

Although initial health behavior change is not easy, maintaining behavior change over time is perhaps more difficult because it requires ongoing commitment and effort. Although the timeline varies according to different theories and types of behavior, 6 months is often used as a threshold of transition from starting to maintaining behavior change (34). *Relapse prevention* is an ongoing process in which efforts are made by the individual engaging in behavior change to prevent a return to an undesirable behavior (24). Relapse prevention research and interventions have evolved from initial efforts linked to addiction and now extend to a variety of health behaviors including physical activity. In terms of exercise, the relapse prevention model's goal is to prevent an individual from returning to an inactive lifestyle after establishing a regular exercise routine. Relapse prevention incorporates various techniques, many of which are also used during the initial behavior change process. For example, goal setting, self-monitoring, and rewards are often used in both the initiation of behavior change and relapse prevention processes. Although full relapse is undesirable and highly problematic, individuals engaging in behavior change are encouraged to plan for brief lapses in behavior. Maintaining a perfect diet or exercise plan is almost impossible. Therefore, a healthy approach is to expect lapses to occur and to have a plan in place to restart the desired behavior change immediately (18). A significant challenge to long-term behavior change is the common perspective that a single lapse in behavior means that all hope is lost and that returning to prior unhealthy behaviors is the natural next step. The primary goal is preventing a relapse but an important secondary goal is being ready to respond when lapses occur. Health fitness professionals should aim to encourage their clients and patients to develop specific plans for how they will prevent relapse and also how they will handle lapses when they occur.

HOW TO   Perform a Motivational Interview

First: Complete the readiness ruler.

On the following scale, indicate your readiness to increase your physical activity level.

0	1	2	3	4	5	6	7	8	9	10
Not Ready										Fully Ready

Second: Complete the change grid.
Use the grid below to list and describe your thoughts and feelings about changing and increasing your level of exercise. The grid should be completed in numerical order.

	Pros	Cons
Maintaining Current Activity	1	2
Increasing Activity	4	3

Instructions and Tips
Readiness and motivation for change is dynamic and will vary over time. The readiness ruler can be completed at different points in time to allow for measurement of change over time. Alternatively, a single measurement time point could ask the client to rate his or her level of readiness at some point in the past and compare that value to readiness today. Changes toward lesser or greater readiness can be utilized to initiate conversation about what is behind the change and what factors led to the change and/or what could impact readiness in the future.

The change grid provides an opportunity for the client to explore his or her motivations and ambivalence toward change. Clients should be encouraged to provide thoughtful entries that can be used as talking points. Completing the sections in order allows the client to flow away from a position that does not support change behavior toward a final position that can provide a launch point for further communication and potential commitment to change.

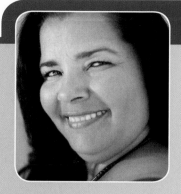

The Case of Brenda

Submitted by **Joyce Dendy, MS, RD, ACSM-HFS, Z-Health Movement Performance Specialist (R, I, S, T), Affirmative Fitness, Waltham, MA**

This case describes how MI is used to effect change over time with a 52-year-old client.

Narrative

Brenda is a 52-year-old married woman who has two children in college and is actively involved in the care of her aging parents. She left her job as an attorney more than 9 years ago. Brenda has gained 30 lb over the past 3 years because of an increase in sedentary behaviors and a lack of routine in her day. With her role as caretaker and a history of anxiety, she found it increasingly difficult to "find" the time to exercise and to consider her health needs. Brenda was active in high school, where she played basketball and softball. In college, she played varsity basketball and did some occasional running.

Brenda has been working with a training and performance coach/registered dietitian/certified exercise physiologist for the past 6 years, meeting with her twice a month. During this period, Brenda has worked with her coach at clarifying her long-term goals, identifying barriers, and planning and completing her weekly exercise, specifically spinning and tai chi.

Weight History

Height: 5 ft 9½ in
Heaviest weight: 180 lb
Current weight: 165 lb
Goal weight: 155 lb
Lowest weight: 138 lb
Pregnancy weight: 195 lb

Medical History

Postmenopausal, anxiety, tinnitus
No history of coronary artery disease, hypertension, diabetes mellitus, cancer, smoking
No surgeries
Bone density — NA
Labs: complete blood count and lipid profile: normal; vitamin D <30 ng $\cdot$ mL^{-1}
Medications/supplements: vitamin D

Eating Habits

Three meals per day plus snacks. Brenda eats mostly organic foods and avoids meat and chicken; protein sources include fish, dairy, eggs, cheese, Greek yogurt, nuts, and legumes; vegetables and greens are from a farmers market or home grown; she limits sugar and sweet intake; beverages include decaffeinated tea, water, about two glasses (6–8 oz) of wine in the evening.

Physical complaints: neck and upper back pain due to tension and left knee pain with squatting and lunging
Sleep: approximately 7 hours a night, reports sleeping well throughout the night
Respiration: paradoxical breathing, upper chest breathing pattern, mouth breathing
Social support: serves on multiple committees, organizes group gatherings with friends, belongs to a book club and a singing group, serves as a trainer/coach, and so on

Objective

Utilizing MI strategies, the coach guides, listens, and elicits information from the client to encourage the process of change. (Please note that this was a conversation that took place as coach and client over the span of several months after we had spent a significant amount of time together.)

Conversation 1

Brenda: I really want to lose the weight I've gained, but don't think I'll ever be able to lose it.

Coach: What makes you say that?

Brenda: I've always heard that being postmenopausal makes it harder to lose the weight.

Coach: So, tell me about what your eating habits are like.

Brenda: [See diet history, eating habits.]

Coach: It sounds like you eat really healthy and have good knowledge about nutrition.

Brenda: I really think I do, but I just don't know what to do.

Coach: What have you tried in the past to help lose weight?

Brenda: I don't like diets. I just try to eat healthy, but it's not coming off. I eat healthy foods like salads, maybe my portion size is too big, I don't know.

Coach: What are your thoughts about keeping a food diary so that we could get a good sense of what's going on?

Brenda: I don't want to do food records! (Breathing rate and anxiety level go up.)

Coach: I hear what you're saying. They can be really time-consuming, especially when you've got a lot going on.

Brenda: I'd prefer to see if we could do this without food records.

Coach: OK. Sounds like food records are not the right plan for you now. Let's see if you can identify foods or beverages that are contributing extra calories. What foods or beverages, if any, would you say are contributing extra calories?

Brenda: Wine. I could easily cut back on this. I'm drinking two glasses per night with my husband.

Coach: Sounds like a great way to save some calories! I wouldn't want you to miss out on the social benefits of spending time with your husband. So what beverage(s) would be a good replacement?

Brenda: I think a cup of tea would be best (client solution).

Coach: How would that work for you?

Brenda: I think having tea instead of wine is fine.

Coach: Give it a whirl over the next week and let me know how it goes!

Conversation 2 (2 wk later)

Coach: How did your goal of cutting down on your wine consumption go?

Brenda: I cut back to having it only one or two nights a week. And I actually lost a few pounds.

Coach: Nice job! How did you feel about not having the wine at night?

Brenda: I found the nights that I didn't drink the wine I actually felt better in the morning.

Coach: Sounds like this is something you wouldn't have been aware of if you had continued to drink the wine at night.

Brenda: I didn't realize it, but it really makes a difference. But I really want to lose this weight!

Coach: You really are committed to making changes that make a difference you can see! [reinforcing change talk]

Coach: Let me summarize where we are at. Last time we met, we talked about the challenges to monitoring your food intake. I know that keeping a food record is something you prefer not to do and eating healthier is not where you want to focus right now and because you are already eating healthy foods. Does this sound right?

Brenda: Yes, that's right.

Coach: The question then becomes "Where do we go from here?" Most people tend to focus on the food, but focusing on a few small behaviors can make a huge impact on weight loss. So, let's take a look at this "menu of behaviors" I brought for you.

Menu of behaviors
Become a conscious eater.

Do not eat in the car.

Do not eat in front of the TV.

Eat all meals and snacks sitting down.

Take smaller bites.

Put your fork down between bites.

Take several breaths before eating.

Brenda: WOW! I have a tendency to eat while I'm standing up, especially when I'm cooking; I eat off my plate as I'm walking to the table before I sit down; and I frequently grab a handful of almonds when I'm stressed and I eat them while I walk through the kitchen. And I definitely don't put my fork down between bites either!

Coach: Well, it sounds like you've hit on some things that are contributing to extra calories. Which one do you think would be the biggest priority for you?

Brenda: I really think I need to eat all my meals and snacks seated. That way I can stop myself if I'm not really hungry and I'm eating just because I'm stressed (commitment).

Coach: Great! We have a plan!

Follow-Up

A few months later, Brenda had lost a total of 13 lb without keeping a food dairy. She continues to work on the repetition of these habits. Over the past year, she has kept the weight off and has even been able to lose a few more pounds. Gaining confidence in her ability to create change has motivated her to work on other goals.

A Message from the Coach

This was a real client with a common problem, the inability to make change happen to reach a goal. Reflecting back on my experience of working with clients over the past 20 years, I learned that to facilitate behavior change, my communication skills needed to change. I had plenty of education and knew all the reasons why people needed to change their behaviors. And most people know they would be healthier by exercising more, losing weight, getting more sleep, eating healthier foods, and so on. Accepting that the ideas and solutions for change need to come from the client is really important. But knowing how to recognize the clues to ambivalence and how to get the client to "argue for change" by guiding him or her through a conversation (DARN-C) about his or her Desires, Abilities, Reasons, and Needs for change, and ultimately getting someone to Commit, is just the beginning. Changing behavior takes time, patience, trial and error, and repetition on both the coach's and client's parts.

> ### QUESTIONS
> - Define MI and describe how the coach used this approach with his or her client.
> - With guidance from the coach, the client was able to identify several antecedents that were preventing her from losing weight. Define antecedent and consequence and identify them from this conversation.
> - What is ambivalence? When someone is ambivalent, what "stage of change" is this person at? From the given conversation, what statement from the client provides a clue to the coach to know this?

References

1. Coyle D. *The Talent Code: Greatness Isn't Born. It's Grown. Here's How.* New York (NY): Bantam Books; 2009. 258 p.
2. Goulston M. *Just Listen: Discover the Secret to Getting Through to Absolutely Anyone.* New York (NY): AMACOM; 2010. 256 p.
3. Patterson K, Grenny J, Maxfied D, McMillan R, Switzler A. *Change Anything: The New Science of Personal Success.* New York (NY): Business Plus; 2011. 288 p.
4. Prochaska JO, Norcross J, Diclemente C. *Changing for Food: A Revolutionary Six-Stage Program for Overcoming Bad Habits and Moving Your Life Positively Forward.* New York (NY): Avon Books; 1994. 304 p.
5. Rollnick S, Miller W, Butler C. *Motivational Interviewing in Health Care: Helping Patients Change Behavior (Applications of Motivational Interviewing).* New York (NY): Guilford Press; 2008. 210 p.

EXERCISE IS MEDICINE CONNECTION

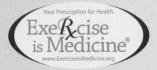

Turner-McGrievy GM, Beets MW, Moore JB, Kaczynski AT, Barr-Anderson, Tate DF. Comparison of traditional versus mobile app self-monitoring of physical activity and dietary intake among overweight adults participating in an mHealth weight loss program. *J Am Med Inform Assoc.* 2013;20(3):513–18.

There exists an old idea that one of the best ways to improve a behavior is to monitor that behavior. It seems that paying close attention to and recording the things we do tends to produce behavior changes in a desirable direction. This principle has been demonstrated in a variety of contexts including diet and physical activity, and the clear message from this research is that tracking and monitoring activity produces notable increase in total exercise (28). Importantly, this old idea has been applied to new technologies such as smartphones. A recent study of overweight adults enrolled in a 6-month weight loss intervention indicates that participants were more likely to report exercise when assigned to the mobile app monitoring group when compared to the group that self-monitored using a paper journal. These differences were significant. Mobile app participants reported more than twice as much exercise and concluded the study with a lower body mass index than their paper journal counterparts. It seems the convenience provided by the mobile phone method combined with our insatiable appetite to use technology made a meaningful difference on outcomes. Although excessive use of media and screens can negatively impact physical activity, the results of this study make clear that technology can be leveraged in a positive manner and encourage the utilization of exercise as medicine for healthful living.

SUMMARY

The adoption and maintenance of healthful behaviors, such as exercise, is no easy task. Demands of work, family, friends, and other aspects of life place limits on the time and energy typically needed to engage in recommended amounts of physical activity. The realities of these life challenges have led to the development of numerous physical activity interventions that aim to increase the rate of exercise adoption and adherence. The intervention ideas provided within this chapter are based on sound health behavior change theories and evidence made available through scientific research. Each intervention approach can provide great benefit to health fitness professionals in the pursuit of methods that can provide profound and lasting benefit for a wide array of clients and patients.

STUDY QUESTIONS

1. What is self-monitoring? Provide two examples.
2. What does the acronym SMART stand for in the context of goal setting?
3. What are the four types of social support? Provide examples of each.
4. What is motivational interviewing? Describe its four guiding principles.
5. What is relapse prevention? Provide physical activity examples.

REFERENCES

1. Armitage CJ, Conner M. Efficacy of the theory of planned behaviour: a meta-analytic review. *Br J Soc Psychol.* 2001;40 (Pt 4):471–99.

2. Baumeister RF, Vohs KD, Tice DM. The strength model of self-control. *Curr Direct Psychol Sci.* 2007;16:351–55.

3. Carver CS, Harmon-Jones E. Anger is an approach-related affect: evidence and implications. *Psychol Bull.* 2009;135(2): 183–204.

4. Carver CS, Scheier MF. *On the Self-Regulation of Behavior.* New York (NY): Cambridge University Press; 2001. 460 p.

5. Case MA, Burwick HA, Volpp KG, Patel MS. Accuracy of smartphone applications and wearable devices for tracking physical activity data. *JAMA.* 2015;313(6):625–26.

6. Driediger MV, McKay CD, Hall CR, Echlin PS. A qualitative examination of women's self-presentation and social physique anxiety during injury rehabilitation. *Physiotherapy.* 2015;102(4):371–76.

7. Friese M, Messner C, Schaffner Y. Mindfulness meditation counteracts self-control depletion. *Conscious Cogn.* 2012; 21(2):1016–22.

8. Friese M, Wänke M. Personal prayer buffers self-control depletion. *J Experimental Social Psychol.* 2014;51;56–9.

9. Gailliot MT, Baumeister RF. The physiology of willpower: linking blood glucose to self-control. *Pers Soc Psychol Rev.* 2007;11(4):303–27.

10. Green SH, Glanz K. Development of the perceived nutrition environment measures survey. *Am J Prev Med.* 2015; 49(1):50–61.

11. Haber MG, Cohen JL, Lucas T, Baltes BB. The relationship between self-reported received and perceived social support: a meta-analytic review. *Am J Community Psychol.* 2007;39 (1–2):133–44.

12. Hart EA, Leary MR, Rejeski WJ. The measurement of social physique anxiety. *J Sport Exerc Psychol.* 1989;11(1):94–104.

13. Hausenblas HA, Fallon EA. Exercise and body image: a meta-analysis. *Psychol Health.* 2006;21(1):33–47.

14. Heesch KC, Mâsse LC. Lack of time for physical activity: perception or reality for African American and Hispanic women? *Women Health.* 2004;39(3):45–62.

15. Hekler EB, Buman MP, Grieco L, et al. Validation of physical activity tracking via android smartphones compared to ActiGraph accelerometer: laboratory-based and free-living validation studies. *J Med Internet Res.* 2015;3(2):e36.

16. Kahn EB, Ramsey LT, Brownson R, et al. The effectiveness of interventions to increase physical activity: a systematic review. *Am J Prev Med.* 2002;22(4 Suppl):73–107.

17. Kang M, Marshall SJ, Barreira TV, Lee JO. Effect of pedometer-based physical activity interventions: a meta-analysis. *Res Q Exerc Sport.* 2009;80(3):648–55.

18. Knapp DN. Behavioral management techniques and exercise promotion. In: Dishman RK, editor. *Exercise Adherence: Its Impact on Public Health.* Champaign (IL): Human Kinetics; 1988. p. 203–35.

19. Kooiman TJ, Dontje ML, Sprenger SR, Krijnen WP, van der Schans CP, de Groot M. Reliability and validity of ten consumer activity trackers. *BMC Sports Sci Med Rehabil.* 2015;7(1):24.

20. Kyllo LB, Landers DM. Goal setting in sport and exercise: a research synthesis to resolve the controversy. *J Sport Exerc Psychol.* 1995;17(2):117–37.

21. Leary MR. Self-presentational processes in exercise and sport. *J Sport Exerc Psychol.* 1992;14(4):339–339.

22. Locke EA, Latham GP. Building a practically useful theory of goal setting and task motivation: a 35-year odyssey. *Am Psychol.* 2002;57(7):705–17.

23. Marcus BH, Williams DM, Dubbert PM, et al. What we know and what we need to know: a scientific statement from the American Heart Association Council on nutrition, physical activity, and metabolism (subcommittee on physical activity); Council on cardiovascular disease in the young; and the Interdisciplinary Working Group on quality of care and outcomes research. *Circulation.* 2006;114(24): 2739–52.

24. Marlatt GA, George WH. Relapse prevention: introduction and overview of the model. *Br J Addict.* 1984;79(3):261–73.

25. Marquez DX, Jerome GJ, McAuley E, Snook EM, Canaklisova S. Self-efficacy manipulation and state anxiety responses to exercise in low active women. *Psychol Health.* 2002;17:783–91.

26. Martins RK, McNeil DW. Review of motivational interviewing in promoting health behaviors. *Clin Psychol Rev.* 2009;29(4):283–93.

27. McAuley E, Talbot HM, Martinez S. Manipulating self-efficacy in the exercise environment in women: influences on affective responses. *Health Psychol.* 1999;18(3):288–94.

28. Michie S, Abraham C, Whittington C, McAteer J, Gupta S. Effective techniques in healthy eating and physical activity interventions: a meta-regression. *Health Psychol.* 2009; 28(6):690–701.

29. Miller WR, Rollnick S. *Motivational Interviewing: Preparing People for Change.* New York (NY): Guilford Press; 2002. 428 p.

30. Nolan M, Mitchell JR, Doyle-Baker PK. Validity of the Apple iPhone®/iPod Touch® as an accelerometer-based physical activity monitor: a proof-of-concept study. *J Phys Act Health.* 2014;11(4):759–69.

31. Parks SE, Housemann RA, Brownson RC. Differential correlates of physical activity in urban and rural adults of various socioeconomic backgrounds in the United States. *J Epidemiol Community Health.* 2003;57(1):29–35.

32. Physical Activity Guidelines Advisory Committee. *Physical Activity Guidelines Advisory Committee Report, 2008.* Washington (DC): U.S. Department of Health and Human Services; 2008. 683 p.

33. Polzien KM, Jakicic JM, Tate DF, Otto AD. The efficacy of a technology-based system in a short-term behavioral weight loss intervention. *Obesity.* 2007;15(4):825–30.

34. Prochaska JO. *Systems of Psychotherapy: A Transtheoretical Analysis.* Homewood (IL): Dorsey Press; 1979. 407 p.

35. Rhodes RE, Kates A. Can the affective response to exercise predict future motives and physical activity behavior? A systematic review of published evidence. *Ann Behav Med.* 2015; 49(5):715–31.

36. Rodgers WM, Brawley LR. The influence of outcome expectancy and self-efficacy on the behavioral intentions of novice exercisers. *J Appl Soc Psychol.* 1996;26(7):618–34.

37. Rollnick S, Miller WR, Butler CC. *Motivational Interviewing in Health Care: Helping Patients Change Behavior*. New York (NY): Guilford Press; 2008. 210 p.

38. Rubak S, Sandbaek A, Lauritzen T, Christensen B. Motivational interviewing: a systematic review and meta-analysis. *Br J Gen Pract*. 2005;55(513):305–12.

39. Sabiston CM, Pila E, Pinsonnault-Bilodeau G, Cox AE. Social physique anxiety experiences in physical activity: a comprehensive synthesis of research studies focused on measurement, theory, and predictors and outcomes. *Int Rev Sport Exerc Psychol*. 2014;7(1):158–83.

40. Sears SR, Stanton AL. Expectancy-value constructs and expectancy violation as predictors of exercise adherence in previously sedentary women. *Health Psychol*. 2001;20(5):326–33.

41. Sharkey JR, Johnson CM, Dean WR, Horel SA. Association between proximity to and coverage of traditional fast-food restaurants and non-traditional fast-food outlets and fast-food consumption among rural adults. *Int J of Health Geogr*. 2011;10:37.

42. Shilts MK, Horowitz M, Townsend MS. Goal setting as a strategy for dietary and physical activity behavior change: a review of the literature. *Am J Health Promot*. 2004;19(2):81–93.

43. Strecher VJ, Seijts GH, Kok GJ, et al. Goal setting as a strategy for health behavior change. *Health Educ Q*. 1995;22(2):190–200.

44. Tice DM, Baumeister RF, Shmueli D, Muraven M. Restoring the self: positive affect helps improve self-regulation following ego depletion. *J Exper Soc Psychol*. 2007;43:379–84.

45. Tice DM, Bratslavsky E. Giving in to feel good: the place of emotion regulation in the context of general self-control. *Psychol Inquiry*. 2000;11:149–59.

46. Tice DM, Bratslavsky E, Baumeister RF. Emotional distress regulation takes precedence over impulse control: if you feel bad, do it! *J Pers Soc Psychol*. 2001;80:53–67.

47. Tudor-Locke C, Burkett L, Reis JP, Ainsworth BE, Macera CA, Wilson DK. How many days of pedometer monitoring predict weekly physical activity in adults? *Prev Med*. 2005;40(3):293–8.

48. Tudor-Locke C, Craig CL, Aoyagi Y, et al. How many steps/day are enough? For older adults and special populations. *Int J Behav Nutr Phys Act*. 2011;8:80.

49. Tudor-Locke C, Craig CL, Beets MW, et al. How many steps/day are enough? For children and adolescents. *Int J Behav Nutr Phys Act*. 2011;8:78.

50. Tudor-Locke C, Craig CL, Brown WJ, et al. How many steps/day are enough? For adults. *Int J Behav Nutr Phys Act*. 2011;8:79.

51. Tudor-Locke C, Schuna JM. Steps to preventing type 2 diabetes: exercise, walk more, or sit less? *Front Endocrinol*. 2012;3:142.

52. Uchino B. *Social Support and Physical Health: Understanding the Health Consequences of Relationships*. New Haven (CT): Yale University Press; 2004. 234 p.

53. Umstattd MR, Baller SL, Hennessy E, et al. Development of the Rural Active Living Perceived Environmental Support Scale (RALPESS). *J Phys Act Health*. 2012;9(5):724–30.

54. Wilcox S, Castro C, King AC, Housemann R, Brownson RC. Determinants of leisure time physical activity in rural compared with urban older and ethnically diverse women in the United States. *J Epidemiol Community Health*. 2000;54(9):667–72.

55. Williams DM, Dunsiger S, Ciccolo JT, Lewis BA, Albrecht AE, Marcus BH. Acute affective response to a moderate-intensity exercise stimulus predicts physical activity participation 6 and 12 months later. *Psychol Sport Exerc*. 2008;9(3):231–45.

56. Wing RR, Tate D, LaRose JG, et al. Frequent self-weighing as part of a constellation of healthy weight control practices in young adults. *Obesity*. 2015;23:943–49.

57. Zheng Y, Klem ML, Sereika SM, Danford CA, Ewing LJ, Burke LE. Self-weighing in weight management: a systematic literature review. *Obesity*. 2015;23(2):256–65.

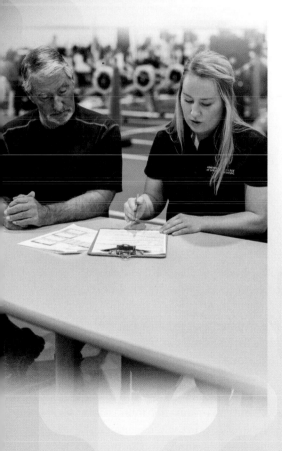

- To examine the effects of stress on health behaviors (including physical activity), well-being, and physical health.

- To evaluate the role of exercise and how it may be utilized effectively to manage acute and chronic stress.

- To identify the role of other techniques and resources in effective stress management.

INTRODUCTION

Psychological stress is an enduring and relevant issue for the health care and fitness professional. For instance, a wide swath of society reports being stressed, as determined by the Stress in America investigation (6). This report, published annually by the American Psychological Association, found that during the financial crisis of the late 2000s, this score was greater than 6 (on a 1–10 scale, with 10 being "a great deal of stress") (6). Although the average score has dropped to just under 5 in 2014 — indicating improving conditions — it remains a reasonably high level of stress. This report also corroborates a large literature that has generally found stress to negatively impact health. Specifically, stress has been linked with the common cold, development of chronic illness, including cardiovascular disease and stroke, and worsening of autonomic diseases, such as multiple sclerosis (MS), and premature death (31). How stress and health are connected is complex but likely involves the effects of stress on motivation for and practice of health behaviors both positive (*e.g.*, exercise and physical activity) and negative (*e.g.*, illicit drug use). Exercise, on the other hand, is typically a productive way to cope with stress, and a growing literature indicates that exercise programs have a positive impact on perceptions of stress. Many other stress management techniques have also been successfully utilized, such as mindfulness meditation, biofeedback, and massage. Lastly, it goes without saying that this concept is also personally relevant because exercise professionals — like anyone else — are not immune to the effects of stress.

 ## Definition and Characteristics of Stress

Stress is a popular term in today's vocabulary, used in regular, everyday language (109). People often use the word stress to express uncomfortable situations in life, with phrases such as "I feel stressed out" or "my job is stressful," and the word is often used to refer to pressure or tension (109). In fact, if you search books for these terms (https://books.google.com/ngrams; used January 13, 2017), it is clear that use of the words "stressful" and "stressed out" are still exponentially increasing, indicating a clear and continued relevance for today's society. Likewise, "stress" ranks in the top 2,100 of English words currently used, more common than words like "actions," "improved," "milk," and "spot" (http://www.wordcount.org; used January 13, 2017).

From a scientific perspective, however, stress is defined as the *process* by which one responds to an environmental demand that is perceived as threatening (109). Understanding the interaction between the environment and the person is important — essentially, stress occurs whenever an environmental demand taxes one's resources (68). This discrepancy between demands and resources elicits a physiological response that compensates for the disturbance and restores equilibrium (homeostasis). The specific pattern of responses may be physical (*e.g.*, increased heart rate or blood pressure), behavioral (*e.g.*, increased movement, such as pacing), psychological (*e.g.*, emotional distress), or a combination of these reactions (109). If demands exceed resources over a long period of time, one's well-being may be endangered, and the inability of the body to cope properly and restore homeostasis after exposure to a stressor can result in biological or psychological damage (119). Stress encompasses this full process — from demand to response and recovery. As such, it is important to consider the component parts.

The stimulus, or environmental demand, is known as a stressor. Stressors have a diverse set of sources and characteristics. To start, the source of a stressor can come from within the person (*e.g.*, a health problem), the family (*e.g.*, divorce), the community (*e.g.*, crime, traffic), or the society (*e.g.*, civil unrest). Stressors vary in intensity, from mild (*e.g.*, waiting in a long line) to severe (*e.g.*, witnessing the 911 tragedy). Stressors differ in their time course, from infrequently to very often. For example, chronic stress is often thought of as the steady accumulation of minor, everyday challenges, such as daily demands from clients or patients at work (90). Chronic stress could also be described as the long-term grinding kind of stress, and some examples of this might be poverty, demanding jobs with long work hours, or poor relationships (133). The duration of a stressor can also be acute, as in an immediate "fight or flight" response (*e.g.*, seeing a snake). The duration of the stressor is not always easy to determine. For example, a major life event, such as experiencing a car wreck, may in itself only last seconds, but the repercussions may be long-lasting. Stressors that are severe, occur often, and of longer duration are considered to be the most impactful and potentially damaging. However, even small incidents in everyday life (*i.e.*, daily hassles) such as giving a speech, encountering heavy traffic, or misplacing keys can be perceived as stressful and possibly have a larger effect as they occur consistently over time. That is, recent minor life events, major life events, and traumatic events can add up to form *cumulative adversity*. Thus, any single stressor or event may not be considered a significant disturbance in isolation, but the additive effect of these may be damaging (130).

Importantly, not all stressors are perceived as negative; indeed, some stress is considered favorable and adaptive. Good stress, or eustress, is considered to be a pleasant and stimulating experience that promotes growth, development, and improvement in performance (93). An example of this type of stress might be a marriage, addition to the family, or a job promotion (109). Conversely, bad stress or distress is negative and more likely to be disruptive. An example of this type of stress could include being diagnosed with an incurable illness or loss of employment. However, the perception that an event is stressful depends entirely on the individual and his or her appraisal process and resources needed to meet the demand. These will be addressed in the next section on the appraisal of stress.

Appraisal of Stress

According to the transactional model of stress and coping, the impact of a stressor is largely based on one's cognitive appraisal of two components, namely, the event's threat (primary appraisal) and availability of resources (secondary appraisal) (28,67,68). In primary appraisal, individuals gauge both their susceptibility to and the severity of the threat by asking questions such as "What does this mean to me?" and "Will I be in trouble?" The significance of a stressor is further refined by one's expectations of future harm and potential for achieving growth, mastery, and additional resources. These appraisals may, therefore, result in perceptions of positive challenge instead of negative threat (113). For example, a sedentary person starting a new exercise routine may perceive a bout of exercise as unsafe and thus injurious, or he may think of it as fairly benign, fun, and challenging. With secondary appraisal, one evaluates his or her resources to control and cope with the stressor to either alter the situation or at least manage the emotional reaction. For secondary appraisal, individuals evaluate (a) their resources available to cope with the stressor (perceived control over the threat), (b) their emotional reaction (perceived control over feelings), and, finally, (c) their ability to deal effectively with the resources concerning the burden of stress (coping self-efficacy) (51). For example, exercise may be less threatening if a new exerciser perceives that she has adequate resources to deal with the experience (*e.g.*, plenty of water, time to take breaks, someone to ask for help), the ability to manage these resources (*e.g.*, use of a smartphone application, ability to approach someone for guidance), and the ability to manage emotions (*e.g.*, minimize feelings of hurt or pain). Each of these is a part of the coping process — a process that is critical for understanding the impact of a given demand on each person's response.

Coping

Coping is what people do to alleviate, eliminate, or manage stress, and this term has as many meanings as the term *stress*. Coping activities are geared toward decreasing the person's appraisal of (or concern of) the discrepancy between the demands of the situation and the resources of the person (113). Coping is an ongoing, dynamic process that involves continuous appraisals and reappraisals of the shifting person–environment relationship (68). That means that coping reflects our efforts to both manage the demands of a situation as well as our response to those demands. In general, to neutralize or reduce stress, a person will attempt to change the environment, their perception of it, or the meaning of the stressor. The transactional model of stress and coping suggests that appraisals influence and predict the specific coping processes implemented during a stressful event (68). According to the original model, coping efforts were conceptualized in two dimensions, problem management (*i.e.*, problem-focused coping) and emotional regulation (*i.e.*, emotion-focused coping).

Problem-Focused Coping

In problem-focused coping, the person attempts to modify the nature of the stressor by either reducing the demands of the stressful situation or expanding his or her resources to deal with it (113). This type of coping may include actively seeking out information, talking with a professional or friend to get advice on how to handle the problem, or drawing from previous experience and knowledge to brainstorm, weigh alternatives, and make plans — all in an attempt to resolve the problem (51). Examples of problem-focused coping in everyday life would be negotiating an extension on an assignment, learning a new skill (*e.g.*, time management, assertiveness training), making a new relationship with someone who has expertise in the problem area, or seeking out a less stressful job (113). This type of coping is most often used when people believe that either the personal resources or the demands of the situation are changeable (68), thereby resulting in the perception of control and self-efficacy (51).

Emotion-Focused Coping

Emotional regulation is a more passive coping effort where the person attempts to control or manage the emotional response to a stressful event, particularly one that is difficult to change. In this type of coping, people engage in behaviors to distract their attention from the problem or to simply make themselves feel better. In the 2015 Stress in America report, nearly one-half of respondents endorsed exercise/walking to deal with stress. Respondents also endorsed listening to music, watching TV, surfing the Internet, napping/sleeping, eating, drinking alcohol, and smoking to manage stress (in that order). As can be seen in this list, not all emotion-focused coping would be considered unproductive or negative. Some are positive pursuits which help a person endure a temporary period of emotional distress. The key difference from problem-focused coping is that the person is trying to modify his or her emotional response rather than dealing with the challenge. People tend to use emotion-focused coping when they believe that the circumstances they are facing are fixed and they cannot change their stressful condition (68). When a stressor is appraised as uncontrollable and highly threatening, individuals often adopt disengaging or passive coping strategies (134). One may attempt to alter thoughts about the stressful situation: denying, distancing, and avoiding the situation (51). Unfortunately, escape-avoidance behavior (*e.g.*, hiding feelings, refusing to think about illness or situation) has been associated with higher levels of psychological distress and poorer quality of life (10,138). Accepting responsibility (which involves acknowledging the role one has played in the situation and trying to make things right) and positive reappraisal (which involves choosing to create a positive meaning from the situation rather than a negative meaning) are more effective techniques. Recent evidence indicates that suppressing thoughts about

HOW TO	**The Experience of Stress and Coping Associated with Fitness Testing**

One common stressor in the health and fitness setting is the stress of receiving a fitness or body composition assessment. For some, this may be a time of excitement (*e.g.*, eustress) about starting (or completing) a training regimen. For others, facing objective data about their lack of physical conditioning may elicit feelings of threat and dread (*e.g.*, distress). Feedback about one's fitness and performance may be most intimidating for individuals lacking adequate baseline fitness and training experience. In a study investigating the response to body composition testing with dual-energy x-ray absorptiometry (DXA), all participants responded with a decline in positive affect (*e.g.*, enthusiasm, high energy, alertness) (44). Clearly, seeing an image that depicts your body fat may create a sense of displeasure for anyone. However, an increase in negative affect (*e.g.*, distress, anger, guilt) was only observed for overweight and obese individuals, for whom feedback about body fat may have been a particularly threatening experience. Later research (45) suggests that this negative emotional response may actually undermine future motivation for exercise and diet. Specifically, those with a negative response reported eating significantly greater amounts calorically dense and highly palatable foods in the week following testing (*i.e.*, ice cream) (45). This suggests that fitness professionals must be aware of the potential of their feedback to clients to increase stress and undermine their goals of an active, healthy lifestyle. Sometimes, negative feedback is important, but it is just as important to help the client cope with this information through problem-focused (*e.g.*, choosing an appropriate exercise program) and emotion-focused (*e.g.*, encouragement, comparison to former clients who improved) efforts.

the stressful event and the experience of the event have no positive impact on coping with feelings (142). Conversely, reappraising the emotional stimulus and using cognitive techniques like perspective taking are the most effective (142).

Depending on the individual and the situation, a person may be more inclined to engage either in problem-focused or in emotion-focused coping (47,48). However, both may be necessary and therefore will be used in combination with each other not only to manage emotions in the short term but also engage in active, problem solving. Exercise, such as a short walk around the block, is an excellent way to help temporarily manage distress (41). Once the person is more calm and focused, it is easier to initiate efforts to deal with the challenge.

The Response to Stress

Stress has a combined and interrelated impact on the physiological and psychological aspects of a person, including bodily systems, mental processes (*e.g.*, distress, negative affect), and behaviors. The physiological and psychological response of a person to a stressor is called *strain*. Strain, if severe or prolonged, can negatively affect the functioning and health of a person, increase illness vulnerability, and worsen disease progression and activity (90).

When an event or stimulus exceeds one's capacity (*e.g.*, is stressful), the body elicits an immediate response to counteract the disturbance and restore homeostatic balance. The stress response is similar across species and is, therefore, often referred to as the general adaptation syndrome. This response has three main stages of varied and undefined duration, although the specific response depends on the characteristics of the individual (*e.g.*, fitness, personality) and their appraisal, among other factors. If stressors begin to accumulate — and recovery is inadequate — a person may begin to experience excessive wear and tear or *allostatic load* where stress responses become dysregulated and ineffective. The next sections will describe both the general adaptation syndrome and allostatic load model in more detail (92).

General Adaptation Syndrome

The physiologic stress response of the body was first theorized by Hans Selye (118), who later became known as the father of stress research. Selye conducted experiments that exposed animals to various and diverse homeostatic challenges such as heat, cold, infection, and toxic substances and objectively measured physiological changes. The reaction to each stressor varied respectively according to its unique characteristics, but his primary finding was an underlying nonspecific response pattern that was consistent across the different stressors. This stereotypical response pattern of stress was coined the general adaptation syndrome (GAS).

The GAS consists of three broad stages, each with a wide variety of nonspecific and specific responses, all working together to restore homeostasis and ensure the survival of the organism. The first stage is called the *alarm reaction*, where the stressor is first recognized by the system and a fight-or-flight response is initiated (118). The second stage is that of *resistance*, where a cascade of cardiovascular, metabolic, hormonal, and immune changes is generated as a compensatory stress reaction (113). During this stage, some compensatory reactions may include the release of glucocorticoids (*e.g.*, cortisol), the activation of the hypothalamic–pituitary–adrenal (HPA) axis, and changes in autonomic neurotransmitters and inflammatory cytokines (92). The last stage is that of *exhaustion*, when the organism has depleted all biochemical substrates and additional resources and is no longer able to mount a defense to the stressor (118). If the stressor continues and activation of these systems is extended for a long period, the bodily systems can eventually break down and result in dysfunction of major organs (*e.g.*, heart or brain). In extreme situations, stress-related exhaustion has the capacity to result in death (118). On the basis of GAS, the impact of repeated stress exposure can be problematic because individuals who remain in the resistance phase have difficulty withstanding additional challenges (118). For example, there is evidence that those experiencing higher levels of chronic, unremitting stress have difficulty recovering from strenuous resistance exercise, taking two to four times as long to recover as those reporting lower levels of chronic stress (125,126) (see "Exercise is Medicine Connection").

EXERCISE IS MEDICINE CONNECTION

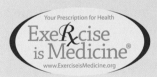

Your Prescription for Health
Exe**R**cise is Medicine®
www.ExerciseisMedicine.org

Stress and Recovery, Implications for Exercise and Adaptation

How people respond to a bout of exercise is also impacted by the experience of stress in their lives. The stress response can essentially be divided into two phases, reactivity and recovery (return to homeostasis). The physical and metabolic stress of exercise results in decrements of function initially. For instance, after completing a vigorous bout of resistance training, muscles that have been exercised will be fatigued and unable to generate high force. Such a response is typically followed by quick rebound and adaptation, but these processes and the speed of recovery can vary greatly between individuals, from 24 to 96 hours for recovery. Chronic psychological stress includes things like changing jobs, poor performance in a class, and ending a relationship. College students who reported higher chronic stress also had much slower recovery from heavy resistance training (125,126). That is, even though they did the same challenging bout of exercise — multiple repetitions on a leg press machine — they needed almost 4 days to fully recover from the activity. In contrast, a person reporting lower stress recovered in about 1 day. Such an effect may help to account for why some individuals respond to exercise with positive adaptations, whereas others have little to no change (83). Indeed, those reporting higher chronic stress have been shown to gain less strength over a multi-month resistance training program (16). Some of this may be due to interference from the stress response. That is, higher cortisol levels may undermine recovery. It may also be due to how these people cope with stress (*e.g.*, problems with sleep, or change in diet). Regardless, it is important for fitness professionals to be aware of the stress of their clients and how this might impact their training.

Allostasis and Allostatic Load Model

Allostasis is the ability to achieve stability through change, and the allostatic load model refers to the rapid activation of bodily systems to cope with a stressor and restore homeostasis as effectively and efficiently as possible (90). In regard to allostasis, all of the systems in the body are involved, including the autonomic nervous system and HPA axis along with the cardiovascular, immune, and metabolic systems (90). However, if the body does not compensate well and the wear and tear of repeated stressors on the body accumulates (*i.e.*, allostatic load), then there is an increased risk of the development of physical ailments (91). Overactivity of the allostatic systems, where there is limited time for rest and restoration, can increase the risk of cardiovascular disease (75). Sometimes, the body is unable to stop or shut off the stress response even after the stressor has ended. When this occurs, the systems can be driven to exhaustion resulting in the breakdown of feedback mechanisms and overexposure to stress hormones such as cortisol (75). Stress, chronic and acute, minor and severe, can have an impact on the functioning of an individual. Likewise, any accumulation of a certain type of stressor or combination of various stressors can be damaging to one's health (104). This explains the link between stress and health outcomes, which are detailed in the following text.

The Effects of Stress on Health

Stress has consistently been related to poor physical and mental health (93,130). The physical changes in response to chronic or intense stress can lead to, contribute to, or worsen life-threatening and life-altering conditions such as myocardial infarction, stroke, cancer, or autonomic diseases. In the Stress in America report, respondents disclosed that stress was impacting their health to such a degree that the report was entitled "Paying with Our Health" (6). The American Institute of Stress (3) has compiled a list of several signs and symptoms of excessive stress (Table 13.1), and this list includes physical, emotional, and behavioral responses and conditions. Some of these symptoms are relatively mild, such as blushing and headaches, whereas others are serious, such as social isolation and excessive drug use. The American Psychological Association (4) notes that there are not always symptoms associated with the experience of stress. For instance, some symptoms may be camouflaged by medications. The following sections describe some of the most common stress-related health problems.

Digestive Issues

Ulcers, inflammatory bowel disease, and irritable bowel syndrome are all disorders in the digestive tract that are influenced by stress (113). Ulcers are due to an increase in gastric juices and erosion of the lining of the stomach or upper small intestine. Inflammatory bowel disease may involve inflammation of the colon and small intestine, whereas irritable bowel syndrome may involve diarrhea, constipation, and abdominal pain (113). The connection between stress and digestive tract problems has been linked to alternations in bacterial growth in the gut, but many other mechanisms likely play a role (89).

Headaches

Intense headaches can also be a physical disorder that results from exposure to chronic stress. The two most common recurrent headaches are migraines and tension-type headaches (72,105). Migraines are typified by intense throbbing and pulsating sensations in the head, often accompanied by sensations of nausea and sensitivity to stimuli. Stress is the most common trigger for the development of migraines but may also magnify the effects of migraines (114). Tension-type headaches are the result of the contraction and tightening of muscles in the neck and head, which is a common reaction of persons under stress (113). In both cases, the strain of the headache itself is a stressor, necessitating a coping response, the selection of which may have effects on choices to be physically active or sedentary (66).

Table 13.1	Signs and Symptoms of Excessive Stress

1. Frequent headaches, jaw clenching, or pain
2. Gritting, grinding teeth
3. Stuttering or stammering
4. Tremors, trembling of lips, hands
5. Neck ache, back pain, muscle spasms
6. Light-headedness, faintness, dizziness
7. Ringing, buzzing, or popping sounds
8. Frequent blushing, sweating
9. Cold or sweaty hands, feet
10. Dry mouth, problems swallowing
11. Frequent colds, infections, herpes sores
12. Rashes, itching, hives, "goose bumps"
13. Unexplained or frequent "allergy" attacks
14. Heartburn, stomach pain, nausea
15. Excess belching, flatulence
16. Constipation, diarrhea
17. Difficulty breathing, sighing
18. Sudden attacks of panic
19. Chest pain, palpitations
20. Frequent urination
21. Poor sexual desire or performance
22. Excess anxiety, worry, guilt, nervousness
23. Increased anger, frustration, hostility
24. Depression, frequent, or wild mood swings
25. Increased or decreased appetite
26. Insomnia, nightmares, disturbing dreams
27. Difficulty concentrating, racing thoughts
28. Trouble learning new information
29. Forgetfulness, disorganization, confusion
30. Difficulty in making decisions
31. Feeling overloaded or overwhelmed
32. Frequent crying spells or suicidal thoughts
33. Feelings of loneliness or worthlessness
34. Little interest in appearance, punctuality
35. Nervous habits, fidgeting, feet tapping
36. Increased frustration, irritability, edginess
37. Overreaction to petty annoyances
38. Increased number of minor accidents
39. Obsessive or compulsive behavior
40. Reduced work efficiency or productivity
41. Lies or excuses to cover up poor work
42. Rapid or mumbled speech
43. Excessive defensiveness or suspiciousness
44. Problems in communication, sharing
45. Social withdrawal and isolation
46. Constant tiredness, weakness, fatigue
47. Frequent use of over-the-counter drugs
48. Weight gain or loss without diet
49. Increased smoking, alcohol, or drug use
50. Excessive gambling or impulse buying

Source: Adapted with permission from http://www.stress.org/stress-effects/.

Cardiovascular and Metabolic Diseases and the Role of Cortisol

Unresolved, chronic stress profoundly affects the cardiovascular system, including the heart, blood vessels, and blood itself (124). High levels of stress have been associated with abnormally enlarged hearts and hypertension (115). These changes in the heart and blood vessels can increase cardiovascular reactivity to a stressor, which is considered a risk factor for the development of coronary heart disease (84,121). Persons under stress have higher concentrations of activated platelets (82,100) and more triglycerides, free fatty acids, and lipoproteins in the blood (76,99,141), which promote the development of plaques in the arteries or atherosclerosis leading to increased blood pressure and increased likelihood of myocardial infarction and stroke (113). Corticosteroids, specifically cortisol, are released in response to a stressful event (especially social stressors), and high concentrations of cortisol in the blood over time can increase the risks of cardiovascular disease (75,76). In addition, by blocking the uptake of glucose from the cells, high levels of cortisol increase insulin resistance and can lead to the development of Type 2 diabetes (76). Cortisol also contributes to the accumulation of fat in the abdominal region, and this visceral fat is readily released into the bloodstream. Overall, stress can have a major impact on the functioning of the cardiovascular and metabolic systems and can lead to the development and progression of cardiovascular pathologies.

Immune Suppression, Cancer, and Multiple Sclerosis

The immune systems of persons exposed to chronic, severe stress are often suppressed, rendering a person more vulnerable to infections and susceptible to contracting a disease (29). In fact, Selye observed that animals exposed to a stressor had a reduction in the size of immune system organs, such as the thymus gland (74,118). The sympathetic nervous system activity and the release of cortisol after a stressful event suppress the immune system, which limits the number of lymphocytes that are activated in response to a viral challenge (74). For example, among mice exposed to repeated restraint stress, there was a decrease in the production of antibodies and activation of T cells in response to the influenza virus (120). Among humans who were exposed to the common cold virus, those who had high stress developed cold symptoms at nearly twice the rate of who had low stress (33). Similarly, psychological stress has been correlated with a reduction in and activity of natural killer (NK) cells, which combat cancerous tumor cells and monitor neoplastic (new and abnormal) growth (52,55,73). NK cell activity is considered to be important to survival rates in certain types of cancers, specifically breast cancer (70). Experiencing major social stressors in the previous 5 years, such as marital divorce, infidelity, quarreling, and financial problems, has been associated with an increased risk or likelihood of being diagnosed with cervical cancer (36). There is a lack of evidence in well-controlled studies linking stress with the onset of cancer; however, specific stressors — such as loss of social support — have been found to influence the course of cancer (133). Depression, stress, and trauma have all adversely affected disease progression in patients with HIV, and negative beliefs and expectations about the disease and one's future are associated with declines in helper T cells (CD4) and the onset of AIDS (69,117). Finally, there is a significant association between stressful life events and relapse incidence of MS (96). In one study, the majority of MS relapses were associated with one or more stressful life events occurring in the 6 weeks prior (1). Overall, the functioning of the immune system in fighting off viruses, infections, cancer, and autonomic diseases can be severely compromised because of stress.

Stress and Psychological Functioning

The impact of stress is not limited to the physical body. Stress can affect psychological well-being, cognitive function, emotion (*e.g.*, distress, negative moods), social involvement, and behavior, such as physical activity and sedentarism (129). There are several psychological conditions that can be influenced by chronic stress such as anxiety, depression, fatigue, insomnia, and burnout, and these conditions can have a profound negative impact on quality of life.

Psychological Distress, Depression, and Burnout

Chronic stress has been shown to promote psychological distress and the development of psychological disorders (64,133). Research studies have shown that people who report exposure to chronic stress in their marriage, household functioning, parenting, or jobs have an increased likelihood of being psychologically distressed (101). Chronic stress is a greater predictor of depressive symptoms than acute stress, and if it is experienced over 2 years or more, it may lead to the development of depression (94). In addition, chronic stress of any type can magnify the impact of even minimal life events on clinical depression (23). Persons who continually deal with exposure to high levels of occupational stress can develop a psychological response called burnout. Burnout is characterized by physical, mental, and emotional exhaustion (109). Burnout is defined as a debilitating psychological condition brought about by unrelieved work stress, which results in (a) depleted energy reserves, (b) lowered resistance to illness, (c) increased dissatisfactions and pessimism, and (d) increased absenteeism and inefficiency at work (109). Employees who experience burnout may develop a variety of symptoms, including overall job dissatisfaction, lack of energy and insomnia, tension headaches, ulcers, and dysregulated cortisol responses (107,109).

Cognition

High levels of cortisol associated with long or extreme exposure to stress have been related to cognitive impairment, specifically in spatial memory tasks (20,76,110). This may be because the elevated levels of glucocorticoids (*i.e.*, cortisol) are associated with shrinkage and toxic degeneration of the brain's memory center, the hippocampus, in which loss of neurons and their connectivity occurs (77–79,85,112). Burnout symptoms (described earlier) have been associated with cognitive failures in everyday life, increased inhibition errors, and variability in performance on attention tasks (140). Fortunately, exercise has the opposite effect, promoting memory and cognitive performance and delaying the onset of dementia (56).

 ## Healthy Stress Management

Although stressful events are unavoidable in daily life, the majority of people would prefer to limit or manage the amount of exposure to stress. Currently, there is no drug that can be taken or ritual that can be performed to make people "immune" to stress and stressors, but there are several strategies for coping and managing stress. Both cognitive and behavioral approaches exist for decreasing the negative impact of stress. Not all strategies work for everyone, but all play a role in preventing or reducing stress and stress reactivity.

Exercise: Breaking the Link between Stress and Health Problems

Although the bulk of this chapter has focused on the negative impact of stress, it is encouraging that the majority of studies demonstrate that exercise may neutralize this impact (26,49,130). For example, men who report increased levels of exercise behavior also reported fewer health problems across all levels of reported lifetime exposure to stress (130). Likewise, a study of college students with high stress and low levels of leisure physical activity experienced more physical symptoms and anxiety than did those students engaging in high levels of physical activity (47). Given this, it is important to more fully explore the relationship between exercise and stress.

Exercise

Physical exercise is one of the most cited means of managing stress (135). This recommendation is found in any number of news reports, magazine articles, and blogs. Why would exercise be so effective at managing stress? As was illustrated in the earlier discussion of the GAS and the alarm reaction, the stress response is a set of physiological changes that disrupt homeostasis as it readies the body for action — fight or flight. Unfortunately, most stress is psychological in nature (*e.g.*, exams, relational problems). Not only are these generally not reduced through physical action — they can be made worse if the action is misplaced. This mismatch between the form of stress and the body's reaction can lead to a long-duration disruption of homeostasis that undermines physical and mental health. Thus, one way to think about coping with stress is to find a physical action that can make use of the alarm reaction.

Acute bouts of exercise have been shown to effectively serve this role and reduce the stress response. One of the best examples of this is the ability of a single bout of exercise to reduce feelings of anxiety and other negative moods. The benefit of exercise for state anxiety is very consistent and occurs with nearly all forms of activity — especially those of moderate to low intensity (43,102). Although the benefit of exercise to improve mood and reduce stress also applies to resistance exercise (14), one should be cautious with high-intensity resistance exercise. Continuous exercise above lactate threshold has consistently been shown to reduce mood during exercise (42), which may serve to undermine its effectiveness for stress management. A closer examination of this effect has revealed that high-intensity exercise may increase somatic anxiety during exercise, but cognitive aspects of anxiety remain unaltered and both reduce during recovery (19).

What is especially interesting is that exercise may also be of benefit to those who are living with chronic mental health conditions. For example, exercise is sufficient to help manage anxiety and mood in those who are clinically depressed (15). In fact, for those with a history of depression, as little as 15 minutes of self-selected cycle exercise was enough to improve mood (88). In addition, exercise training has been associated with reductions in clinical levels of ongoing stress (7). Studies have shown a significant reduction in stress across a range of conditions, from panic disorder (22) to posttraumatic stress disorder (PTSD) (40), and in a variety of populations, including methadone-maintained drug abusers (38). Chronic occupational stress (49) and perceived stress (98) also improve with several months of aerobic training.

Although there is no well-accepted mechanism to explain this effect, it has been suggested that the improvement in managing stress may be due to the ability of exercise to improve positive emotions, which in turn are reduced by sedentary behaviors (57). This, in turn, allows for the development of other psychological resources to combat the experience of stress (57). For example, 20 minutes of low- to moderate-intensity treadmill exercise appears to be sufficient to reduce sensitivity to anxiety (21). Moreover, a bout of exercise, especially higher doses of activity (either high intensity or long duration) can actually reduce a person's physiological response to a later stressor (53). That is, on the days that a person completes a bout of exercise, he or she can expect to have less physiological response to stress for the next hour or two than if he or she had been sedentary.

Interestingly, despite the benefits of exercise on perceptions of stress, the experience of stressors impedes efforts to be physically active (129). For example, those reporting high levels of chronic stress experience dampened responses to exercise — lower pleasure and arousal but higher ratings of perceived exertion (RPEs) and pain, which may be a signal of dysregulation (80,128). Not surprisingly, those who are less habitual in their exercise routines respond to periods of stress with less physical activity (80). In contrast, those who have strong exercise habits appear to be resilient in the face of stress and maintain their levels of activity (80). This may be due to the use of exercise as a form of coping. Regardless, those who are inconsistently active — and are likely to need help from an exercise professional the most — appear to be the least likely to adhere to an exercise program. This may impact how the exercise prescription should be presented to these individuals. For example, among highly active individuals, enjoyment is the primary motive behind exercise, whereas only a small percentage of highly active individuals report stress management as a reason they exercise (127). Branding exercise for its ability to enhance fun, enjoyment, and challenge may be more important than advocating its therapeutic effects on mental and physical health (116).

HOW TO   Rate Chronic Perceived Stress

The most common instrument used to assess perception of chronic stress is the 10-item version of the *Perceived Stress Scale* (PSS-10), which measures stress perceptions over the previous month (30,32,34).

Brief Instructions and Tips

1. The questions in this scale ask you about your feelings and thoughts during the last month.

2. Beside each item, indicate the frequency of these feelings and thoughts (0 = never, 1 = almost never, 2 = sometimes, 3 = fairly often, and 4 = very often).

3. The best approach is to answer fairly quickly. That is, don't try to count up the number of times you felt a particular way that month but rather choose the option that seems like a reasonable estimate.

4. After completing the questions, use the table called "Perceived Stress Scale Scoring" to determine your score.

Question	Never	Almost Never	Sometimes	Fairly Often	Very Often
1. How often have you been upset because of something that happened unexpectedly?	0	1	2	3	4
2. How often have you felt that you were unable to control the important things in your life?	0	1	2	3	4
3. How often have you felt nervous and "stressed"?	0	1	2	3	4
4. How often have you felt confident about your ability to handle your personal problems?	0	1	2	3	4
5. How often have you felt that things were going your way?	0	1	2	3	4
6. How often have you found that you could not cope with all the things that you had to do?	0	1	2	3	4
7. How often have you been able to control irritations in your life?	0	1	2	3	4
8. How often have you felt that you were on top of things?	0	1	2	3	4
9. How often have you been angered because of things that happened that were outside of your control?	0	1	2	3	4
10. How often have you felt difficulties were piling up so high that you could not overcome them?	0	1	2	3	4

Perceived Stress Scale Scoring

PSS scores are obtained by reversing responses (*e.g.*, 0 = 4, 1 = 3, 2 = 2, 3 = 1, and 4 = 0) to the four positively stated items (items 4, 5, 7, and 8) and then summing across all scale items.

Item	Your response (0–4)	Reverse score needed?	Final item score
1		No	
2		No	
3		No	
4		Yes	
5		Yes	
6		No	
7		Yes	
8		Yes	
9		No	
10		No	
		Grand total score →	

Interpretation and Normative Values

The scores can range from 0 to 40, and higher scores reflect a higher level of perceived stress. High scores on the PSS-10 questionnaire have been associated with increased difficulty in making lifestyle changes, such as adopting physical activity, and increased susceptibility to stress-induced illness (129). Men in the United States have an average score of about 12 and women have an average of about 14, but scores significantly vary by race or ethnicity (*i.e.*, African Americans average about 15), age (*i.e.*, people 29 years and younger have the highest reported stress), and education (*i.e.*, less educated people are more stressed) (30,34).

Other Modifiers or Buffers of Stress

Enhancing Social Support

Stress is typically perceived when demands outweigh resources. A key resource is social support. When social resources are low, stressors may be particularly dire. In contrast, evidence indicates that social support has a buffering effect on the harmful physical and mental effects of stress exposure (136). It also enhances well-being and health, regardless of stress levels (18). People typically seek out and rely on help and comfort from friends, neighbors, classmates, coworkers, significant others, and health professionals, including fitness professionals (123,139).

Four types or functions of social support exist (59):

- *Emotional support* — the provision of empathy, love, trust, and caring (*e.g.*, actively listening to concerns)
- *Instrumental support* — the provision of tangible aid and services that directly meet a need (*e.g.*, providing services at no additional cost to client when they are experiencing a traumatic stressor)
- *Informational support* — the provision of advice and information concerning the problem (*e.g.*, understanding why an issue is causing significant stress)
- *Appraisal support* — the provision of information useful for self-evaluation purposes such as constructive feedback and affirmation (*e.g.*, helping client brainstorm possible solutions to a problem)

All types of support may be offered by a fitness professional. However, given the situation and client, some types of support are more important and appropriate than others. The matching hypothesis suggests that social support is most beneficial when it meets the needs caused by a stressful event (35). Consider this real-life scenario. A patient of a certified clinical exercise physiologist (CEP) experienced traumatic flooding of his home midway through a training phase. The CEP provided an ideal amount of social support: expressing empathy and genuine concern, placing the training sessions on hold (with no penalty), and providing tips on maintaining fitness when staying out of town. Social aspects of exercise (*e.g.*, walking with a friend) were emphasized. Later, the CEP provided feedback on reinitiating a serious routine once the client was ready. A referral was also made to a social worker, who provided additional assistance, helped the client to strengthen existing relationships, expand his social network and develop new relationships, and get involved in a self-help group. All of these actions improved social support resources (54,59,113,132) and helped the client to manage his experience of a stressful event without sacrificing his health goals.

The mechanism for how social support improves health and well-being is not clear. Social support may improve coping responses by reducing uncertainty and unpredictability about a stressful situation. This would, in turn, promote a greater sense of personal control and the use of problem-focused coping methods (54). It may also be that social support merely relieves some of the stressor-related demands through a sharing of the burden. Regardless, the many forms of social support are an important contributor to the ability of people to cope with stress.

Improving Personal Control and Self-Efficacy

As alluded to earlier, another psychosocial factor that modifies the evaluation of stress is personal control (9,95,137). There is evidence that people who have a strong sense of personal control experience less of a negative response, or strain, with stressors, compared with those who feel they have no control over their lives (93,131). Individuals who believe that they personally have control over their lives are considered to have an internal locus of control. On the other hand, individuals who believe that their lives are dictated by forces outside of themselves, such as destiny, fate, or faith, have an external locus of control (107,111). These two areas of control have a major impact on health and health practices. For instance, those with a more internal sense of control are more persistent in their exercise behavior. Based on how it may impact health, sense of personal control may be further divided into four different types (113):

1. *Informational control* — when a person can glean knowledge about the stressful event and the potential consequences of the situation
2. *Cognitive control* — when a person can use thought processes and strategies to manipulate and modify the impact of the stressor
3. *Decisional control* — when a person can choose between different courses of action
4. *Behavioral control* — when a person can take concrete action to reduce the impact of stress

When people perceive that they have a good sense of control, they feel like they are able to effectively make decisions and execute a plan of action to produce the outcome desired (86,113). This points to another aspect of personal control, self-efficacy, which is the belief or conviction that one can successfully execute the behavior required to produce the outcomes desired (11). When encountering a challenging situation, a person will actively evaluate his or her ability (*i.e.*, efficacy) to properly execute behaviors and determine if they think that they can be successful in handling an activity (108). Generally speaking, people who are highly efficacious show less psychological and physiological strain in the face of a stressor than those who are less efficacious (12,13,58). Goal setting and preplanning for stressors are useful strategies help to boost self-efficacy to regulate one's behaviors in the face of demanding situations (50).

Nonexercise Techniques for Reducing Stress

Although it is critical for the exercise professional to understand the role of exercise as a stress management tool, there are numerous nonexercise techniques that are also successful in helping people cope with stress, reduce arousal and promote relaxation (103). These include progressive muscle relaxation, deep breathing, biofeedback, meditation, mindfulness, and massage (among many others). Each of these areas takes months to years of persistent practice to master, and several, such as massage, have their own certifications and credentialing. However, aspects of each technique may be learned within a short period of time, and thus has utility for the exercise professional. Various techniques may also be combined to suit different people and needs (61). To incorporate stress management techniques into a fitness program, one might begin with time during the cool down and stretching period after exercise when the focus is on relaxation and recovery (87,124).

Diaphragmatic Breathing and Body Scans

Breathing exercises are the easiest and fastest methods to induce the relaxation response, with capability to relieve symptoms of stress and anxiety, including headaches, muscle tension, irritability, and fatigue (39). Diaphragmatic breathing, or breathing from the stomach (as opposed to the chest) is superior for the experience of these benefits. This consists of deep breaths into the lungs and exhaling as the diaphragm contracts and relaxes. Beginners to this practice first must become aware of their normal breathing habits, often while lying down with one hand on the abdomen and another on the chest. Usually a *body scan* is also employed, where a person consciously examines the entire body, usually starting at the toes and upward toward the scalp. Once awareness has been achieved, the practitioner can assume a "dead man" pose, lying with arms and legs spread and palms facing upward, scanning the body for tension and relaxing. Then, one may focus the attention on the breath, breathing in through the nose and out through the mouth slowly and in a rhythmic fashion. Even short bouts of diaphragmatic breathing can provide immediately stress relief. Practice over a longer period (*i.e.*, 30–60 min) in the recovery period of exercise has even been shown to decrease free radical production and cortisol (87).

Progressive Muscle Relaxation

Progressive muscle relaxation is a technique that teaches people how to focus on certain muscle groups and alternatively contract and relax these muscles, focusing on the sensation of relaxation (39,60). This helps the individual to identify areas of the body that tighten and hold tension when they are under stress (*e.g.*, jaw clamps shut, shoulders tighten up, and fingers cramp). Once identified, feelings of tension can be targeted and neutralized. With practice, whenever a person feels tension rising in these areas, he or she can stop what he or she is doing for 5–10 minutes, breathe deeply, tighten (5–7 s) and relax the affected muscles (20–30 s), repeat systematically, and then return to his or her work (39,133). Researchers have postulated that progressive muscle relaxation may additionally promote feelings of calmness and generate pleasant thoughts in the individual, which counteract negative feelings and thoughts associated with stress (103).

Biofeedback

Biofeedback is a method of increasing control over bodily processes, such as heart rate, muscle tension, or sweating, in response to a stressor (37,133). Biofeedback has been useful in treating stress-related health problems, such as chronic muscle tension headaches (25). The procedure involves attaching sensors to the body that provide immediate biophysiological feedback on how a person's body is responding to a stressor (*i.e.*, seeing fluctuations in heart rate or electrodermal activity). This process helps patients to recognize when their body is engaged in a stress response. Individuals are then encouraged to modify their bodily response to the stressor. For instance, one may be asked to slow down a speeding heart rate by blocking out all sounds and breathing deeply until the heart rate reduces and returns to normal. This practice helps individuals gain awareness of and attain voluntary control over their bodily response to a stressor.

Massage

Massage is the external application of pressure to muscles and tendons that can range from smooth, light pressure to deep kneading motion, depending on technique, the purpose of the massage, and individual's preference. Deep tissue massage has been an effective method for reducing stress, muscle tension, pain, and asthma symptoms and has been shown to boost immune function (46,113). The deep tissue massage is the application of forceful, penetrating pressure that is applied to the muscles and joints by a trained massage therapist. Breast cancer patients in the earlier stages of the disease have shown positive results after 3 weeks of massage therapy, such as a decrease in anxiety, depression, and anger and an improvement in mood (55). These patients also showed a boost in their dopamine and serotonin levels and number of NK immune cells and lymphocytes, which could potentially promote a better and faster recovery (55).

Meditation and Prayer

Meditation is an exercise of the mind in which the individual actively focuses on calming and quieting the body while keeping the mind alert (109). There are several forms of meditation: (a) mantra meditation focuses on sounds and phrases, and the same word or verse is repeated over and over again to promote concentration; (b) yantra meditation uses a visual image, and the person focuses on that image to eradicate distracting thoughts from the mind; and (c) transcendental meditation incorporates breathing, visualization, relaxation, and repetition (109). Transcendental meditation has been shown to reduce stress and improve mental and physical health by decreasing blood pressure, heart rate, respiratory response, and stress hormone production (17,81). Use of meditation has also been associated with improved lactate recovery after exercise (122). An alternative to meditation is the practice of prayer, which has been associated with facets of recovery from illness and improved health outcomes (2).

Mindfulness

Mindfulness is the discipline of paying attention to the present moment in a deliberate (purposeful) and nonjudgmental manner (63). It is especially useful during periods of stress, when the mind often dwells on and is clouded by past experiences, current frustrations and hurts, and potential dire consequences. The practice of mindfulness is useful for restoring the mind–body connection, bolstering emotional balance, and enhancing functioning at work and in relationships (24). By being in the present moment, without worry about the future or preoccupation with the past, one may observe automatic emotions and behaviors with greater clarity and perspective. This permits development of a deeper awareness about thoughts and feelings, body sensations, and habitual stress reactions, which in turn encourages more healthy choices about health behaviors (63). Mindfulness is more effective than relaxation practices for reducing ruminations and distracting thoughts, enhancing positive states of mind (61), and increasing sense of control (8). To facilitate these changes, practitioners practice acceptance, trust, patience, nonjudgment, having a beginner's mind (*i.e.*, curiosity), nonstriving, and letting go (63) even during daily activities like putting on one's workout clothes, walking into the gym, and preparing the post-workout meal. Mindfulness can also be performed during physical exercise, such as walking, by focusing more on (a) the present-moment experience of moving, (b) bodily sensations (such as sweating, the heart rate, breathing), and (c) emotional reactions to such perceptions (such as excitement, fear, pain) (106). Some of these exercise sensations and emotions are uncomfortable, but these would be observed and approached with openness and self-compassion and not judged or avoided. Furthermore, attention is not paid to goals, striving, and competition, which can detract from the experience and render exercise less enjoyable.

Yoga and Martial Arts

Some individuals may experience greater stress management with exercise programs that incorporate breath control, mindful movements, and meditative practices. Yoga and martial arts, such as tai chi and qigong, incorporate all of these elements. Mindful exercise practices have been shown to promote numerous health benefits, such as increases in positive emotions, dampened cortisol and cardiovascular reactivity, and lower inflammatory responses to stress (27,62,71,97). Research indicates that those who regularly practice yoga have substantially reduced serum interleukin 6 levels (one of the primary inflammatory cytokines) compared with novice yoga attendees (65). Sessions of yoga, tai chi, or other martial arts performed routinely are effective for reducing symptoms of stress and improving sense of well-being (27,71,97).

Referring a Client or Patient to a Psychologist (Reviewed by Lydia R. Malcolm, PhD, University of Miami)

Exercise professionals, such as personal trainers, often find themselves as confidants to their clientele. Consequently, conversations about stressful experiences are quite common. Although these are to be expected, occasionally clients may deal with stress poorly or in an inappropriate manner. They may (a) display a number of symptoms, such as those in Table 13.1; (b) communicate feelings of distress, worry, anxiety, or other mental health problems; or (c) verbally expresses a need for support. Under such conditions, referral to a mental health professional may be advisable. When referring a client make sure to be empathetic. Consider using language outlined in Table 13.2. The American Psychological Association provides a number of resources, including a mental health professional locator (http://locator.apa.org/), if a referral is accepted. Most importantly, if a person is suicidal or discusses hurting themselves in any way, get professional help immediately.

Table 13.2	Suggested Remarks When Making a Referral to a Mental Health Professional	
Step	**Action**	**Suggested Remark**
1	Start by broaching the topic with a general observation.	"You seem to have a lot of stress."
2	Normalize the context.	"I see a lot of people who are dealing with _____ [fill in the blank]."
3	Emphasize strengths.	"It's good that you are doing some healthy things, such as exercising [and anything else you know they are doing] to help you manage this situation."
4	Suggest that they seek out additional support.	"I know some of my clients have found that getting some extra support to help with [stress, sadness, anxiety, grief, etc.] has been helpful."
5	Obtain permission to make a referral.	"Would you like me to make a recommendation?"
6	If they deny needing additional help keep the option available for future need.	"It sounds like now might not be a good time for you to go to therapy. You can always contact me at a later date for the information."

The Case of Terry

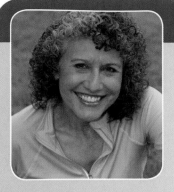

Submitted by **Matthew Stults-Kolehmainen, PhD, EP-C, Yale-New Haven Hospital, New Haven, CT, Teachers College Columbia University, New York, NY**

Terry is a middle-aged woman attempting to lose weight. Her chief complaint is chronic stress, and she has a history of mild depression. She was referred to an integrated health center by her primary care physician to meet with a licensed psychologist and an American College of Sports Medicine (ACSM) Certified Exercise Physiologist^{SM} *(EP-C).*

Narrative

Terry is a 55-year-old African American woman was referred to an integrated health center in a mid-sized urban city by her primary care physician. She is in the obese category for body mass index (BMI) even after numerous attempts to lose weight. She also continues to smoke 5–6 times a day, despite repeated warnings from her doctor. She works full-time and teaches elementary students at a local urban magnet school. Her job requires long hours at work, grading on the weekends, and can be very stressful. She suffers from mild depression (diagnosis is depressive disorder not otherwise specified), which has minimally improved since her husband died 3 years ago. In particular, she reports that she has difficulty experiencing pleasure from things she used to enjoy. She has a good relationship with her adult daughter, who lives locally.

Before her husband became sick, she reported that she and her husband were very active hikers and walked daily. During her last attempt to be physically active, she maintained a personal training program (mostly resistance training, 2 times a week) for 8 weeks until her apartment was broken into, disrupting her routine. She finished a 12-week program but with great struggle. She has been inactive for about a year. Fortunately, she is metabolically healthy (*e.g.*, normal cholesterol and blood sugar), and her only other complaint is some mild symptoms of arthritis. She has no family history of cardiovascular disease.

Based on her clinical intake and interest to lose weight and increase fitness, she was assigned to a licensed psychologist and exercise physiologist (ACSM EP-C) for further evaluation, risk stratification, and treatment. At intake, she reported that her goals were to lose 15 lb (returning to weight 3 yr ago; approximately 165 lb), increase fitness, improve her mental well-being, and maintain independence going into retirement.

Health Fitness Examination

Screening Tools and Outcome Measures:
PSS-10: Terry scored 20 (see box earlier for an interpretation).
Centers for Epidemiology Depression Scale (Revised): Terry scored 19 and did not meet or exceed the cut-off for major depression based on other criteria.
Risk Stratification: moderate (*i.e.*, obesity, smoking, sedentarism, age)

Vitals

Age: 55 years; resting HR: 64 bpm, 66 bpm (second visit); resting BP: 119/63 mm Hg, 124/64 mm Hg (second visit); height: 64 in; weight: 178.5 lb, 180.8 lb (second visit); BMI: 30.6, 31.0 (second visit)

Cardiorespiratory Fitness and Body Composition

YMCA Submaximal Cycle Ergometer Test predicted aerobic capacity = 29 mL · kg^{-1} · min^{-1}, 45th percentile for age and gender.
Body fat estimated with bioelectrical impedance (Tanita model TBF − 300 WA) = 40.0%, 39.8% (second visit)
Waist circumference = 99.5 cm, 99.0 cm (second visit)
Hip circumference = 110.4 cm, 109.5 cm (second visit)

QUESTIONS

- What testing and outcome measures may be appropriate in this case besides health fitness testing?
- Are there indications for use of exercise in clients with chronic stress and mild depression?
- How might an exercise program be structured and what resources may be needed for a client such as Terry?

References

1. American College of Sports Medicine. *ACSM's Guidelines for Exercise Testing and Prescription*. 9th ed. Philadelphia (PA): Lippincott Williams & Wilkins; 2014. 456 p.
2. Carek PJ, Laibstain SE, Carek SM. Exercise for the treatment of depression and anxiety. *Int J Psychiatry Med*. 2011;41(1):15–28.
3. Lavie CJ, Milani RV, O'Keefe JH, Lavie TJ. Impact of exercise training on psychological risk factors. *Prog Cardiovasc Dis*. 2011;53(6):464–70.
4. Stults-Kolehmainen M, Malcolm LR, DiLoreto J, Gunnet-Shoval K, Rathbun EI. Psychological interventions for weight management: a primer for the allied health professional. *ACSM Health Fitness J*. 2015;19(5):16–22.

SUMMARY

The APA's *Stress in America* reports from 2007 and 2015 demonstrate that stress continues to be a problem in American society (5,6). Whether a person feels stressed or not, stress is an everyday facet of life that must be managed. The perception of an event as stressful greatly depends on the person and his or her perceived resources to deal with the stressors. Situations that are perceived to be stressful may result in a variety of physical and mental symptoms, including burnout, fatigue, headaches, gastrointestinal problems, muscular pain, and greater risk for infections. Long-term chronic stressors can increase the risk of cardiovascular disease, heart attacks, stroke, and cancer. Contrary to popular belief, stress is not always negative. Stress can act as a positive challenge that encourages individuals to rise to the occasion and possibly even face their fears or anxieties. This chapter has offered and explained a wide variety of methods for buffering and decreasing the negative impact of stress on the individual. Some tactics and strategies focus on changing the psychological perception of a stressor and others on decreasing the physiological response to a stressor. Exercise interventions are primarily an example of the latter, and only 10–15 minutes of moderate aerobic activity, such as a brisk walk, may provide stress-relieving benefits (41). A challenge for the health and fitness professional is to minimize the psychological toll of exercise itself, which may be perceived as yet another task added to an already full plate. Indeed psychological stress is associated with impaired efforts to be physically active (129). Perhaps by focusing on an individual's preferences and maximizing his or her exercise enjoyment, the full benefits of exercise may be realized. Another strategy would be prescribing exercise regimens with additional meditative qualities, such as mindful walking, yoga, or tai chi (97). A multifaceted approach to stress and exercise may magnify results but does require the exercise practitioner to be more mindful of the complex attributes of the stress experience.

STUDY QUESTIONS

1. Understanding stress: What is stress? How is stress different from *stressors*? Are all stressors bad? What are some examples of good stress? What is the feeling of being *stressed out* and how does it relate to distress?

2. Why are some people apparently immune to stress when they encounter a demanding situation? Explain the two coping mechanisms that can be implemented to minimize the impact of stress. Exercise is which of these?

3. Discuss the consequences of stress on the development and progression of disease and evidence that exercise may buffer this relationship.

4. Before encountering a stressful event, how can a person can prepare himself or herself to ideally handle the event and avoid becoming stressed? Discuss some of the strategies for weakening the impact of stress.

5. What are examples of healthy stress management? Discuss three techniques or approaches for handling and decreasing perceived stress, the potential benefits of each, and how they might be integrated into a fitness program.

REFERENCES

1. Ackerman KD, Heyman R, Rabin BS, et al. Stressful life events precede exacerbations of multiple sclerosis. *Psychosom Med.* 2002;64(6):916–20. doi:10.1097/01.psy.0000038941.33335.40.

2. Ai AL, Dunkle RE, Peterson C, Bolling SF. The role of private prayer in psychological recovery among midlife and aged patients following cardiac surgery. *Gerontologist.* 1998;38(5): 591–601.

3. American Institute of Stress. 50 common signs and symptoms of stress [Internet]. Fort Worth (TX): American Institute of Stress; [cited 2015 Sept 29]. Available from: http://www.stress.org/stress-effects/

4. American Psychological Association. Six myths about stress [Internet]. Washington (DC): American Psychological Association; [cited 2015 Sept 29]. Available from: http://www.apa.org/helpcenter/stress-myths.aspx

5. American Psychological Association. Stress in America [Internet]. Washington (DC): American Psychological Association; [cited 2013 Nov 7]. Available from: www.stressinamerica.org

6. American Psychological Association. Stress in America: paying with our health 2015 [Internet]. Washington (DC): American Psychological Association; [cited 2015 Jun 29]. Available from: www.stressinamerica.org

7. Asmundson GJG, Fetzner MG, DeBoer LB, Powers MB, Otto MW, Smits JAJ. Let's get physical: a contemporary review of the anxiolytic effects of exercise for anxiety and its disorders. *Depress Anxiety.* 2013;30(4):362–73. doi:10.1002/da.22043.

8. Astin JA. Stress reduction through mindfulness meditation. Effects on psychological symptomatology, sense of control, and spiritual experiences. *Psychother Psychosom.* 1997;66(2):97–106.

9. Averill JR. Personal control over aversive stimuli and its relationship to stress. *Psychol Bull.* 1973;80(4):286–303. doi:10.1037/h0034845.

10. Baider L, Perry S, Sison A, Holland J, Uziely B, DeNour AK. The role of psychological variables in a group of melanoma patients: an Israeli sample. *Psychosomatics.* 1997;38(1):45–53.

11. Bandura A. Self-efficacy: toward a unifying theory of behavioral change. *Psychol Rev.* 1977;84(2):191–215. doi:10.1037/0033-295x.84.2.191.

12. Bandura A, Reese L, Adams NE. Microanalysis of action and fear arousal as a function of differential levels of perceived self-efficacy. *J Pers Soc Psychol.* 1982;43(1):5–21. doi:10.1037/0022-3514.43.1.5.

13. Bandura A, Taylor CB, Williams SL, Mefford IN, Barchas JD. Catecholamine secretion as a function of perceived coping self-efficacy. *J Consult Clin Psychol.* 1985;53(3):406–14. doi:10.1037/0022-006x.53.3.406.

14. Bartholomew JB, Moore J, Todd J, Todd T, Elrod CC. Psychological states following resistance exercise of different workloads. *J Appl Sport Psychol.* 2001;13(4):399–410. doi:10.1080/104132001753226265.

15. Bartholomew JB, Morrison D, Ciccolo JT. Effects of acute exercise on mood and well-being in patients with major depressive disorder. *Med Sci Sports Exerc.* 2005;37(12):2032–7. doi:10.1249/01.mss.0000178101.78322.dd.

16. Bartholomew JB, Stults-Kolehmainen MA, Elrod CC, Todd JS. Strength gains after resistance training: the effect of stressful, negative life events. *J Strength Cond Res.* 2008;22(4):1215–21. doi:10.1519/JSC.0b013e318173d0bf.

17. Benson H, Rosner BA, Marzetta BR, Klemchuk HP. Decreased blood-pressure in borderline hypertensive subjects who practiced meditation. *J Chronic Dis.* 1974;27(3):163–9. doi:10.1016/0021-9681(74)90083-6.

18. Berkman LF, Glass T. Social integration, social networks, social support, and health. In: Berman LF, Kawachi I, editors. *Social Epidemiology.* New York (NY): Oxford University Press; 2000.

19. Bixby WR, Hatfield BD. A dimensional investigation of the State Anxiety Inventory (SAI) in an exercise setting: cognitive vs. somatic. *J Sport Behav.* 2011;34(4):307–24.

20. Borcela E, Pérez-Alvarez L, Herreroa AI, et al. Chronic stress in adulthood followed by intermittent stress impairs spatial memory and the survival of newborn hippocampal cells in aging animals: prevention by FGL, a peptide mimetic of neural cell adhesion molecule. *Behav Pharmacol.* 2008;19(1):41–9.

21. Broman-Fulks JJ, Berman ME, Rabian BA, Webster MJ. Effects of aerobic exercise on anxiety sensitivity. *Behav Res Ther.* 2004;42(2):125–36. doi:10.1016/s0005-7967(03)00103-7.

22. Broocks A, Bandelow B, Pekrun G, et al. Comparison of aerobic exercise, clomipramine, and placebo in the treatment of panic disorder. *Am J Psychiatry.* 1998;155(5):603–9.

23. Brown GW, Harris T. *Social Origins of Depression: A Study of Psychiatric Disorder in Women.* New York (NY): Free Press; 1978. 399 p.

24. Brown KW, Ryan RA, Creswell JD. Mindfulness: theoretical foundations and evidence for its salutary effects. *Psychol Inq.* 2007;18(4):211–37.

25. Budzynsk T, Stoyva JM, Adler CS, Mullaney DJ. EMG biofeedback and tension headache: controlled outcome study. *Psychosom Med.* 1973;35(6):484–96.

26. Carmack CL, Boudreaux E, Amaral-Melendez M, Brantley PJ, de Moor C. Aerobic fitness and leisure physical activity as moderators of the stress-illness relation. *Ann Behav Med.* 1999;21(3):251–7. doi:10.1007/bf02884842.

27. Chong CSM, Tsunaka M, Tsang HWH, Chan EP, Cheung WM. Effects of yoga on stress management in healthy adults: a systematic review. *Altern Ther Health Med.* 2011;17(1):32–8.

28. Cohen F, Lazarus RS. Coping and adaptation in health and illness. In: Mechanic D, editor. *Handbook of Health, Health Care, and the Health Professions.* New York (NY): Free Press; 1983. 806 p.

29. Cohen S, Frank E, Doyle WJ, Skoner DP, Rabin BS, Gwaltney JM. Types of stressors that increase susceptibility to the common cold in healthy adults. *Health Psychol.* 1998;17(3):214–23.

30. Cohen S, Janicki-Deverts D. Who's stressed? Distributions of psychological stress in the United States in probability samples from 1983, 2006, and 2009. *J App Soc Psychol.* 2012;42(6):1320–34. doi:10.1111/j.1559-1816.2012.00900.x.

31. Cohen S, Janicki-Deverts D, Miller GE. Psychological stress and disease. *JAMA.* 2007;298(14):1685–7.

32. Cohen S, Kamarck T, Mermelstein R. A global measure of perceived stress. *J Health Soc Behav.* 1983;24(4):385–96.

33. Cohen S, Tyrrell DAJ, Smith AP. Psychological stress and susceptibility to the common cold. *N Engl J Med.* 1991; 325(9):606–12.

34. Cohen S, Williamson G. Perceived stress in a probability sample of the United States. In: Spacapam S, Oskamp S, editors. *The Social Psychology of Health: Claremont Symposium on Applied Social Psychology*. Newbury Park (CA): Sage; 1988. p. 31–67.

35. Cohen S, Wills TA. Stress, social support, and the buffering hypothesis. *Psychol Bull*. 1985;98:310–57.

36. Coker AL, Bond S, Madeleine MM, Luchok K, Pirisi L. Psychosocial stress and cervical neoplasia risk. *Psychosom Med*. 2003;65(4):644–51.

37. Critchley HD, Melmed RN, Featherstone E, Mathias CJ, Dolan RJ. Brain activity during biofeedback relaxation: a functional neuroimaging investigation. *Brain*. 2001;124:1003–12. doi:10.1093/brain/124.5.1003.

38. Cutter CJ, Schottenfeld RS, Moore BA, et al. A pilot trial of a videogame-based exercise program for methadone maintained patients. *J Subst Abuse Treat*. 2014;47(4):299–305. doi:10.1016/j.jsat.2014.05.007.

39. Davis M, Eshelman ER, McKay M. *The Relaxation and Stress Reduction Workbook*. Oakland (CA): New Harbinger Publications; 2008. 336 p.

40. Diaz AB, Motta R. The effects of an aerobic exercise program on posttraumatic stress disorder symptom severity in adolescents. *Int J Emerg Ment Health*. 2008;10(1):49–59.

41. Ekkekakis P, Hall EE, VanLanduyt LM, Petruzzello SJ. Walking in (affective) circles: can short walks enhance affect? *J Behav Med*. 2000;23(3):245–75. doi:10.1023/a:1005558025163.

42. Ekkekakis P, Parfitt G, Petruzzello SJ. The pleasure and displeasure people feel when they exercise at different intensities: decennial update and progress towards a tripartite rationale for exercise intensity prescription. *Sports Med*. 2011;41(8): 641–71. doi:10.2165/11590680-000000000-00000.

43. Ensari I, Greenlee TA, Motl RW, Petruzzello SJ. Meta-analysis of acute exercise effects on state anxiety: an update of randomized controlled trials over the past 25 years. *Depress Anxiety*. 2015;32(8):624–34. doi:10.1002/da.22370.

44. Faries MD, Boroff CS, Stults-Kolehmainen M, Bartholomew JB. Does a visual representation impact the affective response to body composition testing? *Pers Individ Dif*. 2011; 50(4):502–5.

45. Faries MD, Kephart W, Jones EJ. Approach, avoidance and weight-related testing: an investigation of frontal EEG asymmetry. *Psychol Health Med*. 2015;20(7):790–801. doi:10.1080/ 13548506.2014.959530.

46. Field TM. Massage therapy effects. *Am Psychol*. 1998;53(12): 1270–81.

47. Folkman S, Lazarus RS. Coping as a mediator of emotion. *J Pers Soc Psychol*. 1988;54(3):466–75. doi:10.1037/0022-3514 .54.3.466.

48. Folkman S, Lazarus RS, Dunkelschetter C, Delongis A, Gruen RJ. Dynamics of a stressful encounter: cognitive appraisal, coping, and encounter outcomes. *J Pers Soc Psychol*. 1986;50(5):992–1003. doi:10.1037/0022-3514.50.5.992.

49. Gerber M, Pühse U. Do exercise and fitness protect against stress-induced health complaints? A review of the literature. *Scand J Public Health*. 2009;37(8):801–19. doi:10 .1177/1403494809350522.

50. Gilson TA, Heller EA, Stults-Kolehmainen MA. The relationship between an effort goal and self-regulatory efficacy beliefs for Division I football players. *J Strength Cond Res*. 2013;27(10):2806–15. doi:10.1519/JSC.0b013e31828151ca.

51. Glanz K, Schwartz MD. Stress, coping, and health behavior. In: Glanz K, Rimer B, Viswanath K, editors. *Health Behavior and Health Education: Theory, Research, and Practice*. 4th ed. San Francisco (CA): Jossey-Bass; 2008. p. 211–36.

52. Glaser R, Rice J, Stout JC, Speicher CE, Kiecoltglaser JK. Stress depresses interferon production by leukocytes concomitant with a decrease in natural killer cell activity. *Behav Neurosci*. 1986;100(5):675–8. doi:10.1037/0735-7044.100.5.675.

53. Hamer M, Taylor A, Steptoe A. The effect of acute aerobic exercise on stress related blood pressure responses: a systematic review and meta-analysis. *Biol Psychol*. 2006;71(2):183–90. doi:10.1016/j.biopsycho.2005.04.004.

54. Heaney CA, Israel BA. Social networks and social support. In: Glanz K Rimer BK, Viswanath K, editors. *Health Behavior and Health Education: Theory, Research, and Practice*. 4th ed. San Francisco (CA): Jossey-Bass; 2008. p. 189–210.

55. Hernandez-Reif M, Ironson G, Field T, et al. Breast cancer patients have improved immune and neuroendocrine functions following massage therapy. *J Psychosom Res*. 2004;57(1):45–52. doi:10.1016/s0022-3999(03)00500-2.

56. Hillman CH, Erickson KI, Kramer AF. Be smart, exercise your heart: exercise effects on brain and cognition. *Nat Rev Neurosci*. 2008;9(1):58–65. doi:10.1038/nrn2298.

57. Hogan CL, Catalino LI, Mata J, Fredrickson BL. Beyond emotional benefits: physical activity and sedentary behaviour affect psychosocial resources through emotions. *Psychol Health*. 2015;30(3):354–69. doi:10.1080/08870446.2014.973410.

58. Holahan CK, Holahan CJ, Belk SS. Adjustment in aging: the roles of life stress, hassles, and self-efficacy. *Health Psychol*. 1984;3(4):315–28. doi:10.1037/0278-6133.3.4.315.

59. House JS. *Work Stress and Social Support*. Reading (MA): Addison-Wesley; 1981. 156 p.

60. Jacobson EJ. *Progressive Relaxation*. Chicago (IL): University of Chicago Press; 1938. 493 p.

61. Jain S, Shapiro SL, Swanick S, et al. A randomized controlled trial of mindfulness meditation versus relaxation training: effects on distress, positive states of mind, rumination, and distraction. *Ann Behav Med*. 2007;33(1):11–21. doi:10.1207/ s15324796abm3301_2.

62. Jin PT. Efficacy of tai chi, brisk walking, meditation, and reading in reducing mental and emotional-stress. *J Psychosom Res*. 1992;36(4):361–70. doi:10.1016/0022-3999(92)90072-a.

63. Kabat-Zinn J. Mindfulness-based interventions in context: past, present, and future. *Clin Psychol Sci Pract*. 2003;10(2):144–56. doi:10.1093/clipsy/bpg016.

64. Kahn JR, Pearlin LI. Financial strain over the life course and health among older adults. *J Health Soc Behav*. 2006;47(1):17–31.

65. Kiecolt-Glaser JK, Christian L, Preston H, et al. Stress, inflammation, and yoga practice. *Psychosom Med*. 2010;72(2):113–21. doi:10.1097/PSY.0b013e3181cb9377.

66. Lake AE. Headache as a stressor: dysfunctional versus adaptive coping styles. *Headache*. 2009;49(9):1369–77. doi:10.1111/j .1526-4610.2009.01516.x.

67. Lazarus RS. *Stress and Emotion: A New Synthesis*. New York (NY): Springer; 1999. 340 p.

68. Lazarus RS, Folkman S. *Stress, Appraisal and Coping*. New York (NY): Springer; 1984. 456 p.

69. Leserman J. Role of depression, stress, and trauma in HIV disease progression. *Psychosom Med*. 2008;70(5):539–45. doi:10.1097/PSY.0b013e3181777a5f.

70. Levy SM, Herberman RB, Lippman M, D'Angelo T, Lee J. Immunological and psychosocial predictors of disease recurrence in patients with early-stage breast cancer. *Behav Med.* 1991;17(2):67–75.

71. Li AW, Goldsmith CA. The effects of yoga on anxiety and stress. *Altern Med Rev.* 2012;17(1):21–35.

72. Lipton RB, Silberstein SD, Stewart WF. An update on the epidemiology of migraine. *Headache.* 1994;34(6):319–28. doi:10.1111/j.1526-4610.1994.hed3406319.x.

73. Locke SE, Kraus L, Leserman J, Hurst MW, Heisel JS, Williams RM. Life change stress, psychiatric symptoms, and natural killer cell activity. *Psychosom Med.* 1984;46(5):441–53.

74. Lovallo WR. *Stress & Health: Biological and Psychological Interactions.* 2nd ed. Thousand Oaks (CA): Sage Publications; 2005. 279 p.

75. Lundberg U. Coping with stress: neuroendocrine reactions and implications for health. *Noise Health.* 1999;1(4):67–74.

76. Lundberg U. Stress hormones in health and illness: the roles of work and gender. *Psychoneuroendocrinology.* 2005;30(10):1017–21. doi:10.1016/j.psyneuen.2005.03.014.

77. Lupien SJ, de Leon M, de Santi S, et al. Cortisol levels during human aging predict hippocampal atrophy and memory deficits. *Nat Neurosci.* 1998;1(1):69–73. doi:10.1038/271.

78. Lupien SJ, Evans A, Lord C, et al. Hippocampal volume is as variable in young as in older adults: implications for the notion of hippocampal atrophy in humans. *Neuroimage.* 2007;34(2):479–85. doi:10.1016/j.neuroimage.2006.09.041.

79. Lupien SJ, Lecours AR, Lussier I, Schwartz G, Nair NPV, Meaney MJ. Basal cortisol-levels and cognitive deficits in human aging. *J Neurosci.* 1994;14(5):2893–903.

80. Lutz RS, Stults-Kolehmainen MA, Bartholomew JB. Exercise caution when stressed: stages of change and the stress-exercise participation relationship. *Psychol Sport Exerc.* 2010;11(6):560–7. doi:10.1016/j.psychsport.2010.06.005.

81. MacLean CRK, Walton KG, Wenneberg SR, et al. Effects of the transcendental meditation program on adaptive mechanisms: changes in hormone levels and responses to stress after 4 months of practice. *Psychoneuroendocrinology.* 1997;22(4):277–95. doi:10.1016/s0306-4530(97)00003-6.

82. Malkoff SB, Muldoon MF, Zeigler ZR, Manuck SB. Blood-platelet responsivity to acute mental stress. *Psychosom Med.* 1993;55(6):477–82.

83. Mann TN, Lamberts RP, Lambert MI. High responders and low responders: factors associated with individual variation in response to standardized training. *Sports Med.* 2014;44(8):1113–24. doi:10.1007/s40279-014-0197-3.

84. Manuck SB. Cardiovascular reactivity in cardiovascular disease: "once more unto the breach." *Int J Behav Med.* 1994;1(1):4–31. doi:10.1207/s15327558ijbm0101_2.

85. Marin MF, Lord C, Andrews J, et al. Chronic stress, cognitive functioning and mental health. *Neurobiol Learn Mem.* 2011;96(4):583–95. doi:10.1016/j.nlm.2011.02.016.

86. Marshall GN. A multidimensional analysis of internal health locus of control beliefs: separating the wheat from the chaff? *J Pers Soc Psychol.* 1991;61(3):483–91.

87. Martarelli D, Cocchioni M, Scuri S, Pompei P. Diaphragmatic breathing reduces postprandial oxidative stress. *J Altern Complement Med.* 2011;17(7):623–8. doi:10.1089/acm.2010.0666.

88. Mata J, Hogan CL, Joormann J, Waugh CE, Gotlib IH. Acute exercise attenuates negative affect following repeated sad mood inductions in persons who have recovered from depression. *J Abnorm Psychol.* 2013;122(1):45–50. doi:10.1037/a0029881.

89. Mayer EA. The neurobiology of stress and gastrointestinal disease. *Gut.* 2000;47(6):861–9. doi:10.1136/gut.47.6.861.

90. McEwen BS. Protective and damaging effects of stress mediators. *N Engl J Med.* 1998;338(3):171–9.

91. McEwen BS, Stellar E. Stress and the individual. Mechanisms leading to disease. *Arch Intern Med.* 1993;153(18):2093–101. doi:10.1001/archinte.153.18.2093.

92. McEwen BS, Wingfield JC. The concept of allostasis in biology and biomedicine. *Horm Behav.* 2003;43(1):2–15. doi:10.1016/s0018-506x(02)00024-7.

93. McFarlane AH, Norman GR, Streiner DL, Roy RG. The process of social stress: stable, reciprocal, and mediating relationships. *J Health Soc Behav.* 1983;24(2):160–73. doi:10.2307/2136642.

94. McGonagle KA, Kessler RC. Chronic stress, acute stress, and depressive symptoms. *Am J Community Psychol.* 1990;18(5):681–706. doi:10.1007/bf00931237.

95. Miller SM. Controllability and human stress: method, evidence and theory. *Behav Res Ther.* 1979;17(4):287–304. doi:10.1016/0005-7967(79)90001-9.

96. Mohr DC, Hart SL, Julian L, Cox D, Pelletier D. Association between stressful life events and exacerbation in multiple sclerosis: a meta-analysis. *Br Med J.* 2004;328(7442):731–3. doi:10.1136/bmj.38041.724421.55.

97. Naves-Bittencourt W, Mendonça-de-Sousa A, Stults-Kolehmainen M, et al. Martial arts: mindful exercise to combat stress. *Eur J Hum Mov.* 2015;34:34–51.

98. Norris R, Carroll D, Cochrane R. The effects of physical activity and exercise training on psychological stress and well-being in an adolescent population. *J Psychosom Res.* 1992;36(1):55–65. doi:10.1016/0022-3999(92)90114-h.

99. Patterson SM, Matthews KA, Allen MT, Owens JF. Stress-induced hemoconcentration of blood-cells and lipids in healthy women during acute psychological stress. *Health Psychol.* 1995;14(4):319–24. doi:10.1037/0278-6133.14.4.319.

100. Patterson SM, Zakowski SG, Hall MH, Cohen L, Wollman K, Baum A. Psychological stress and platelet activation: differences in platelet reactivity in healthy-men during active and passive stressors. *Health Psychol.* 1994;13(1):34–8. doi:10.1037/0278-6133.13.1.34.

101. Pearlin LI, Schooler C. Structure of coping. *J Health Soc Behav.* 1978;19(1):2–21. doi:10.2307/2136319.

102. Petruzzello SJ, Landers DM, Hatfield BD, Kubitz KA, Salazar W. A meta-analysis on the anxiety-reducing effects of acute and chronic exercise. Outcomes and mechanisms. *Sports Med.* 1991;11(3):143–82.

103. Peveler RC, Johnston DW. Subjective and cognitive effects of relaxation. *Behav Res Ther.* 1986;24(4):413–9. doi:10.1016/0005-7967(86)90006-9.

104. Pike JL, Smith TL, Hauger RL, et al. Chronic stress alters sympathetic, neuroendocrine, and immune responsivity to an acute psychological stressor in humans. *Psychosom Med.* 1997;59(4):447–57.

105. Pothmann R, Frankenberg SV, Muller B, Sartory G, Hellmeier W. Epidemiology of headache in children and ad-

olescents: evidence of high prevalence of migraine. *Int J Beh Med.* 1994;1(1):76–89. doi:10.1207/s15327558ijbm0101_5.

106. Prakhinkit S, Suppapitiporn S, Tanaka H, Suksom D. Effects of Buddhism walking meditation on depression, functional fitness, and endothelium-dependent vasodilation in depressed elderly. *J Altern Complement Med.* 2014;20(5):411–6. doi:10.1089/acm.2013.0205.

107. Pruessner JC, Hellhammer DH, Kirschbaum C. Burnout, perceived stress, and cortisol responses to awakening. *Psychosom Med.* 1999;61(2):197–204.

108. Rodgers WM, Sullivan MJL. Task, coping, and scheduling self-efficacy in relation to frequency of physical activity. *J App Soc Psychol.* 2001;31(4):741–53. doi:10.1111/j.1559-1816.2001.tb01411.x.

109. Rout UR, Rout JK. *Stress Management for Primary Health Care Professionals.* New York (NY): Kluwer Academic; 2002. 201 p.

110. Sandi C, Davies HA, Cordero MI, Rodriguez JJ, Popov VI, Stewart MG. Rapid reversal of stress induced loss of synapses in CA3 of rat hippocampus following water maze training. *Eur J Neurosci.* 2003;17(11):2447–56. doi:10.1046/j.1460-9568.2003.02675.x.

111. Sandler IN, Lakey B. Locus of control as a stress moderator: the role of control perceptions and social support. *Am J Community Psychol.* 1982;10(1):65–80. doi:10.1007/bf00903305.

112. Sapolsky RM, Krey LC, McEwen BS. The neuroendocrinology of stress and aging: the glucocorticoid cascade hypothesis. *Endocr Rev.* 1986;7(3):284–301

113. Sarafino EP. *Health Psychology: Biopsychosocial Interactions.* 4th ed. New York (NY): John Wiley & Sons; 2002. 688 p.

114. Sauro KM, Becker WJ. The stress and migraine interaction. *Headache.* 2009;49(9):1378–86.

115. Schnall PL, Pieper C, Schwartz JE, et al. The relationship between 'job strain,' workplace diastolic blood-pressure, and left-ventricular mass index: results of a case-control study. *JAMA.* 1990;263(14):1929–35. doi:10.1001/jama.263.14.1929.

116. Segar ML, Eccles JS, Richardson CR. Rebranding exercise: closing the gap between values and behavior. *Int J Behav Nutr Phys Act.* 2011;8:14. doi:10.1186/1479-5868-8-94.

117. Segerstrom SC, Taylor SE, Kemeny ME, Reed GM, Visscher BR. Causal attributions predict rate of immune decline in HIV-seropositive gay men. *Health Psychol.* 1996;15(6):485–93. doi:10.1037/0278-6133.15.6.485.

118. Selye H. *The Stress of Life.* New York (NY): McGraw-Hill; 1956. 324 p.

119. Selye H. *The Stress of Life.* 2nd ed. New York (NY): McGraw-Hill; 1976. 515 p.

120. Sheridan JF, Dobbs CM. Stress, viral pathogenesis, and immunity. In: Glaser R, Kiecolt-Glaser J, editors. *Handbook of Human Stress and Immunity.* San Diego (CA): Academic Press; 1994. p. 101–23.

121. Sherwood A, Turner JR. Hemodynamic responses during psychological stress: implications for studying disease processes. *Int J Behav Med.* 1995;2(3):193–218. doi:10.1207/s15327558ijbm0203_1.

122. Solberg EE, Ingjer F, Holen A, Sundgot-Borgen J, Nilsson S, Holme I. Stress reactivity to and recovery from a standardised exercise bout: a study of 31 runners prac-

tising relaxation techniques. *Br J Sports Med.* 2000;34(4):268–72.

123. Stetler CA, Miller GE. Social integration of daily activities and cortisol secretion: a laboratory based manipulation. *J Behav Med.* 2008;31(3):249–57. doi:10.1007/s10865-007-9143-2.

124. Stults-Kolehmainen MA. The interplay between stress and physical activity in the prevention and treatment of cardiovascular disease. *Front Physiol.* 2013;4:346. doi:10.3389/fphys.2013.00346.

125. Stults-Kolehmainen MA, Bartholomew JB. Psychological stress impairs short-term muscular recovery from resistance exercise. *Med Sci Sports Exerc.* 2012;44(11):2220–7. doi:10.1249/MSS.0b013e31825f67a0.

126. Stults-Kolehmainen MA, Bartholomew JB, Sinha R. Chronic psychological stress impairs recovery of muscular function and somatic sensations over a 96-hour period. *J Strength Cond Res.* 2014;28(7):2007–17. doi:10.1519/JSC.0000000000000335.

127. Stults-Kolehmainen MA, Ciccolo JT, Bartholomew JB, Seifert J, Portman RS. Age and gender-related changes in exercise motivation among highly active individuals. *Athl Insight.* 2013;5(1):45–63.

128. Stults-Kolehmainen MA, Lu T, Ciccolo JT, Bartholomew JB, Brotnow L, Sinha R. Higher chronic psychological stress is associated with blunted affective responses to strenuous resistance exercise: RPE, pleasure, pain. *Psychol Sport Exerc.* 2016;22:27–36.

129. Stults-Kolehmainen MA, Sinha R. The effects of stress on physical activity and exercise: a systematic review. *Sports Med.* 2014;44(1):81–121. doi:10.1007/s40279-013-0090-5.

130. Stults-Kolehmainen MA, Tuit K, Sinha R. Lower cumulative stress is associated with better health for physically active adults in the community. *Stress.* 2014;17(2):157–68. doi:10.3109/10253890.2013.878329.

131. Suls J, Mullen B. Life change and psychological distress: the role of perceived control and desirability. *J App Soc Psychol.* 1981;11(5):379–89. doi:10.1111/j.1559-1816.1981.tb00830.x.

132. Taylor RL, Lam DJ, Roppel CE, Barter JT. Friends can be good medicine: an excursion into mental health promotion. *Community Ment Health J.* 1984;20(4):294–303. doi:10.1007/bf00757078.

133. Taylor SE. *Health Psychology.* 8th ed. New York (NY): McGraw-Hill; 2012. 576 p.

134. Taylor SE, Kemeny ME, Aspinwall LG, Schneider SG, Rodriguez R, Herbert M. Optimism, coping, psychological distress, and high-risk sexual-behavior among men at risk for acquired-immunodeficiency-syndrome (AIDS). *J Pers Soc Psychol.* 1992;63(3):460–73. doi:10.1037/0022-3514.63.3.460.

135. Thayer RE, Newman JR, McClain TM. Self-regulation of mood: strategies for changing a bad mood, raising energy, and reducing tension. *J Pers Soc Psychol.* 1994;67(5):910–25. doi:10.1037/0022-3514.67.5.910.

136. Thoits PA. Mechanisms linking social ties and support to physical and mental health. *J Health Soc Behav.* 2011;52(2):145–61. doi:10.1177/0022146510395592.

137. Thompson SC. Will it hurt less if I can control it? A complex answer to a simple question. *Psychol Bull.* 1981;90(1):89–101. doi:10.1037/0033-2909.90.1.89.

138. Trask PC, Paterson AG, Hayasaka S, Dunn RL, Riba M, Johnson T. Psychosocial characteristics of individuals with non-stage IV melanoma. *J Clin Oncol*. 2001;19(11): 2844–50.

139. Umberson D. Family status and health behaviors: social control as a dimension of social integration. *J Health Soc Behav*. 1987;28(3):306–19. doi:10.2307/2136848.

140. Van der Linden D, Keijsers GPJ, Eling P, Van Schaijk R. Work stress and attentional difficulties: an initial study on burnout and cognitive failures. *Work Stress*. 2005;19(1):23–36. doi:10.1080/0267837050065275.

141. Vitaliano PP, Russo J, Niaura R. Plasma-lipids and their relationships with psychosocial factors in older adults. *J Gerontol Ser B Psychol Sci Soc Sci*. 1995;50(1):P18–P24.

142. Webb TL, Miles E, Sheeran P. Dealing with feeling: a meta-analysis of the effectiveness of strategies derived from the process model of emotion regulation. *Psychol Bull*. 2012;138(4):775–808. doi:10.1037/a0027600.

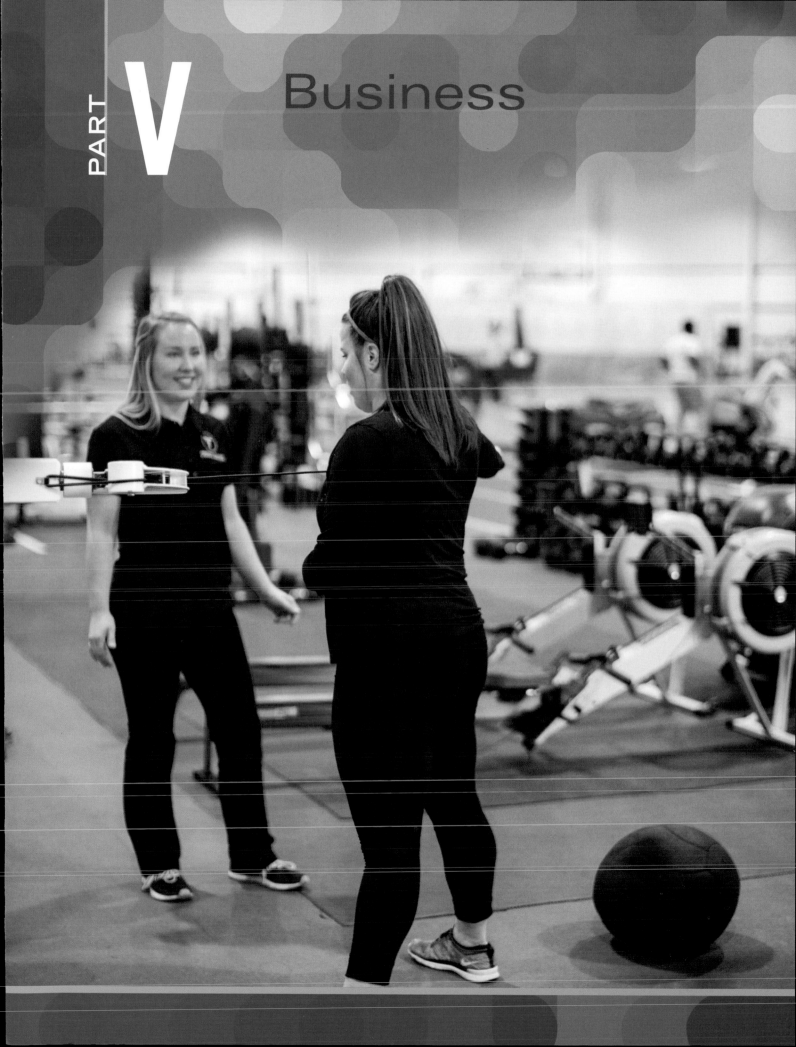

PART **V** Business

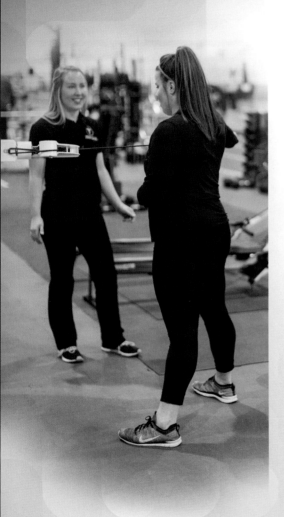

14 Legal Structure and Terminology

OBJECTIVES

- To understand basic concepts of the law and legal system.

- To understand the potential for legal liability and areas of primary concern.

- To appreciate the significance of industry standards and guidelines.

- To become acquainted with risk management strategies.

- To become acquainted with administrative responsibilities.

INTRODUCTION

What is the relevance of understanding the law and legal system by the certified exercise physiologist (EP-C)? With the recognition that the EP-C is a more qualified instructor than those typically found within the fitness industry, it is understandable that he or she will be held to a higher "standard of care." Therefore, it is incumbent on the EP-C to be knowledgeable of the basic structure and function of our legal system. Being aware of how this system may be used either as an asset or as a liability to the client–instructor relationship enables the EP-C to take advantage of protective mechanisms afforded by the system and to avoid pitfalls that can threaten not only the safety of their clients but also the livelihood of the EP-C.

The EP-C who trains within a fitness facility will most likely find that an injured party will pursue a claim against the facility rather than the EP-C because the facility is viewed as having more extensive financial resources. Nevertheless, claims have been filed jointly against facilities and instructors wherein multiple judgments have been rendered.

In this chapter, the EP-C is exposed to those tenets of the standard of care that are promulgated by industry leaders and available to protect the instructor. The focus will be on essential client services and, more importantly, protective actions that help insulate the EP-C against litigation while simultaneously promoting professionalism.

The Law and Legal System

The EP-C must be knowledgeable about the basic concepts of the law and the legal system. Along with this is the accompanying terminology that will provide the EP-C with insight into issues affecting his or her business and potential exposure to liability. The EP-C needs to understand the various divisions of the law, and especially the division of civil law, where tortuous and contract claims are areas within which the EP-C is most likely to become legally embroiled. The anatomy of a lawsuit should be understood such that the EP-C can navigate the sequence of legal proceedings and requirements to successfully support or defend a negligence claim or contract violation.

The EP-C must understand that negligence is defined as one's failure to act, or as more likely will be the case, one's substandard performance. There are four elements of a negligence claim that must be documented to bring a successful suit against the EP-C. If in fact these elements are substantiated, then the court can assess monetary damages against the EP-C. Each element will be discussed in more detail later in this chapter.

The EP-C needs to be aware of those varied situations wherein an instructor may create a risk of insult, injury, or possibly death, as these all present a potential case of negligence. There exists a myriad of settings to be considered when determining one's susceptibility to a negligence lawsuit, and these areas of vulnerability can primarily be found within the five stages of the instructor–client relationship. In short, if the EP-C can remember the acronym STEPS (Fig. 14.1), this will be helpful in avoiding the distressing experience of litigation. By being attentive and applying the standard of care to the details of each one of these five steps, the EP-C can successfully navigate through potentially litigious waters (3).

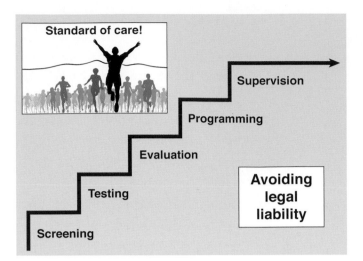

FIGURE 14.1. STEPS to success: avoiding legal liability.

 ## Primary Sources of Law

The primary sources of law can be divided into four categories: (a) constitutional law, (b) statutory law, (c) case law, and (d) administrative law. The federal government and all states have constitutions that not only provide the authority for government but also define how it will function and what its responsibilities are. Statutory laws or legislative laws are enacted by mandates from federal, state, and municipal governments, and this codification of law imposes duties or restrictions on individuals. However, in the case of the Good Samaritan law, immunity is granted to those persons who in good faith try to protect, serve, and tend to others who are injured or ill. It should be noted, though, that the Good Samaritan law does not apply to the EP-C while on the job. Case law, sometimes referred to as common law, is based on decisions of courts and administrative tribunals. Common law is founded on unwritten law (not codified) and is based on customs and general usages, whereas case law is based on reported judicial decisions of selected lower and appellate courts. Administrative law is found within specialized bodies or agencies that have been granted lawmaking power to regulate specific activities. Federal agencies such as the Occupational Safety and Health Administration (OSHA), along with numerous state agencies, draft and enforce regulations that impact a wide range of individuals and entities, including fitness instructors and health facilities (6). Primary sources of law then are official bodies with the authority to make laws that can affect the legal rights of citizens.

In addition, our system of jurisprudence is subdivided into the two domains of criminal law and civil law, both of which dispose the citizenry to act in a way that benefits society. Whereas criminal law governs the conduct of both individuals and groups toward society as a whole, civil law pertains to personal responsibilities that an individual or a group must observe when dealing with other individuals or groups. This division of law addresses expressed grievances and judicial remedies between individuals, between an individual and a group, or between groups.

When individuals or groups violate criminal laws, they are subject to the penalties for misdemeanors and felonies, including fines, imprisonment, or both. Although the EP-C is less likely to violate criminal law, there is the possibility that he or she could be charged with the unauthorized practice of medicine or unauthorized practice of an allied health field such as physical therapy or dietetics. For example, after screening a client for resting blood pressure, the EP-C cannot diagnose him or her as hypertensive, as such a diagnosis remains only within the purview of a licensed physician. It could also be considering encroaching upon the realm of physical therapy by conducting postural analyses and providing corrective exercises, or encroaching upon the field of dietetics by providing clients with specific meal plans to correct nutritional deficiencies. The EP-C could be found guilty of committing a first-degree misdemeanor that not only is punishable by a severe fine but also could be punishable by imprisonment. Therefore, it is especially wise for the EP-C, and any other unlicensed provider, to remain well within his or her scope of practice.

When individuals or groups violate civil law, they are subject to the jurisprudence of civil courts that adjudicate noncriminal cases. Civil lawsuits handle disputes between individuals, organizations, businesses, and governmental agencies wherein two parties, the plaintiff (*e.g.*, the injured party or representative of an injured or deceased individual) and the defendant (*e.g.*, the EP-C and/or the facility that he or she represents), present their cases for litigation (6). Whereas criminal law requires that a prosecutor provide proof beyond a reasonable doubt to find the defendant guilty, civil law only requires that the plaintiff demonstrate that the preponderance of the evidence supports his or her claim to find the defendant liable. This again emphasizes that the EP-C should stay within the stated scope or practice, as to avoid any potential issues of negligence that may lead to litigation.

When considering lawsuits against instructor personnel and fitness facilities, the plurality of such cases falls within the domain of civil law. The typical civil law violation falls under the categories of either tort law or contract law.

Tort Law

A tort is a breach of legal duty amounting to a civil wrong or injury for which a court of law will provide compensation/damages. Therefore, tort law governs the legal rights and obligations between individuals as well as between collective bodies in relationship to injuries, deaths, or civil wrongdoings (5). A tort by definition is a wrongful act, whether intentional or accidental, from which an insult, injury, or death occurs to another person or perhaps an organization that sustains pecuniary damage. The individual or group that is injured or sustains pecuniary damage is known as the plaintiff, whereas the individual or group responsible for the tortuous act is known as the defendant or tortfeasor. When an injury, death, or wrong is documented and attributed to the defendant, a remedy, usually in the form of a financial judgment, is then levied against the defendant. This levy, applied by the civil court, provides relief to the plaintiff. A tort does not include a breach of contract that also can lead to adjudication and compensation in the form of monetary damages.

Torts do include all negligence cases as well as intentional wrongdoings that result in injury or death. There also exists a tort due to "no fault" conduct. Therefore, tortuous acts are divided into the following three categories: (a) intentional misconduct, (b) negligent conduct, and (c) "no fault" conduct. "No fault" conduct falls under the category of strict liability and relates to ultrahazardous activities and product liability that will not be addressed in this chapter (6). An intentional tort is indicative of an act that willfully caused an injury, a death, a financial distress, or a damaged reputation. Because it is extremely difficult to document an intentional tort, courts typically give the benefit of doubt to the defendant and presume that the tort is one of negligence.

Negligence

When considering the lawsuits filed against fitness facilities and/or fitness instructors, the overwhelming majority are suits alleging negligence. The definitions of "negligence" and "standard of care" are similar in that they both are concerned with prudence and caution in dealing with clients. Standard of care refers to the application of a degree of prudence and caution required by an individual or organization that owes a duty of care. As it relates to the fitness industry, the standard of care is the degree of care that a reasonably prudent fitness instructor or reasonably prudent facility management would utilize under similar circumstances. A failure to exercise that degree of care utilized by prudent instructors or management represents negligence. The failure to do, or the failure to avoid, that which the prudent instructor would have done or not done may lead an individual to becoming liable for negligence. As a certified practitioner, the EP-C will be held to a higher standard than most other instructors. Figure 14.2 provides an image of the components of negligence.

FIGURE 14.2. Minimizing negligence through risk management.

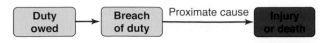

For the plaintiff to prosecute a successful tort claim, four basic elements of negligence must be well documented (8). First, a legal duty must be established from the relationship between the client and the EP-C, a duty in which the EP-C is required to provide safe and effective instruction without exposure to risks that could be the cause of injury and, perhaps, even death. Second, a breach of that legal duty, which is either substandard performance or a failure to act, is determined to have taken place. Third, the breach of duty owed was the factual or proximate cause of the injury or death. Fourth, the negligent act or failure to act resulted in well-documented damages or losses to the plaintiff, both economic damages (*e.g.*, medical costs and lost wages) and noneconomic damages (*e.g.*, pain and suffering).

EP-Cs can use three major risk management strategies to lessen the chances of becoming embroiled in legal liability with a negligence tort. First, the EP-C must adhere to the standard of care in the screening process, fitness profiling, evaluation, programming, and supervision of clients. Second, the EP-C must use waivers and assumption of risk forms in varied venues of the client–instructor relationship. Third, the EP-C must ensure that he or she has purchased appropriate liability insurance for the activities in which his or her client is engaged.

Regarding adherence to the standard of care, the grasp of safe and effective fitness practices is dealt with in other chapters within this resource manual. However, the prudent and cautious EP-C is unlikely to be faced with litigation because of his or her commitment to providing such safe and effective practices. This is the first line of defense in risk management. Waivers and assumption of risk forms provide a second line of defense and must be understood in light of their implementation and limitations.

Protective legal documents exist in different forms, of which the three most common are informed consent, agreement to participate, and prospective waivers or releases. However, before discussing the legal protection each of the above documents provides, it is necessary to review the three major causes of injury or death associated with physical activity:

- *Inherent:* injuries due to accidents that are not preventable and are no one's fault
- *Negligence:* injuries due to the fault of the defendant (sometimes the plaintiff)
- *Extreme forms of negligence:* injuries due to the gross negligence, willful and wanton, or reckless conduct of the defendant (5)

When lawsuits are filed due to an inherent injury such as a sprained ankle on a fitness facility's basketball court, an informed consent or agreement to participate provides the best legal protection by strengthening what is termed an assumption of risk defense. For this reason, informed consents are utilized prior to fitness testing or exercise programming and participation. Therefore, despite the fact that the client has been advised and warned of the risks, he or she declares that the risks are understood, appreciated, and voluntarily assumed. Although this defense is generally upheld in court for injuries due to inherent causes, it is sometimes used unsuccessfully be defendants for various reasons; for example, the injury was due to negligence of the defendant or the plaintiff did not fully understand and appreciate the inherent risks prior to participation. Chapter 2 of this textbook covers preparticipation screening in greater detail.

When lawsuits are filed due to negligence on the part of the instructor, a prospective waiver or release provides the best legal protection to thwart potential liability. Within the waiver, there exists an "exculpatory" clause explicitly stating that the instructor is released from liability due to any negligence. This clause is designed to document that the client has relinquished his or her right to pursue litigation. The validity of waivers to provide protection from negligent torts is determined by state law, which can vary greatly from state to state. In some states, waivers provide no protection from liability due to negligence, whereas in other states, lenient, moderate, or rigorous requirements (4) must be upheld to protect the instructor from negligence.

To ensure that waivers and releases are legally binding, EP-Cs should engage legal counsel to draft their exculpatory forms, recognizing that state laws not only vary but also change periodically. Therefore, if the EP-C has been using waivers or releases for an extended period, it is wise to have legal counsel review the forms to ensure that they remain compliant with current law. Frequently, the EP-C can obtain samples of waivers and releases from seminars or copies in texts such as American College of Sports Medicine (ACSM) *Health/Fitness Facility Standards and Guidelines* (11). Although this may save the cost of hiring a lawyer, the EP-C should be aware that these documents might not be applicable and legally enforceable in their state.

When lawsuits are filed due to extreme or gross negligence, there are generally no protective legal documents. A few states may permit the use of a waiver or release to provide such protection, but this is rarely the case (4). Extreme forms of negligence exist when the defendant is aware of the potential danger and risk of an activity or exercise but fails to warn the client and instead allows the performance of that activity or exercise. In such cases, punitive damages may be awarded, and normally, liability insurance policies will not cover the instructor who is liable of extreme negligence.

As discussed, protective legal documents are an important line of defense for the EP-C in that they can provide evidence in a court of law that the client was made aware of risks but decided to assume such risks as outlined. In addition, an exculpatory clause may provide a defense in case of an inadvertent lapse in the EP-C's performance related to either an act of commission or an act of omission. Frequently, protective legal documents in the form of prospectively signed waivers or exculpatory agreements may prevent a claim from going forward, as a judge can dismiss a case through a pretrial motion termed a summary judgment.

Insurance Coverage

As previously stated, liability insurance is an important component of an EP-C's risk management strategy. There are multiple types of insurance coverage available to the EP-C; however, those of interest should be "general" and "professional" liability insurance that affords protection from negligence claims. The EP-C can obtain a general liability insurance policy, which protects from "ordinary" negligence, from a commercial general liability firm, or CGL (2).

Professional liability insurance (PLI), also called professional indemnity insurance (PII) but more commonly known as errors and omissions (E&O), protects individuals who provide professional advice and service as part of their job responsibility. This insurance is similar to malpractice insurance purchased by physicians. When the EP-C is employed in a health care provider setting, he or she is more likely to be regarded as conducting professional services and, therefore, should have PII. However, because CGL firms may attempt to avoid a payoff by claiming their policy excludes coverage for "professional services," the EP-C should hold both general and PLI (6).

The last line of defense in risk management is the possession of both general and PLI. With this coverage, the EP-C can be assured that an untoward event at work resulting in a negligence claim will not dampen his or her future but that he or she can continue to enjoy a personally rewarding and financially secure career as a fitness professional.

Federal Laws

Key laws, in which both employers and EP-Cs should be well versed, include those pertaining to sexual harassment, workplace safety, and maintaining privacy of clients and employees. Each of these is critical to promoting a safe and inviting environment and conducting business in the most professional manner possible. Ideally, legal counseling will be retained to make sure the place of business is in compliance with the various aspects of each law.

Sexual Harassment

The definition of sexual harassment is any kind of intimidation, browbeating, bullying, or coercion of a sexual nature; the inappropriate promise of promotions in exchange for sexual favors; or the threat of loss of job security for failure to provide such favors (10). Both sexes may be guilty of sexual harassment, although, more often, complaints are lodged against men. The EP-C could be the victim of sexual harassment by peers as well as superiors; of course, the EP-C could also be accused of sexual harassment in relation to clients. Sexual harassment is a form of sex discrimination and as such can lead to litigation.

Title VII of the Civil Rights Act of 1964 prohibits sex discrimination in the workplace, and since that time, the courts have extended this prohibition to include sexual harassment. In 1980, the U.S. Equal Employment Opportunity Commission amended its "Guidelines on Discrimination Because of Sex" to include sexual harassment and helped solidify judicial acceptance of this cause of action (10).

Sexual harassment could include a range of behaviors from seemingly mild transgressions and annoyances to actual sexual abuse or sexual assault. In some circumstances, sexual harassment may be not only unethical but also illegal and, therefore, a violation of criminal law. In the workplace, sexual harassment is a form of illegal employment discrimination. For many fitness facilities, preventing sexual harassment among personnel and defending employees from sexual harassment charges have become key goals of managers.

The EP-C must be aware that charges of sexual harassment by clients can be made against him or her, and therefore, the EP-C needs to choose his or her words carefully, to be cautious with touching as in assisting and spotting clients, and to avoid any suggestion of impropriety. For example, when the male EP-C is conducting body fat testing with skinfold calipers within the confines of a testing center, it would be wise to have a female employee assisting, thereby ensuring that no unjust accusations may be directed against the examiner.

OSHA Guidelines

Under the U.S. Department of Labor, the OSHA is the principal federal agency charged with the enforcement of safety and health legislation in the workplace. In an effort to improve worker safety, OSHA has established regulations that have some specific implications for the fitness industry. The health code relating to blood-borne pathogens presents a formidable challenge to facility managers and often their EP-Cs who, as a result of their higher level of certification, are assigned the task of implementing a safety policy to prevent the possibility of employees contracting HIV and hepatitis B and C viruses.

EP-Cs frequently become responsible for understanding, recognizing, and dealing with the blood-borne pathogen threat inherent within fitness center operations, especially during an emergency response. There are potential dangers for pathogen exposure to both staff and members, and therefore, the EP-C may have to educate employees how to protect not only themselves but also their members through necessary preventive techniques.

EP-Cs should become familiar with OSHA's published guidelines that provide directives on the training and record-keeping procedures of how to avoid and handle blood-borne pathogens. To adequately protect both staff and members, the EP-C may need to educate facility employees on the following:

- What is a blood-borne pathogen?
- What is meant by *occupational exposure* to blood-borne pathogens?
- What are potential infectious materials and how to prevent exposure to them?
- What are the possible methods of disease transmission and how can they be controlled?
- What protective equipment is required to safeguard the first responder in an emergency situation? (3)

An explanation of the stated concerns along with additional information of interest is available from OSHA, with regional offices located throughout the country that can provide fitness facility personnel with written materials and advice on how to meet OSHA requirements and how to improve workplace safety. Furthermore, the International Health, Racquet and Sportsclub Association (IHRSA), the professional trade association of the fitness industry, has published a briefing paper for its member facilities regarding the OSHA blood-borne pathogens requirements (9). Failure to meet OSHA's legally enforceable standards may result in facility citations and penalties.

Besides blood-borne pathogens, employees and perhaps even facility members may be exposed to potentially hazardous substances such as swimming pool chemicals and cleaning agents. Therefore, the EP-C may be assigned the task of advising facility employees, including independent contractors, of potentially harmful materials other than blood-borne pathogens. This may be accomplished through the posting of placards, notices, and memoranda. To this end, the ACSM's *Health/Fitness Facility Standards and Guidelines*, indicates under Appendix B, Supplement 5, that "The OSHA Hazard Communication Standard requires you to develop a written hazard communication program" (11).

HIPAA Guidelines and Recommendations

Under the U.S. Department of Health and Human Services, the Health Insurance Portability and Accountability Act (HIPAA) of 1996 was established to protect the privacy of health information. The Office for Civil Rights is provided the legal authority to enforce the HIPAA Privacy Rule, a rule that protects the privacy of an individual's identifiable health information. The HIPAA Security Rule sets national standards for the security of electronically protected health information and also for the confidentiality of such information (12).

HIPAA requires that all information gathered about a client's health status must be kept confidential in the fitness facility. The EP-C will frequently oversee the health screening process and therefore needs to guarantee that all information from medical histories, physical exam reports, and lifestyle questionnaires are only available to the appropriate individuals and that this information will be properly maintained and secured.

The HIPAA Privacy Rule provides federal protections for personal health information held by covered entities such as health care providers, health plans, and health care clearinghouses. The rule gives patients an array of rights regarding the privacy of their information. Concurrently, the Privacy Rule is balanced by permitting the disclosure of personal health information that is required by legitimate health care professionals for patient care. Although fitness facilities are not technically listed as covered entities, because they have access to members' health information, they have an obligation to guarantee the confidentiality, integrity, and security of that information, or they could be found in violation of the Privacy Rule.

 ## Client Rights and Responsibilities

The EP-C is expected to have a mature grasp of instructor–client relations and what it means to provide professional service to his or her clientele. The EP-C should know what is included in the rights of the client, such as making informed choices and knowing how to voice grievances. Likewise, it is often the duty of the EP-C to ensure that clients in turn know their responsibilities to the facility and instructor, which could mean being truthful about their health history and assisting in keeping the workout environment safe.

Client Rights

Clients have the right to receive quality service that is provided in a respectful manner without offensive or defamatory remarks or any form of discrimination. Clients should be provided with an overview of services provided and what would be typical health and fitness requirements to safely participate in these physical activities. This information allows clients to make informed choices about services and programs that would be suitable to their needs and capabilities.

Clients have the right to know the qualifications of staff members and the educational requirements met to achieve different certifications. Client should be well informed about any activities in which they will be exposed and any inherent risks as well as risks created through the inability to carry out activities as directed by instructors.

Clients not only have the right to an appropriate health screening but also have the necessity to be screened prior to physical activity. In addition, they have the right for a thorough orientation to the facility, operation of equipment to be used, and physical activity programs available, while also being advised of how to respond to potential emergencies within the facility.

Clients have a right to timely responses to their requests and inquiries along with reasonable continuity and coordination of any services provided. Any charges for services should be openly disclosed and discussed, and if there are any complaints, clients have a right to know how to voice their grievances about services provided or omitted.

In line with the HIPAA Privacy Rule as well as described in ethical statements published by ACSM and other professional organizations, clients have the right to expect confidentiality regarding health information that is disclosed to facility staff. In addition, if there is other personal and financial information shared with a facility, it must be handled discreetly and securely.

Client Responsibilities

Clients have the responsibility to give accurate information about their physical and mental health, any substance abuse, or any other conditions or circumstances that could adversely impact their physical activity programming. If during activities clients experience pain or any injuries, it is their responsibility to report such concerns to instructor personnel in a timely and forthright manner.

Clients are to assist instructor personnel in maintaining a neat and safe environment, such as in putting weights back in their racks or not leaving clothing or bottles on the floor where they could become a hazard to others. This means respecting not only the workout areas but also other areas such as lounges or locker rooms.

Personal training clients are responsible for notifying their trainers well in advance if they cannot make appointments or if appointments need to be rescheduled. Likewise, clients should also notify facilities well in advance if they have to suspend a membership. If clients' addresses or phone numbers have changed, facilities must be advised. Clients are responsible for working with their instructors or trainers in reviewing, planning, or changing programs to ensure that programs meet their needs, capabilities, and schedules. In this respect, clients should also be quick to inform instructors or trainers if they are having any concerns or problems with the service being provided.

Both IHRSA and the ACSM have addressed a facility's responsibilities to its membership and therefore the rights to be anticipated by clients (9,11). Both IHRSA's *Standards Facilitation Guide* and ACSM's *Health/Fitness Facility Standards and Guidelines* publications outline important responsibilities addressing preactivity screening, orientations, education, and supervision of membership; risk management; and emergency policies. These responsibilities, and more, are owed to the client; in addition, there are responsibilities outlined that the member/client has to the facility and its staff.

Contract Law

The law of contracts governs agreements that are enforceable in court. Contracts are agreements pertaining to the legal rights and obligations between individuals as well as between collective bodies. The contract is a stipulation to which both parties consent and recognize as legally enforceable. This agreement or promise gives rise to a legal obligation that one will perform or not perform some activity or venture. An offer is proposed by one party and then accepted by the other. In effect, there exists a promised exchange between the parties, and this promised exchange may be written, oral, and even implied. This agreement or promised exchange within the health and fitness industry usually amounts to a service (availability of a facility and exercise instruction) for money (financial remuneration). Examples of contracts used in the health fitness field are (a) employment contracts for employees and independent contractors, (b) informed consents, (c) waivers, and (d) membership contracts.

Employer and Employee Rights and Responsibilities

When individuals are hired by a facility to work as an EP-C, there is in effect a contract regarding the rights and responsibilities of the employee. The employee has agreed to perform certain services for which he or she will be remunerated. And the employee has the recognizable expectation that he or she will be treated with a degree of propriety and decorum while in the conduct of his or her service, whether it be from fellow workers, management, or even clientele.

Employers and employees have responsibilities to each other, and they should expect their rights to be upheld while their responsibilities are met. Regarding employee rights, one expects that he or she will be presented with a well-defined job description and that there will be periodic reviews of work performance with accompanying critiques and recommendations for improvement or, hopefully, recognition for exemplary performance.

Employees can expect that the provision of their terms and conditions of employment will be explicitly spelled out. They can expect that the terms and conditions will set forth what their primary and secondary duties are, to whom they are accountable, their rates of pay, and other entitlements such as vacation time, health benefits, sick leave, and the like.

Employees can expect that there will be no discrimination of any kind (to include sexual harassment) and that there will be equal opportunities for advancement with appropriate pay adjustments. Equal opportunity legislation mandates that all employees must receive the same pay and same work conditions for carrying out the same or similar work. There are also specific laws relating to gender, racial, and disability discrimination (15).

Employees are expected to conduct their services in a manner that has regard to the safety of others, both staff and clientele. In this vein, employees have a serious obligation to educate clients about the safe operation of exercise equipment, in addition to the safety practices involved with all physical activities that clients perform not only in the facility but also outside of the facility.

Regarding OSHA requirements, employees must be advised and have every right to expect that management will caution them about any potential hazards, whether of a physical or chemical nature. This caution may be delivered through verbal warnings or written and posted notices that are readily observable. As previously stated, there exist specific regulations about the manner in which potentially harmful substances should be used, stored, and recognized by both staff and clientele, and this information should be clearly posted for all to see.

In light of the stated requirements, employers are expected to abide by numerous regulations such as providing safe equipment, carrying out regular maintenance and safety checks, ensuring the training of employees in health and safety issues, and carrying out a risk assessment to assess the dangers of the unique work environment within fitness facilities. In short, during their employment, workers can anticipate that management will place a priority on their health and safety.

Employers and employees are expected to meet minimum legal requirements in the area of health and safety at work, as well as minimum standards and conditions related to hours, pay scales, and the treatment of people in the workplace. Along with rights for employees, there are corresponding responsibilities such as the expectation that employees will work in a safe manner and will have regard for the safety of their colleagues and clientele. In addition, employees are responsible for conducting all their relations with management, fellow workers, and clientele with the respect and decorum, reflecting ethical and collegial behavior.

Federal Employment Laws

When in a position to hire personnel, the EP-C must understand the myriad laws that govern hiring. These laws cover issues related to civil rights, disabilities, and more; such laws are continually changing. It is not legally defensible to simply claim that a hiring law changed and you were unaware. Instead, similar to what was mentioned regarding earlier federal laws, legal counsel should be retained to ensure complete compliance with all local, state, and federal hiring laws.

Hiring and Prehiring Statutes

There are federal employment regulations or statutes regarding the hiring and prehiring of individuals and related regulations that apply to the fitness industry and other industries. The two important federal laws that prohibit employment discrimination related to preemployment inquiries include the Civil Rights Act of 1964 and the Americans with Disabilities Act (ADA) of 1990.

The Civil Rights Act of 1964 prohibits discrimination on the basis of race, color, gender, religion, and national origin (14). Therefore, unfair inquiries related to the stated characteristics or preferences within job application forms, preemployment interviews, or any type of inquiry made of job applicants are unlawful. Questions that appear to take a candidate's race; creed; color; national origin; age; gender; marital status; or any physical, mental, or sensory handicap into consideration for discriminatory purposes must be avoided. However, these rules do not prevent employers from asking questions to determine which candidates are most qualified to perform the specific functions or tasks of a given job. These rules were developed to prevent characteristics or conditions that have nothing to do with an individual's ability to perform the job from influencing the process of candidate selection. Understandably, certain physical and mental conditions in addition to personality traits would prevent some individuals from successfully performing various staff duties within a fitness facility, including exercise instruction.

The ADA prohibits employment discrimination on the basis of disabilities or perceived disabilities (14). The ADA addresses the "Dos and Don'ts" regarding preemployment inquiries, specifically those questions to be avoided at the preoffer stage. This means that employers cannot directly ask whether an applicant has a particular disability or ask questions that are closely related to disability issues at any time during the hiring process. The reason for this prohibition is that this information has been used in the past to exclude applicants with disabilities prior to an evaluation of their ability to perform the job.

Both the Civil Rights Act and the ADA make it clear that anyone involved in the interviewing process must avoid asking unfair preemployment questions. Interview questions are considered fair only when they specifically relate to an individual's ability to perform the actual duties of the job. Within the fitness industry, there are many staff positions that can be handled by individuals with disability. In addition, there are individuals with disability who can carry out many of the functions of an EP-C and, in some cases, may be the ideal candidate to offer classes for individuals with disability.

In light of the ADA, it is unfortunate that many barriers still exist that prevent individuals with disability from participating in mainstream society. Sadly, too many fitness facilities cannot accommodate individuals with disability, even though federal requirements mandate such accommodation. In addition to limited accessibility to the fitness facility as a whole, which in itself is an impediment to hiring, it is not uncommon to find rooms within the facility so overcrowded with exercise equipment that individuals who use a wheelchair cannot maneuver between machines nor have proper access to them, which is a clear violation of the ADA.

There are two other federal employment regulations related to hiring, which bear mentioning, background checks and drug testing. A background investigation is normally the process of researching criminal records, commercial records, and, in some cases, financial records of an individual. Background checks are frequently requested by employers interviewing job applicants, especially applicants pursuing positions that require high security or substantial trust, such as in a schools, hospitals, financial institutions, airports, and government. As background checks are normally conducted by government agencies or private enterprises for a fee, most fitness facilities conduct their own checks and are principally interested in criminal history and past employment verification. Such checks allow management to also evaluate qualifications such as education and certifications, along with character.

However, although a fitness facility may want more information on an applicant than that stated earlier, management does not have unlimited rights to investigate an applicant's background and personal life. As employees have a right to privacy in certain areas of their life, they can take legal action if they feel these rights have been violated. Consequently, it is essential that management understand what is permitted when doing further investigation on a potential employee's background and work history.

Under the Federal Trade Commission's Fair Credit Reporting Act (FCRA), applicants must give written permission to prospective employers if employers wish to obtain applicants' credit reports (7). If an employer decides not to hire an applicant or to promote an existing employee based on his or her credit report, then that applicant or employee must be provided a copy of the report, so he or she may challenge the veracity of the report. Statutes regulating the use of investigations of credit reports vary from state to state, and some states have very serious restrictions on obtaining credit reports.

As stated earlier, although fitness facilities have a vested interest in an applicant's potential criminal past, the extent to which a facility's management may consider one's criminal history in making a hiring decision varies from state to state. Owing to this wide variation, management should consult a lawyer or do further legal research on state laws before probing into whether or not an applicant does in fact have a criminal past.

The Drug-Free Workplace Act of 1988 and the mandatory guidelines for federal drug testing programs were specifically designed for federal employees with certain sensitive occupations relating to safety and security (14). Although the Act only applied to federal employees, many state and local governments followed suit and adopted similar programs under state laws and drug-free workplace programs. However, challenges to drug testing arose based on contested violations of the fourth and fifth amendments to the constitution. Generally, applicants are deemed to have a lesser expectation of privacy than current employees, and therefore, employers do enjoy greater freedom to test applicants without the same concerns of constitutional violations being invoked.

Drug testing may be of interest to the fitness facility not only because non–drug users make better employees but also because some facilities may insist that staff, particularly instructors, not engage in the use of steroids or other quasi-illegal performance-enhancing drugs. Although employers rightfully argue that the safety of clientele and coworkers may depend on the alertness of fellow employees and that employers will be liable if an employee under the influence of narcotics or alcohol injures a staff member or client, there are understandable concerns about the invasion of one's privacy. This idea of invasion of one's privacy is not only of concern to the American Civil Liberties Union (ACLU) but also deeply upsetting to many Americans who value their rights and privacy of person and property.

Owing to the stated concerns, there has been the tendency to limit the type and extent of drug testing in the workplace. Specifically, some states have found their courts more restrictive than the federal legislature in regard to preemployment drug testing as well as ongoing drug testing in the workplace. Consequently, it is essential that before designing a drug-free workplace with a testing program, management not only familiarize itself with both state and federal regulations but also secure legal counsel specializing in labor relations and law.

An additional federal regulation and requirement related to prehiring and hiring is the Equal Pay Act of 1963, which prohibits different pay rates on the basis of gender (15). This act was necessitated because over the years, women have received lower wages for the exact same duties performed by men. Another employment regulation is the Age Discrimination in Employment Act (ADEA), which prohibits discrimination on the basis of age for people older than 40 years (15). Yet, another necessary regulation is the Immigration Reform and Control Act of 1986 (IRCA), which requires all employers to complete an employment eligibility verification form on individuals hired after November 6, 1986 (15).

These are but a few of the important requirements that employers need to address when hiring staff for their fitness facilities. In order to be thoroughly versed with prehiring and hiring requirements, employers should visit the U.S. Department of Labor Web site and search under the "Hiring" section for information related to these and numerous other concerns such as affirmative action, the hiring of veterans and foreign workers, and the employment of workers younger than 18 years (13).

Facility Policies and Procedures

A fitness facility's policies and procedures represent a type of contract with employees as the applicant is agreeing to abide by such policies and procedures as a term of his or her employment. The development and implementation of policies and procedures provides businesses, such as fitness facilities, with operational uniformity and consistency. The adherence to policies and procedures is recognized to be one of the most important keys to profitability within a business. Policies and procedures are guidelines as well as mandates to the daily operation of a facility, and observing these assists employees in becoming more proficient because of the implied consistency of practice. This consistency, and proficiency, is noted by members and engenders greater confidence in the staff as a whole.

There are numerous policies and procedures related to the efficient conduct of business and financial operations within a facility. Unfortunately, many facilities fail to develop a comprehensive policy and procedure manual, and instead, it is the responsibility of the EP-C to work with management to develop and implement such a manual. Once developed, the number 1 priority of any facility should be the health and safety of its membership. Within this context of health and safety, there are certain policies and procedures that should take precedence: membership screening, fitness testing, orientations, instructor qualifications, supervision, equipment maintenance, facility cleanliness, and emergency procedures.

Screening members through health risk appraisals is essential to determine whether they are ready for the stress of exercise or whether medical clearance is needed. The health risk appraisal is the procedure by which a facility can identify those members who are at an increased risk for experiencing exercise-related cardiovascular incidents as well as musculoskeletal problems and the consequent need for physician referral before exercise programming can commence. Therefore, this appraisal should be completed and a review for potential risk concluded prior to finalizing a membership agreement and paying for services (3). The current standard of care dictates that screening procedures be practiced without exception. Additionally, it should be noted that too frequently abbreviated screening devices such as the Physical Activity Readiness Questionnaire (PAR-Q) are utilized when more comprehensive health risk appraisals are warranted.

Although it is possible for facilities to require that all members undergo a fitness assessment in conjunction with their health appraisal, it is typical that most facilities only offer and, hopefully, encourage members to avail themselves of this valuable service. There are numerous advantages for the member who participates in such an assessment or fitness profile. The real advantage to the facility, however, is the ability to design safer and more effective programs for clientele, thereby minimizing the chances of injuring a client or creating an untoward incident and consequently lessening the potential for litigation, an obvious priority for any facility.

Managers have a primary responsibility to ensure that facility members receive a formal and comprehensive orientation related to the effectiveness and safety in exercise programming. During the orientation, members should be apprised of the advantages of personal training, to include fitness profiling, which will enhance their chances of program success. Other program services and benefits can be outlined with appropriate cautionary notes regarding one's preparedness for some of the more demanding activities. A walk-through of the facility highlighting both aerobic and resistance equipment should be available, with an emphasis on equipment operation and safety concerns. There are numerous topics to be covered during the orientation, and these should be explicitly detailed in the procedure manual.

Of paramount importance are policies relating to instructor qualifications, particularly regarding education, certifications, and prior work experience. However, it is important to remember that although instructors may possess appropriate education, certification and experience requirements and, therefore, appear qualified, this does not guarantee effective and safe training on their part. Too often, apparently qualified instructors demonstrate poor judgment and a lack of common sense thereby endangering their clients. In effect, they may be certified and qualified but not justified in their actions (1).

In addition to the required knowledge, skills, and ability, instructors must be evaluated and advised on their interpersonal relations with fellow workers and members. Hiring policies must be clear as to which qualifications are most desirable and which qualifications meet minimal requirements. Performance reviews, along with continuing education expectations, should also be clearly detailed in the policy and procedure manual.

Policies regarding supervisory responsibilities ensure that personnel are always available to assist members having difficulty with equipment operation or the technique of specific exercises. Floor supervisors must be aware of potentially unsafe activities and alert to their anticipated implementation. Safe floor monitoring also requires that equipment is arranged in a manner that allows for all areas to be readily visible by personnel on duty and that there are no blind spots in which a member could become endangered without being observed.

Policies regarding equipment maintenance should be in writing and regularly observed. There are general, everyday maintenance requirements and inspections that can be carried out by staff members such as checking cables, pull–pin security, loose belts, gated snap hooks, and so on, along with the routine cleaning and wiping down of equipment. Policies regarding equipment should also include timely and proper reporting of any defects to be listed in maintenance and repair logs. Posted warnings or out-of-order signage is to be visibly secured on inoperable equipment if the equipment cannot be removed from the floor. Besides in-house inspection and cleaning, management should have service contracts with outside vendors who are certified in the inspection and repair of equipment. In addition to regularly scheduled appointments for servicing aerobic and resistive equipment, vendors should also be available for short notice or emergency calls.

Policies regarding facility cleanliness not only lead to member satisfaction and retention but also, more importantly, lead to hygienic safety that can lessen the potential for litigation. An undercover investigation of fitness facilities indicated that "gyms" are some of the most likely environments for the transmission of germs (2). Accordingly, management needs to establish policy and procedures for daily equipment cleaning and hiring a professional cleaning service for nightly or early morning operations. Increased awareness of germ transmission has led many fitness facilities to provide members with clean towels and, more recently, with antiseptic spray bottles, germicidal wipes, paper towel dispensers, and antibacterial hand gel throughout the exercise floor. However, this cannot take the place of policies requiring regular and thorough cleaning provided by staff and professional services.

Of all facility policies, the emergency policy, and particularly the emergency medical policy, is the most consequential. It is incumbent on management to develop a written, venue-specific emergency response plan to deal with any reasonably foreseeable untoward event within the facility. The emergency plan's primary purpose is to ensure that minor problems do not escalate into major incidents and that major incidents do not intensify to fatal events. Possible emergencies could be fires, floods, tornadoes, earthquakes, hurricanes, severe storms, bomb threats, and even terrorist activities.

However, the most likely emergency is a "Code Blue" or "member down," indicating that a client is having a heart attack, stroke, or some other potentially fatal event. This emphasizes the need for an emergency response plan to include an explicit medical emergency policy in which all staff must be well versed. Such a policy dictates that sufficient staff members are certified in first aid and CPR with AED. Another important consideration, too often overlooked, is the availability of supplemental oxygen that is probably one of the most important steps that can be taken in treating the suspected heart attack. Additionally, in the case of a sudden cardiac arrest, an oxygen source attached to a resuscitation mask dramatically increases the chance of survival (3).

A well-rehearsed emergency response plan guarantees a timely response in carrying out the multiple duties expected of staff, such as who coordinates the scene, who are first and assistant responders, who takes charge of crowd control, who meets and directs paramedics to the scene, and who is responsible for securing the member's file along with notifying the nearest relative. If these policies and procedures are lax, or staff rehearsal is not frequent, the potential for litigation increases exponentially. Therefore, anticipative management is considered not only imperative but also "good insurance" (6).

SUMMARY

The key to the health and safety of facility members is the availability of knowledgeable, skilled, and conscientious fitness instructors capable of establishing a safe exercise environment. This requires that staff members at all levels must not only be appropriately qualified to carry out their respective duties but also be sufficiently motivated to do the job to the best of their abilities.

Today, however, the public is beginning to hold health facilities and fitness instructors more accountable than in the past. As a result, there has been an upsurge in the number of personal injury lawsuits against facilities and instructors along with a concurrent rise in the costs of relevant liability insurance. Even with the obvious deterrent of prospectively executed waivers and releases, the public appears more willing to take their grievances to court.

The current escalation of litigation is a reflection of a serious industry problem regarding client expectations and service delivery. Too frequently, individuals are injured as a result of certified instructors not being truly qualified professionals, and too often, individuals die while pursuing a healthier lifestyle because of insufficient screening, ineffective instruction, improper supervision, and/or an inadequate emergency response.

To lessen the possibility of litigation, facility personnel must be capable of thoroughly screening potential members, providing suitable fitness tests, evaluating health assessments and fitness profiles, designing appropriate exercise programs, and attentively supervising member activities. In addition, staff should constantly be aware of potentially dangerous situations and be empowered with the responsibility as well as the accountability to immediately correct hazardous conditions and respond effectively to emergency situations. This can only occur if management is knowledgeable about the field of exercise science and if instructors are properly qualified.

EP-Cs are typically placed in positions of not only conducting fitness programming but also managing facility operations. Therefore, their knowledge of exercise science must be complemented with a well-rounded knowledge of the many different areas within which management and personnel can become legally embroiled. Too often, the many administrative and legal concerns of a health/fitness facility have gone unrecognized or have been misunderstood. The truly knowledgeable EP-C recognizes the numerous responsibilities in managing and operating a facility that is totally committed to the health, fitness, and safety of its membership as well as the professionalism of the health and fitness industry

STUDY QUESTIONS

1. What are those incidents in which an EP-C would most likely become legally embroiled?
2. Identify major risk management strategies to lessen the chances of litigation.
3. What is the last line of defense in risk management?
4. List some of the municipal, state, and federal administrative requirements in the hiring of personnel and the operation of a fitness facility.
5. List various roles of responsibility in handling a medical emergency such as a sudden cardiac arrest.

REFERENCES

1. Abbott A. Fitness professionals: certified, qualified and justified. *Exerc Stand Malpract Rep.* 2009;23(2):17, 20–22.

2. ABC News. Is your health club unhealthy? [Internet]. New York (NY): ABC News; [cited 2005 Jan 13]. Available from: http://abcnews.go.com/Primetime/Fitness/story?id =410907

3. Bates M, editor. *Health Fitness Management.* 2nd ed. Champaign (IL): Human Kinetics; 2008. 400 p.

4. Cotten D, Cotten M. *Legal Aspects of Waivers in Sport, Recreation and Fitness Activities.* Canton (OH): PRC Publishing Inc.; 1997. 206 p.

5. Earle R, Baechle T, editors. *NSCA's Essentials of Personal Training.* Champaign (IL): Human Kinetics; 2004. 688 p.

6. Eickhoff-Shemek J, Herbert D, Connaughton D. *Risk Management for Health/Fitness Professionals.* Philadelphia (PA): Lippincott Williams & Wilkins; 2009. 407 p.

7. Federal Trade Commission Web site [Internet]. Washington (DC): Federal Trade Commission; [cited 2016 Sep]. Available from: http://www.ftc.gov

8. Franklin B, editor. *ACSM's Guidelines for Exercise Testing and Prescription.* 6th ed. Philadelphia (PA): Lippincott Williams & Wilkins; 2000. 368 p.

9. International Health, Racquet & Sportsclub Association. *IHRSA's Standards Facilitation Guide.* 2nd ed. Boston (MA): International Health, Racquet & Sportsclub Association; 1998.

10. Paul E. Sexual harassment as sex discrimination: a defective paradigm. *Yale Law Policy Rev.* 1990;8(2):333–65.

11. Tharrett S, Peterson J. *ACSM's Health/Fitness Facility Standards and Guidelines.* 4th ed. Champaign (IL): Human Kinetics; 2012. 256 p.

12. U.S. Department of Health and Human Services Web site [Internet]. Washington (DC): U.S. Department of Health and Human Services; [cited 2017 Feb 7]. Available from: http://www .hhs.gov

13. U.S. Department of Labor. Hiring issues [Internet]. Washington (DC): U.S. Department of Labor; [cited 2017 Feb 7]. Available from: https://www.dol.gov/general/topic/hiring

14. U.S. Department of Labor Web site [Internet]. Washington (DC): U.S. Department of Labor; [cited 2017 Feb 7]. Available from: http://www.dol.gov

15. U.S. Equal Employment Opportunity Commission Web site [Internet]. Washington (DC): U.S. Equal Employment Opportunity Commission; [cited 2017 Feb 7]. Available from: http://www.eeoc.gov

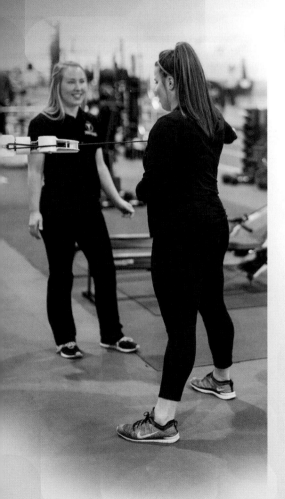

15 Leadership and Management

OBJECTIVES

- To address similarities and differences of leadership and management.

- To discuss the past, present, and future of leadership and management research.

- To describe several established leadership behaviors, theories, and styles.

- To identify application of practical management techniques for the certified exercise physiologist (EP-C).

- To discuss organizational development and strategic planning.

INTRODUCTION

The context of the health and fitness industry is often complex and volatile and, like most other industries, is constantly changing. There is a steady stream of changing regulations, evolving accreditation standards, emerging or reorganized regulatory agencies, new research, and an onslaught of fitness fads. In addition to satisfying many stakeholders (*e.g.*, clients and fitness club owners and peers), there is now the need to have and develop sufficient leadership and managements skills for sustained success.

Leadership has become a fundamental behavior expected of all EP-Cs regardless of their work context. As the practice of exercise physiology becomes more closely associated with the mainstream health care industry, leadership practices within the profession and during the socialization process become critical. In 1998, the Pew Health Professions Commission recommended that all health professionals in the 21st century, whether they seek management positions or not, should practice leadership (31). In other words, leadership behaviors have not only become an industry standard but also become a professional standard that transcends the work place. Leadership, apart from management, should be practiced consistently and intentionally. The aim of this chapter is to instill a sense of responsibility in the EP-C to introduce and cultivate a working leadership philosophy into their professional practice.

Defining Leadership and Management

The construct of leadership has hundreds of nuances, anecdotes, gradations, and theories. So much literature exists on leadership and its development, making it difficult to sort through and implement. In the past, many of the concepts and ideas concerning organizational effectiveness and motivation focused solely on management techniques. Recently, however, there has been a clear swing toward leadership competencies as a means of achieving organizational effectiveness and employee motivation. Management and leadership, whether independent of each other or in combination, are necessary within the health fitness industry (21). There are clear differences between leadership and management (29) that can be summarized as in leadership, *people* are led; in management, *resources* are managed. Often, the EP-C might fall into the trap of wanting to manage people, and this is an important and central skill set for the EP-C; however, management should not be a substitute for leadership. The temptation to manage people is because it is perceived as easier than leading. For example, managing might lead to "punishing" by enforcing established policies and procedures, whereas leading may involve discussion, negotiation, and established new ways of operating.

Operational Definitions

Operationally, leadership is the ability to facilitate and influence others (*i.e.*, superiors, peers, and subordinates) to make recognizable strides toward shared and unshared objectives (21). Management is the ability to use organizational resources to accomplish predetermined objectives (21). Leadership transcends the workplace, whereas management is often confined to the workplace. For example, in a health and fitness setting, leadership is demonstrated when the EP-C motivates and inspires clients or patients to make needed lifestyle changes. However, management in this situation may require the EP-C to add additional or longer training days, make a referral to other health professionals, or schedule additional consultations. This would require having a well-organized, managed schedule and referral system in place.

Management and leadership are not always different. In fact, it is not unusual for them to have similar outcome objectives and for both to project power and use influence. However, the differences between leadership and management may best be delineated in the examination of intended outcomes and processes (45). The intended outcome of leadership is typically change, vision casting, and innovation; the intended outcome of management is predictability, vision implementation, and maintaining the efficient status quo. These two constructs often require different techniques and operate from fundamentally different frameworks. Dye and Garman (9) describe management as the "science" of mitigating risk, whereas "leadership is the art of taking risks." Therefore, leadership tends to use vision casting, alignment, meaningful communication, self-reflection, and self-assessment to develop willing followers, whereas management uses "planning, organizing, controlling, and coordinating," regardless of its subordinate's willingness (17). Stated another way, management is a function or role within an organization, and leadership is a relationship between the follower and the leader, regardless of the organizational context (24). Any time something occurs despite the context, complexity is involved. This further helps us to distinguish between management and leadership. Leadership takes place in a complex environment where boundaries and borders are not clearly delineated. With leadership, there are many variables to consider in the decision-making process (this is also true of management); however, in leadership, those variables are not easily separated. On the other hand, management is often understood as complicated (as opposed to complex), which means it also has many variables, but often, those variables can be separated and operate independent of each other. This is not true with leadership, as we have already mentioned they are interdependent and are not easily separated.

Another distinguishing factor is that management is required when problems arise of a technical nature, which requires preestablished policies and procedures to be enacted, whereas leadership is required when problems do not have preestablished solutions and instead require adaptability, critical thinking, creativity, and innovation (14).

Although management and leadership are generally accepted as distinct, they are not necessarily exclusive, as both need to exist to efficiently operate at health/fitness facility. Therefore, the EP-C should be able to manage a facility (budget, mitigate risk, use policy and procedures, etc.) while also leading people (inspire, communicate, motivate, exhibit empathy and ethical behavior, etc.). Figure 15.1 is an adaptation of a relationship matrix for the integration of leadership and management — the higher the value, the greater the competency. Table 15.1 outlines the central tendencies that differentiate leadership and management.

Evidence-Based Management

One way to make the process of management more effective is a relatively new concept of evidence-based management. As EP-Cs, we are familiar with the concept of evidence-based practice, but the rapid growth and complexity of the health care system has required the introduction of evidence-based management. Evidence-based management is helpful in that it allows the EP-C to use the best available management research combined with the practitioner's experience and stakeholder expectations. The ultimate outcome of evidence-based management is to make efficient and reliable decisions. Evidence-based management is a decision-making process that considers equally three inputs. Input number 1 is the best available research. Of course, the key is "best available," which implies that the EP-C knows how to evaluate and consume the *best* research, not just *any* research. Because leadership and management tend to be social sciences, it may be necessary for EP-Cs to familiarize themselves with nonexperimental or social scientific study design techniques in order to evaluate this research accurately. The second input is the personal experience of the EP-C. Of course, this does not mean clinical experience, but decision making and management

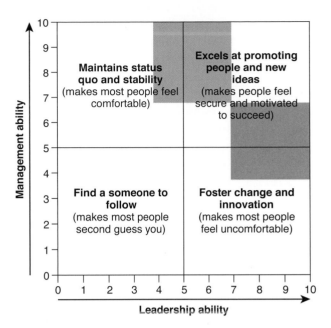

FIGURE 15.1. Integrating leadership and management. (From Kutz MR. *Leadership and Management in Athletic Training: An Integrated Approach.* Baltimore [MD]: Lippincott Williams & Wilkins; 2010. 331 p.)

Table 15.1	Differences between Leadership and Management
Leadership's Tendencies	**Management's Tendencies**
▪ Change-oriented	▪ Predictable
▪ Vision caster	▪ Vision implementer
▪ Innovates	▪ Maintains status quo
▪ Motivated to take risk	▪ Motivated to analyze risk
▪ Influence/authority transcends the organization	▪ Influence/authority confined to within the organization
▪ Solves unexpected and novel problems with creativity	▪ Solves known and technical problems with established policy and procedure
▪ Proactive	▪ Reactive
▪ Focus on long term	▪ Focus on short term
▪ Identifies opportunities	▪ Identifies obstacles
▪ Idea- and person-centered	▪ System and plan centered
▪ Shares information freely	▪ Shares "need to know" information
▪ Uses interpersonal skills to handle conflict	▪ Uses precedent, policy, procedure to handle conflict
▪ Places emphasis on team accomplishments	▪ Places emphasis on individual performance
▪ Works to prevent conflict or problems	▪ Works to solve existing conflicts or problems

experience. When this is lacking, say in the instance of a novice, the EP-C may have the tendency to overrely on research for input. To mitigate that risk, seek opportunities to lead and manage even if that means volunteering outside of your employer, professional organization, or even health care. Valuable leadership and management experience can be gained from involvement in civic and social organizations. The third input for effective evidence-based management is understanding and knowing stakeholder expectations. This means the EP-C must be familiar with the values and desires of several stakeholders. Stakeholders can be patients or clients, but they can also be physicians, coworkers, other allied health care professionals, and administrators. It is important when learning to manage (and lead) that these three inputs be considered. When one strives to integrate all three inputs equally, decision making in the outcomes of decisions improves.

 # Leadership: Past, Present, and Future

Although leadership theory is dynamic and continually evolving, four major models of leadership theory are consistently referenced in the literature: classical, transactional, visionary, and organic (1,2). Collectively, these four leadership models serve as a philosophical foundation from which leadership is practiced.

Through the early 1970s, the classical model dominated leadership theory. Under this model, a leader's power or influence was considered innate and having a vision was not considered necessary to ensure follower support. Often, a leader's influence was based on fear or respect. A leader's position or placement was rarely challenged. Of course, as workers became more skilled and knowledgeable, this model became less popular and was less able to motivate subordinates.

Transactional Model

The transactional model also began to gain popularity in the 1970s and signaled the era of the manager. Under this model, vision was neither necessary nor articulated. Instead, influence was based on contractual negotiations of rewards and punishments between the leader and subordinates. Considerable effort was taken by transactional leaders to create "environments" conducive to management intervention. In other words, the focus was on the manager's ability to generate policies and procedures that capitalized on productivity and efficiency. This model rewarded management for generating systems where a manager could intervene. Productivity was considered an outcome of "good" management, and any role employees had in productivity was minimized.

Visionary Model

The visionary model emerged shortly thereafter (mid-1980s) and still has many proponents today, although it has lost some popularity. Visionary leadership (also called charismatic or transformational leadership) involves the leader using emotion to inspire and create buy-in of the followers. It is also interesting to note that with the entrance of visionary model, the language changed from "subordinates" to "followers." Within this model, vision became fundamental and followers were encouraged to contribute to the leader's vision.

Organic Model

The most recent model, organic, tends to overlap with visionary. The organic leadership model centers on a collective vision of the group as a team. A vision is important, but it is not "owned" only by the leader, instead the vision is created collectively and the leader helps implement the will of the team. Influence is based on the relationship and mutuality of the team and the endorsement of a leader. Organizational charts from an organic model tend to look like an amoeba instead of the pyramid shape of the other models. It is from a leadership development standpoint where the organic model is most unique. In the previous three models, leadership development occurs by traditional means. In traditional leadership development, it is the responsibility of external institutions (*e.g.*, a university) to socialize its members and provide formal leadership instruction. However, within the organic model, leadership development is grass roots. That means, leadership development takes place within the organization and socialization occurs as one is practicing their profession and not *before* they enter the profession. This, of course, has huge implications for hiring leaders. Whereas in the other models leaders would be searched for from outside and imported, in an organic model, leaders are look to and developed from within.

Leadership Theory and Model

As new and more research emerges, leadership models and theories will continue to evolve. As this evolution occurs, there will always be the temptation for leaders to operate out of multiple models, some of which are in conflict with each other. For example, having a personal belief that leadership is something people are born with and is innate (classical model) is very different from the open leadership development programs to anyone interested (organic model) or soliciting feedback on strategic plans from nonleaders (visionary model). Applying different leadership models during the practice of management or leadership is contradictory. However, mixing leadership behaviors or styles is encouraged. It is appropriate to transition between or mix leadership styles when confronted with new or novel problems or situations. For example, in a situation or with certain personnel, a leader may have to demonstrate servant leadership and then use a path–goal approach, or situational style in a different situation.

The seminal work of Ralph Stogdill (38) in the 1950s identified 1,800 separate leadership behaviors. Stogdill was eventually able to identify the two key behaviors that were rated by the vast majority of subordinates as critical to leadership: "initiating structure" and "consideration" (8). Initiating structure means organizing and defining relationships in a group (8). Consideration is defined as the degree to which the leader creates an environment of emotional support, warmth, friendliness, and trust (8). These two constructs have served as the foundation for much of how leadership is practiced and understood.

Leadership Behaviors and Theories

Trait Theory

The "great man" (or woman) theory promoted the idea that being a "superior leader" is an issue of genetics; it is in fact the idea that one is born to lead and has an innate set of leadership qualities and abilities (38). The "great man" ideology still has proponents today; for example, a popular leadership book states, "Leadership cannot be manufactured. It cannot be mustered up. It's an innate gifting" (25).

Trait theory postulates two forms — (a) leadership traits are innate or a divine endowment (*i.e.*, great man theory) or (b) an individual can awaken dormant traits over time (44). Regardless if leadership is innate, divine endowment, or learned, those who might have innate leadership ability still must improve their leadership ability through years of practice and experience (9).

Situational Leadership Theory

Situational leadership was originally developed by Blanchard and Hersey in the 1960s. Situational leadership's purpose is to open up communication and to increase the quality and frequency of conversations about performance and development (16). Situational leadership suggests that leadership style is adapted by the leader on the basis of the leader's "diagnosis" of

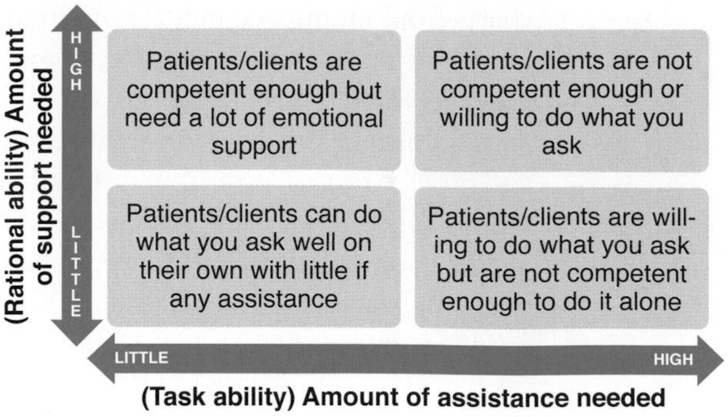

FIGURE 15.2. Situational leadership. (Reproduced with permission from Kutz MR. Toward a conceptual model of contextual intelligence: a transferable leadership construct. *Leadersh Rev.* 2008;8:18–31.)

the "development level" of the subordinate (16). The development level or "situation" of a subordinate is based on a relationship between two factors: competence and commitment (16). For example, subordinates with high competence and high commitment (*i.e.*, experts) warrant delegation with little supervision (*i.e.*, a "leader who empowers them to act independently, affirming and confirming their decisions") (30). On the other hand, subordinates who demonstrate low competence but high commitment warrant direction aimed at "developing competence" (16) (Fig. 15.2).

Path–Goal Leadership Theory

Path–goal theory was popularized by House in the 1970s and is a modification of contingency or situational leadership. It involves the leader setting a path to a specific goal for a specific member or team on the basis of that member's personality or team's dynamics (8). Path–goal theory is about how leaders motivate employees to accomplish their designated goals (30). It draws heavily on motivational theory and emphasizes how the leader's style is influenced by both the work setting and subordinates (30).

Transformational and Transactional Leadership

Burns (6) identified two types of leadership: transformational and transactional. Transformational leadership can be summarized as that which inspires and motivates others. Followers are influenced by the leader's creativity, admiration, and respect (6). Transformational leaders give respect and admiration to their followers and are likewise typically admired and respected by their followers. Transformational leadership is considered similar to charismatic or visionary leadership (8).

Transformational leaders give "individual attention, inspire others to excel and stimulate people to think in new ways" (19). Stated another way, transformational leadership fosters innovation in coworkers and followers. There are five "practices" associated with transformational leadership: "challenging the process, inspiring a shared vision, enabling others to act, modeling the way, and encouraging the heart" (19).

Transactional leaders view leadership as the process of "exchanging one thing for another" (6). Often, transactional leadership comes down to exchanging rewards (salary and benefits) for performance or work (6). Transactional leaders operate under different circumstances and from a different motivation than transforming leaders. Burns (6) pointed out the divergent nature of the two leadership types. Transactional leadership is about the "individual interest" of the leader and is not concerned with the "collective interest of followers"; on the other hand, transformational leadership concerns itself with the follower's interests (6). "The transactional leader's behavior closely resembles that of a manager" (19). It should be noted that transformational leadership is preferred by followers but is not necessarily the most efficient style.

Lewin's Leadership Styles

In 1939, Kurt Lewin identified three styles of leadership that were commonly used in the decision-making process of managers: autocratic, democratic, and laissez-faire (23). In the autocratic style, the leader makes decisions on his or her own and typically does not consult with others. Autocratic style often results in the highest level of discontentment among subordinates and followers. An autocratic style typically only works well in an "emergency" situation.

In the democratic style, the leader involves his or her peers and subordinates in the decision-making process. One often-misunderstood aspect of democratic leadership is that consensus or the will of the followers should override the leaders. However, true democratic leadership may still make the unpopular decision; in this style, the leader always reserves the authority to make the ultimate decision. The democratic style is often highly valued by followers. However, a democratic style can be challenging when there are wide ranges of opinions.

The third style is laissez-faire, which virtually eliminates any leadership involvement in decision making. In other words, followers usually make their own decisions. This is problematic because the "leader" is still ultimately responsible for the group's decisions. This style can work when followers take ownership of the process and are competent and willing to make decisions. However, this style was found to be the least rewarding and often showed low morale of followers.

Servant Leadership

Servant leadership theory was introduced by Greenleaf in the early 1970s, and it shares many traits with transformational leadership (43). The one major difference is that in the decision-making process of servant leadership, the individual's interest is considered. Although transformational leadership implies that the organization is considered first, servant leadership establishes that organizational performance is secondary to the relationship between the leader and the follower (43). The servant leader is said to be a servant first and leader second. Leading and directing are part of their roles and functions, but that role and function is secondary to the desire or need to promote others.

Leader–Member Exchange Theory

Leader–member exchange (LMX) theory centers on the "interactions" between the leader and the follower (30) and was intended to help establish a more mature leadership relationship (12). LMX theory is based on vertical dyad research, which establishes *in-groups* and *out-groups* (30). In-groups are those leader–follower relationships that allow for subordinate's roles to be expanded and negotiated; out-groups are those leader–follower relationships based purely on formal contract and predefined roles (30). Followers falling into the in-group category tend to achieve more and receive more of the leader's time and attention (30). Out-group members do what they are told and stick to formal procedures. Typically, out-group members are treated fairly by leaders but do not get "special attention." Current LMX research is based on how the leader can make relationships with every subordinate so that each one feels he or she is part of the in-group (30).

Emotional Intelligence

Although more of a concept than a theory, emotional intelligence (EI) is recognized as a set of skills (*i.e.*, street smarts) that include awareness of self and others and the ability to handle emotions and relationships (4,12,34). EI is the capacity to reason about emotions and use emotions to enhance thinking (26). EI includes the ability to accurately perceive emotions, to access and generate emotions to assist thought, to understand emotions and emotional knowledge, and to effectively regulate emotions (26,34).

HOW TO   **Identify Emotional Intelligence**

Emotional intelligence is a trait that works closely with social, practical, and personal intelligence and allows leaders to accurately perceive others feelings and emotions. To recognize someone with high levels of emotional intelligence, you should note the following four factors.

Internal Factors
1. *Self-awareness*: someone who is aware of his or her own emotions and feelings
2. *Self-management*: someone who can regulate his or her own emotions and feelings

External Factors
1. *Social awareness*: someone who displays empathy, or is aware of others emotions and feelings
2. *Relationship management*: someone who can successfully regulate emotional aspects of work-related relationships

Theoretically, EI involves the relationship between cognition and emotion and works closely with other intelligences such as social, practical, and personal (26). Practicing EI involves four critical skills. Those skills are as follows: (a) being able to recognize and perceive emotions of others, (b) using emotions to assist (not hinder) thoughts and thinking, (c) ability to analyze and understand emotions, and (d) managing personal emotions based on personal goals, self-knowledge, and social awareness (26).

Goleman (11) has written extensively on the topic of EI and has popularized its concept. Successful leaders have a high emotional quotient (EQ), which appears to be directly related to EI. In fact, leaders with very high expertise and technical knowledge (*i.e.*, high IQ) fail in certain leadership initiatives because of low EQ (10). The "How to Identify Emotional Intelligence" box shows key elements that must be present to identify a leader with EI.

Contextual Intelligence and Three Dimensional Thinking

Contextual intelligence (CI) is also a concept that has great implications for leadership and management. CI has been described by researchers in psychology, education, and athletic training, as well as by intelligence theorists as the ability to adapt or respond appropriately to any number of different contexts, where the context is determined by environmental factors and stakeholder values (13,22,36,39). CI is a cluster of individual leadership skills that are integrated and demonstrated simultaneously (Table 15.2). Sternberg (36) is recognized as introducing the term *contextual intelligence* as a subtheme of practical intelligence. CI is typically associated with tacit knowledge (41,42) and is closely associated with wisdom gained from experience; however, recently strategies for teaching and learning CI have also emerged (13,20). As opposed to academic intelligence, often measured by IQ, CI has been shown to be the best predictor of success in real-life performance situations (18,37).

CI requires the integration of knowledge gained from a person's total experiences. In other words, problems are solved or solutions are generated on the basis of knowledge built from all experiences (direct and indirect), and this does not exclude experiences that might seem to be unrelated or irrelevant. For the contextually intelligent leader, solutions are based on the use of knowledge acquired in the past and the present, combined with what is currently anticipated about the future. This phenomenon has been described as thinking in three dimensions or 3D (20).

The 3D-thinking model of CI is the simultaneous integration of three distinct time orientations: hindsight, insight, and foresight (20). Lessons learned from the past are referred to as hindsight. Hindsight requires accurately reflecting on the past and ensuring that the lessons learned from the past are always being reevaluated for new lessons. Therefore, hindsight requires

Table 15.2	Leadership Skills Associated with Contextual Intelligence
Future-minded	Has a forward-looking mentality and sense of direction and concern for where the organization should be in the future
Influencer	Uses interpersonal skills to ethically and noncoercively affect the actions and decisions of others
Mission-minded	Understands and communicates how the individual performance of others influences subordinate's, peer's, and supervisor's perception of how the mission is being accomplished
Socially responsible	Expresses concern about social trends and issues (encourages legislation and policy when appropriate) and volunteers in social and community activities
Embraces new ideas	Promotes diversity in multiple contexts, aligns diverse individuals by creating and facilitating diversity, and provides opportunities for diverse members to interact in nondiscriminatory manner
Multicultural leadership	Can influence and affect the behaviors and attitudes of peers and subordinates in an ethnically diverse context
Diagnoses context	Knows how to appropriately interpret and react to changing and volatile surroundings
Change agent	Has the courage to raise difficult and challenging questions that others may perceive as a threat to the status quo Proactive rather than reactive in rising to challenges, leading, participating in, or making change (*i.e.*, assessing, initiating, researching, planning, constructing, and advocating)
Constructive use of influence	Demonstrates the effective use of different types of power in developing and demonstrating influence
Intentional leadership	Assesses and evaluates own leadership performance and is aware of strengths and weaknesses Takes intentional action toward continuous improvement of leadership ability Has an action guide and delineated goals for achieving personal best
Critical thinker	Cognitive ability to make connections, integrate, and make practical application of different actions, opinions, and information
Consensus builder	Exhibits interpersonal skill and convinces other people to see the common good or a different point of view for the sake of the organizational mission or values by using listening skills, managing conflict, and creating win-win situations

intentionally applying lessons learned from the past in every new context the EP-C may find him or herself. Accurately understanding the present is referred to as insight. Insight is knowing what to do in the moment you are in right now, the present. Insight occurs after the convergence of hindsight and foresight. Foresight is being able to accurately articulate the future. Not any future, but your future. It is simply the ability to answer the questions what sort of future are you hoping for and how specifically are you going to accomplish it. Once hindsight and foresight began working together, insight is a natural consequence (20). The CI model has a lot of promise for helping leaders learn to manage complex and ambiguous environments while still bringing the

Table 15.3	Obstacles and Solutions for Contextual Intelligence	
Obstacle to Contextual Intelligence	**Description**	**Recommended Solution**
The pace of change	Change often happens so quickly that there is no time to respond without some element of guesswork or reflexive reaction.	Intentionally "extract" lessons from any and all experiences and be prepared to apply those lessons in seemingly unrelated situations or events.
Complexity	The ever-increasing number of external and internal variables that have an impact on people and organizations	Realize that as complexity increases, the amount of information/data required for accurate decision making decreases.
Learned behavior	Past success often creates incredible obstacles to adapting or responding to changing contexts. People are often strongly biased by their existing knowledge and rarely can interpret what they see without that bias.	Adopt a new commitment to learn what informs the behaviors and attitudes of self, others, society, and the organization. Do not rely as heavily on precedent or actions that lead to previous success.
Inappropriate orientation to time	Most people when faced with a decision will disproportionately pull and apply information from one of three time orientations (past, present, and future), rarely are all three time orientations consulted proportionately.	One solution is to think in 3D. Thinking in 3D requires a proportionate awareness of how the past, present, and future are influencing the current context.

most value to stakeholders. However, practicing CI and its related 3D-thinking framework is not without its obstacles. Specifically, there are four obstacles to CI that need to be addressed. Those four obstacles (20) are presented in Table 15.3.

 ## Management Techniques

Management techniques are viewed as distinct from leadership styles, skills, or behaviors. The term *technique* was chosen because it implies that something can be implemented by anyone in a position to do so and does not necessarily require any prerequisite skill for the technique to be used. Therefore, management techniques can be applied even if one does not possess leadership skills or demonstrate leadership behaviors. Obviously, the management techniques can be improved, or applied with greater success, if combined with appropriate leadership skills in the management application or implementation.

Management Grid (Blake and Mouton)

The management grid is intended to measure the relationship between one's concern for people and production. The grid allows a manager to identify which of five major styles he or she belongs to better utilize his or her management skills. In addition, the grid takes into account the leader's concern for people and the concern for production. For the concern of people, the leader considers the needs of team members and their interests when deciding how best to accomplish goals. For the concern of production, the leader emphasizes efficiency and productivity when deciding how best to accomplish goals. The five major styles identified by Blake and Mouton are as follows:

1. *Improvised management*: a low concern for people and production. The manager's main motivation is to stay out of trouble and maintain the status quo. Effort is at a minimum, and they are satisfied to simply pass orders from superiors.
2. *Country-club management*: high concern for employees but low concern for production. The goal of the manager is to satisfy needs of employees and provide a friendly atmosphere.
3. *Authoritarian management*: high concern for production and efficiency but low concern for employees. Managers often perceive personal needs as irrelevant or perhaps even harmful to goals. Often, authority is used to coerce subordinates to meet goals.
4. *Middle-of-the-road management*: moderate concern for production and employee satisfaction.
5. *Team or democratic management*: high concern for both production and morale. Team or democratic managers often try to develop committed work groups and focus.

Scientific Management (Frederick W. Taylor)

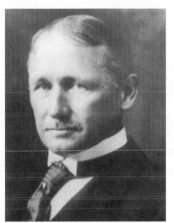

Scientific management is the organization and supervision of jobs and duties based on the manager's direct observation of the job. The manager's job was to create rules and procedures on how to do a given job that replaced "rule of thumb," and these were based strictly on the manager's direct and "scientific" observation of that job. Any deviation from the manager's scientifically prescribed procedures is punished. Scientific management's basic tenet was that monetary payment was the only motivation employees needed. In fact, when Taylor published *The Principles of Scientific Management* in 1911, he suggested that sole responsibility of the organization rests with the manager and that only the manager needed to be concerned with working conditions and outcomes. According to Taylor, a manager's responsibility was to provide detailed and specific instructions on how to do the assigned task and that the organization was more important than the individual (27,33). Scientific management is no longer a popular model; however, remnants of it can be seen in bureaucratic and transactional behaviors. Eventually, the presuppositions that framed scientific management were rejected, but Taylor's contribution to management practice has served as a foundational framework for much of what is practiced today.

Bureaucratic Model of Management (Max Weber)

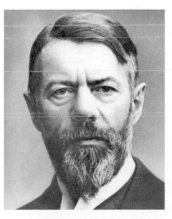

Bureaucratic structures are typically formalized and centralized, have a firm hierarchy, and divide labor between specialists (8). Bureaucracy requires standardized rules in the forms of policy and procedure. The benefit of bureaucracy is with an unskilled labor force because it creates a reference point for action and reduces variability. However, critics of bureaucratic management point out that minimized variability is not as effective with today's knowledgeable workers (8). Weber believed bureaucracy to be a set of official functions bounded by rules with a clear division of labor and qualification replaced favoritism as the basis of selection for certain jobs. Bureaucracy, as Weber showed, leveled the playing field for many workers and increased their social equality. Although today elements of bureaucratic management remain, even Weber was able to foresee the risk of bureaucracy and warned of the potential for the organization to dominate policy and individuals.

Total Quality Management (W. Edwards Deming)

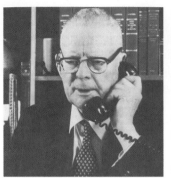

Originally adopted and practiced in Japan, total quality management (TQM) was not favored in the United States until the United States began to fall behind in global competition (44). Deming described TQM as 14 separate aspects of quality management, including such points as "create consistency of purpose for the improvement of product and service," "cease dependence on inspection to achieve quality," and "put everyone in the company to work to accomplish the transformation" (42).

One additional point that is consistently used by EP-Cs as they work with clients and customers toward reaching their goals is to "remove barriers that rob people of pride and workmanship."

Management by Objective (Peter Drucker)

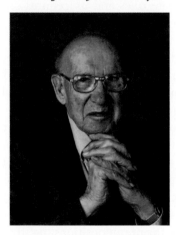

Management by objective (MBO) was the idea that preestablished objectives should be used in the appraisal of every aspect of an organization and that performance relies on defining and assessing those objectives and requires collaboration, strategic planning, and goal setting (28). MBO seeks employee buy-in and participative decision making for departmental or organizational objectives. It is not uncommon that MBO managers allow, and even require, employees to develop their own career or job development action plan.

For MBO objectives to work, they must be SMART (specific, measurable, achievement oriented, realistic, and time-oriented). Drucker believed that every goal or objective must have each of these five elements of SMART in order to be actionable. Finally, MBO requires appraisal, which is routine clarification and assessment of progress toward previously agreed on goals and objectives. Participating in MBO appraisals is an involved process that includes identifying obstacles that have been hindrances to employees accomplishing their objectives and creating new ones once original objectives have been met.

Motivator-Hygiene Theory (Fredrick Herzberg)

The motivator-hygiene theory was first popularized in business management and states that there are factors that contribute separately to both job satisfaction and dissatisfaction (21). Job satisfaction elements are also known as motivators, which when present add to employee satisfaction. These might include work that is intellectually challenging, recognition of superior performance, and increasingly greater levels of responsibility. Hygiene factors are those that when not present increase worker dissatisfaction. They may include status, job security, salary, and fringe benefits. Hygiene factors do not give satisfaction, but if they are absent, they result in dissatisfaction.

A career as an EP-C can serve as a highly satisfying one; there is often a high degree of responsibility and intellectually challenging work. However, there may be hygiene factors, salary and job security, that in spite of the motivators, may lead the EP-C to become dissatisfied.

Theory X and Y (Douglas McGregor)

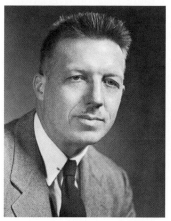

McGregor was a management professor who proposed that human motivation is based on one of two tendencies, which he called X and Y as part of his Theory X and Theory Y of human motivation and management. Theory X is the assumption that most people (followers) are inherently lazy and if given the chance will try to avoid work (21). Belief in Theory X has a profound effect on how a leader would choose to motivate his or her employees. For example, managers who subscribe to Theory X would need to closely monitor and supervise their employees, likely employing a high degree of micromanagement.

Theory Y is the assumption that employees are self-motivated, desire responsibility, and exercise self-direction (21). Managers who hold to Theory Y tend to believe that if given the chance, employees will be creative and productive. Therefore, managers who subscribe to Theory Y often delegate and share responsibility and can be more transformational leaders.

Behavioral Approach (Mary Parker Follet)

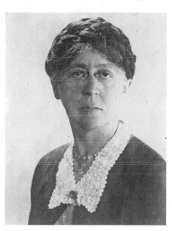

Mary Parker Follett introduced the behavioral model of management and is perhaps the single greatest contributor to how management practice is understood today. Follett was a political scientist and is credited with advancing the democratic style of management. Follett was a "management philosopher" and believed that an organization was a microcosm of society (27,33). The behavioral model of management placed a large emphasis on the individual's ability to define and shape his or her own roles and life and was the precursor to what eventually became known as human resource management (27,33). Within this model, communication flowed both up and down (vertically), as opposed to the more traditional horizontal communication pathways of the time. Follett was a pioneer who suggested that leadership could be learned, and anyone who did not learn leadership would always remain in a subordinate position. Follet also emphasized how important it was for followers to realize the necessity of the instructions for a job rather than follow instructions blindly or mindlessly. Leaders need to understand the jobs themselves and need to be able to communicate the short- and long-term aspects of the job from the worker's perspective.

 ## Organizational Behavior

Understanding the fundamental management techniques and certain theories of leadership provides a foundation for understanding or effectively navigating organizations. Organizational behavior, similar to human resource management, is the capacity to understand, explain, and improve the attitudes and behaviors of individuals and groups within organizations (7). This brings clarity to why the EP-C must be equipped to practice both leadership and management. Many organizational interactions require dealing with human resources, which ultimately require mastery of leadership skills, abilities, and behaviors. Dealing with non–human resources (budgets, facilities, information and knowledge, etc.) requires correct application of different management techniques, with the understanding that there may be overlap or integration of leadership and management.

Colquitt presents an integrated model of organizational behavior that includes five major elements (7):

1. *Individual outcomes*: These are what happens as a result of the other four elements and include job performance and commitment to the organization. For the EP-Cs, this would represent competency (*i.e.*, proficiency toward EP-Cs exam content outline) and commitment (to his or her customers and employer).

2. *Individual mechanisms*: These consist of five areas that directly impact individual outcomes: (a) job satisfaction — how EP-Cs feel about their job when not at the job as well as how well they feel in their day-to-day operations, (b) stress — dealing with the psychological responses to the demands of the job, (c) motivation — the energy EP-Cs put into their work, (d) trust and ethics — how EP-Cs believe their employer handles business in terms of honesty and integrity, and (e) learning and decision making — how EP-Cs acquire and apply new knowledge and continuing education for their job.

3. *Individual characteristics*: These include EP-Cs' abilities or skills (*i.e.*, how well they could do their job respective to the expectations and complexity of the job) and personality.

4. *Group mechanisms*: These include how leadership uses power and implements different leadership styles within the EP-C's organization.

5. *Organizational mechanisms*: These include the larger concepts of organizational culture and structure.

EP-Cs should consider all five of these elements when diagnosing how well they fit into an organization while also realizing that these elements play a critical role in their own individual and organizational success.

Strategic Planning

Strategic planning is another major component of good leadership and management. It is the process of diagnosing the organization's external and internal environments and includes deciding on a vision and mission, developing overall goals, creating and selecting general strategies to be pursued, and allocating resources to achieve the organization's goals (15). Strategic thinking requires conceptualizing the past, present, and future from the organization's and stakeholder's vantage point. This requires understanding the relevant history of the decision at hand, including the factors that helped or hindered the process up until the present day. Also important is to account for relevant present-day activities that occur locally, professionally, or globally (*i.e.*, perceptions, new research, and changing regulations or reforms). Only after historical information and present-day environment have been evaluated can the process of planning for the future begin. Planning for the future must include innovation and a willingness to navigate change.

The overall strategic process is multifaceted process that includes delineating organizational, stakeholder, and individual values; creating vision and mission statements; setting goals and objectives; doing program analysis; and establishing a decision-making process. Therefore, planning is a fundamental aspect of leadership and management, including in the health and fitness context, and should include the following steps:

■ *Determining stakeholders*: All enterprises in every industry across the globe have stakeholders. Stakeholders are anyone affected by the actions or plans of an organization, department, or individual. For example, the stakeholders for the EP-C in a private health club might include the manager, members, clients, other employees, vendors, sales department, and the neighborhood or community where the club is located. A fundamental component to proper planning is to realize that all decisions and actions are likely to affect most if not all stakeholders.

- *Delineating values*: Values are those practices or attitudes that are predetermined to be celebrated (19). Values are a list of ideals that the organization focuses its time, attention, and resources on; later, it will be these very values that guide the vision and mission statements. Delineating values, therefore, serves a critical role in any organization.

- *Creating a vision*: "Without a vision people perish" (35). A clear and articulate vision is essential for the successful operation of any enterprise and is an ideal image of the future one seeks to create (19,35). It is the goal or direction an organization, individual, or team strives toward. This concept of vision suggests an orientation toward the future, and a key leadership practice is to visualize an ideal future (5). The EP-C can facilitate the advancement of his or her industry and profession by maintaining a clear and articulate vision.

- *Drafting a mission*: Mission statements expand on the vision by adding "how" the vision will be accomplished. There is a fundamental difference between vision and mission: The vision statement is future-oriented, and the mission statement is oriented toward current services and conditions — visions challenge; missions anchor (32). The mission statement keeps the EP-C focused on who is being served and how to best serve them. A clearly defined mission can help drive leadership decisions and actions (3,40).

- *Establishing goals and objectives*: Goals and objectives are critical to tie together all the planning. Objectives are dynamic end points that can stated quantitatively (we want to sell 25% more memberships) or qualitatively (we want to be the best fitness center in the city). The EP-C should strive to create SMART goals, each with a realistic objective. Once goals and objectives are identified, actions can be taken toward implementing the strategy. Figure 15.3 is an overall schematic of the strategic planning process.

After strategy is implemented, it is necessary to evaluate the progress. Evaluation is most commonly done with an SWOT analysis (strengths, weaknesses, opportunities, and threats). Strength and weaknesses are internal factors that identify the good and the bad of what is happening that can be controlled and changed within the organization by leaders and managers. The opportunities and threats are external factors that cannot be controlled. Strengths and opportunities are considered positive, whereas weaknesses and threats are typically negative. All strategic plans must be evaluated regularly, and the EP-C should be familiar with the stages of strategic planning and how to perform an SWOT analysis.

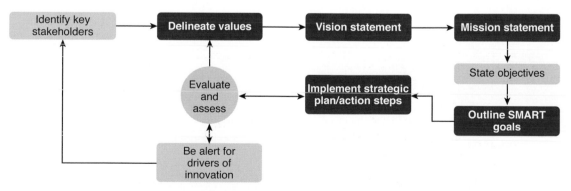

FIGURE 15.3. Strategic planning process. (Reproduced with permission from Kutz MR. Contextual intelligence: overcoming hindrances to performing well in times of change. *Develop Learn Organ.* 2011;25[3]:8–10.)

The Case of Jeanie

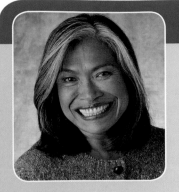

Submitted by **Carol Jean Dale, ACSM EP-C, North Mississippi Medical Center — Pontotoc Wellness Center, Pontotoc, MS**

Jeanie Dale, an EP-C manager and a 25-year veteran of hospital-based wellness operations, has used varying styles of management during the constantly changing outcomes-based expectations for the industry. For Jeanie, management is not just about efficiency but about empowering people to care about their work and the work of others.

Narrative

I work at the Pontotoc Wellness Center, a medical fitness center located in Pontotoc, Mississippi, and at a satellite facility of North Mississippi Medical Center (NMMC), located in Tupelo, Mississippi. NMMC was the 2006 recipient of the Malcolm Baldrige Quality Award, the nation's highest presidential honor for organizational performance excellence. As a manager, I walk a fine line to ensure safety and a rigorous standard of care while introducing commercially relevant current trends and meeting the needs of our stakeholders. We want to serve diverse populations while being able to provide the more resource-demanding special populations that are referred by our Exercise is Medicine (EIM) program.

Initially, we had a medical board of physicians who helped our team set up our EIM program so that we could all be clear about the expectations that the physicians had for us serving their patients. We looked at ease of entry into the program, safety, and reducing physician time. We also considered the educational, nutritional, and exercise components of our services to make it affordable to the clients referred. The referral system has now broadened from physicians to other health care practitioners such as physical therapists, behavioral psychologists, nurse practitioners, and professionals from specialty programs such as our cancer clinics, cardiac, gastric bypass, and pulmonary rehabilitation. The EIM program is a successful venture and continuing to thrive and develop.

I encourage my team to submit ideas for excellence for our department. Although our mission and vision are rooted in the mission of the institution, the organizational plans for wellness services are in continual development. We implemented a dynamic evaluation involving a 90-day action plan process to assess our progress toward achieving our annual goals and outcomes. This organic style of leadership is practiced system-wide and is encouraged by our director of wellness services. The collection of good ideas from everyone helps find the best idea for a particular circumstance and also improves morale of the team at our wellness center.

We also use tools that evaluate our team by having coworkers give feedback to each employee on what we do well and what improvements we need. Because our field is emerging, we need to empower dynamic independent thinkers who can be an important bridge in preventing disease and reducing risk factors. These frontline professionals will directly impact future health care costs and serve to bridge the gap from rehabilitation into improved functional capacity and healthier lifestyles. The transformational leadership style that I try to demonstrate is primarily to encourage individuals to work with autonomy, commitment, and care to improve the quality of life of clients and coworkers. The EIM program provides a framework for us to work as a team to challenge mediocrity and implement evidence-based practices within the context of a medical fitness facility.

QUESTIONS

- Provide an example of management and an example of leadership in the implementation of the EIM program.
- How does Jeanie exemplify transformational leadership style?
- Which of the approaches to management and leadership align most closely with the way Jeanie manages the team at Pontotoc Wellness Center?

SUMMARY

Leadership and management are separate constructs that have overlapping outcomes. The two are equally valuable aspects of performance for EP-Cs, particularly as they seek to advance their career. Leadership is a relationship with people that is based on the ethical use of influence, whereas management accomplishes goals and objectives by controlling and organizing resources. Leadership research and theory has evolved from a classical approach, which is based on giftedness of the leader, to an organic model, which is a grassroots approach in which everyone can demonstrate leadership. Once EP-Cs have a grasp on the differences between leadership and management and on the framework for developing their own philosophical underpinnings, they will be well on their way to making a lasting and meaningful difference in their organization and the lives of their customers.

STUDY QUESTIONS

1. Explain why leadership research and theory are important in developing sound leadership practices across different contexts.
2. What are some key applications of an EP-C in regard to the different leadership concepts and theories discussed in this chapter?
3. How can CI be used to increase leadership effectiveness in the health and fitness industry?
4. What are the primary differences between leadership and management and how might these differences be seen in the day-to-day operation of a health/fitness facility?
5. Describe which management techniques might be easiest and most difficult to implement in health/fitness facility.

REFERENCES

1. Antonakis J, Cianciolo A, Sternberg R. *The Nature of Leadership*. Thousand Oaks (CA): Sage; 2004. 448 p.

2. Avery G. *Understanding Leadership*. London (United Kingdom): Sage; 2004. 328 p.

3. Bart C, Hupfer M. Mission statements in Canadian hospitals. *J Health Organ Manag*. 2004;18(2–3):92–110.

4. Bolman LG, Deal TE. *Reframing Organizations*. San Francisco (CA): Jossey-Bass; 2003. 483 p.

5. Brown MG. Improving your organization's vision. *J Qual Particip*. 1998;21(5):18–21.

6. Burns JM. *Leadership*. New York (NY): Harper and Row; 1978. 530 p.

7. Colquitt JA, Lepine JA, Wesson MJ. *Organizational Behavior: Improving Performance and Commitment in the Workplace*. New York (NY): McGraw-Hill; 2010. 630 p.

8. DuBrin AJ. *Leadership: Research Findings, Practice, and Skills*. New York (NY): Houghton Mifflin; 2004. 538 p.

9. Dye CF, Garman AN. *Exceptional Leadership: 16 Critical Competencies for Healthcare Executives*. Chicago (IL): Health Administration Press; 2006. 227 p.

10. Fullan M. *Leading in a Culture of Change*. San Francisco (CA): Jossey-Bass; 2001. 176 p.

11. Goleman D. Leadership that gets results. *Harv Bus Rev*. 2000; 78(2):78–90.

12. Graen GB, Uhl-Bien M. Relationship-based approach to leadership: development of leader–member exchange (LMX) theory of leadership over 25 years: applying a multi-level multi-domain perspective. *Leadersh Q*. 1995; 6:219–47.

13. Hays KF, Brown CH. *You're On! Consulting for Peak Performance*. Washington (DC): American Psychological Association; 2004. 328 p.

14. Heifetz R. Anchoring leadership in the work of adaptive progress. In: Hesselbein F, Goldsmith M, editors. *The Leader of the Future 2*. San Francisco (CA): Jossey-Bass; 2006. p. 73–84.

15. Hellriegel D, Jackson SE, Slocum JW. *Management: A Competency-Based Approach*. Cincinnati (OH): South-Western Thomson Learning; 2002. 561 p.

16. Hersey P, Blanchard KH, Johnson DE. *Management of Organizational Behavior: Leading Human Resources*. Upper Saddle River (NJ): Prentice Hall; 2001. 516 p.

17. Kent T. Leading and managing: it takes two to tango. *Manag Decis*. 2005;43(7/8):1010–7.

18. Knight W, Moore M, Coperthwaite C. Institutional research: knowledge, skills, and perceptions of effectiveness. *Res High Educ*. 1997;38(4):419–33.

19. Kouzes JM, Posner BZ. *The Leadership Challenge*. San Francisco (CA): Jossey-Bass; 1995. 416 p.

20. Kutz MR. *Contextual Intelligence: Smart Leadership in a Constantly Changing World*. Raleigh (NC): Lulu Press; 2015. 192 p.

21. Kutz MR. *Leadership and Management in Athletic Training: An Integrated Approach*. Baltimore (MD): Lippincott Williams & Wilkins; 2010. 331 p.

22. Kutz MR. Toward a conceptual model of contextual intelligence: a transferable leadership construct. *Leadersh Rev*. 2008;8:18–31.

23. Lewin K, Lippitt R, White RK. Patterns of aggressive behavior in experimentally created "social climates." *J Soc Psychol*. 1939;10:271–99.

24. Maccoby M. Understanding the difference between management and leadership. *Res Technol Manag*. 2000;43:57–9.

25. Maxwell JC. Foreword. In: Kouzes J, Posner B, editors. *Christian Reflections on the Leadership Challenge*. San Francisco (CA): Jossey-Bass; 2004. p. x.

26. Mayer J, Salovey P, Caruso D. Emotional intelligence: theory, findings, and implications. *Psychol Inq*. 2004;15(3):197–215.

27. Miller T, Vaughan B. Messages from the management past: classic writers and contemporary problems. *SAM Adv Manag J*. 2001;66(1):4–20.

28. Muczyk J, Reimann B. MBO as a complement to effective leadership. *Acad Manag Exec*. 1989;3(2);131–8.

29. Nellis SM. Leadership and management: techniques and principles for athletic training. *J Athl Train*. 1994;19(4):328–35.

30. Northouse PG. *Leadership: Theory and Practice*. Thousand Oaks (CA): Sage; 2004. 360 p.

31. O'Neil EH; for the Pew Health Professions Commission. *Recreating Health Professional Practice for a New Century*. San Francisco (CA): Pew Health Professions Commission; 1998. 142 p.

32. Pointer D, Orlikoff J. *The High Performance Board: Principles of Nonprofit Organization Governance*. San Francisco (CA): Jossey-Bass; 2002. 208 p.

33. Robinson D. Management theorists: thinkers for the 21st century? *Train J*. 2005:30–1.

34. Salovey P, Mayer JD. Emotional intelligence. *Imagin Cogn Pers*. 1990;9(3):185–211.

35. Senge P. Leadership in living organizations. In: Hesselbein F, Goldsmith M, Somerville I, editors. *Leading Beyond the Walls*. San Francisco (CA): Jossey-Bass; 1996.

36. Sternberg RJ. *Beyond IQ: A Triarchic Theory of Human Intelligence*. New York (NY): Cambridge University Press; 1985. 411 p.

37. Sternberg RJ. Intelligence and wisdom. In: Sternberg RJ, editor. *Handbook of Intelligence*. New York (NY): Cambridge University Press; 2000. p. 631–50.

38. Stogdill RM. *Handbook of Leadership*. New York (NY): Free Press; 1974. 613 p.

39. Teremzini PT. On the nature of institutional research and the knowledge and skills it requires. *Res High Educ*. 1993;34(1):1–9.

40. Umbdenstock R, Hageman W, Amundson B. The five critical areas for effective governance of not-for-profit hospitals. *Hosp Health Serv Adm*. 1990;35(4):481–92.

41. Wagner R. Practical intelligence. In: Sternberg RJ, editor. *Handbook of Intelligence*. New York (NY): Cambridge University Press; 2000. p. 380–95.

42. Wagner RK. Tacit knowledge in everyday intelligent behavior. *J Pers Soc Psychol*. 1987;52(6):1236–47.

43. Winston B, Patterson K. An integrated definition of leadership. *Int J Leadersh Stud*. 2005;1(2):6–66.

44. Yoder-Wise P. *Leading and Managing in Nursing*. St. Louis (MO): Mosby; 2003. 612 p.

45. Yukl GA. *Leadership in Organizations*. Englewood Cliffs (NJ): Prentice-Hall; 2002. 508 p.

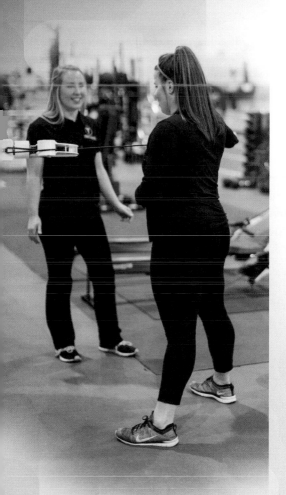

16

General Health Fitness Management

OBJECTIVES

- To know the basics of human resource management, including the procedures necessary to recruit and staff a fitness facility.

- To recognize the relationship between employee training and development and employee performance and retention.

- To identify basic financial statements and their components.

- To recognize revenues, expenses, and different budgets and budget processes.

- To understand the basic elements of the standards and guidelines relating to facility operations and management.

INTRODUCTION

This chapter provides an overview of some general responsibilities involved in managing a fitness-based facility. Although a manager should have knowledge and experience in the fitness industry, management positions also require expertise in human resources, financial planning, and facility operations. The role of the manager as a steward of human resources in identifying staffing needs, recruiting, hiring, and empowering employees as valuable assets is covered. Basic financial principles relating to the operation of a fitness center and an overview of facility management and operations are also presented.

 ## Human Resource Management

One of the most important aspects of any fitness-based business is the team of individuals providing services to the customer. To ensure repeat business, it is critical to build a team of highly qualified individuals who can create strong relationships with customers while providing a friendly and motivating environment.

Staffing and Recruiting

Because every fitness facility is structured differently, the first step to staffing is to determine the service requirements. This will then dictate the types and number of positions needed at different levels throughout the organization. This process should consider the following questions: How many people will it take to complete a job? What staff-to-member ratio will provide sufficient customer service? What responsibilities will be held by each type of position? How many hours will the facility be in operation each day of the week? What is the membership market? These are just some of the key questions that will help a manager determine the appropriate staffing needs (2).

Types of Positions

Regardless if a facility is corporate, commercial, hospital, or community-based, similar positions appear in each type of organization. In its *Occupational Outlook Handbook*, the Bureau of Labor Statistics reports that "recreational worker" roles ranging from fitness instructor to exercise physiologist are growing from at an above to almost double the average employment growth rate (5). According to the *2010 Fitness Salary Survey*, conducted by the American Council on Exercise (ACE), the seven most common job titles in the fitness industry are (a) personal trainer, (b) group fitness instructor, (c) fitness director, (d) advanced health and fitness specialist, (e) Pilates instructor, (f) group fitness director, and (g) club owner. Table 16.1 provides sample job roles for a few of these positions.

Employee versus Independent Contractor

Many positions in the health fitness industry are filled by hiring employees or independent contractors. According to the Internal Revenue Service Publication 15-A (8), an individual is an independent contractor if the person for whom the services are performed can only control the result of the work but not the means or methods of accomplishing the result. An employee is an individual who performs services for a client/business that has control over the details of how the services are performed (6). A manager must review the tasks and responsibilities of each job to determine whether it is more appropriate to hire an employee into a position or use an independent contractor, as different situations dictate different practices (Table 16.2) (12).

Table 16.1	Common Positions in the Fitness Industry
Job Position	**Job Roles**
General manager	Develops core values; creates and implements strategic plan; develops relationship with complimentary business services; oversees annual budget and marketing development and distribution; and manages all on-site directors
Fitness director	Creates and implements member fitness programs; markets fitness services; encourages members to achieve fitness goals through offered programs and services; and oversees on-site fitness employees, including personal trainers and group fitness instructors
Group fitness director	Responsible for creation and implementation of group exercise programs; oversees all on-site group fitness instructors
Personal trainer	Markets and sells personal training packages; leads one-on-one or group personal training sessions; performs initial evaluations and reassessments; conducts fitness orientations for all new members; and supervises members while circulating fitness floor
Group fitness instructor	Teaches group-based exercises classes and programs for members

Table 16.2	Factors Defining Employees and Independent Contractors	
Factors	**Employees**	**Independent Contractors**
Behavior control	Subject to the business' instructions about when and where to do work, how to perform the job tasks, what equipment or tools to use, who can assist with the work, where to purchase supplies, what order or sequence to follow, etc.	Typically make their own decisions about how and when to do work, where to purchase supplies/services, maintain their own office or workspace off-site, use personal tools and equipment, etc.
	May be trained to perform services in a particular manner	Use their own methods to complete tasks
Financial control	Most expenses incurred while working for the business are reimbursed	Typically have unreimbursed expenses that occur while work is being completed
	Uses facility and tools owned and maintained by business	Has a significant investment in the facilities/tools used in performing services for someone else
	Work for the business, typically does not market their services/skills to other businesses	Free to seek out business opportunities, advertise, and maintain public business location, and are available to work in the relevant market
	Generally guaranteed a regular wage by hour per week or other period of time	Often paid a flat fee or on a time and materials basis for the job
Type of relationship	Receive employee benefits, such as insurance, pension plan, vacation pay, sick time, etc.	Do not received employee benefits from client
	Indefinite relationship	Relationship lasting for a specific project or period
	Provide services that are a key aspect of regular business activity	Typically provide a one-time service, or service on as-needed basis

Exempt versus Nonexempt

Another consideration for managers when recruiting is whether an employee should be considered exempt or nonexempt. An exempt employee is one who is paid a base salary on a scheduled (weekly, biweekly, monthly, etc.) basis and is typically not eligible for overtime pay. A nonexempt employee is paid on an hourly basis and is usually eligible for overtime pay. Having nonexempt positions can impact financial planning, as overtime pay may pose a significant burden on a facility's budget (7). In addition, it is important not to impose unreasonable working hours on exempt employees, knowing they do not need to be paid overtime. Otherwise, you may hurt morale and increase employee turnover.

Job Descriptions

Detailed job descriptions are important to the staffing and recruiting process for both the interviewer and potential candidates. During the recruiting process, job descriptions define the skills necessary to complete the job and serve as a guide for questions to ask during the interview. Ultimately, this leads to the selection of the best candidate for the position. Once a position has been filled, the job description becomes a guide for employees around which they can base their performance. A detailed job description (see box titled "How to Create a Job Description") should include the job title, main purpose of the job, responsibilities of the job, required skills, reporting structure, conditions of employment, and performance measures. Once detailed job descriptions have been written, recruiting efforts can begin (12).

Recruiting

Recruiting refers to the process of finding and attracting new employees. Solid, well-planned recruiting efforts lead to a simplified selection process, allowing a manager to fill positions quickly and with ease.

Recruiting Strategies

The most effective recruiting strategies help fill positions quickly while limiting the cost to the employer. Print and virtual advertising, such as listings posted in the "Help Wanted" sections in local or regional newspapers and advertisements submitted to major Internet job search engines, targets general populations and increases the number of people who see the position yet decreases the likelihood of reaching qualified candidates. Many companies use professional agencies to save time while recruiting, especially for higher level management positions, but this method can be considerably costlier than others. Internal recruitment, moving or promoting a current employee, can significantly decrease recruitment cost and training time, as the applicant is already familiar with the company and facility. Internal hiring also gives current employees additional work incentive to strive for a higher position. Of course, this method also leaves the company with a new vacancy, although typically at a more entry-level position, which tends to be less costly to recruit for and easier to fill. Employee referral is another low-cost recruiting strategy and gives current employees an opportunity to help the company reach competent applicants, as they often know best the skills required for the position. Colleges and universities have career services centers where current and former students can search local job positions and can be targeted particularly if there is an academic major in health and fitness (7). Many academic institutions offer internship opportunities for students to gain hands-on experience for academic credit. Internship programs allow a company to provide training to students and screen potential future employees. Students who participate in internships tend to have higher grade point averages and are more motivated to find employment after graduation (9).

HOW TO	Create a Job Description

Creating a job description involves more than just writing down whom you want to hire. There are plenty of variables to consider if you want to attract an outstanding pool of applicants and hire the best possible person for the job. Following is the description of key items to consider when drafting a job description for a general fitness manager.

Position Overview

This is the section that will give potential applicants a general sense of the hierarchy within the facility and where they will fit into that scheme. A typical position overview could look like this:

Responsible for supervising the performance of all employees and contractors; deliver first class fitness experience to all members; monitor all facility expenses and revenue; meet monthly, quarterly, and annual goals. This position reports to the regional vice president.

Job Responsibilities

Job responsibility is the key to a good job description. It is critical to lay out the specific key aspects of the job so that the applicants know what is expected of them and so that the employer has a solid basis of evaluation. It may not be necessary to list each and every responsibility or potential responsibility, and if not, you should at least state "other responsibilities as they apply" to indicate the list is not comprehensive. The "other responsibilities" should be discussed during any interviews. The responsibilities could look like this:

Supervisory: Oversee all facility employees including personal trainers, group exercise instructors, front desk staff, spa services staff, and maintenance staff; recruit, hire, and train all staff in facility; and conduct performance reviews and create development plans for each employee.

Facility Operations: Manage all facility services (group exercise, personal training, day care program); track operating expenses and revenues while monitoring budget guidelines; oversee maintenance and purchase of equipment; coordinate group exercise and personal training programs and schedules; manage employee payroll and benefits; participate and manage daily operations including floor supervision, class instruction, and fitness appointments when appropriate; develop marketing strategies; determine individual and team goals; and review goals on a monthly, quarterly, and annual basis.

Position Credentials

This category can also be called "qualifications," "skills required," or any number of other words or phrases that makes it clear that this is the background expected of all serious applicants. It is critical to list everything here that you feel necessary to be competitive for this position, as eliminating a candidate based on something not listed can turn into a legal issue regarding inappropriate hiring practices. A typical Credentials section could look like this:

High School diploma required, bachelor's degree preferred; 5+ years of relevant work experience; experience in working in a team environment with the ability to delegate workload and responsibilities; competence in management skills including quality management, risk management, and achievement of goals; strong verbal and written communications; time management and organizational skills; ability to design, deliver, and evaluate programs and services; provide exceptional customer service; knowledge of fitness management software; experience in the performance of fitness assessments; basic computer literacy; budget tracking and management experience; current CPR/AED and first aid certification; current fitness certification from an accredited organization (*e.g.*, ACSM, ACE, and AFAA)

Employee Status

This section is relatively straightforward and indicates the working hours, including if the position is salaried or hourly. The status section could look like this:

40 hours per week; salaried, exempt

Attracting the Right Candidates

The key to recruiting is to advertise open positions in areas frequented by the types of individuals needed for that specific job. Positions requiring certifications such as personal trainers or group exercise instructors can be recruited on the career services site at top fitness-related organizations, such as American College of Sports Medicine (ACSM) and ACE. These groups often keep their career services pages limited to individuals already certified, thereby preventing exposure of the job posting to individuals without a baseline qualification. Setting up a booth at the regional conference for a professional organization provides an exposure to local job opportunities for seasoned professionals seeking a change in employment and young professionals ready to enter the field. However, this can come at a great expense.

Selection Process

Once a number of applications have been compiled from recruiting efforts, the selection process can begin. Selection is the process of sorting through the applicants to find qualified individuals who will be taken through the interview process. Depending on the size of a facility, a manager may create a search committee to screen and interview potential candidates. The search committee comprises individuals from key areas within the facility; for example, the group exercise director may have a unique role in the hiring of individuals who may be needed to teach group exercise. Forming a committee also allows for greater collaboration among employees. The first step a manager or committee must take is to create a checklist or matrix of the qualifications and responsibilities needed for the position. Each resume and cover letter should be reviewed within the matrix, looking for past experiences and knowledge that match the crucial items outlined on the matrix. Checking professional references also provides insight into the work habits and skills of the applicant. Applicants whose resumes, cover letters, and references pass the matrix test should be contacted to start the interview process. Sometimes, in larger organizations, the human resources department conducts this initial screening and works with the hiring manager to select the most suitable candidates to interview.

Interview Process

A multiple-stage interview process should be applied to each candidate who passes the initial selection process. The first interview may be by telephone. Telephone interviews provide a glimpse of the candidate's interpersonal skills and ability to be prepared. Telephone interviews also allow a search committee to conduct several interviews remotely without incurring additional costs. In situations where a search committee is not warranted, and when the first interview is not by telephone but in person, the immediate supervisor for the position should conduct this interview. The supervisor can gain insight into the candidate's knowledge, skills, experience, and attitude. This interview should be structured with the supervisor using a preplanned checklist of questions to ensure that all necessary information is collected and that all questions asked are legally acceptable. Chapter 14 provides references for employers to check the legality of questions used in the hiring process. A second interview should include team members with whom the applicant will be working. For example, if there is a personal trainer position available, the applicant should be interviewed by the other personal trainers in the facility in an open, team format. The primary focus of the team interview should be on personality and team dynamics to ensure that the applicant is an appropriate fit to the current team in place (12).

Once all candidates have completed the interview process, they should be ranked by both the position's immediate supervisor and the employees in the department in which the open position exists. In the case when there is a search committee, the chair of the committee makes a recommendation to the hiring manager based on the discussion and vote of the committee. In some cases, more than one name can be submitted and the hiring manager makes the final decision. Once the candidates are ranked, an offer should be extended to the applicant with the highest rank first (12).

Compensation

Compensation is not limited to wages. When offering a position to a candidate, it is important to outline the additional benefits that may be included with employment. Organizations vary greatly on what types of supplemental benefits can be offered to augment wages. Some organizations provide professional development funds for employees to support conference attendance or the cost of obtaining additional specialty certifications. Other organizations provide partial or whole health care, dental, vision, or mental health benefits. In addition, child or adult care opportunities, flexible schedules, vacation time, or incentives to earn additional income all provide an attractive package for candidates. For some employees, job security and work–life balance are equally as important as salary (4). Providing opportunities for advancement and professional development aids in recruiting and maintaining a satisfied and qualified workforce.

Employee Orientation, Development, and Training

New employee orientation is important to any facility, as a well-planned orientation will make onboarding easier for the new individual as well as the current staff and members. According to a study published by the Society for Human Resource Management (SHRM) in 2011, more than 80% of organizations have either formal or informal onboarding programs or practices. These programs are used to reduce an employee's uneasiness and anxiety that comes with starting a new position, to prepare the employee to start his or her new position, and to create a strong and positive relationship between the new employee and the organization. If an orientation is effective and successful, it will reduce training time, lower costs related to training, and decrease absenteeism and tardiness (11).

Techniques used to deliver critical orientation information will vary on the basis of position, learning style of the new employee, and teaching style of the immediate supervisor or human resources representative. Regardless of the technique used, new employee orientations should include an overview of both company and facility policies as well as teach the new employee job-related skills.

Company orientations, often conducted by a Human Resources or employee personnel department representative, should include the following:

- *The structural and cultural organization of the company, facility, and department*: A discussion should be held regarding the mission statement of the organization, as well as its importance to the new employee and his or her position, and the organizational culture and the expectation it creates. Any employee in a fitness facility must understand the hierarchy and chain of command that exists within the organization, from chief executive officer (CEO) to general manager, fitness director to personal trainers, maintainers, and desk staff.
- *Human resource policies and procedures applicable to all employees*: Although information about benefits and compensation is often provided when a position is offered, new employees must be equipped with all company/facility policies and procedures that apply to them and their position. A human resources associate or manager should discuss pay, absenteeism and tardiness, benefits, and the processes the employee needs to follow to access him or her as well as highlight key areas in the employee handbook, such as job performance and reviews.

Job-specific orientation, typically conducted by an immediate supervisor or department mentor, should the following:

- *Informing the employee of specific job responsibilities and expectations*: A written job description should be given to the new employee, outlining job tasks and responsibilities. At this point, a time frame should be decided on by the new employee and immediate supervisor regarding when the individual will be able to perform the job tasks independently, signifying the completion of the orientation sessions. A probationary period may be used to ensure employee performance in a timely manner.

- *Laying out the workspace to be used by the new employee*: An aquatic exercise class instructor would need an in-depth tour of the pool area and changing rooms, whereas a certified exercise physiologist (EP-C) will need to be shown where equipment is kept, places to find paperwork for members, and a tour of the entire facility before working independently.
- *Including an introduction to immediate coworkers*: Meeting coworkers will allow a new employee to settle in to his or her position quickly and will provide the employee with potential mentors as he or she gains more experience. Group exercise instructors often gain valuable information from other instructors, including member preferences, equipment issues, and class structure — a benefit they will not get from spending time with employees in unrelated positions (9).

Performance Management and Employee Retention

During the onboarding process, new employees should be equipped with the knowledge of what is expected of someone in their position. Expectations must be clearly defined by an organization and the position's immediate supervisor in order for an employee to be successful. For example, if employees on the membership sales team do not know that they are expected to sell 50 memberships each month, they will be frustrated when they are disciplined or penalized for selling only 30 memberships. Unknown expectations create a sense of uneasiness among employees, and this can lead to poor performance and increased turnover. Instead, make it clear what each employee's specific expectations are and revise them when needed.

Setting Goals

Expectations should be set with employees on an annual basis, emphasizing the commitment a company has to its employees' development over time. Annual goals give employees insight into where the company plans to be in a year as well as provide them guidance as to how they can help the company succeed. It is the responsibility of a manager to meet with each employee, explain the goals of the company, and help the employee determine how his or her position can contribute to the accomplishment of those goals (7).

Goal setting should be a collaboration between the employee and the immediate supervisor. It is important to maintain a distinction between ongoing tasks or responsibilities and goals targeted to improve company standing. Goals should be specific, measurable, achievable, relevant, and time-based — five qualities known as the SMART criteria for goal setting (Table 16.3).

Table 16.3	SMART Goal-Setting Principle
Specific	A specific goal answers the questions "Who?" "What?" "Where?" "When?" and "Why?" and has a much greater chance of being accomplished because it has definition.
Measureable	Goals must be stated with either a quantitative or qualitative assessment. To determine if a goal is measurable, ask "How much? How many? What determines success?"
Attainable/achievable	The goal must be attainable given the employee/employer resources.
Relevant	Goals need to relate to an employee and his or her position and hold some significance or meaning.
Time-based	A goal needs a time frame in which to be accomplished.

Performance Appraisals

Many companies conduct formal annual performance appraisals. Some managers, fearing conflict or confrontation, prefer this method to be an informal process. In reality, regularly scheduled evaluations give the manager an opportunity to gather both positive and negative feedback about employees over the course of the year and make an informed decision about employee's progress. However, this technique of analyzing and critiquing an employee's performance does not replace day-to-day performance management and can sometimes lead to negative experiences for both the employee and the immediate supervisor. For example, a manager observes a front desk employee ignoring members as he or she enters the facility. If the manager waits months before telling the employee that he or she needs to be acknowledging members while signing in, the employee will continue to perform incorrectly, and the manager will become increasingly frustrated. Instead, feedback, both positive and negative, should be delivered to employee on both a regular and as-needed basis (7).

Formal performance appraisals should be held annually, giving the employee and the immediate supervisor a chance to assess the goals set at the beginning of the review year as well as providing the opportunity for the discussion of future goals. Performance evaluation forms should be completed by the employee first and then by the immediate supervisor. Using this method allows a supervisor to understand how the employee thinks he or she has been performing. Performance evaluation forms should include sections for the following:

1. Employee strengths
2. Employee weaknesses
3. Goals from the review period, with explanations of achievement or challenges that were met in the process of achieving success
4. Company-defined skills and competencies

All reviews, whether informal or formal, should be documented by the immediate supervisor, acknowledged by the employee, and kept in the employee's folder (7).

Employee Retention

An effective performance appraisal process can positively affect employee retention. A Gallup Survey completed in 2006 revealed that 32% of employees voluntarily leaving their jobs did so for career advancement/promotional opportunities, whereas another 17% left because of management and general work environment. More frequent performance checks can help maintain strong relations between an immediate supervisor and his or her employees, improving the company's retention rates (10). Additionally, other more informal employee morale activities are beneficial for employee retention.

Section Summary

The EP-C in management positions will typically find themselves involved in staffing or restaffing their facility. It is imperative for the EP-C to understand the recruiting, selection, and hiring processes and to collaborate with the appropriate departments (*i.e.*, human resources and talent acquisition). Good team dynamics and hardworking and dedicated employees are important to running a successful fitness facility.

Risk Management

As the fitness industry continues to grow, the EP-C has a great opportunity to work in a variety of settings and make a powerful difference in people's lives. More professional opportunities, however, increase expectations of responsible professional conduct, which means greater potential for liability for failing to act responsibly. Today's EP-C must understand these areas of risk exposure and the legal issues and industry standards and guidelines that surround them, and be able to deliver services confidently and proactively.

Risk management is a critical area of concern to any EP-C manager and is an initial and ongoing process to identify relevant risks associated with the delivery of a service. This process occurs through the application of various techniques intended to recognize, eliminate, reduce, or transfer risk through the implementation of operational strategies to the program activities designed to benefit both the patients and the program (1).

The role of the EP-C manager in creating and maintaining a safe work environment is critical to the success of any fitness facility. It is important to develop a comprehensive and effective risk management plan that minimizes unsafe conditions and practices while maximizing safety by establishing policies and procedures that address safe practices and protect the assets of the company.

Standards and Guidelines for Risk Management and Emergency Procedures

The ACSM has identified eight fundamental standards relating to risk management and emergency procedures (14) (Table 16.4). Because the EP-C may offer services in a variety of locations, including

Table 16.4	ACSM Standards and Guidelines for Risk Management and Emergency Procedures

1. Facility operators must have written emergency response policies and procedures, which shall be reviewed regularly and physically rehearsed at least twice annually. These policies shall enable staff to respond to basic first aid situations and emergency events in an appropriate and timely manner.

2. Facility operators shall ensure that a safety audit is conducted, which routinely inspects all areas of the facility to reduce or eliminate unsafe hazards that may cause injury to employees and health/fitness facility members or health/fitness facility users.

3. Facility operators shall have a written system for sharing information with members and users, employees, and independent contractors regarding the handling of potentially hazardous materials, including the handling of bodily fluids by the facility staff in accordance with the guidelines of the Occupational Safety and Health Administration (OSHA).

4. In addition to complying with all applicable federal, state, and local requirements relating to automated external defibrillators (AEDs), all facilities (*i.e.*, staffed or unstaffed) shall have as part of their written emergency response policies and procedures a public access defibrillation (PAD) program in accordance with generally accepted practice, as highlighted in this section.

5. AEDs in a facility shall be located within a 1.5-min walk to anyplace an AED could be potentially needed.

6. A skills review, practice sessions, and a practice drill with the AED shall be conducted a minimum of every 6 mo, covering a variety of potential emergency situations (*e.g.*, water, presence of a pacemaker, medications, and children).

7. A staffed facility shall assign at least one staff member to be on duty during all facility operating hours who is currently trained and certified in the delivery of cardiopulmonary resuscitation (CPR) and in the administration of an AED.

8. Unstaffed facilities must comply with all applicable federal, state, and local requirements relating to AEDs. Unstaffed facilities shall have as part of their written emergency response policies and procedures a PAD program as a means by which either members and users or an external emergency responder can respond from time of collapse to defibrillation in 4 min or less.

Table 16.5	Guidelines for Risk Management and Emergency Procedures

1. Facilities should use waivers of liability and/or assumption of risk documents with all facility members and users.

2. A facility that delivers or prescribes physical activity programs, primarily or exclusively, to members and users who are considered at an elevated risk for experiencing a health-related event because of their participation in physical activity (*e.g.,* users older than 50 y, individuals with coronary risk factors, diabetes, or clinical obesity) should have a medical director, a medical liaison, or a medical advisory committee provide assistance in reviewing the facility's physical activity screening and programming protocols as well as its emergency response protocols.

3. Facilities should provide the appropriate level of supervision and monitoring for each of the physical activity areas in the facility.

4. All physical activity areas should have a clock, a chart of target heart rates, and a chart depicting ratings of perceived exertion to enable members and users to monitor their level of physical exertion.

5. A facility should extend to each employee and staff the opportunity to receive training and certification in first aid and the use of CPR and an AED.

6. Facilities should have an incident report system that provides written documentation of all incidents that occur within the facility or within the facility's scope of responsibility. Such reports should be completed in a timely fashion and maintained on file, according to the regulatory statute of limitations for the location in which the facility does business.

a health and fitness facility, the outdoors, or a client's home, basic precautions should be taken to ensure that every exercise setting is safe.

Developing an emergency response policy includes the organization of a risk management team. A risk management team might consist of a health care professional, a local emergency medical service professional, and key staff members. The emergency response policy should include the procedures for responding to critical incidents such as sudden cardiac arrest or heat illness as well as less life-threatening incidents requiring first aid. Emergency response policies also need to include evacuation procedures in case of fire or natural disaster. The risk management team is charged with the responsibility of training and practicing the emergency response plan so that every employee is prepared in the event of an emergency. Table 16.5 provides additional suggestions for the development and implementation of emergency response plans. The EP-Cs who are sole proprietors of a fitness business or provide in-home training should also have written emergency policies and procedures.

Risk Management Summary

Risk management is an initial and ongoing process to identify relevant risks associated with the delivery of a service. This occurs through the application of various techniques to identify, eliminate, reduce, or transfer those risks through the implementation of operational strategies to the program activities designed to benefit the clients and program. The EP-C is critical in the development of a team of individuals working together to establish and maintain a safe environment for both employees and clients. Although a clearly defined written emergency plan is essential, cultivating meaningful relationships with members and developing a vigilant attitude around safety will create an atmosphere of security and well-being for all. The EP-C may also be responsible for facility operations that extend beyond the acute emergency situations.

Facility Management and Operations

Fitness facilities vary greatly in square footage, usage, equipment, layout, and member access. However, there are several key principles of facility management that pertain to every facility regardless of capacity. *ACSM's Health/Fitness Facility Standards and Guidelines* provide critical information required both to meet industry benchmarks and to comply with NSF International facility accreditation standards. The EP-C may be involved in different aspects of facility management. Therefore, a brief description of the role of the EP-C from the perspective of operations and equipment usage will be presented.

Operations

In addition to human resource functions relating to scheduling and supervision, facility operations may involve a great variety of tasks relating to supervision of members, access of equipment for members and guests, temperature control, music and sound functions, information technology, and overall facility maintenance. The EP-C must always consider the well-being of all members and staff and the overriding principle of creating a safe workplace. Although facility-dependent, there are certain operating standards that should be included within all facilities: monitoring entrance/exit and usage of the facility; maintaining proper water temperature and chemical balance for saunas, steam rooms, and/or whirlpools; and employing appropriate supervision for youth programing (14).

The standards are written to ensure that expectations regarding supervision, responsibility, and duty are clearly defined. Facilities that are nontraditional in the hours of operation such as 24-hour access sites also have an obligation to provide clear policies and procedures around supervision and access. In addition, creating a safe workplace involves relevant and thoughtfully placed signage that communicates the expectations, responsibility, risks, and actions required to maintain a successful fitness operation. It is also important to consider the policies and procedures around equipment and supplies.

Equipment

Although it is the responsibility of every member and employee to respect equipment, the EP-C may be charged with the task of calibrating, inspecting, and maintaining equipment. There are several key questions to ask when considering the care and use of equipment. An equipment checklist is presented below:

1. Is the equipment being used for the purpose it was designed?
2. Is the preventive maintenance schedule adequate given the equipment usage?
3. Is the manufacturer's warranty reasonable given the equipment usage?
4. Is the equipment thoughtfully and safely positioned within the facility?
5. Is the equipment stored properly?
6. Is the equipment being replaced on a reasonable usage cycle?
7. Is the equipment reflective of the mission and character of the facility?
8. Is the equipment user-friendly?

In addition to the responsibility to provide clean and well-functioning equipment to clients, the EP-C has a responsibility to provide clear instructions about the use and misuse of equipment. Empowering members with the knowledge of the variety of uses of fitness equipment enables clients to adjust exercise routines and develop additional strategies for adherence and success.

The EP-C must understand potential areas of risk exposure and the industry standards and guidelines that surround these facility operations to deliver services confidently and to proactively manage risk. The professionalism that such vigilance requires increases the personal and professional rewards of life as a fitness professional while also ensuring lasting business success. The most successful EP-C will always keep in mind that his or her top priority is to protect the best interests of the participant at all times and in all ways. Protecting the client also means acting with financial integrity.

Fiscal Management

For any fitness facility, accurate financial planning and management are crucial to succeeding in the industry. Fitness managers need a basic understanding of accounting and financial processes to create facility budgets and financial forecasts; the list below defines key accounting terms:

Accounts payable: money the business owes to another individual or business
Accounts receivable: money owed to the business by individuals or businesses
Asset: any property owned by a business that has monetary value
Balance sheet: a financial statement that presents the assets, liability, and equity of a business at a specific point in time
Budget: a plan forecasting expected income and expenses for a given period
Capital: money, goods, land, or equipment that is used to produce other goods and services
Cash flow: movement of money in and out of a business through the collection of revenue and payments of expenses
Depreciation: a decline in the value of any given asset over a period, often because of wear and tear, or age
Equity: the monetary value of a property or an interest in a property in excess of claims or liens against it
Income statement: a financial statement that includes the revenue, expenses, and net income/loss of a business for a specified period
Liability: a debt owed to an individual or business
Net income: gross income less expenses, representing the profit of a business for a specific period
Variance: the difference between an expected and an actual result

Accounting is the process of recording and summarizing business and financial transactions and analyzing, verifying, and reporting the results. These financial records provide information needed to make decisions about the future state of the business.

Basic Accounting Terminology and Principles

A standard method of recording business transactions is necessary to maintain accurate records. The most common methods used in the fitness industry are cash accounting and accrual accounting. In cash accounting, transactions are recorded when money is actually received or paid out. Using this method, membership dues would be recorded on the day the payment was received from the member. In contrast, accrual accounting requires transactions to be recorded when they occur. Therefore, membership dues would be recorded on the day a membership payment is considered due regardless of if the payment has been received. Accrual accounting tends to be the preferred method in the fitness industry, as it portrays a more accurate depiction of the financial operations of the business (7,8).

Financial Statements

Financial statements provide a financial summary of a business to owners, accountants, and lending institutions. Balance sheets and profit and loss statements are two of the most important financial statements a manager needs to understand.

Balance Sheet

A balance sheet (Fig. 16.1) indicates the financial status of a business at any given time and is separated into assets, liabilities, and owner's equity. In order for a balance sheet to be accurate, the total assets must always be equal to the total liabilities plus total equity (3).

1. Assets are anything a company owns that has monetary value (*i.e.*, cash, buildings, land, and equipment). Assets are typically divided into two categories: current (short-term) and fixed (long-term). Current assets are those that can and are expected to be turned into cash within the next 12 months. Examples of current assets include the following:

   ■ Cash and cash equivalents
   ■ Inventory
   ■ Accounts receivable
   ■ Prepaid expenses

Balance Sheet for ABC Fitness Center June 30, 20XX		
Assets		
Current assets		
Cash	200,000	
Cash equivalents	90,000	
Inventory	25,000	
Accounts receivable	130,000	
Total current assets	$445,000	
Fixed assets		
Equipment	845,000	
Building	1,500,000	
Land/property	675,000	
Accumulated depreciation		200,000
Total fixed assets	$2,820,000	
Total assets	$3,265,000	
Liabilities		
Current liabilities		
Accounts payable		115,000
Accrued expenses		65,000
Deferred taxes		9,500
Total current liabilities		$189,500
Non–current liabilities		
Notes payable (bank)		1,650,000
Others		120,000
Total non–current liabilities		$1,770,000
Total liabilities		$1,959,500
Owner's equity		
Capital stock		985,000
Retained earnings		215,500
Paid in capital		105,000
Total owner's equity		$1,305,500
Total liabilities and owner's equity		$3,265,000

FIGURE 16.1. Sample balance sheet.

Fixed assets are those that have been acquired for long-term use by the business. These assets include the following:

- Property (land and buildings)
- Equipment
- Office furniture

2. Liabilities are financial obligations or credits owed by the business. Liabilities are defined as current (short-term) or noncurrent (long-term).
   Current liabilities are debts the business is obligated to pay within the next 12 months. Examples include the following:

- Accounts payable
- Income taxes
- Accruals
- Deferred revenue, rent, or taxes

Noncurrent liabilities are debts and expenses that are not due in the next 12 months. Examples include the following:

- Future payments on loans
- Deferred revenue, rent, or taxes

3. Owner's equity is the owner's investment in the business plus any profits or minus any losses. How equity appears on a balance sheet is determined by how the business was established — either as a corporation, limited liability corporation, partnership, or sole proprietorship.

Profit and Loss Statement

A profit and loss statement, also referred to as an income statement (Fig. 16.2), summarizes the financial performance over a specific time (month, quarter, or year). This financial tool includes actual expenses and revenues in the stated time frame as well as a look at how those numbers compare with a year-to-date plan. Revenues are primarily generated by membership sales, fitness programs, and miscellaneous profit centers, whereas expenses reflect the costs incurred to collect revenue and operate the facility.

Budgeting

Effective financial management relies on a well thought-out budget, created to lay out the allotment of funds spent or brought in by departments and programs. Budgeting, the process of coordinating resources and expenditures required for business functions, is essential for any business to survive. Budgets span a minimum of one fiscal year (typically January 1 to December 31 or July 1 to June 30). It is beneficial to a business to be conservative when estimating revenues and liberal when predicting expenses. Underestimating expenses or overestimating sales can put a business in a challenging position, where expenses cannot be paid and profits will not be made.

Types of Budgets

Two of the most common budget processes in the health and fitness industry are zero-based and trend-line. Zero-based budgeting is the process often used when opening a new facility or when making significant changes in operation of an existing facility. This process uses assumptions of business expenses and revenues to develop a budget rather than relying on previous years' actual numbers. Trend-line budgeting is the most common process used and involves using previous years' financial data to develop the budget for the current and upcoming years. This process makes the assumption that facility expenses and revenues will continue on the trend seen over the past years (7).

ABC Fitness Center Income Statement for the quarter ending March 31, 20XX

	Actual Year to Date	Forecast YTP	Variance
Revenue			
Membership dues	$397,500	$357,750	$39,750
Enrollment fees	$21,000	$26,250	($5,250)
Personal training	$315,965	$280,860	$35,105
Pilates instruction	$1,527	$2,290	($763)
Pro shop	$2,384	$1,500	$884
Miscellaneous	$11,934	$10,000	$1,934
Total revenue	**$750,310**	**$678,650**	**$71,660**
Expenses			
Payroll and benefits			
Wages	$124,876	$130,000	($5,124)
Commission	$32,000	$30,000	$2,000
Payroll costs	$22,478	$23,400	($922)
Benefits	$18,433	$20,000	($1,567)
Total payroll and benefits expenses	*$197,787*	*$203,400*	*($5,613)*
Fitness			
Locker room supplies	$4,765	$4,500	$265
Equipment maintenance	$5,500	$7,000	($1,500)
Entertainment fees	$1,254	$1,200	$54
Total fitness expenses	*$11,519*	*$12,700*	*($1,181)*
Utilities			
Electricity	$95,988	$100,000	($4,012)
Gas	$17,934	$16,000	$1,934
Water	$16,223	$15,000	$1,223
Total utilities expenses	*$130,145*	*$131,000*	*($855)*
Other			
Advertising	$9,241	$11,500	($2,259)
Office supplies	$1,329	$2,000	($671)
Landscaping	$23,925	$33,320	($9,395)
Total other expenses	*$34,495*	*$46,820*	*($12,325)*
Fixed			
Depreciation	$73,453	$75,680	($2,227)
Insurance	$126,177	$123,725	$2,452
Total fixed expenses	*$199,630*	*$199,405*	*$225*
Total expenses	*$573,576*	*$593,325*	*($19,749)*
Pretax operating income	**$176,734**	**$85,325**	**$91,409**

FIGURE 16.2 Sample income statement.

Creating a Budget

Once the method of creating the budget has been determined, there are four main steps to follow to develop a complete and accurate budget:

1. *Determine budget expectations*: Any limitations must be determined before starting the development of a budget. Limitations may include restrictions to keep overall expenses close to the previous year's budget or even possibly to cut the expenses to a percentage less than the previous year.
2. *Forecast revenues*: Using previous years' data, a manager can estimate the revenue coming into the facility for the next fiscal year. It is important to include any new sources of revenue that may not have existed in the previous year (*i.e.*, usage fees from a new child care facility opening in the next fiscal year).
3. *Forecast expenses*: Determine operating costs for the upcoming year, making sure to include percentage increases for salaries, increases in maintenance and repairs as equipment ages, etc.
4. *Project profits and losses*: Comparing revenue and expense streams will determine the overall profits or losses for the projected budget. Revisit the first step to ensure that the profits/losses fall within the limitations set for the budget.

It is important to remember that a budget is only a tool; it is a map to follow throughout the fiscal year to ensure the facility can continue to operate and potentially provide a profit. A manager must revisit the budget on a monthly or quarterly basis, reviewing the year-to-date revenue and expenses. On the basis of the direction the finances are headed, adjustments may need to be made for the rest of the fiscal year to stay on track financially (7).

Income Management

All revenue, which is reported on the income statement, must be diligently tracked throughout the year. Areas of revenue include the following:

- *Membership dues*: Membership and entrance fees are generally a facility's main sources of revenue, accounting for 75% to 80% of total revenue (8).
- *Fitness center*: This category would include fees for fitness programs, personal training, specialty group exercise sessions, and locker/towel rentals.
- *Food and beverage*: Often a small profit center, facilities have started to include a snack/smoothie bar as an incentive to members.
- *Other services*: Depending on the type and size of the facility, a spa department offering services such as massage, youth center, on-site child care, or a pro shop selling clothing or fitness equipment can provide other sources of revenue.

Controlling and tracking accounts receivable is critical to the survival of a fitness facility. Decisions must be made on how to collect and manage revenue streams (12). Managing accounts receivables can be a time-intensive task, and most fitness organizations use software programs or third-party systems to facilitate the collection of revenue.

The collection of revenue will be fairly straightforward in most instances; however, all businesses must have procedures in place for delinquent accounts. Aged trial balance reports, listing all outstanding balances by category (1–30 d, 31–60 d, 61–90 d, and 90+ d), should be run on a scheduled basis to facilitate the collection of funds (7).

Expense Management

Expenses are nearly as important to a company's financial stability as revenue. If spending is out of control, revenue streams may not be enough to keep a business functioning while still producing a profit. Expenses can be broken down into variable or fixed categories. Variable costs are those that fluctuate on the basis of usage of resources or participation in a program. Possible variable expenses include payroll, benefits, employee education and training, supplies, marketing, equipment maintenance and repairs, and inventory. Fixed expenses are those that are relatively consistent year after year and include insurance, rent, property tax, management fees, and principal and interest owed on any debts or loans (13).

It should be the goal of any manager to eliminate excess spending in any areas within his or her control. Fixed expenses often cannot be negotiated, but most variable expenses can be effectively reduced by following a few guidelines:

1. Obtain at least three quotes from different vendors to find the right price for the best product. Be sure to repeat this process on a regular basis for any items that may be purchased repeatedly to ensure the cost reflects industry norms. Negotiate with vendors to get the best deal on goods and services.
2. Eliminate unnecessary expenses. Examine every cost center and determine its expendability. Fill empty spaces or cost center with profit centers (*i.e.*, make an office or storage closet into a massage room).
3. Contract out services (*i.e.*, landscaping) to limit staff usage, equipment and training expenses, and liability concerns.
4. Use internal resources when possible. A business may prefer to hire a few part-time employees to create and publish all marketing efforts instead of signing a contract with a marketing firm.

Regardless of the methods used, managers must constantly review the budget to keep expenses in control and within the parameters set at the beginning of the fiscal year (7).

Section Summary

Using budgeting and financial planning skills, an EP-C can successfully manage a facility's profits and losses. Exposure to different types of facilities will allow managers to develop a variety of financial skills, enhance their ability to accurately forecast a facility's budget, and provide their investors with an annual profit.

A Day in the Life of an EP-C Manager

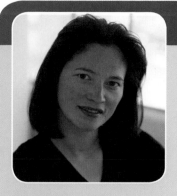

Submitted by **Nancy Hudson, ACSM EP-C, Baystate Health Employee Fitness Center, Springfield, MA, and Teresa Fitts, DPE, ACSM EP-C, FACSM, Westfield State University, Westfield, MA**

This case focuses on the myriad roles of EP-Cs who manage facilities. An interview with a health fitness manager is presented.

Background

Based in Springfield, Massachusetts, Baystate Health is a multi-institutional, integrated health care delivery organization serving a population of nearly one million in western New England. With more than 10,000 employees, Baystate Health is the largest private employer in western Massachusetts. Baystate Health's charitable mission is to improve the health of the people in our communities every day, with quality and compassion. The Baystate Health Employee Fitness Center serves the employee population and acts in collaboration with the Department of Health, Wellness & Worklife Solutions. Nancy Hudson, EP-C, was interviewed to learn more about her role as a manager.

> **Interviewer:** Tell me a little about your role as a manager?
>
> **Nancy:** In my position as the supervisor of the Baystate Health Employee Fitness Center, I play a key role to support program design and delivery of wellness and fitness programs for our health system's employees to help build a culture of health and fulfill the organization's charitable mission. The primary role of my position is to effectively and efficiently manage the employee fitness center operation. As the supervisor of a hospital-based facility, I am required to wear many hats and possess a wide range of management skills, including human resource management, financial management, and facility management.
>
> **Interviewer:** Can you tell me more about what you do in terms of human resources?
>
> **Nancy:** My role as a human resource manager includes hiring new staff, training, mentoring, staff development and engagement, performance management, policy development, and compensation management. I also develop the schedule of staffing coverage for the fitness center and for group exercise classes.
>
> **Interviewer:** While no 2 days are alike, what might you do on a typical day?
>
> **Nancy:** You are right, there is no such thing as a typical day! One thing I love about my job is that no 2 days are the same. However, let me give you a snapshot of my day last week:

5:15 AM — Open the fitness center. Turn on equipment and check to make sure that the area is clean and orderly.
5:30 — Greet members.
5:40 — Read and respond to e-mails from the previous day.
6:15 — Review the schedule of staff coverage for the week and make adjustments if necessary; e-mail or speak to staff regarding changes in the schedule.
6:30 — Update the fitness center's Web site with current program information.
6:45 — Sign off on payroll.

7:00 — Do a walk-through of the fitness center, ensuring the facility and locker rooms are clean and well stocked with supplies and towels.

7:45 — Prepare for a business meeting with the manager of compensation to review the job descriptions for the staff position we will be hiring.

8:00 — Call my recruiter to determine necessary paperwork to fill a staffing shortage. Fill out a temporary staffing position request and submit for approval.

8:30 — Meet with the manager of compensation.

9:00 — Call the equipment repair vendor to provide a cost estimate on the replacement of two treadmill belts; review operating budget and expenses to determine timing of repair.

9:05 — Begin developing a group exercise class schedule for the fourth quarter of the fiscal year; gather staff interest and feedback on my initial thoughts and ideas; e-mail Independent Contractors to discuss their availability for teaching specialty classes and create a basic framework for the group exercise schedule.

9:30 — Travel to management meeting to develop enterprise-wide strategic fitness and wellness initiatives.

11:30 — Provide a tour of the facility and enroll a new member; schedule a fitness assessment and exercise orientation with staff member.

12:00 PM — Spend time on the fitness floor talking to members and encouraging them to sign up to participate in an enterprise-wide, team-based physical activity challenge.

12:45 — Lead staff in a discussion to develop retention and recruitment strategies; delegate responsibilities.

1:45 — Check and respond to e-mails/voicemail.

2:00 — Leave for the day.

Interviewer: Sounds like a busy day! If you had to name the favorite part of your day, what would it be?

Nancy: I really like the challenge of using our resources to meet the member's needs. The Exercise is Medicine (EIM) initiative is really exciting. We are continually looking for new ways to collaborate and grow. EIM has opened up many opportunities for us.

Interviewer: How would you describe your greatest challenge?

Nancy: My background is in fitness. I needed to learn and get experience in management and financial accounting. Baystate is a great organization, so I was able to get the training and support I've needed to succeed.

QUESTIONS

- How does Nancy's role as manager change throughout the day?
- How did Nancy distinguish between different types of staff?

SUMMARY

Managing a fitness-based facility requires experience across many specialties. As discussed in this chapter, managers need expertise not only in the fitness industry but also in human resources and financial planning in order to be able to maintain an attractive and lucrative facility.

Customer service is such an important draw for potential customers in the fitness industry, such that a manager must make it a top priority to hire and develop a team of individuals with strong communication skills and a positive attitude toward their clients. Building the team and their skills is an ongoing managerial responsibility, as training and development must continually be available to keep staff up-to-date with industry standards and to provide customers with the best experience possible.

Finances touch all aspects of managerial decision making. As such, it is critical to plan and implement budgets when developing a team, creating programs, deciding on marketing tactics, and more. Managers need to take an active role in budget creation to ensure that the facility is run according to the expectations set for by the company. Finally, the development and knowledge of skills in areas other than fitness are crucial for any manager's success in this industry, which can be found throughout other chapters in this text.

STUDY QUESTIONS

1. Provide an example of how employee recruitment strategies utilized by a corporate fitness center may differ from a local commercial fitness center.
2. How can the professional development of employees' impact budget decisions? What are some strategies to empower employees to gain additional experience without putting a strain on financial resources?
3. Describe the difference between a trend-line budget and a zero-based budget? When is one budget process more appropriate to utilize?

REFERENCES

1. American College of Sports Medicine. *ACSM's Guidelines for Exercise Testing and Prescription*. 10th ed. Philadelphia (PA): Wolters Kluwer; 2018.

2. Bates M, editor. *Health Fitness Management*. 2nd ed. Champaign (IL): Human Kinetics; 2008. 400 p.

3. Bauer TN. *Onboarding New Employees: Maximizing Success* [Internet]. Alexandria (VA): Society for Human Resource Management; 2010 [cited 2011 Nov]. Available from: http://www.shrm.org/about/foundation/products/Pages/OnboardingEPG.aspx

4. Bokorney J. Security trumps salary for today's engineers. *Eval Eng.* 2009;48(4):14–7.

5. Bureau of Labor Statistics, U.S. Department of Labor. *Occupational Outlook Handbook, 2014-15 Edition, Athletic Trainers and Exercise Physiologists* [Internet]. [cited 2015 Oct 5]. Available from: http://www.bls.gov/ooh/healthcare/athletic-trainers-and-exercise-physiologists.htm

6. Collins J, Porras J. *Built to Last: Successful Habits of Visionary Companies*. New York (NY): Harper Business, Division of Harper Collins Publishers; 1994. 368 p.

7. Herbert DL, Herbert WG, Herbert TG. *Legal Aspects of Preventive, Rehabilitative and Recreational Exercise Programs*. 4th ed. Canton (OH): PRC Publishing, Inc.; 2002. 508 p.

8. Internal Revenue Service, U.S. Department of the Treasury. *Publication 15-A: Employer's Supplemental Tax Guide*. Washington (DC): Internal Revenue Service; 2016.

9. Knouse S, Tanner J, Harris E. The relation of college internships, college performance, and subsequent job opportunity. *J Empl Couns.* 1999;36(1):35.

10. Paychex, Inc. *Exempt vs. Non-Exempt: Identifying Employee Classification*. [Internet]. Rochester (NY): Paychex, Inc.; 2008 [cited 2011 October]. Available from: http://www.paychex.com

11. Perkins T. Basic accounting principles for fitness professionals. *IDEA Fitness J.* 2008;5(7):75.

12. Rockhurst University Continuing Education Center, Inc. *How to Avoid Making a Terrible Hiring Mistake — Participant Notebook*. [Internet]. Mission (KS): National Seminars Training; [cited]. Available from: www.nationalseminarstraining.com

13. Spurga RC. *Balance Sheet Basics*. New York (NY): Penguin Group; 2004. 176 p.

14. Tharrett S, McInnis K, Peterson JA. *ACSM's Health/Fitness Facility Standards and Guidelines*. 4th ed. Champaign (IL): Human Kinetics; 2007. 256 p.

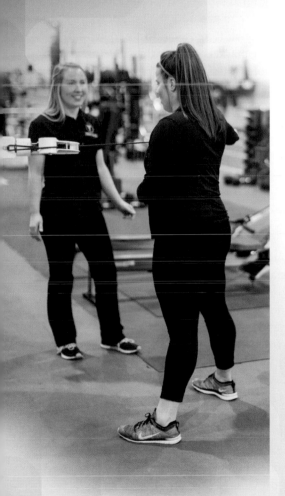

Marketing

- To identify the different aspects of the marketing mix, including the five Ps.
- To recognize the concepts behind the acquisition of new clients and/or participants.
- To apply marketing strategies to business development and growth.

INTRODUCTION

This chapter is designed to provide the certified exercise physiologist (EP-C) with a basic understanding of the marketing mix as it relates to the EP-C's specific job profile. An overview of the marketing mix and the application of the strategies that may be used to promote health and fitness services and products will be presented.

 ## Marketing Basics

The marketing mix represents a basic building block of marketing for the EP-C. At its core, marketing is a function of the aspects that make up product, place, price, and promotion, also known as the four Ps. However, the fitness industry lends itself to one additional "P," representing "people." Knowing and understanding the customers, stakeholders, and target markets enables the EP-C to apply a tailored marketing strategy to increase revenues and promote fitness efficiently and effectively. Below is a breakdown of the five Ps:

1. People (not formerly considered part of the marketing mix)
2. Place
3. Product
4. Price
5. Promotion

People

The first function relating to people involves learning more about the individuals and groups who will be served by fitness-related businesses and services. Understanding the demographic, psychographic (attitudes, values, and opinions), and physical activity attributes of potential customers enables the EP-C to employ deliberate marketing strategies and build sustainable relationships. For example, once the EP-C decides to establish a fitness business, a demographic analysis needs to be performed to better understand the people most likely to frequent the facility. Demographic analyses can provide public information about people residing in any specific geographic area. Researchers have found that individuals who reside within 1- to 5-mile radius of a fitness or recreational facility tend to be more physically active and thus become a target audience (3,13). Alternatively, a demographic analysis can be performed for an entire trade area or city in an attempt to learn more about a broader client base. Either way, the goal is to evaluate data that can provide information necessary to make good decisions with regard to successful marketing practices. A demographic search can be performed with a variety of online resources, including the United States Census Bureau, which is updated every 10 years, providing easily accessed, reliable data, at no cost (http://2010.census.gov/2010census/).

Because of the vast amount of information available, finding a trade area and requesting demographic data can be overwhelming. Therefore, it is important to distinguish which data are relevant to both the industry and the product. In the health and fitness industry, the major factors to examine in a demographic profile are number of people, number of households, household income, and gender breakdown.

The Centers for Disease Control and Prevention (CDC) also provides important information about the exercise and leisure-time habits of individuals. Accessing and synthesizing CDC information enables the EP-C to consider both demographic profiles of a particular area and epidemiological data relating to a particular population. For example, almost regardless of the region of

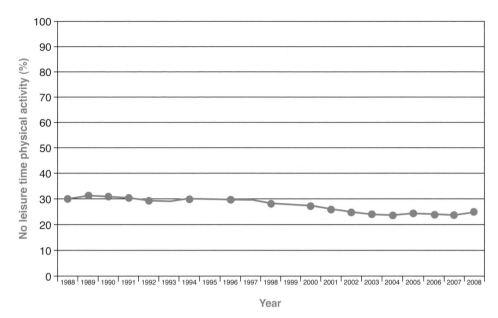

FIGURE 17.1. No leisure-time physical activity 1998 to 2008. (Reproduced from CDC Physical Activity Statistics. Available from: http://www.cdc.gov/nccdphp/dnpa/physical/stats/leisure_time.htm.)

the country, approximately 25% of all adults in the United States perform no leisure-time physical activity (Fig. 17.1). This segment of the population may be a very difficult target for a new EP-C.

However, the remaining 75% of adults are active and therefore more likely to respond to physical activity marketing. In addition, given that the target population should specifically include those living within 1–5 miles of a potential location (21), the EP-C can quickly assess the number of potential customers willing to purchase some type of health and fitness services. Having demographic and epidemiological data enables the EP-C to make informed decisions about possible services and programs to develop and promote these programs effectively.

Successful program development requires an ability to distinguish between trends and fads. Several organizations provide reliable survey data to help make informed decisions about program development. The annual American College of Sports Medicine (ACSM's) Worldwide Survey of Fitness Trends provides information about the top 20 fitness trends within a historical perspective (24). Listed below are the top 20 fitness trends for 2016 (24).

1. Wearable technology
2. Body weight training
3. High-intensity interval training
4. Strength training
5. Educated, certified, and experience fitness professionals
6. Personal training
7. Functional fitness
8. Fitness programs for older adults
9. Exercise and weight loss
10. Yoga
11. Group personal training
12. Worksite health promotion
13. Wellness coaching
14. Outdoor activities
15. Sport-specific training
16. Flexibility and mobility rollers

17. Smart phone exercise apps
18. Circuit training
19. Core training
20. Outcome measurements

The International Health, Racquet & Sportsclub Association (IHRSA) also provides research reports on industry data and fitness club trends (www.ihrsa.org).

Although these data may seem plentiful, more information is usually needed to determine whether a program can be successful, including issues related to possible competitors and market demand in a particular area. Data about people alone are not enough to develop a comprehensive marketing plan. Therefore, product development and implementation is the next critical component of the marketing mix.

Product

Product can be both tangible (selling a membership) and nontangible (helping someone achieve a fitness goal). Possibly, the most common product of EP-Cs is personal training services, which can include something to sell (*i.e.*, training sessions) or something to achieve (*i.e.*, increase strength), or both. The EP-C might work in a clinical, community, corporate, or private setting, and each of these will determine the type of product available. The product may be an incentive program, educational series, or community-based boot camp class. Regardless of product type, it is important for EP-Cs to recognize themselves and their services as an integral part of the product, so they can appropriately market the product in the best possible way. The skills and knowledge required to become an EP-C must not be undervalued by the individual who has attained them. As a matter of principle, marketing success begins with believing in the value of the product. Every EP-C must first believe in himself or herself.

Practically, one approach might include viewing the product in a different way than originally thought. What is the intention of a client purchasing a fitness-related product and what does the consumer want or expect from the product? The top reasons cited for joining a fitness center are consistently reported as improving health and fitness and improving appearance (16). The job of the EP-C is to market themselves as a professional with the skills and knowledge to help the client achieve these exact results. Although the EP-C is continually educating clients about evidence-based practices, it is important not to sell a product purely for the sake of the sale without regard for client interest. Where the product is located can play a pivotal role in the sales and marketing process.

Place

Place refers to where the product can be purchased and/or delivered. For most EP-Cs, the service will be delivered out of a particular physical location such as a commercial, corporate, private fitness facility, or clinic. However, others may elect to conduct in-home or online personal training services with their clients. In addition, current market practices dictate the need for creating a virtual environment to deliver personal training services over and above the brick and mortar setting. The EP-C will need to identify how to properly market his or her services, within a specific environment, whether that be cyberspace, a fitness center, or a client's home.

By clearly defining "place," the EP-C can better understand his or her market. For instance, if the place is a private fitness center, considerations must be made for the physical environment of the club in terms of how the product is perceived. It is important to consider the impact a place, including physical location or Web site, can have on the perceived value of the product (7). An easily navigated Web site and/or impeccably clean training studio set forth an image of professionalism, organization, and quality. Consideration should be given to any sensory perception of the

| **HOW TO** | Develop an Incentive Program Incorporating Exercise is Medicine |

As a grassroots effort, Exercise is Medicine (EIM) is a scientifically sound tool that can be used to promote fitness and wellness. As an educational initiative endorsed by many major health, medical, and fitness organizations, EIM initiatives can reach a broad base of consumers across several levels of expertise and engagement. Although the objectives of this program may go beyond a single incentive program, EP-Cs can focus on one aspect of health, for example, blood pressure, or choose to create a broader connection between fitness and disease prevention. The following are examples of ways to incorporate EIM into programmatic incentives. Creating a team to develop the EIM strategy is the first place to start.

Step 1: Develop Objectives

The vision of EIM to make physical activity and exercise a standard part of a global disease prevention and treatment medical paradigm can be adopted as the vision of any fitness facility.

Objective 1: Increase awareness among members, staff, and the local medical community about EIM Initiatives.

Objective 2: Increase member usage of fitness testing programs 25%.

Objective 3: Increase membership of health care professionals 10%.

Step 2: Develop Strategies to Address Objectives

Objective 1: Increase awareness of EIM.

> *Strategy 1*: Create an EIM team comprised facility members, human resources representatives, local medical professionals, and local educators.

> *Strategy 2*: Provide free blood pressure screening to provide initial information about the connection between exercise and the prevention of hypertension.

> *Strategy 3*: Provide members with a blood pressure form they can bring to their primary care physician.

Objective 2: Increase membership of health care professionals 10%.

> *Strategy 1*: Provide trial or discounted memberships to health care professionals.

> *Strategy 2*: Invite health care professionals to "lunch and learn" sessions.

> *Strategy 3*: Develop a strategic partnership with Institute of Lifestyle Medicine (www.instituteoflife stylemedicine.org) to provide educational incentives to health care professionals.

Step 3: Develop an EIM Incentive Program Action Plan

On the basis of the objectives and strategies listed earlier, develop an action plan to implement the strategies. The resources available for the implementation of an EIM initiative are numerous and are listed at www.exerciseismedicine.org.

Action item: Using the theme of May is EIM month, prepare news releases and other media information relating to exercise and disease prevention to send to local newspapers.

Action item: Develop a reward system for members who access fitness assessment programming.

Action item: Host "lunch and learn" series for local medical professionals to network and share ideas about exercise as a disease prevention tool.

Action item: Connect with local college or university to enlist kinesiology students as ambassadors of EIM message.

Action item: Use social media to create opportunities to provide information about EIM.

Action item: Organize fitness-related event as culminating EIM month activity.

Step 4: Evaluation

Schedule a meeting of the EIM team as soon as possible after event to discuss ways in which the objectives were met.

Develop simple questionnaire for members about effectiveness of EIM campaign.

Follow up with medical professionals about effectiveness of EIM campaign.

place where the product will be delivered. Sensitivity to scents, appropriate music, and comfortable temperatures are just a few of the many factors that relate to a customer's perception of the product as related to the place of delivery. Facility attractiveness and operation has been identified as a key component for customer satisfaction (17). Interconnected with place is the function of price, which involves not only the actual costs of operation but also the perceptions of quality and value.

Price

Determining the appropriate price of the product is multifaceted and critical to the success of any business (3). Basic issues affecting price include cost of developing and/or delivering, profit margin, and market value (real and perceived).

Cost of delivery — The most important factor is the cost of delivering the service. Cost includes marketing, materials (*e.g.*, paper or online), equipment, facility, and the time value of the EP-C. Unless subsidized, the price must at least cover the costs of delivery. It is important to be comprehensive in calculating these costs so as not to under- or overprice the product.

Acceptable profit margin — The cost as noted earlier includes everything except a profit, which is one of the ultimate goals of delivering the product. Therefore, the price above the cost of delivery becomes the actual profit margin. The higher the margin, the more profitable the business. However, set the margin too high, and the product becomes unaffordable to many and overall profit may suffer. An acceptable profit margin varies depending on the type and goals of the business (not for profit vs. for profit) and what the current market will bear. If there are similar products being offered locally, the profit margin should be set with due consideration to competitors pricing. If the price is set too high, many potential customers will be tempted to patronize a lower priced competitor. If the price is too low, people may be skeptical of the product's quality. Therefore, thoroughly assessing what the local market will bear in terms of overall price becomes critical to the success of the product.

Market value — Another important pricing factor is the balance between perceived value and actual demand for a product. A product with high demand, yet low perceived value ("yes we want it, but we are not willing to pay much for it"), may have to be priced very differently than a product with low demand but great perceived value (a select few want it and are willing to pay handsomely for it). Ideally, develop a product that falls somewhere in the middle such that reasonable demand exists and the product is perceived as valuable. Researchers have found that the consumer behaviors of fitness center members have shifted in the perceptions of the costs associated with fitness club memberships (25), which further emphasize value and perception. In the past, members paid only for programs they would consume. Today, members are more likely than ever to try a new program (26). This may be in part due to the variety of membership options available and the increased popularity of nontraditional programming.

Like many other industries, the pricing of fitness-related services also varies according to region. Facilities located on the West Coast may be able to set pricing at a much higher rate than their midwest counterparts, which may largely be a function of cost of living differences. Another issue influencing pricing is the demand for access to fitness facilities, and given the West Coast has higher rates of physical activity participation, the demand is also naturally higher. Of course, demand and price are linearly related, which is then reflected in the average income of the EP-C (Fig. 17.2).

EP-Cs who develop marketing plans that incorporate an appreciation of the customer (people) with an understanding of the product and recognition of the perceptions related to price and value are able to apply myriad promotional strategies to achieve and sustain successful business practices.

Promotion

As the fifth "P" in the marketing mix, promotion is an ever-expanding and complex process of educating, presenting, and engaging stakeholders so that consumer loyalty and sustained relationships

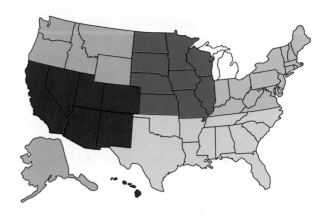

Northwest
PT (FT) - $56,000
PT (PT) - $20.00

GFI (FT) - $77,000
GFI (PT) - $22.00

Northcentral
PT (FT) - $46,000
PT (PT) - $23.00

GFI (FT) - $42,000
GFI (PT) - $28.00

Northeast
PT (FT) - $52,000
PT (PT) - $27.00

GFI (FT) - $56,000
GFI (PT) - $25.00

Southwest
PT (FT) - $60,000
PT (PT) - $28.00

GFI (FT) - $56,000
GFI (PT) - $26.00

Southeast
PT (FT) - $53,000
PT (PT) - $27.00

GFI (FT) - $47,000
GFI (PT) - $25.00

FIGURE 17.2. Average income of personal trainers and group exercise/fitness instructors by geographic region. (Data: https://www .acefitness.org/salary/docs/ACE_SalarySurvey.pdf.)

develop, grow, and are maintained. Following a brief explanation of branding, this section will provide a limited overview of promotional strategies related to the following areas:

1. Advertising
2. Referrals
3. Direct mail/e-mail
4. Internet
5. Business to business (B2B)
6. Sponsorship
7. Personal sales
8. Public relations

Branding

While considering the five Ps, the EP-C can also evaluate strategies for reaching the appropriate target market with a suitable message. Deciding how to package the message helps determine the best marketing strategies to implement. Branding is an important consideration for the EP-C to convey. What is it not what it is about the product or services that makes them special, unique, or different from other products in the same industry? Why should a potential customer want to purchase fitness services or memberships from you or your facility as opposed to someone else? The EP-C working privately has to be able to answer questions about his or her education, experience, and ability in a way that can be successfully branded. If the EP-C is employed in a corporate or clinical setting, what is the mission and vision of the organization? What distinctive qualities does the organization have that enables the fitness services to serve a special niche, fulfill a unique need, or carry a particular association? Once these questions are answered, the EP-C will have a clearer picture of how to brand the product. As an intangible, brand development is often accomplished by focusing on the health and wellness outcomes associated with fitness. Incorporating vicarious achievement and nostalgia have been found to build brand loyalty (8). In addition, the concept of building a "brand community" has been proposed as an effective mechanism to engage stakeholders both physically and virtually (5). A second consideration in marketing is the image being portrayed. Many fitness professionals create a logo, trade character, or image that relates in some way to health, wellness, and exercise. The logo is another tool to create brand awareness that can be used on business cards and other marketing materials. Increasing brand recognition builds brand loyalty within the target market of potential customers. Creating a professional and unique brand enables the EP-C to employ marketing strategies across multiple mediums with a comprehensive design that is easily recognized and identified by stakeholders and potential customers.

Advertising

Advertising can be both a general and a targeted approach to spreading the word about a product. Commonly used advertising mediums in the health and fitness industry include print media such as newspapers, trade magazines, television, radio, and billboard. Social media and directed use of the Internet is fast becoming an effective advertising medium (9). The EP-C may consider using one or more of these resources to advertise, although cost needs to be considered. Each advertising medium has unique pros and cons that will vary depending on the goals of the promotion, available resources, and breadth of the marketing plan (23). In addition, word-of-mouth recommendations have long been considered a highly successful means of promoting products and services, especially in the fitness industry.

Referral

The business of fitness has traditionally been a face-to-face process, although online options are becoming increasingly popular. A rapport built with faithful clientele is deep and long-lasting. Consequently, one of the most effective ways to market services to new clients is to ask for referrals from existing clients. Existing clients are the best sales team because they have experienced the impact of incorporating fitness into their lifestyle and the role a particular EP-C can play in bringing about positive change over a period. When clients do refer a new prospect who then becomes a client, it is important to recognize the referring member with some type of reward. A free personal training session or group exercise goes a long way toward future referrals.

Direct Mail/E-mail

Direct mail is an expensive but effective method of reaching a target market because of the ability to select the specific households to pursue. Traditionally, direct mail efforts produce a return rate between 1% and 3%. E-mail marketing has been found to be effective in reaching specific customers with similar interests (20). The key for creating effective e-mail blasts is to compile a list of potential customers. The EP-C can build an e-mail list through referrals, existing clients, and, if permissible, club e-mail listings. A good e-mail blast can be a powerful message and include images, videos, and coupons that are tailored to a specific type of customer. Typical response rates from e-mail blasts run between 5% and 15%. E-mail marketing has also been found to be an effective strategy for health promotion and behavior change (19). Therefore, carefully crafting the e-mail message is critical to the success of any program or promotion (17). Virtual exchanges provide another opportunity for an EP-C to connect with a client or potential client. Facebook, Twitter, and other social network sites provide outstanding mediums to promote the EP-C's services.

Internet

Integrated marketing strategies that include e-mail communications and a Web site presence have been found to be more effective than print messages alone (14,18). Web site development, however, can be complex or simple. Trade magazines relating to health fitness management and Internet businesses offer excellent advice on the choices and process of launching a health fitness Web site (2). A simple Web site would include basic information about the product, place, price, and promotions. More dynamic Web sites can provide a virtual tour and engage a client at a personal level. Interactive Web opportunities can also be developed using social media tools.

Social media can be an excellent marketing tool when used correctly. Facebook, Twitter, and other Internet sites have proven useful in referral-based businesses such as fitness because potential clients can make contact quickly and ask questions with relative anonymity. Social media sites can provide an opportunity for exchanges about topics that may be uncomfortable to discuss in face-to-face settings (9,10).

Business to Business

Like client referrals, B2B referrals can be a very inexpensive and powerful way to reach a target audience. Taking the extra time to meet business owners in the area can pay huge dividends in terms of reaching new prospects. The key to developing strategic relationships in the community is to seek out businesses and individuals whose client bases overlap. Some ways to connect with other business professionals may be to attend a chamber of commerce event, host an open house, serve on a city or town committee, or volunteer and/or sponsor a local road race or event. Bartering for services is also an excellent way to build relationships with other professionals. B2B associations provide opportunities for collaboration and growth that can increase profitability with minimal use of resources.

Sponsorship

Sponsorship has been found to be an effective means of promoting fitness-related products and growing B2B connections. Many small business owners seek ways to encourage physical activity for employees (22). Sponsorship enables the EP-C to allocate resources toward a specific event and particular target market. Sponsorship also provides an opportunity for the EP-C to practice good citizenship by being actively involved in a local community. Sponsorship builds brand recognition with vendors, participants, and spectators; provides a means of distributing print and media communications; and actively engages current fitness club members in the prospect of participating in a cause-related activity. Research has found that corporations primarily use sponsorship as a means of seeking exclusivity and raising public awareness and a positive image (4). Effective sponsorships include an evaluation on the return on investment that enables the sponsor to negotiate tailored packages that best meet the needs of those involved (28). Table 17.1 provides an illustration of the cost/benefit breakdown of common marketing tools.

Personal Sales

When evaluating the performance of fitness center employees, sales revenues are often included in the employee evaluation process (27). Most academic programs do not provide extensive sales training for students majoring in exercise science or kinesiology. However, fitness-related majors tend to be more physically active and appreciate the relationship of physical activity to greater quality of life (12). Translating that personal experience to the sale of health and fitness is the key to success for the EP-C. Having confidence in the value of the fitness product is important to conveying a genuine attitude. Research cites empathy, ego drive, high energy level, integrity, an

Table 17.1	Cost/Benefit Breakdown of Common Marketing Tools		
Method	**Type**	**Cost**	**Impact**
Advertising	Internet	Low	Moderate/high
	Television	High	High
	Radio	High	Moderate
	Newspaper/magazine	Moderate	Low
Personal contact	Referrals	Free	High
B2B	Chamber of commerce	Low	High
Sponsorship	Event/cause marketing	Moderate	High

ability to learn, positive self-image, and an ability to forge relationships as critical characteristics of successful salespeople (15). To be a maven about a product (1) has also been cited as a significant quality to possess. A maven salesperson is described as someone who has an expertise in a given area or subject, is passionate about the subject, and wants to share that knowledge with others. Confidence in the product coupled with an ability to find and follow leads can lead to a successful career for an EP-C.

FINDING LEADS

In sales, a lead is defined as someone who fits the profile of a target market and has shown an interest in the product or service. The marketing and advertising process is designed almost entirely to help identify leads through e-mail, phone calls, or Web site inquiries. Ideally, leads are individuals who have been exposed to one of the marketing mediums described above and have indicated a desire for more information about the product or service for sale. Each lead is a potential client. For this reason, it is imperative to have a system of managing leads, as each phone call, e-mail, or Web site inquiry that comes in is a potential customer. To be successful, the EP-C will develop an organizational plan to include the lead on a spreadsheet and contact the person as soon as possible. The spreadsheet should include all relevant information about the lead, including home address, e-mail address, phone number, and any other personal details the lead provided when he or she responded to the marketing campaign. The more information gathered about the lead, the more personalized response can be provided. The lead spreadsheet should also include the date of each attempted contact and the eventual status of the lead.

QUALIFYING PROSPECTS

Once a solid lead list is in place, the goal is to turn those leads into prospects. A lead becomes a prospect when he or she has expressed a need for the fitness product or service after an initial contact has been made. Qualifying prospects is a process that involves talking to the prospect and learning as much about the potential client as possible. The key to qualifying the prospect is (a) asking open-ended questions that will allow the EP-C to learn the maximum amount possible about the individual ("What do you see as the next action steps?" "What is your timeline for implementing/purchasing this type of service/product?" "What concerns do you have?"), (b) listening to the potential client's responses and remembering relevant information, and (c) helping the prospect realize that what you offer can meet the needs they have expressed. Essentially, the goal is to become familiar with the individual and learn why they are interested in the services and products being promoted.

THE ART OF THE DEAL

Many EP-Cs will be able to positively impact their own compensation by attracting and closing new clients. Learning and adhering to specific sales guidelines should improve closing percentages and overall success.

Closing the deal is an extension of the "qualifying prospects" strategies. At this stage, the EP-C will have adequate knowledge of the demographic, psychographic, exercise motivations, and activity goals of the potential client. The key to an effective close is to connect the fitness product or service with a need the prospect mentioned during the qualifying process. For example, a prospect may have identified a need to engage a personal trainer because they have little knowledge in the area of strength training. An appropriate closing strategy would be to reiterate this need verbally to the prospect and then highlight how personal training with you will enhance the prospect's strength training knowledge base. Once the prospect confirms that this benefit serves his or her personal need, the sale is likely to occur. Typically, many needs are uncovered during the prospect qualification process. If possible, try to highlight a second benefit that can be met with the fitness services being promoted and ask the prospect to confirm that the benefit exists. Complimenting a potential customer and engaging in active listening have been found to increase sales of add-on features of fitness equipment (6).

After the prospect has acknowledged at least two needs that can be met with the services being promoted, the groundwork is in place to ask for the sale. At this point, it is important to have some options for the prospect to consider. When asking for the sale, highlight two or three options that fit the prospect needs that were previously identified. The final step is to actually ask the question: "Which of these packages would be the best fit for you?" The framing of this question allows for a positive "either/or" response rather than a "yes or no" response. With proper preparation by really trying to understand where the client is coming from (empathy) and engaging in active listening, the sales process is often more an educational opportunity for both the EP-C and the client to learn and understand in greater depth about the challenges and opportunities available for individuals choosing active lifestyles.

Public Relations

Unlike costly advertising, public relations strategies provide an opportunity to promote fitness products and services using minimal financial resources. Although advertising is effective in communicating information about a product or service, public relations gives potential customers an opportunity to consider the product or service at a more emotional level (11). Public relations can be used in several ways from writing a news release to announce a new program or service to writing a weekly column or blog in a local paper or Web site about exercise and physical activity. Both examples provide an opportunity to gain exposure, build brand community, and increase consumer confidence. Although public relations has traditionally been part of a print communication process, online media outlets often utilize expert bloggers to support different content areas. The EP-C is qualified and capable of serving as a valuable resource for disseminating evidence-based information about fitness and exercise. Writing is therefore a prerequisite proficiency for preparing quality promotional materials. Seven suggestions for writing simple and effective news releases are provided (19):

1. Identify and address the target audience.
2. Keep it simple and short (never longer than a page).
3. The basics of who, what, when, where, why, and how belong in the first short paragraph.
4. Use short paragraphs and emphasize one major point in each paragraph.
5. Avoid acronyms and technical jargon.
6. With permission, quote authority.
7. Careful and deliberate.

Careful and deliberate use of public relations can support other promotional efforts by providing positive exposure that may create opportunities for future ventures and collaborations.

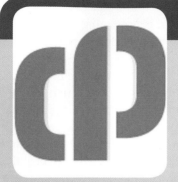

The Case of the Continuum Performance Center

Submitted by **Chris Worrell, ACSM EP-C, NSCA-CSCS, and Geoff Sullivan, ACSM EP-C, NSCA-CPT, Continuum Performance Center, East Longmeadow, MA**

A team of certified professionals reinvented themselves to develop a unique brand identity and create a fitness business that defines success by individual client achievement.

Narrative

The Continuum Performance Center (CPC) was created by industry professionals who worked within the confines of an outdated commercial system and witnessed countless active individuals become turned off by the membership structure of "gyms." CPC centers all of its programming around the active individual or those who truly desire to become recreationally involved in activity and movement on a deeper level.

CPC opened its doors with one employee-owner and has grown to support three full-time and one part-time nationally certified employees who are referred to as "coaches." Within one calendar year, CPC has grown its "subscriber" (title for members) base from 9 unique subscribers to over 160 subscribers who actively train at the facility at least one time every 14 days.

CPC's floor plan is unique in its design. Although constant functional movements are promoted to all subscribers in all training areas at all times, CPC has separate training spaces, totaling 50 square feet. The north end of CPC is dedicated for group programming in a more functional training environment with a large tie into TRX Suspension Training. The south end of CPC offers a more traditional strength environment, but CPC coaches still place a large emphasis on movement.

Branding: Don't Talk About It, Be About It

CPC established itself as the alternative to traditional fitness facilities through its tag line: Don't talk about it. Be about it. By using challenge-oriented Facebook posts, dynamic uploaded video on Vimeo and YouTube, and an information stream from Constant Contact to relay tips, advice, and reminders, CPC has grown 200% within its first year of business. On a daily basis, CPC gets more than 50 hits on Facebook and Twitter and has an 88% open rate on their Constant Contact campaigns. CPC relies solely on social media and e-mail communication with its subscribers to deliver inspiration, motivation, and information. Subscribers have come primarily through word-of-mouth sales and Facebook "shares."

To keep subscribers involved, CPC rotates programming on a consistent basis to keep interest and motivation high. By having subscribers take ownership of the space and the offerings, it allows CPC to grow at a consistent and positive rate.

Collaboration

Through the CPC 1,500 (a muscular endurance challenge involving 1,500 repetitions of five exercises), TRX Training, and partnerships with other like-minded area small business such as Fit to Ride and Heartsong Yoga Center, members are able to connect to others and take on a physical and mental challenge in a safe, supervised, and challenging environment.

CPC is a neighborhood place for regular people trying to incorporate exercise that is fun, challenging, and variable into their busy lives. Subscribers are from every walk of life, but they have one thing in common — they *want* to be healthy and they've made a commitment to be well. CPC's commitment to the community doesn't stop with its subscribers or other businesses. Giving back to the community is essential to the organizations growth and the core to the mission. Partnering with organizations such as The Western Massachusetts Food Bank, Toys for Tots, and the American Red Cross, CPC sets a standard of community involvement that resonates with CPC subscribers.

Using social media has enabled CPC to not only reach a broader base of subscribers but also gain critical feedback about what are the "likes" and "dislikes" of any given demographic. As CPC grows, we hope to continue to be about it and not just talk about it!

QUESTIONS

- How does CPC develop the tangible and intangible aspects of their product?
- How has CPC branded itself?
- How does CPC sell its brand?

SUMMARY

This chapter focused on the marketing mix and strategies the EP-C can use when initiating and developing a marketing plan for health and fitness-related products, services, and programs. An overview of the five Ps of people, place, product, price, and promotion was provided. Examples of how the EP-C could apply strategies to different promotional programs were also presented. Several aspects of the promotions function of marketing were discussed in the context of the experience of the EP-C. In addition to personal selling, B2B promotions, sponsorship, and social media promotions, a brief overview of the benefits and uses of public relations as a marketing tool was provided. As a health fitness professional, the EP-C is uniquely qualified to act both as an advanced personal trainer and as a manager. As the fields relating to health fitness expand, knowledge and skills relating to management, marketing, and business also expand. The EP-C is well positioned to serve in a managerial role, seeking additional training when necessary and building on the competencies and skills inherent in the professional nature of the field.

STUDY QUESTIONS

1. How does advertising differ from public relations? What are the similarities and differences?
2. Explain the five Ps of marketing.
3. What role does the mission and vision of an organization have on the development and implementation of fitness services and products?

REFERENCES

1. Adidam P. Mavenness: a non-explored trait of quality sales-people. *Paradigm.* 2009;13(1):6–7.

2. Alsac B. Maximizing your social media investments. *IDEA Fitness J.* 2010;7(7):42–7.

3. Bates M. *Health Fitness Management: A Comprehensive Resource for Managing and Operating Programs and Facilities.* 2nd ed. Champaign (IL): Human Kinetics; 2008. 381 p.

4. Copeland R, Frisby W, McCarville R. Understanding the sport sponsorship process from a corporate perspective. *J Sport Manag.* 1996;10(1):32–48.

5. Devasagayam P, Buff C. A multidimensional conceptualiza-tion of brand community: an empirical investigation. *Sport Mark Q.* 2008;17(1):20–9.

6. Dunyon J, Gossling V, Willden S, Seiter JS. Compliments and purchasing behavior in telephone sales interactions. *Psychol Rep.* 2010;106(1):27–30.

7. Ferrand A, Robinson L, Valette-Florence P. The intention-to-repurchase paradox: a case of the health and fitness industry. *J Sport Manag.* 2010;24(1):83–105.

8. Filo K, Funk D, Alexandris K. Exploring the role of brand trust in the relationship between brand associations and brand loyalty in sport and fitness. *Int J Sport Manag Mark.* 2008;3(1/2):39–57.

9. Frimming RE, Polsgrove MJ, Bower GG. Evaluation of a health and fitness social media experience. *Am J Health Educ.* 2011;42(4):2–7.

10. Gold J, Lim M, Hocking J, Keogh L, Spelman T, Hellard M. Determining the impact of text messaging for sex-ual health promotion to young people. *Sex Transm Dis.* 2011;38(4):247–52.

11. Hoyle LH. *Event Marketing: How to Successfully Promote Events, Festivals, Conventions and Expositions.* New York (NY): Wiley; 2002. 4 p.

12. Huddleston S, Mertesdorf J, Araki K. Physical activity be-havior and attitudes toward involvement among physical education, health and leisure services pre-professionals. *Coll Stud J.* 2002;36(4):555–73.

13. Kaczynski A, Henderson K. Environmental correlates of physical activity: a review of evidence about parks and rec-reation. *Leisure Sci.* 2007;29(4):315–54.

14. Marshall A, Owen N, Bauman A. Mediated approaches for influencing physical activity: update of the evidence on mass media, print, telephone and website delivery of interventions. *J Sci Med Sport.* 2004;7(1 Suppl):74–80.

15. Mayer D, Greenberg H. What makes a good salesman? *Harv Bus Rev.* 2006;84(7/8):164–71.

16. Mullen S, Whaley D. Age, gender and fitness club mem-bership: factors related to initial involvement and sustained participation. *Int J Sport Exerc Psychol.* 2010;8(1):24–35.

17. Papadimitriou D, Karteroliotis K. The service quality expec-tations in private sport and fitness centers: A reexamination of the factor structure. *Sport Mark Q.* 2000;9(3):157–64.

18. Parrott M, Tennant L, Olejnik S, Poudevigne M. Theory of planned behavior: implications for an email-based physical activity intervention. *Psychol Sport Exerc.* 2008;9(4):511–26.

19. Perry DJ. Writing for the media. *Tech Commun.* 1992;39(4):638–42.

20. Reed J. Examining the impact of an email campaign to promote physical activity and walking in adult women six-weeks and one-year post-intervention. *CHPER—SD J Res.* 2009;4(1):64–9.

21. Roux A, Moore L, Evenson KR, et al. Availability of recre-ational resources and physical activity in adults. *Am J Public Health.* 2007;97(3):493–9.

22. Suminski R, Poston W, Hyder M. Small business policies toward employee and community promotion of physical activity. *J Phys Act Health.* 2006;3(4):405–14.

23. Tharrett SJ, Peterson JA. *Fitness Management.* 2nd ed. Monterey (CA): Healthy Learning; 2008. 579 p.

24. Thompson W. Worldwide survey of fitness trends for 2016: 10th Anniversary edition. *ACSM Health Fitness J.* 2015;19(6):9–18.

25. Wang B, Wu C, Quan W. Changes in consumers behavior at fitness clubs among Chinese urban residents — Dalian as an example. *Asian Soc Sci.* 2008;4(10):106–10.

26. Wang H, Lin H. An investigation into exercisers at fitness clubs in Dalian. *J Phys Educ Issue.* 2000;14(4):22–4.

27. Wen-Yu C, Yuan-Duen L, Tsai-Yuan L. Performance eval-uation criteria for personal trainers: an analytical hierarchy process approach. *Soc Behav Pers Int J.* 2010;38(7):895–905.

28. Zinger J, O'Reilly N. An examination of sports sponsorship from a small business perspective. *Int J Sport Mark Sponsorsh.* 2010;11(4):283–301.

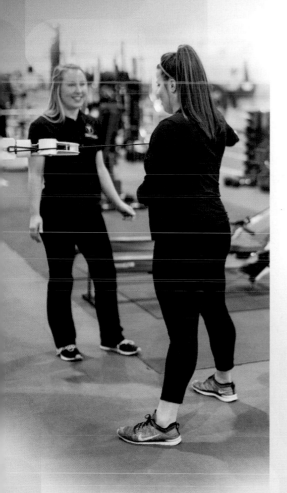

18 Professional Behaviors and Ethics

OBJECTIVES

- To briefly trace the historical development and identify the breadth of Certified American College of Sports Medicine (ACSM) Professionals.

- To identify the settings and skills defined in the scope of practice of the exercise physiologist.

- To distinguish boundaries of professional practice between the exercise physiologist and other allied health professionals.

- To encourage the use of referral tools for clients outside the scope of practice.

- To demonstrate behaviors that meet professional standards.

INTRODUCTION

Ethics, as a branch of philosophy, can be viewed as an abstract concept focusing on morals and values that inform decisions and behaviors. Ethics is also defined in terms of systematic rules or principles governing right conduct. Each practitioner, upon entering a profession, is invested with the responsibility to adhere to the standards of ethical practice and conduct set by the profession (23,25). Professional ethics, as it is presented in this chapter, is immensely practical. An initial examination of the historical context with which American College of Sports Medicine (ACSM) first offered certifications provides an opportunity to consider the development of the profession and the demand for standards of practice. As certified professionals, it is critical to understand the expectations articulated in our code of ethics. To apply the code of ethics to specific challenges facing the certified exercise physiologist (EP-C), the concept of scope of practice is operationalized through several research-based examples. In addition, a useful tool to assist the EP-C in ethical decision making relating to scope of practice is provided. Professional ethics encompasses professional practices relating to honesty with others by identifying conflicts of interest as well as disseminating evidence-based information. Professional ethics also includes personal practices relating to responsibility and accountability by staying current and maintaining a certification as well as demonstrating personal behaviors that exemplify the professional nature of the EP-C. The need for qualified, competent, and engaged fitness professionals is well documented (27). Professional ethics is the foundation for continuing the tradition of excellence initiated and sustained by the founders and fellows of ACSM.

Therefore, this chapter provides a basic overview of professional ethics as applied to the practice of the EP-C. A brief overview of the role ACSM has played in the development of fitness-related certifications is presented, along with a close examination of the ACSM Code of Ethics, with particular focus on the scope of practice for the EP-C. Additional areas related to conflict of interest, developing evidence-based practices, maintaining certification, and defining professional behaviors are examined.

History

Eleven physicians, physiologists, and physical educators founded the American College of Sports Medicine (ACSM) in 1954 to provide a professional society for individuals sharing a common interest in health and fitness. As part of ACSM's efforts to gain new interest, growth, and visibility, the College hosted an "Invitational Conference on Implementation of ACSM's Exercise Testing and Exercise Prescription Guidelines" in Aspen, Colorado, in December 1974. Here, a small group of ACSM members finalized plans for a proposed certification process for Exercise Program Directors and Exercise Leaders. In May 1975, ACSM's Guidelines for Graded Exercise Testing and Exercise Prescription were first published. The following month at Pennsylvania State University,

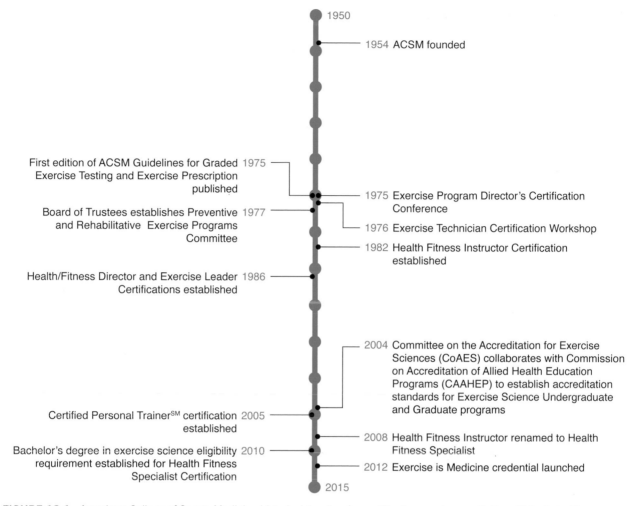

1950

1954 ACSM founded

First edition of ACSM Guidelines for Graded 1975
Exercise Testing and Exercise Prescription
published

1975 Exercise Program Director's Certification
Conference

Board of Trustees establishes Preventive 1977
and Rehabilitative Exercise Programs
Committee

1976 Exercise Technician Certification Workshop

1982 Health Fitness Instructor Certification
established

Health/Fitness Director and Exercise Leader 1986
Certifications established

2004 Committee on the Accreditation for Exercise
Sciences (CoAES) collaborates with Commission
on Accreditation of Allied Health Education
Programs (CAAHEP) to establish accreditation
standards for Exercise Science Undergraduate
and Graduate programs

Certified Personal Trainer(SM) certification 2005
established

2008 Health Fitness Instructor renamed to Health
Fitness Specialist

Bachelor's degree in exercise science eligibility 2010
requirement established for Health Fitness
Specialist Certification

2012 Exercise is Medicine credential launched

2015

FIGURE 18.1. American College of Sports Medicine historical timeline for certifications and accreditation. (Adapted with permission from Berryman JW. *Out of Many, One: A History of the American College of Sports Medicine.* Champaign [IL]: Human Kinetics; 1995. 283 p.)

ACSM held its first Exercise Program Director's Certification Conference, with 35 professionals earning the first-ever ACSM certification. Later, in September of 1975, 20 individuals were certified by ACSM as exercise specialists. The Exercise Test Technician certification began the following year, 1976, with 92 individuals earning certification. ACSM's Health/Fitness Instructor certification (now EP-C) started in 1982, followed by the Health/Fitness Director and Exercise Leader certifications in 1986 (12). In the 20 years since, ACSM certifications have evolved, and as part of this evolution, some certifications are no longer offered, some are new, and some have been dramatically redefined. All of these changes, however, are a tribute to ACSM's commitment to reflect the current state of the fitness and wellness industry. Figure 18.1 provides a basic timeline as it relates to the development of ACSM certifications, particularly the EP-C.

Accreditation

In 2004, ACSM collaborated with six other leading fitness organizations to establish the Committee on the Accreditation for the Exercise Sciences, or CoAES. CoAES is responsible for establishing standards and guidelines for academic programs that prepare students seeking employment in the health, fitness, and exercise industry. In addition, CoAES establishes and implements a process of self-study, review, and recommendation for all exercise science–related academic programs seeking accreditation through the Commission on Accreditation of Allied Health Education Programs (CAAHEP). Today, there are four postsecondary program accreditations through CAAHEP: Associate or Certificate in Personal Fitness Training, Bachelor of Science in Exercise Science, Master of Science in Applied Physiology, and Master of Science in Clinical Exercise Physiology. Accreditation, like certification, is a critical component for ensuring a consistent and standardized set of knowledge and skills, which is essential for industry professionals and is conveyed to students through their academic experience.

The need for certified professionals who are competent and proficient in a subject area and who are evaluated through the successful completion of a psychometrically sound, objective examination has grown exponentially. ACSM currently offers five primary certifications and four specialty certifications, with more than 30,000 ACSM-certified professionals practicing worldwide. The clinical certifications (Table 18.1) (5) include the Registered Clinical Exercise Physiologist® (RCEP) and the Certified Clinical Exercise Physiologist® (CEP). The fitness certifications (see Table 18.1) include the Certified Exercise Physiologist[SM] (EP-C), the Certified Personal Trainer[SM] (CPT), and the Group Exercise Instructor[SM] (GEI). In addition, ACSM offers four specialty certifications that focus on serving individuals with unique needs: ACSM/ACS Certified Cancer Exercise Trainer[SM] (CET), ACSM/NCPAD Certified Inclusive Fitness Trainer[SM] (CIFT), ACSM/NSPAPPH Physical Activity in Public Health Specialist[SM] (PAPHS), and ACSM/ARP Certified Ringside Physician® (CRP).

What was for many years known as the Health/Fitness Instructor certification was renamed the Health Fitness Specialist, or HFS, in 2008. The eligibility requirements of the HFS were changed in 2010 to limit the certification to those holding a Bachelor of Science degree in Kinesiology, Exercise Physiology, or Exercise Science. In 2015, the name was changed again to Certified Exercise Physiologist or EP-C. The change in the education prerequisite evolved to better support the job tasks associated with this profession. The changes in the name of the certification resulted from a commitment on the part of ACSM to adopt a uniform professional title for degreed exercise professionals that aligns with positive perceptions and name recognition by both internal and external constituencies (4). Attainment of the ACSM EP-C certification implies specialized training and competencies for degreed individuals to pursue careers in university, corporate, commercial, hospital, and community settings, serving healthy individuals and individuals with controlled conditions released for independent physical activity. The Exercise is Medicine (EIM) credential provides further support for the unique characteristics of the ACSM EP-C.

The EIM credential was developed and launched in 2012 to support the EIM initiative and provide health care providers with an identifiable exercise professional qualified to work with different clients (17). A description of the three-tiered EIM credential is presented in Exercise is Medicine Connection.

Committee on the Certification and Registry Board

The Committee on the Certification and Registry Board (CCRB), a volunteer committee comprised of ACSM members, oversees the process of regularly reviewing and revising the job definition, eligibility requirements, and scope of practice for each certification. In addition, each certification undergoes a rigorous external review through the National Commission for Certifying Agencies (NCCA). The NCCA is a nonprofit, external certifying agency whose mission is to safeguard public safety and well-being through the assessment and evaluation of professional competencies and standards. The NCCA provides accreditation to a broad range of professions, including nursing, respiratory therapy, and counseling. The guiding principle of advancing health through science, education, and medicine that inspired the early community of ACSM members is kept alive today by the ACSM-certified professionals who adhere to the ACSM's Code of Ethics through the personal and professional responsibility they practice.

EXERCISE IS MEDICINE CONNECTION

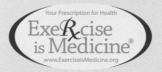

The EIM credential contains three levels based on the health status of the patient referrals. All three levels require exercise professionals to be certified by an NCCA accrediting organization. Those with formal education in exercise science (BS or MS degree) are able to qualify for the higher levels of certification.

Level 1: Individuals at Low or Moderate Risk

NCCA-accredited fitness professional certification

Successful completion of the EIM credential course and EIM credential examination

EIM course and examination exempt for NCCA-accredited fitness certification and approved BS/BA in Exercise Science/Exercise Physiology/Kinesiology

Level 2: Individuals at Low, Moderate, or High Risk Who Have Been Cleared for Independent Exercise

Approved BS/BA in Exercise Science/Exercise Physiology/Kinesiology

NCCA-accredited fitness professional certification

Successful completion of the EIM credential training course and EIM credential examination

EIM course and examination exempt for certifications with an emphasis on special populations (ACSM EP-C, ACSM CEP, ACSM RCEP, ACE Advanced Heath Fitness Specialist)

Level 3: Individuals at Low, Moderate, or High Risk, Requiring Clinical Monitoring

Approved MS/MA Exercise Science/Exercise Physiology/Kinesiology *or* approved BS/BA in Exercise Science/Exercise Physiology/Kinesiology plus 4,000 hours of experience in a clinical exercise setting

NCCA-accredited clinical exercise certification

EIM credential course and EIM credential examination exempt for those with ACSM CEP or ACSM RCEP

Organizations with NCCA-Accredited Health Fitness and/or Clinical Exercise Certifications

- Academy of Applied Personal Training (AAPTE)
- ACTION certification (ACTION)
- American College of Sports Medicine (ACSM)
- American Council on Exercise (ACE)
- National Academy of Sports Medicine (NASM)
- National Council for Certified Personal Trainers (NCCPT)
- National Council on Strength and Fitness (NCSF)
- National Exercise and Sports Trainers Association (NESTA)
- National Exercise Trainers Association (NETA)
- National Federation of Professional Trainers (NFPT)
- National Strength and Conditioning Association (NSCA)
- The Cooper Institute (CI)

Table 18.1	Current Levels of ACSM Certifications
Registered Clinical Exercise Physiologist® (RCEP)	Health care professional with a master's degree in exercise science, exercise physiology, or kinesiology who utilizes scientific rationale to design, implement, and supervise exercise programming for those with chronic diseases, conditions and/or physical shortcomings. Services provided by an RCEP include, but are not limited to, individuals with cardiovascular, pulmonary, metabolic, orthopedic, musculoskeletal, neuromuscular, neoplastic, immunologic, and hematologic disease.
Certified Clinical Exercise Physiologist® (CEP)	Health care professional with a bachelor's degree in exercise science, exercise physiology, or kinesiology who conducts preparticipation health screening, maximal and submaximal graded exercise tests, and performs strength, flexibility and body composition tests for patients and clients challenged with cardiovascular, pulmonary, and metabolic diseases and disorders, as well as with apparently healthy populations.
Certified Exercise Physiologist^SM (EP-C)	Health and fitness professional with a bachelor's degree in exercise science who performs preparticipation health screenings, conducts physical fitness assessments, interprets results, develops exercise prescriptions, and applies behavioral and motivational strategies to apparently healthy individuals and individuals with medically controlled diseases and health conditions.
Certified Personal Trainer^SM (CPT)	Fitness professional with a high school diploma who plans and implements exercise programs for healthy individuals or those who have medical clearance to exercise. The CPT facilitates motivation and adherence as well as develops and administers programs designed to enhance muscular strength, endurance, flexibility, cardiorespiratory fitness, body composition, and/or any of the motor skills related components of physical fitness.
Certified Group Exercise Instructor^SM (GEI)	Fitness professional with a high school diploma who works in a group exercise setting with apparently healthy individuals and those with health challenges, who have been cleared by their physicians for independent exercise to enhance quality of life, improve physical fitness, manage health risk, and promote lasting health behavior change

 ## ACSM Code of Ethics

The ACSM Code of Ethics states, "The principal purpose of the College is the generation and dissemination of knowledge concerning all aspects of persons engaged in exercise with full respect for the dignity of people" (3). The Code is further defined by four standards:

Section 1: Members should strive continuously to improve knowledge and skill and should make available to their colleagues and the public the benefits of their professional expertise.
Section 2: Members should maintain high professional and scientific standards and should not voluntarily collaborate professionally with anyone who violates this principle.
Section 3: The College, and its members, should safeguard the public and itself against members who are deficient in ethical conduct.
Section 4: The ideals of the College imply that the responsibilities of each fellow or member extend not only to the individual but also to society with the purpose of improving both the health and the well-being of the individual and the community (3).

Although each standard implies many personal and public practices that define the professional nature of an EP-C, the following five areas are of great importance:

1. Practicing within one's scope of practice
2. Acknowledging conflicts of interest
3. Providing evidence-based information
4. Maintaining certification
5. Personal characteristics of professional behavior

 ## Scope of Practice

Scope of practice is the range of responsibility that determines the boundaries within which a profession operates (26). Each phrase in a scope of practice is critical in defining what tasks a professional can do, with whom the professional can work, what settings are appropriate, and what type of oversight is necessary. This textbook is devoted to the knowledge and skills that are needed to practice as an EP-C. As such, the text operationalizes the EP-C scope of practice. In other words, if a given practitioner in the field adheres to the job tasks and skills described in this text, then he or she is operating within the boundaries of the defined field of the EP-C, a requirement for practicing ethically sound behavior. The fundamentals of the scope of practice of the EP-C are outlined in the following description developed by the CCRB.

The ACSM EP-C is a health fitness professional with a minimum of a bachelor's degree in exercise science. The EP-C performs preparticipation health screenings, conducts physical fitness assessments, interprets results, develops exercise prescriptions, and applies behavioral and motivational strategies to apparently healthy individuals and individuals with medically controlled diseases and health conditions to support clients in adopting and maintaining healthy lifestyle behaviors. The academic preparation of the EP-C also includes fitness management, administration, and supervision. The EP-C is typically employed or self-employed in commercial, community, military, studio, corporate, university, and hospital settings (2).

The scope of practice is a living document that is regularly reviewed by ACSM's EP-C subcommittee. Each of the ACSM certifications has a subcommittee that operates as part of the CCRB. The components of the scope of practice are verified in a systematic manner through a job task analysis (JTA) of practicing EP-Cs (1). The JTA is a survey sent to EP-C practitioners to gather information about what tasks they are doing in their daily work. On the basis of the survey data, EP-C subcommittee members review the scope of practice, the knowledge and skill statements (KSs), and the content of publications related to EP-C work (such as this textbook) to make sure all are in line with the evolution of the profession.

Defining the scope of what an EP-C does (*e.g.*, risk classification, fitness assessment, exercise prescription, and lifestyle behavior change), the scope of practice also serves as a guide as to what may lie *outside* the boundary of the EP-C's scope. Figure 18.2 and Table 18.2 show that although there may be overlap between scopes of practice of various professionals working with similar clientele as the EP-C, there are distinct areas within which each profession functions. The trick is figuring out where the EP-C practice ends and the practice of another professional begins. The purpose of this section is to provide some examples and guidelines so that EP-C practitioners can make sound decisions to operate within their defined scope of practice. First, a decision tree will be introduced. Practitioners can use the decision tree to check that the tasks they are performing are firmly within the EP-C scope of practice. Then, three scenarios will be presented to delineate the boundaries between some of the professions depicted in Figure 18.2 and Table 18.2.

Consider the following scenarios to better understand the complex and delicate issues that arise when faced with scope of practice decisions.

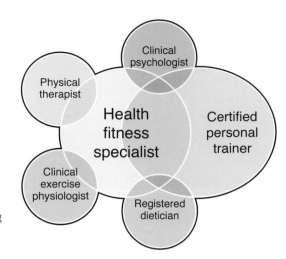

FIGURE 18.2. A visual representation of the overlapping scopes of varying health care, allied health, and health fitness professionals.

Scenario 1

A client asks about recommending a piece of aerobic exercise equipment for his home. The client is a healthy 40-year-old man with hypertension controlled by diet and exercise.

If a practitioner is unsure whether the request in scenario 1 is permitted in his or her scope of practice, then the first place to look might be the most recent EP-C JTA. In the 2011 JTA, under Domain II Exercise Prescription and Implementation, Job Task C states, "Implement cardiorespiratory exercise prescriptions using the FITT framework (frequency, intensity, time and type) for apparently healthy participants based on current health status, fitness goals, and availability of time" (2).

Table 18.2	Areas of Overlapping Scope of Practice between the Certified Exercise Physiologist and Other Professions
Overlap: Certified Exercise Physiologist and	
Personal trainer	Health screening, exercise assessment, and exercise prescription for apparently healthy individuals and for those with health challenges who are capable of independent exercise
Dietician	Promotion of healthy eating, hydration, and energy consumption to optimize; physical performance, recovery from and adaptation to exercise training and competition, and weight management
Clinical, health, and/or counseling psychologist	Promotion of healthy living through behavior change, motivational interviewing, and cognitive restructuring strategies
Clinical exercise physiologist	Adjusting and adapting exercise training for special populations, including those living with chronic diseases and conditions
Physical therapist	Adjusting and adapting exercise training for special populations, including those living with chronic musculoskeletal and neuromuscular conditions

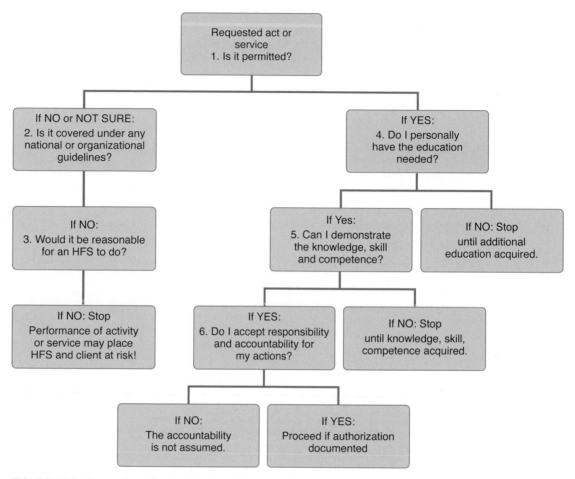

FIGURE 18.3. Scope of practice decision tree. (Adapted with permission from O'Sullivan-Maillet J, Skates J, Pritchett E. American Dietetic Association: scope of dietetics practice framework. *J Am Diet Assoc.* 2005;105[4]:634–40.)

Figure 18.3 shows a decision tree designed to help the EP-C assess whether he or she is practicing within the boundaries of the EP-C scope of practice (29). Because the client has asked for recommendations on a *type* of exercise equipment, this task is clearly permitted. If the client asked about a specific type of equipment that the practitioner was unfamiliar with, then the EP-C must progress further down the decision tree. The EP-C knows the task is permitted but must ask himself or herself question 4 on the decision tree: "Do I personally have the education needed?" If the practitioner is not knowledgeable about that piece of equipment, then he or she needs to gather enough information to advise the client *or* refer the client to someone else with specific knowledge about that particular piece of equipment.

Nutritional counseling is an area with potential overlap for the EP-C, as it is not unusual for clients to request dietary advice (28). The EP-C does have training in basic nutrition, so it seems reasonable that an EP-C should be able to work with clients' diets to some extent. In fact, there are 30 KSs in the most recent JTA related to nutrition and weight management. Most of them are KSs under the job task IIF, "Implement a weight management program as indicated by personal goals that are supported by pre-activity screening, health history, and body composition/anthropometrics" (2). The EP-C should have knowledge of basic nutritional principles related to weight management, should be able to make referrals to scientifically based resources, and should be familiar with ergogenic aids and supplements and their risks and benefits. However, there is no KS indicating that an EP-C should be involved in individual nutritional counseling or therapeutic nutritional advice. Table 18.3 provides clear guidance on what nutritional information is acceptable for an EP-C to share with clients.

Table 18.3	The Practice of Dietetics versus General Nonmedical Nutritional Information
Activity	**Definitions**
Practice of dietetics; limited to licensees[a]	■ Nutritional assessment to determine nutritional needs and to recommend appropriate nutritional intake, including enteral and parenteral nutrition ■ Nutritional counseling or education as components of preventive, curative, and restorative health care ■ Development, administration, evaluation, and consultation regarding nutritional care standards
General nonmedical nutrition information not restricted[b]	Providing information on the following: ■ Principles of good nutrition and food preparation ■ Food to be included in the normal daily diet ■ The essential nutrients needed by the body ■ Recommended amounts of the essential nutrients ■ The actions of nutrients on the body ■ The effects of deficiencies or excesses of nutrients, or food and supplements that are good sources of essential nutrients

[a]Dietetics. Ohio Rev, Code Ann x 4759-2-01(A), 2006.

[b]Dietetics. Ohio Rev, Code Ann x 4759-2-01(M), 2006.

Adapted with permission from Sass C, Eickhoff-Shemek JM, Manore MM, Kruskall LJ. Crossing the line: understanding the scope of practice between registered dieticians and health fitness professionals. *ACSM's Health Fitness J.* 2007; 11(3):12–9.

Scenario 2

The lawsuit *Capati v. Crunch Fitness* provides an instructive example of crossing this line. In 1997, a personal trainer at Crunch Fitness in New York City recommended dietary supplements to Anne Marie Capati. Capati had high blood pressure, and one of the supplements contained Ephedra, contraindicated for those with hypertension. Capati suffered a massive stroke that took her life, hours after a workout at the gym (30,33). This is an extreme example of what can occur when stepping outside the boundary of scope of practice. Even if the consequences are not life-threatening, exceeding one's scope of practice reflects poorly on one's professional practice and calls to question his or her ethics.

If the personal trainer working with Anne Marie Capati had applied the decision tree to his actions, would this tragedy have been avoided? That is difficult to know, however, following the decision tree provides timely and prudent guidance whenever the task at hand is in question. Question 1 asks, Is it permitted, in this example, to recommend a particular supplement for a client who is trying to lose weight? An EP-C would refer to the most current EP-C JTA, whereas the personal trainer working with Capati would refer to the current CPT JTA. In either case, the practitioner would have to answer no to question 2a; the service of recommending specific supplements is not covered under the guidelines for CPTs or EP-Cs. If the practitioner was still unsure, then he could consult the code of ethics for ACSM certified professionals and the licensure laws related to the practice of dietetics in his state. If the answer was still no, then question 3a asks whether it would be reasonable for the practitioner to perform this service. In this case, he might look to position stands, place a call or e-mail to the appropriate certification subcommittee chair, and ask whether the service is routinely performed by other practitioners. In the Capati case, the personal trainer would have found no supporting documentation or practice to support a recommendation of a nutritional supplement to a client.

Looking at this case from a different angle, how might this personal trainer have better handled the query about weight loss supplements? He could have shared evidence-based information about the supplement, including papers that had been published. He could have referred Capati to a registered dietitian, especially because one of the job tasks for the EP-C is to maintain relationships with other health professionals and to have skill in referral to those professionals.

Scenario 3

Another area that has the potential to be unclear is the differences in scopes of practice between the EP-C and the RCEP or CEP.

A 58-year-old woman who is newly diagnosed with heart disease signs up to work with an EP-C at a local fitness facility. She had two stents inserted 6 weeks ago, and her doctor told her to exercise. She has Type 2 diabetes and is taking an oral hypoglycemic drug. The client is obese (body mass index [BMI] $= 35 \text{ kg} \cdot \text{m}^{-2}$) with stage 1 Parkinson disease (PD) and is also taking medication for PD. The EP-C working with her is conscientious, so she has already asked the client to get a referral from a medical doctor (MD), which she has supplied. The referral states, "OK to exercise." The EP-C is unsure as to whether the client should be supervised during exercise and whether she should be scrutinized more closely by a clinical exercise professional. This puts the EP-C at question 2a in the decision tree: Is it covered under any national or organizational guidelines? The EP-C scope of practice defines the population that EP-Cs can work with as "apparently healthy and with controlled conditions released for independent exercise." This client is not apparently healthy as she has a metabolic disease, a cardiovascular disease, and a neuromuscular disease. Are all her diseases in a controlled condition? If the EP-C was unsure, then he or she must conservatively answer no to question 2a and ask herself question 3a: Would it be reasonable for an EP-C to work with a patient who has postsurgical heart disease, with two comorbidities? Even with the MD referral, it would probably be wiser for this client to begin in a cardiac rehab program or other clinically supervised program and then eventually graduate to the services of the EP-C. In a best practice scenario, the EP-C would contact the referring MD and suggest this alternative.

In most day-to-day situations, the tasks of the EP-C will fall squarely within the defined framework for an EP-C. Practicing EP-Cs will not go astray if they are conscientious about using all available professional resources to guide them in scope of practice issues.

Conflict of Interest

Acknowledgment and awareness of potential conflicts of interest are coupled with acting within one's scope of practice as hallmarks of professional ethics. The ACSM Ethics and Professional Conduct Committee has defined conflict of interest as "a significant financial interest in a business or other direct or indirect personal gain or consideration provided by a business that may compromise, or have the appearance of compromising, an ACSM member's professional judgment" (6). Conflict of interest has also been defined in terms of a situation in which financial or other personal considerations have the potential to compromise or bias professional judgment and objectivity (32). An example may be an EP-C who purchases equipment or services from a friend who in return provides a kickback or "refund." The EP-C has not provided fair access for other equipment vendors to bid or offer quotes. In the same way, conflict of interest is apparent in the fitness specialist who will only sell a particular type of nutritional product or clothing without acknowledging the commission base of the sale.

Collaborative models of rehabilitation treatment and fitness training have become more common modes of delivering services to clients. If a company has two divisions in which one provides a referral to the other division for services, this is generally not considered a conflict of interest unless personal gain (commissions) are provided to individual service providers without full disclosure to the customers they serve. In general, the concept of conflict of interest underscores the need to maintain social trust by clearly acknowledging any relationship that may provide personal gain to the professionals involved (13). Disclosure of significant relationships builds client trust and ensures that the professional standards developed to maintain the integrity of the profession are upheld. How information is obtained, discerned, and disseminated is another important aspect of professional ethics.

 ## Providing Evidence-Based Information

The National Academy of Sciences identified evidence-based practice as a critical competency of all heath care practitioners (16,20). Evidence-based practice has been defined in terms of a provision of health care that incorporates the most current and valid research results (19,24). Providing evidence-based information is a critical characteristic for the EP-C to cultivate and develop. Evidence-based information empowers both the client and the EP-C to ask important questions and seek fundamental answers. As a health/fitness professional working with individuals and groups with medically controlled disease, the responsibility to be fully immersed in evidence-based practices is of paramount importance. There are multiple sources of information regarding the explanation and applications of evidence-based practice among allied health and health care providers. Two models of incorporating evidence-based practices among students and young practitioners will be presented.

Amonette, English, and Ottenbacher (8) presented a practical and systematic approach to incorporating evidence-based investigations into the regular practice of the EP-C. The four-step process can be used to disseminate scientifically sound information to clients without reliance on anecdotal myths and falsehoods that are so prevalent in fitness and nutrition.

Step 1: Develop a Question

The EP-C or the client can inspire questions. Client-driven questions provide important information to the EP-C about the level of understanding the client has about his or her physical, emotional, and psychological well-being. Client questions also require that the EP-C engage in active listening.

Step 2: Search for Evidence

Evidence can be found in three ways: personal experience, academic preparation, and research knowledge.

Personal Experience

Although personal experience can provide powerful evidence, it is often anecdotal. An EP-C may have experience with one client that may not be applicable to another client.

Academic Preparation

Supporting personal and professional experience with academic preparation and research knowledge is helpful in the search for evidence. Every EP-C is required to hold a bachelor's degree in exercise science or kinesiology. The discipline and knowledge gained through the process of obtaining that degree provide the EP-C with the tools to seek evidence from appropriate academic sources. However, academic preparation may not always provide the most recent information.

Research Knowledge

Research knowledge is the form of evidence that holds the least amount of bias. With the accessibility of the Internet, peer-reviewed journals can provide ample sources of evidence-based practices that can address a client question. When searching for information, the professional needs to be able to distinguish between quantitative and qualitative research in addition to other types of research studies, for example, a clinical case study or a meta-analysis. In addition, research disseminated at regional and national conferences is cutting-edge and relevant.

Step 3: Evaluate the Evidence

The magnitude of information available makes it difficult to discern appropriate information from inappropriate information. The EP-C needs to be able to discriminate the evidence gathered and make thoughtful decisions about the best way to disseminate information to the client.

Step 4: Incorporate Evidence into Practice

The EP-C can build on his or her knowledge of the scientific foundations of exercise to use the evidence that best answers the original question. Tailoring the information to the client's needs has also been found to be an effective strategy for long-term behavior change (18). A graphic representation of how the four-step process is applied to an exercise prescription is presented in Figure 18.4.

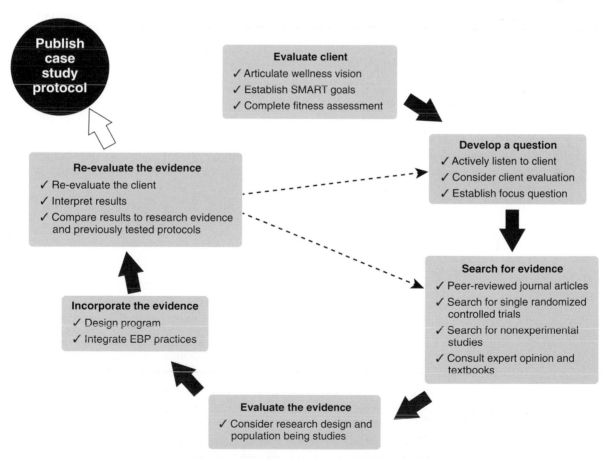

FIGURE 18.4. An example of the application of the evidence-based practice model applied to an individualized exercise prescription. Dashed lines represent alternative or additional steps that may arise. (Used with permission from Amonette W, English K, Ottenbacher K. Nullius in verba: a call for the incorporation of evidence-based practice into the discipline of exercise science. *Sport Med.* 2010;40[6]:449–57.)

A real-life example of the application of the four-step process of evidence-based learning may be found in the "How to Incorporate Evidence-Based Practice" box. Scott, Altenburger, and Kean (34) also provided an example of an effective application of evidence-based clinical decision-making (EBCD) that has been utilized with physical and occupational therapy students and practitioners. The ability to not only know and understand but also actually apply evidence-based learning principles in a relevant context is supported by researchers in a broad range of disciplines from nursing (14) to education (9). Knowing and understanding the process is not enough. Practicing the skill of integrating EBCD in the context of real clients is necessary. The process, which was divided into three phases, is another application of the process outlined earlier by Amonette, English, and Ottenbacher with a similar development and progression.

In Phase 1, the students were introduced to the different types of evidence available and given instruction on how to search for evidence and redesign questions using the PICO format (14): P = population; I = intervention; C = comparison; O = outcome. The therapists generated questions that pertained to real-life problems or practices in their clinics. The student teams selected one question to explore further and seek evidence-based solutions. In phase 2, the students collected evidence and then met with the therapists at the clinic to evaluate the evidence in the context of the question. In phase 3, the students learned about communicating the evidence to the different stakeholders as well as again meeting with the therapists to discuss their findings and get feedback on communication strategies (34).

Although the Scott, Altenburg, and Kean (34) article cited a collaborative arrangement from physical and occupational therapy settings, the application to the EP-C could be made as well. The EP-C who is working as part of a team of trainers can develop and pose questions to one other on the basis of the issues raised by current or past clients. Many fitness facilities also serve as internship sites for students seeking additional practical experience. The EBCD process can be incorporated into the internship experience through case studies, mentoring, and small group discussions. An example of a real-life application of evidence-based learning in a fitness center setting can be found in the case study at the end of this chapter.

Providing evidence-based information enables the EP-C to continue to stay abreast of relevant and important information that impacts the health and well-being of clients. Maintaining the EP-C certification is another mechanism to stay current and involved with the growing fields of fitness and exercise.

 ## Maintaining Certification

A profession is often described as a calling or vocation requiring specialized knowledge, methods, and skills, as well as preparation, in an institution of higher learning, in the scholarly, scientific, and historical principles underlying such methods and skills (22). A profession continuously enlarges its body of knowledge, functions autonomously in formulation of policy, and maintains by force of organization or concerted opinion high standards of achievement and conduct. Members of a profession are committed to continuing education, place service above personal gain, and are committed to providing practical services vital to human and social welfare (29). The purpose of ACSM recertification is to ensure that ACSM certified professionals enhance skills and knowledge above and beyond minimum competence. Periodic recertification occurs through the documentation of required continuing educational activities within the 3-year period following successful passing of an ACSM certification exam.

On the basis of the results from the JTA, along with a comprehensive review of recertification policies and procedures of similar credentials from other organizations, the CCRB determined

HOW TO	**Incorporate Evidence-Based Practice**

You have a new client, a young woman who is apparently healthy and whose primary form of exercise is hot yoga four times a week. She tells you that she heard an interview on the evening news debating whether yoga is an adequate means of gaining aerobic health. She is perplexed because her yoga instructor has assured her that her yoga classes are all she needs for complete fitness (aerobic conditioning, flexibility, and whole body strengthening). Using evidence-based practice, you would follow the following steps.

Formulate a Question

Is yoga an effective means of improving cardiorespiratory endurance in young healthy populations?

Search for Evidence

You are able to find a video of the interview online, so you understand the source of the interview and the statements made.

Personal Experience

You have lots of experience with yoga, although you are not a certified yoga instructor. In some yoga classes, you have experienced physical exertion that seems strong enough to elevate your heart rate. The next time you take a yoga class, you take your heart rate twice during the class.

Academic Knowledge

Because you have a degree in exercise science, you know the FITT Guidelines for minimum physical activity levels required for cardiorespiratory adaptation. You know the physiology of the heart, vessels, and respiratory system and understand the dynamics of how exercise at a defined heart rate maximum can produce cellular changes that manifest to improve aerobic capacity.

Research Knowledge

A search for research related to yoga and cardiorespiratory endurance will reveal the current status of the literature. You carefully assess the quality of the studies you find to formulate your conclusions. Are the studies published in peer-reviewed journals? Are there randomized controlled trials generating consistent data across populations?

Evaluate the Evidence

Even if you are able to get your heart rate in range during your yoga classes, this is not strong enough evidence with which to advise your client. Only by looking further into the current research can you reach a conclusion that has clear evidence behind it. The evidence you find may clearly support the claim in the book or it may refute it. Whatever the outcome, your competence as a health fitness professional and your high ethical standards depend on your ability to educate yourself on the basis of the best evidence available at the time.

Incorporate Evidence into Practice

With an understanding of the strengths and the limitations of the current research related to your question, you can answer your client's question with integrity, and create an exercise program for her that is backed by science.

that a 3-year duration was an appropriate window for a certified professional's recertification (7). EP-C recertification requirements include the following:

1. Accumulate 60 continuing education credits (CECs).
2. Maintain current cardiorespiratory resuscitation (CPR) certification.
3. Pay the required recertification fee.
4. Have the option to repeat the certification exam (current exam prices apply).

Ways to Earn Continuing Education Credits

There are many ways to earn CECs. Continuing education enables the EP-C to build on his or her field experiences and engage in additional networking and scientifically based opportunities that focus and build a professional practice. Table 18.4 provides an overview of ways to earn CECs.

The professional responsibilities of practicing within an appropriate scope of practice, utilizing evidence-based practices, maintaining certification, and adhering to a standard relating to conflict of interest all represent professional ethical behaviors that are informed and nurtured by personal characteristics reflective of a true professional.

Personal Characteristics

Cultivating and developing professional practices that reflect the nature of the EP-C certification are critical to growing respect for and continued growth of the health fitness field. Employers in fields aligned with exercise science have articulated specific personal characteristics desirable in potential employees.

Melton, Dail, Katula, and Mustian (27) interviewed fitness managers from both profit and nonprofit fitness facilities. The managers identified several positive characteristics of personal trainers seeking employment. Trainers who were comfortable interacting and who communicated effectively with a variety of individuals, who had a teachable attitude and aptitude, who were fit or provide evidence of engaging in fit behaviors, and who had the discipline and competence to obtain a relevant degree were seen as valuable employees. Likewise, the fitness managers described personal trainers who were arrogant and overconfident or who acted outside their scope of practice specifically around nutritional advice as a liability for the facility. The managers cited the consequences of such negative behaviors in terms of legal liability as well as loss of members, reputation, and revenue (27).

In comparison, the professional characteristics of athletic trainers have also been examined (21). Some of the defining features of quality athletic trainers include being personable, self-confident, mature, assertive, and enthusiastic (21). Likewise, among recreational staff personnel, characteristics such as patience, fun, creative, passionate, and people-oriented define successful professional behaviors (15). Honest, intelligent, and responsible were the top-rated attributes among nurses (31), as were a positive attitude and overall job satisfaction (35). Health care professionals are further described in terms of respectful, reflective, and socially responsible (11,16). In a white paper focusing on the professional characteristics of pharmacy students, behaviors relating to being accountable, being open to new ideas, and being willing to learn were cited as important to individual success (10). Perhaps one of the most cited characteristics of the helping professions is patience, especially in the role of educator and teacher (36). The EP-C as a helping health care professional can gain insight into the favorable characteristics cited by professionals from related fields.

The acronym WISE (Wisdom, Integrity, Stewardship, and Enthusiasm) provides a helpful summary of personal characteristics and behaviors important to the success of an EP-C.

Wisdom represents the individual seeking answers to sound questions with scientifically based evidence. Integrity signifies the individual respectful of appropriate boundaries while assisting clients in the achievement of holistic and meaningful change. Stewardship represents the individual who values the historical progression of the exercise science professions and acts thoughtfully and professionally as a steward of the future. Enthusiasm denotes the individual whose contagious positive attitude inspires others.

Table 18.4	Ways to Earn Continuing Education Credits	
Obtain a specialty certification.	ACSM/ACS Certified Cancer Exercise Trainer^{SM} (CET)	10 CECs
	ACSM/NCPAD Certified Inclusive Fitness Trainer^{SM} (CIFT)	10 CECs
	ACSM/NSPAPPH Physical Activity in Public Health Specialist^{SM} (PAPHS)	10 CECs
Attend an ACSM Certification workshop.	ACSM Certified Personal Trainer^{SM} 3-Day Workshop	20.75 CECs
	ACSM Certified Personal Trainer^{SM} 1-Day Workshop	7.5 CECs
	ACSM Certified Exercise Physiologist^{SM} Workshop	16.0 CECs
	ACSM Certified Clinical Exercise Specialist Workshop	13.25 CECs
	ACSM Registered Clinical Exercise Physiologist® Workshop	15.0 CECs
Participate in an ACSM or approved provider workshop.[a]	Weight Management for the Fitness Professional (1-d course)	7 CECs
	Behavior Change Strategies for Optimal Client Outcomes (1-d course)	7 CECs
	Business Management for the Fitness Professional (1-d course)	7 CECs
Complete webinars, distance education, other Internet-based continuing education programs on specific clinical or health and fitness related topics.		Varies
Attend professional education meetings from ACSM or other nationally recognized organizations.		Varies
Take continuing education self-tests that offer CECs, CMEs, or CEUs from ACSM or other nationally recognized organizations.	*ACSM's Certified News*, ACSM's quarterly newsletter	4 CECs per issue
	ACSM's Health and Fitness Journal	24 CECs per year
Take and receive a passing grade in a health/fitness or exercise science–related course from an accredited college or university.		10 CECs per credit h[b]
Author or coauthor books, peer-reviewed journal articles, or accepted abstracts.		10 CECs
Teach academic courses; conduct classroom instruction; or present health, fitness, or clinical lectures at an organized professional conference		Varies

[a]A list of approved providers is available at www.acsm.org.

[b]For example, a three-credit-hour course is worth 30 CECs. Course must be health/fitness or clinically related and completed with a grade of "C" or better.

Adapted from American College of Sports Medicine. Renewing your certification [Internet]. Indianapolis (IN): American College of Sports Medicine; [cited 2017 Feb 7]. Available from: http://certification.acsm.org/renew-your-certification

The Case of Marissa, an Undergraduate Intern

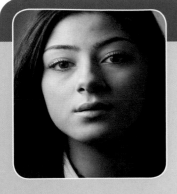

Submitted by **Len Haggerty, Strides Human Performance Institute, Northampton, MA, and Melissa Roti, Westfield State University, Westfield, MA**

Students are often overwhelmed when challenged to complete internships and apply scientific knowledge to real-life situations (2). This case provides an example of how utilizing the EBCD method enables a young student to be guided and instructed in a supportive and safe environment.

Narrative

Len Haggerty, owner of Strides Human Performance Institute, believes that education is a key component of both the undergraduate and the professional experience. Strides Human Performance Institute is a fitness and performance facility that offers adult one-on-one sessions and a wide variety of youth classes. The certified trainers focus on functional, sport-specific movements and high-energy workouts for energy system development. Len offers a highly competitive internship program for qualified young professionals. Part of the internship process is developing and applying evidence-based decision making within the context of the facility.

Marissa Bonito, a Westfield State University senior, is a student-athlete majoring in exercise science and completing her 280-hour internship at Strides. Marissa is an avid runner and is able to focus her evidence-based assignment on an area that is interesting to her. Len provides the structure through an assignment that includes the development of an educational event or program aimed at increasing the understanding of clients on a topic of the intern's choice. Evidence-based decision making provides a framework from which to make appropriate choices for future programming (3,6).

Phase 1: Generating the Questions

Initially, both Len and Marissa generate relevant questions related to running. From that list, Marissa is able to refine the list and apply the PICO format to redesigning the question to seek appropriate evidence. In phase 1, Len is also able to discern and provide feedback on questions that will apply in the context of Strides. Here is an example of a question that follows the PICO format: Does barefoot running reduce injuries compared with traditional running shoe use, in marathon runners? In this case, the *population* is defined as marathon runners; the *intervention* is barefoot running which is *compared* with classic running shoe use. The *outcome* of interest is injury rate.

Phase 2: Gathering the Evidence

Marissa seeks evidence through peer-reviewed journals and works with Len to further evaluate the evidence and the appropriateness of application for the Strides population. Further questions are often generated in this phase.

Phase 3: Communicating the Evidence

After review from Len, Marissa disseminates the information through a blog and presentation that is directed toward both Strides members and individuals in broader running community. During the assessment process, Len and Marissa reflect on the value of the evidence and the benefit of generating and seeking appropriate solutions.

Follow-up

Through written and verbal reflections about the internship experience, Marissa is able to consider ways in which evidence-based learning influenced her ability to make choices about programming that benefit Stride's clients. Marissa is also able to identify ways in which the PICO format would enable her to define questions and seek answers in the future.

QUESTIONS

- What value does the evidence-based decision-making method have outside a clinical setting?
- Would the answers have been different had a different population been under investigation, for example, 5-km runners?
- How can the evidence-based decision-making method empower clients?

References

1. Casey K, Fink R, Jaynes C, Campbell L, Cook P, Wilson V. Readiness for practice: the senior practicum experience. *J Nurs Educ.* 2011;50(11):646–52. doi:10.3928/01484834-20110817-03.
2. Sabas C. The effects of modeling evidence-based practice during the clinical internship. *J Phys Ther Educ.* 2008;22(3):74–84.
3. Scott PJ, Altenburger PA, Kean J. A collaborative teaching strategy for enhancing learning of evidence-based clinical decision-making. *J Allied Health.* 2011;40(3):120–7.

SUMMARY

The EP-C has a personal and professional responsibility to engage in behaviors that "do no harm" (11). After providing a brief history of ACSM certifications, this chapter has reviewed the ACSM Code of Ethics and provided a more in-depth examination of the professional responsibilities and personal characteristics of the EP-C. The professional responsibilities relating to scope of practice, conflict of interest, evidence-based practice, and maintaining certification have been reviewed. Personal characteristics represented by WISE have also been examined in the context of desirable personal characteristics of professionals in the helping professions.

STUDY QUESTIONS

1. The ACSM-certified EP-C is qualified to pursue a career in all EXCEPT _____.
   a. local YMCA
   b. hospital cardiac care unit
   c. university fitness and wellness center
   d. clinical research project related to childhood obesity
2. The ACSM-certified EP-C Scope of Practice includes
   a. exercise testing of a healthy 76-year-old man with mild osteoarthritis.
   b. aerobic training of a 21-year-old woman with acute anorexia.
   c. therapeutic exercise to target a cancer survivor's chronic lymphedema of the left arm.
   d. interpreting a 12-lead ECG of a patient who has coronary artery bypass graft in a phase 2 cardiac rehab program.
3. Henry's business card indicates that he is a certified EP-C working as a manager of an employee wellness center. In addition to his management responsibilities, he functions in the role as a personal trainer at the center for employees who want to pay an extra fee to the center for individualized services. Henry has a side business of selling essential oils and nutritional aids for health and longevity. Discuss whether each example is permissible for Henry to engage in.
   a. Henry has a side business of selling essential oils and nutritional aids for health and longevity.
   b. Henry pins his essential oils business card on a bulletin board in the wellness center where other business cards advertise massage services, nutritional counseling, physical therapy, and acupuncture.
   c. Henry gives his essential oils business card and a free sample to every client he works with at the wellness center.
   d. Henry makes essential oils recommendations within the context of a training session for a client at the wellness center.
   e. Henry makes essential oils recommendations within the context of a training session for a private client.
4. List some ways of maintaining one's EP-C certification.
5. Discuss personal characteristics that you deem important for professional conduct as an EP-C.
6. How do the personal behaviors of an EP-C impact the professional integrity of the field?

REFERENCES

1. American College of Sports Medicine. ACSM Certified Exercise Physiologist^SM job task analysis [Internet]. Indianapolis (IN): American College of Sports Medicine; [cited 2015 Oct 13]. Available from: http://certification.acsm.org/files/file/JTA%20EP-C%20FINAL%202012.pdf

2. American College of Sports Medicine. *ACSM's Guidelines for Exercise Testing and Prescription*. 10th ed. Philadelphia (PA): Lippincott Williams & Wilkins; 2018.

3. American College of Sports Medicine. Code of ethics [Internet]. Indianapolis (IN): American College of Sports Medicine Code of Ethics; [cited 2015 Jul 8]. Available from: http://www.acsm.org/join-acsm/membership-resources/code-of-ethics

4. American College of Sports Medicine. Frequently asked questions: ACSM certification name changes [Internet]. Indianapolis (IN): American College of Sports Medicine; 2015. [cited 2015 Jul 8]. Available from: http://certification.acsm.org/name-change-faqs

5. American College of Sports Medicine. Get certified. 2015. Indianapolis (IN): American College of Sports Medicine; [cited 2015 Oct 13]. Available from: http://certification.acsm.org/get-certified

6. American College of Sports Medicine. *Leadership Manual 2014-2015*. Indianapolis (IN): American College of Sports Medicine. 9 p.

7. American College of Sports Medicine [Internet]. Renewing your certification. Indianapolis (IN): American College of Sports Medicine [cited 2015 Oct 13]. Available from: http://certification.acsm.org/renew-your-certification

8. Amonette W, English K, Ottenbacher K. Nullius in verba: a call for the incorporation of evidence-based practice into the discipline of exercise science. *Sport Med*. 2010;40(6):449–57.

9. Anderson L, Krathwohl D, editors. *A Taxonomy for Learning, Teaching and Assessing: A Revision of Bloom's Taxonomy of Educational Objectives*. New York (NY): Longman; 2001. 336 p.

10. APhA-ASP/AACP-COD Task Force on Professionalism. White paper on pharmacy student professionalism. *J Am Pharm Assoc*. 2000;40(1):96–102.

11. Beach M, Duggan P, Cassel C, Geller G. What does "respect" mean? Exploring the moral obligation of health professionals to respect patients. *J Gen Intern Med*. 2007;22(5):692–5.

12. Berryman JW. *Out of Many, One: A History of the American College of Sports Medicine*. Champaign (IL): Human Kinetics; 1995. 283 p.

13. Brody H. Clarifying conflict of interest. *Am J Bioeth*. 2011; 11(1):23–8.

14. Center for Evidence Based Medicine. *Asking Focused Questions* [Internet]. Oxford (United Kingdom): CEBM; [cited 2015 Oct 13]. Available from: http://www.cebm.net/index.aspx?o=1036

15. Chase D, Masberg B. Partnering for skill development: park and recreation agencies and university programs. *Manag Leisure*. 2008;13(2):74–91.

16. de Cordova PB, Collins S, Peppard L, et al. Implementing evidence-based nursing with student nurses and clinicians: uniting the strengths. *Appl Nurs Res*. 2008;21(4):242–5.

17. Exercise is Medicine. The Exercise is Medicine Credential [Internet]. Indianapolis (IN): American College of Sports Medicine; [cited 2015 Jul 8]. Available from: http://certification.acsm.org/exercise-is-medicine-credential

18. Eyles HC, Mhurchu CN. Does tailoring make a difference? A systematic review of the long-term effectiveness of tailored nutrition education for adults. *Nutr Rev*. 2009;67(8):464–80.

19. Hilton S, Slotnick H. Proto-professionalism: how professionalisation occurs across the continuum of medical education. *Med Educ*. 2005;39(1):58–65.

20. Institute of Medicine. *Crossing the Quality Chasm: A New Health System for the 21st Century*. Washington (DC): National Academies Press; 2001. 360 p.

21. Kahanov L, Andrews L. A survey of athletic training employers' hiring criteria. *J Athl Train*. 2001;36(4):408.

22. Kutz MR. *Leadership and Management in Athletic Training: An Integrated Approach*. Baltimore (MD): Lippincott Williams & Wilkins; 2010. 331 p.

23. Medical Dictionary. Ethics [Internet]. [cited 2015 Oct 13]. Available from: http://medical-dictionary.thefreedictionary.com/ethics

24. Medical Dictionary. Evidence-based practice [Internet]. [cited 2015 Oct 13]. Available from: http://medical-dictionary.thefreedictionary.com/evidence-based+practice

25. Medical Dictionary. Profession [Internet]. [cited 2015 Oct 13]. Available from: http://medical-dictionary.thefreedictionary.com/profession

26. Medical Dictionary. Scope of practice [Internet]. [cited 2015 Oct 13]. Available from: http://medical-dictionary.thefreedictionary.com/scope+of+practice

27. Melton DI, Dail TK, Katula JA, Mustian KM. The current state of personal training: managers' perspectives. *J Strength Cond Res*. 2010;24(11):3173–9.

28. Muth ND. The elephant in the room: nutrition scope of practice: IDEA Fitness Journal, September 2009 [Internet]. [cited 2015 Jul 8]. Available from: http://www.ideafit.com/fitness-library/the-elephant-in-the-room-nutrition-scope-of-practice

29. O'Sullivan-Maillet J, Skates J, Pritchett E. American Dietetic Association: scope of dietetics practice framework. *J Am Diet Assoc*. 2005;105(4):634–40.

30. Perko M, Dennison D. "Does this stuff work?" When health educators discuss dietary supplements. *Int Electr J Health Educ*. 2000;3(1):64–8.

31. Rassin M. Nurses professional and personal values. *Nurs Ethics*. 2008;15(5):614–30.

32. Responsible Conducts of Research Courses Portal. *Conflicts of Interest* [Internet]. New York (NY): Columbia University; [cited 2015 Oct 13]. Available from: http://ccnmtl.columbia.edu/projects/rcr/rcr_conflicts/foundation/index.html#1_1

33. Sass C, Eickhoff-Shemek JM, Manore MM, Kruskall LJ. Crossing the line: understanding the scope of practice between registered dieticians and health fitness professionals. *ACSM Health Fitness J*. 2007;11(3):12–9.

34. Scott PJ, Altenburger PA, Kean J. A collaborative teaching strategy for enhancing learning of evidence-based clinical decision-making. *J Allied Health*. 2011;40(3):120–7.

35. Shields MA, Ward M. Improving nurse retention in the National Health Service in England: the impact of job satisfaction on intentions to quit. *J Health Econ*. 2001;20(5):677–701.

36. Tichenor MS, Tichenor JL. Understanding teachers' perspectives on professionalism. *Profession Educ*. 2004;27(1–2):89–95.

Editors from the Previous Edition of *ACSM's Resources for the Exercise Physiologist, Certified*

FIRST EDITION

Previously titled *ACSM's Resources for the Health Fitness Specialist*

SENIOR EDITOR

Gary Liguori, PhD, FACSM, ACSM-CES
Dean
College of Health Sciences
University of Rhode Island
Kingston, Rhode Island

ASSOCIATE EDITORS

Gregory B. Dwyer, PhD, FACSM, ACSM-PD, ACSM-RCEP, ACSM-CEP, ACSM-ETT, EIM 3
Professor
Department of Exercise Science
East Stroudsburg University
East Stroudsburg, Pennsylvania

Teresa C. Fitts, DPE, FACSM, ACSM-HFS
Westfield State University
Westfield, Massachusetts

Beth A. Lewis, PhD
Associate Professor, Behavioral Aspects of Physical Activity
Director, Undergraduate Studies
University of Minnesota
School of Kinesiology
Minneapolis, Minnesota

Appendix B

Contributors from the Previous Edition of *ACSM's Resources for the Exercise Physiologist, Certified*

FIRST EDITION

Previously titled *ACSM's Resources for the Health Fitness Specialist*

Anthony A. Abbott, EdD, FACSM
Fitness Institute International, Inc.
Lighthouse Point, Florida

Keith Burns, MS
Kent State University
Kent, Ohio

Dino Costanzo, MA, ACSM-RCEP, FACSM, ACSM-PD, ACSM-ETT
The Hospital of Central Connecticut
New Britain, Connecticut

Katrina DuBose, PhD, FACSM
East Carolina University
Greenville, North Carolina

J. Larry Durstine, PhD, FACSM
University of South Carolina
Columbia, South Carolina

Gregory B. Dwyer, PhD, FACSM ACSM-PD, ACSM-CES, ACSM-ETT, ACSM-RCEP
East Stroudsburg University
East Stroudsburg, Pennsylvania

Chris Eschbach, PhD, ACSM-HFS
Valencell, Inc
Raleigh, North Carolina

Avery Faigenbaum, EdD, FACSM
The College of New Jersey
Ewing, New Jersey

Diana Ferris, MS, ACSM-HFS
ACSM/NPAS-PAPHS
Public Health Specialist
Stratford, Connecticut

Teresa C. Fitts, DPE, FACSM, ACSM-HFS
Westfield State University
Westfield, Massachusetts

Charles Fountaine, PhD
University of Minnesota Duluth
Duluth, Minnesota

Benjamin Gordon, MS, ACSM-CES
The University of South Carolina
Columbia, South Carolina

Sarah T. Henes, PhD, RD, LDN
East Carolina University
Greenville, North Carolina

Ernestine Jennings, PhD
Warren Alpert Medical School, Brown University
Providence, Rhode Island

Betsy Keller, PhD, FACSM
Ithaca College
Ithaca, New York

Riggs Klika, PhD, FACSM
Cancer Survivor Center
Aspen, Colorado

Matthew Kutz, PhD, ATC, ACSM-CES
Bowling Green State University
Bowling Green, Ohio

Beth Lewis, PhD
University of Minnesota
Minneapolis, Minnesota

Gary Liguori, PhD, FACSM, ACSM-CES
University of Tennessee Chattanooga
Chattanooga, Tennessee

Sarah Linke, PhD, MPH
University of California, San Diego
La Jolla, California

Randi Lite, MA, ACSM-RCEP
Simmons College
Boston, Massachusetts

Meir Magal, PhD, ACSM-CES
North Carolina Wesleyan College
Rocky Mount, North Carolina

Bess Marcus, PhD, FACSM
University of California, San Diego
La Jolla, California

Jessica Meendering, PhD, ACSM-HFS, ATC
South Dakota State University
Brookings, South Dakota

Laurie Milliken, PhD, FACSM
University of Massachusetts Boston
Boston, Massachusetts

Rob Motl, PhD
University of Illinois
Urbana, Illinois

Mark Nutting, ACSM-HFD, ACSM-HFS
Saco Sport & Fitness
Saco, Maine

Matthew W. Parrott, PhD, ACSM-HFS
H-P Fitness, LLC
Leawood, Kansas

Neal I. Pire, MA, FACSM
Inspire Training Systems
Ridgewood, New Jersey

Deborah Riebe, PhD, FACSM, ACSM-HFS
University of Rhode Island
Kingston, Rhode Island

John M. Schuna, Jr., PhD
Pennington Biomedical Research Center
Baton Rouge, Louisiana

Katie Schuver, MS
University of Minnesota
Minneapolis, Minnesota

John Sigg, PhD
Ithaca College
Ithaca, New York

Madeline Weikert, MS
Human Kinetics
Champaign, Illinois

Molly Winke, PhD
Hanover Colleger
Hanover, Indiana

Index